SECOND EDITION

Mastering Public Health

SECOND EDITION

Mastering Public Health

A Postgraduate Guide to Examinations and Revalidation

GERAINT LEWIS • JESSICA SHERINGHAM
JAMIE LOPEZ BERNAL • TIM CRAYFORD

CRC Press
Taylor & Francis Group
Boca Raton London New York

CRC Press is an imprint of the
Taylor & Francis Group, an **informa** business

CRC Press
Taylor & Francis Group
6000 Broken Sound Parkway NW, Suite 300
Boca Raton, FL 33487-2742

First issued in hardback 2017

Version Date: 20160422

ISBN-13: 978-1-4441-5269-2 (pbk)
ISBN-13: 978-1-138-45997-7 (hbk)

Library of Congress Cataloging-in-Publication Data

Lewis, Geraint H., author.
Mastering public health : a postgraduate guide to examinations and revalidation / Geraint Lewis, Jessica Sheringham, Jamie Lopez Bernal, and Tim Crayford. -- Second edition.
p. ; cm.
Includes bibliographical references and index.
ISBN 978-1-4441-5269-2 (hardcover : alk. paper)
I. Sheringham, Jessica, author. II. Lopez Bernal, Jamie, author. III. Crayford, Tim, author. IV. Title.
[DNLM: 1. Public Health Practice--Great Britain. 2. Public Health--methods--Great Britain. WA 100]

RA412.5.G7
362.10941--dc23 2014015407

Visit the Taylor & Francis Web site at
http://www.taylorandfrancis.com

and the CRC Press Web site at
http://www.crcpress.com

Contents

Section 5 Organisation and Management of Healthcare and Healthcare Programmes 527

Foreword

The work of public health professionals in the United Kingdom has changed enormously since the first edition of this book was published. The four nations have increasingly gone their separate ways. In England, where the magnitude of change has been greatest, the public health function has been fragmented, with the creation of a new executive agency and the transfer of some functions to local government, but there is a considerable uncertainty about the role of those who have previously applied their public health expertise to the delivery of effective and equitable healthcare. The remaining three nations have opted for more integrated models but, in every part of the United Kingdom, neither those working in public health nor the populations they serve are spared the effects of the government's continuing failure to restore economic growth and its choice of austerity as a response to the 2008 economic crisis. Although these are difficult times for public health, the need for a well-functioning public health system has rarely been greater.

The second edition of this book, updated considerably, once again reminds us of the broad scope of public health. The determinants of health stretch from the molecular to the societal. Similarly, the modern public health professional must be able to stretch from new insights into genetics to the health effects of macroeconomic policy. It is not that they should be experts in all of these areas; no one could hope to be. Rather, they will be aware of the scale of the canvas on which they are working, know where to get the information they need, and above all, have the skills to appraise it critically, asking not only whether something will work but whether it will work in the particular circumstances that they face. To do so, they must draw on a wide range of disciplines, including epidemiology, of course, but also economics, sociology, demography, clinical sciences, and political science, among others. They must also have a wide array of personal and organisational skills needed to turn their ideas into reality. They will find all this and more in this book.

The primary purpose of this book is to prepare candidates for the examinations of the UK Faculty of Public Health, something it does admirably, with the new edition incorporating advances in knowledge as well as changes to the faculty's curriculum. There are, of course, many books that cover different parts of the curriculum, but this has the great advantage of bringing it all together in a single volume in which the candidate can find the key elements of knowledge that he or she will need to pass the exams. But it is much more than this and, in a rapidly changing world demanding life-long learning, many experienced practitioners will also find much that is of value here.

The authors of this book are to be congratulated once again for the way in which they have met the need of the next generation of public health professionals (and their trainers), assembling an excellent overview of the essential knowledge required by public health practitioners in a clear and highly readable manner. Although designed primarily for the exams of the UK Faculty, I am confident that it will also be of value to those in training in many other countries.

Professor Martin McKee CBE MD DSc MSc FRCP FFPH FMedSci

Professor of European Public Health

London School of Hygiene and Tropical Medicine

Preface

Six years have passed since we published the first edition of *Mastering Public Health*, so it was high time that we refreshed and updated the text. We were given added impetus to produce a second edition by the whole-scale reorganisation in England of public health and the National Health Service, by the changes that have occurred to the syllabus of the Part A examination for Membership of the Faculty of Public Health (MFPH), but most importantly, by the feedback we received from readers suggesting how we might improve the book. In this second edition, we have therefore attempted to build on what we are told are its key strengths while attempting to address the shortcomings of the first edition and bringing it fully up to date. As a consequence, some sections of the book have changed relatively little compared to the first edition, such as those on statistics and epidemiology. Others, such as those about the organisation of healthcare, have undergone a more radical overhaul.

We believe that *Mastering Public Health* will be useful to anyone studying public health at a postgraduate level. However, we learnt from the feedback on the first edition that many readers appreciated how we organised the book strictly according to the structure of the Part A MFPH syllabus. Although it aids with revision, this dogged approach has certain disadvantages in that it led to duplication in places, and elsewhere material was presented in a less coherent order than we would ideally have chosen. To address these problems, we have introduced signposts in this second edition that are designed to cross-refer the reader to other relevant material within the book and to navigate a more logical route through certain topics, such as health economics and statistics.

As in the first edition, we are incredibly grateful to our panel of expert contributors, to our international editors, and to our publishers. We would also like to thank our former co-author, Kanwal Kalim, for her contributions to the first edition. We were sad that due to work and family commitments, she was unable to work with us on this second edition. In her place, however, we welcome Jamie Lopez Bernal as a new co-author and thank him for his industry, his bright ideas, and his enthusiasm for the book and what it is trying to achieve. Finally, we would like to thank you, our readers, for the invaluable feedback you have provided. Please keep it coming.

Geraint Lewis FRCP FFPH
Chief Data Officer, NHS England

Jessica Sheringham PhD FFPH
Senior Research Associate, University College London

Jamie Lopez Bernal MB BS MSc MFPH
Academic Clinical Fellow, London School of Hygiene and Tropical Medicine

Tim Crayford MB BS MSc FFPH
Chief Medical Advisor, Just Retirement Ltd.

Acknowledgements

We would like to thank the following expert reviewers for their help:

- Dr Araceli Busby, locum consultant in public health at Surrey, Sussex, and Kent, Public Health England
- Helen Crabbe, environmental public health scientist, Centre for Radiation, Chemicals and Environmental Hazards, Public Health England
- Sheila Holmes, radiological assessments scientist, Centre for Radiation, Chemicals and Environmental Hazards, Public Health England
- Alison Iliff, public health specialist, Rotherham Local Authority
- Dr Nora Pashayan, senior clinical lecturer in applied health research, Cancer Research UK Clinician Scientist Fellow, Department of Applied Health Research, University College London
- Dr Simon Turner, senior research associate, Department of Applied Health Research, University College London
- Aris Tyrothoulakis, General manager, Diagnostic Service, NHS Lothian
- Dr Laura Vallejo-Torres, principal research associate in health economics, Clinical Trials Unit, University College London
- Isla Wallace, research associate, Department of Applied Health Research, University College London

We would also like to thank the following international contributors:

- *Australia:* Dr Wendy Scheil, public health physician, SA Health
- *Hong Kong:* Professor Sian M Griffiths, director of the Centre for Global Health, Chinese University of Hong Kong
- *Ireland:* Dr Emer Shelley, consultant in public health medicine, health service executive and senior lecturer in epidemiology, Royal College of Surgeons in Ireland, Dublin
- *Northern Ireland:* Dr Dermot O'Reilly, senior clinical lecturer, Queen's University Belfast
- *Scotland:*
    - Dr Aileen Holliday, health effectiveness coordinator, NHS Forth Valley
    - Dr Sue Payne, public health consultant, NHS Lothian
    - Dr Anne Maree Wallace, director of public health, NHS Forth Valley
- *South Africa:* Dr Stephen Knight, public health medicine physician, University of KwaZulu-Natal
- *Wales:* Dr Nigel Monaghan, consultant in public health/dental public health, Public Health Wales, and visiting professor in public health, University of Glamorgan

List of Abbreviations

ADA	Adenosine deaminase
ADL	Activities of daily living
ADR	Adverse drug reaction
ANOVA	Analysis of variance
APHO	Association of Public Health Observatories
AR	Attributable risk
ARIA	Accessibility/remoteness index of Australia
ARIMA	Autoregressive integrated moving average
BAT	Best available techniques
BBV	Blood-borne virus
BMI	Body mass index
BNF	British National Formulary
BSE	Bovine spongiform encephalopathy
CBA	Cost–benefit analysis
CBT	Cognitive behavioural therapy
CCA	Cost–consequence analysis
CCDC	Consultant in communicable disease control
CCG	Clinical commissioning group
CEA	Cost-effectiveness analysis
CFTR	Cystic fibrosis transmembrane conductance regulator
CHD	Coronary heart disease
CHP	Consultant in health protection
CI	Confidence interval
CIDR	Computerised infectious disease reporting
CJD	Creutzfeldt–Jakob disease
CMA	Cost-minimisation analysis
CMV	Cytomegalovirus
CO	Carbon monoxide
COPD	Chronic obstructive pulmonary disease
COSHH	Control of substances hazardous to health
COVER	Cover of vaccination evaluated rapidly
CPRD	Clinical practice research database
CQC	Care Quality Commission
CQRS	Calculating Quality Reporting Services
CRHD	Chronic rheumatic heart disease
CUA	Cost–utility analysis
CVS	Chorionic villous sampling
DAFNE	Dose adjustment for normal eating
DALY	Disability-adjusted life years
DCSF	Department for Children, Schools and Families
DDD	Defined daily doses
DEFRA	Department for Environment, Food and Rural Affairs
DfID	Department for International Development
DFPH	Diplomate membership of the Faculty of Public Health
DHS	Demographic and Health Surveys
DIPC	Director of Infection Prevention and Control

DNA	Deoxyribonucleic acid
DOT	Directly observed treatment
DRG	Diagnosis-related group
DRR	Drug rehabilitation requirements
DRV	Dietary reference value
DTP	Diphtheria, tetanus, pertussis
DVLA	Driver and Vehicle Licensing Authority
DWI	Drinking Water Inspectorate
EA	Environment agency
EAR	Estimated average requirement
EARSNet	European Antimicrobial Resistance Surveillance Network
EBM	Evidence-based medicine
ECDC	European Centre of Disease Control
EIA	Environmental impact assessment
ELF	Extremely low-frequency
EMF	Electromagnetic field
EPPE	Effective Provision of Pre-School Education
ERSPC	European Randomized Study of Screening for Prostate Cancer
EU	European Union
FAO	Food and Agriculture Organization
FAP	Familial adenomatous polyposis
FAQs	Frequently asked questions
FRR	Familial relative risk
FSA	Food Standards Agency
FSAI	Food Safety Authority of Ireland
FT	Foundation Trust
GIS	Geographic information system
GISRS	Global Influenza Surveillance and Response System
GMS	General Medical Services
GOARN	Global Outbreak Alert and Response Network
GP	General practitioner
GPES	General Practitioner Extraction Service
GPHIN	Global Public Health Intelligence Network
GRADE	Grades of recommendation, assessment, development, and evaluation
GRE	Glycopeptide-resistant enterococci
GSL	General sales list
GUM	Genitourinary medicine
GUMCAD	Genitourinary medicine clinic activity database
HALE	Health-adjusted life expectancy
HARS	HIV/AIDS reporting system
HAV	Hepatitis A virus
HBM	Health belief model
HBV	Hepatitis B virus
HCAI	Healthcare-associated infection
HCV	Hepatitis C virus
HDEC	Health and Disability Ethics Committee
HDV	Hepatitis D virus
HES	Hospital episode statistics
HEV	Hepatitis E virus
HIA	Health impact assessment

HNA	Health needs assessment
HNIG	Human normal immunoglobulin
HNPCC	Hereditary non-polyposis colorectal cancer
HPA	Health Protection Agency
HPCSA	Health Professionals Council of South Africa
HPI	Health poverty index
HPS	Health Protection Scotland
HPSC	Health Protection Surveillance Centre
HPV	Human papillomavirus
HQIP	Healthcare quality improvement partnership
HREC	Human Research Ethics Committee
HRG	Healthcare resource group
HRQoL	Health-related quality of life
HSE	Health service executive
HTML	Hypertext markup language
HUS	Haemolytic–uraemic syndrome
ICD	International Classification of Diseases
ICER	Incremental cost effectiveness ratio
ICHI	International Classification of Health Interventions
ICIDH	International Classification of Impairment, Disabilities, and Handicap
ICM	Infection control manager
ICN	Infection control nurse
ICSEA	Community socio-educational advantage
ICT	Infection control team
ICT	Information and communications technology
IEC	Institutional ethics committee
IHS	Integrated Household Survey
IMC	Integrated marketing communication
IMD	Indices of multiple deprivation
INDEPTH	International Network for the Demographic Evaluation of Populations and Their Health
IPA	Interpretative phenomenological analysis
IQR	Interquartile range
ISD	Information services data
IUGR	Intrauterine growth restriction
IVF	In vitro fertilisation
JCVI	Joint Committee on Vaccination and Immunisation
JSNA	Joint strategic needs assessment
LBW	Low birthweight
LRNI	Lower reference nutrient intake
LSOA	Lower-layer super output areas
MANOVA	Multivariate analysis of variance
MBO	Management by objectives
MBWA	Management by wandering around
MCDA	Multi-criteria decision analysis
MDR-TB	Multidrug resistant tuberculosis
MeSH	Medical Subject Headings
MFPH	Membership of the Faculty of Public Health
MHRA	Medicines and Healthcare Products Regulatory Authority
MINI	Mental illness needs index
MPR	Medication possession ratio

MRSA	Methicillin-resistant *Staphylococcus aureus*
MTB	Mycobacterium tuberculosis
MUST	Malnutrition universal screening tool
NATSAL	National survey of sexual attitudes and lifestyles
NCEPOD	National confidential enquiry into patient outcome and death
NG	Nasogastric
NGO	Non-governmental organisation
NHP	Nottingham health profile
NHS	National Health Service
NNT	Numbers needed to treat
NPP	Negative predictive power
NPV	Negative predictive value
NRAC	National Resource Allocation Committee
NRES	National Research Ethics Service
NRI	Nutritional risk index
NSC	National Screening Committee
NSSEC	National statistics socio-economic classification
OA	Output area
OR	Odds ratio
ORLS	Oxford Record Linkage Study
PACS	Picture and Archiving Communications Systems
PACT	Prescribing analysis and cost
PAF	Population attributable fraction
PAR	Population attributable risk
PARR	Patients at risk of re-hospitalisation
PBMA	Programme budgeting and marginal analysis
PCR	Polymerase chain reaction
PDC	Proportion of days covered
PDP	Personal development plan
PEM	Protein–energy malnutrition
PH	Public health
PID	Pelvic inflammatory disease
PIL	Patient information leaflet
PKU	Phenylketonuria
PLCO	Prostate, lung, colorectal, and ovarian cancer screening trial
PMD	Prescribing Monitoring Documents
PPE	Personal protective equipment
PPP	Positive predictive power
PPV	Positive predictive value
PRI	Population reference intake
PROM	Patient-reported outcome measure
PSA	Public Service Agreement
PSU	Prescribing Support Unit
PU	Prescribing unit
PWS	Private drinking water supplies
QALY	Quality-adjusted life year
QMAS	Quality management and analysis system

QOF	Quality and outcomes framework
QoL	Quality of life
RCT	Randomised controlled trial
RDA	Recommended dietary allowance
REC	Research ethics committee
RIBA	Recombinant immunoblot assay
RIDDOR	Reporting of Injuries, Diseases and Dangerous Occurrences Regulations
RNA	Ribonucleic acid
RNI	Reference nutrient intake
ROC	Receiver operating characteristic
ROP	Retinopathy of prematurity
RRR	Relative recurrence risk
SAQs	Short answer questions
SARS	Severe acute respiratory syndrome
SCID	Severe combined immunodeficiency
SE	Standard error
SEIFA	Socio-economic indexes for areas
SEPA	Scottish Environment Protection Agency
SIDS	Sudden infant death syndrome
SIMD	Scottish index of multiple deprivation
SMR	Standardised mortality ratio
SOA	Super output area
SOPHID	Survey of Prevalent HIV Infections Diagnosed
SPC	Summaries of product characteristics
STI	Sexually transmitted infection
SUS	Secondary Uses Service
TB	Tuberculosis
THS	Thematic household survey
TIA	Transient ischaemic attack
TPFR	Total period fertility rate
TRIPS	Trade Related Aspects of Intellectual Property Rights
UN FCC	United Nations Framework Convention on Climate Change
UNECE	UN Economic Commission for Europe
USAID	US Agency for International Development
UV	Ultraviolet
VDU	Visual display unit
VHF	Viral haemorrhagic fever
VRE	Vancomycin-resistant enterococci
WHO	World Health Organization
WHS	Welsh Health Survey
WNHSS	Welsh Network of Healthy School Schemes
WTP	Willingness-to-pay
XDR-TB	Extreme drug-resistant tuberculosis
YLD	Years lost due to disability
YLL	Years of life lost

Section 1

RESEARCH METHODS

Public health specialists need to understand how health knowledge is generated, not only so they can select and use appropriate research methods for their own work, but also so that they can appraise the quality of published research in order to provide credible professional advice.

Section 1 describes the epidemiological research methods that underpin public health. Epidemiology is key to public health practice because it involves scrutinising data to generate inferences that can be used as the basis of health policy. The validity of public health research therefore relies on the appropriate use of statistics, from the design and collection of data through to the analysis and interpretation stages.

This section also covers qualitative research methods, which are essential for understanding why things happen in the ways that they do. Section 1 ends with a description of healthcare assessment, which draws on a range of research methods in order to evaluate the structure, function, and performance of health systems and services.

1A

Epidemiology

Epidemiology is the study of the distribution and determinants of health and disease in populations. Epidemiological techniques are used to determine the characteristics of **who** becomes ill, **what** diseases affect them, **where** they arise, and **when** they happen. It is the science used to explore the underlying questions of **how** and **why** diseases occur. Epidemiology is therefore fundamental to public health practice because it uses data from large populations to generate meaningful information that can be used as the basis of health policy.

The techniques covered in this chapter are necessary for interpreting the scientific literature and for providing credible professional advice. Public health specialists therefore need to learn how to apply these techniques in order to design and analyse their own simple studies.

1A.1 Health statistics

Use of routine vital and health statistics to describe the distribution of disease in time, place, and person.

Information about a defined population that is collected in a consistent manner for administrative reasons is called **routine data**. Such data may be used to describe the **needs** of and **services** provided to different population groups. Different countries have different sources of routine health data, and the information collected and the frequency of collection will vary. However, almost all countries process their data into **vital statistics**. These indicators describe the most important events in life, such as births, deaths, and migrations.

The two most important vital statistics, which are used across the globe for assessing a population's health, are **life expectancy** and **infant mortality**:

- Life expectancy is the expectation of life from a given age. It is the average number of years that a person can be expected to live.
- Infant mortality is the number of children per 1000 live births who **die in their first year** of life.

Some of the strengths and weaknesses of vital statistics are shown in Box 1A.1.

Box 1A.1 Strengths and weaknesses of vital statistics

Strengths of vital statistics	Weaknesses of vital statistics
Cheap and readily available Almost complete data Contemporary Can be used for ecological studies to develop hypotheses Recorded at regular intervals, so can be used for monitoring trends	Not 100% complete Potential for bias—postmortem inflation of social status; stigmatised diseases under-reported Become out of date—census data only recorded every 10 years

Routine data need to be **reliable**, **valid**, and **complete**. There should therefore be a good reason to begin or stop collecting any item of data.

Some methods of improving the quality of data are shown in Box 1A.2.

Routine statistics in the United Kingdom

The key sources of routine health data in England are listed in Table 1A.1. More details are available in Section 3B.

Box 1A.2 Ways to improve the quality of routine data

Method	Details
Computerised data collation and analysis	Improves the accuracy and timeliness of the collection, preparation, and dissemination of information.
Feedback	Better feedback of data to providers helps maintain their interest and leads to sustained improvements in data quality.
Presentation	Data should be presented in a variety of ways that are meaningful to different groups, such as policymakers, the media, professionals, and the general public.
Training	Improved training for clinical coders and people responsible for data entry helps ensure that definitions and terminology are used consistently.

Table 1A.1 Routine statistics collected in England

Type	Examples	
Demography	Census	
Mortality	Mortality statistics (Office for National Statistics) 10 yearly supplement on occupational mortality	
Morbidity	Primary care	GP clinical codes (Read codes) Clinical practice research database (CPRD)
	Hospital	Hospital episode statistics (HES) Laboratory results
	Registers	Regional cancer registries National childhood cancer register Congenital abnormalities Prostheses Transplants Confidential inquiries
	Other	Notifiable disease statistics General Lifestyle Survey (formerly the General Household Survey)

Mortality indices

UK Mortality data are accurate in the United Kingdom, owing to the legal processes that govern how deaths are registered. Important **mortality indices** are shown in Table 1A.2.

Fertility indices

Measures used to describe the reproductive characteristics of a population are known as **fertility indices** (see Table 1A.3).

Further details are available in Section 3A.8.

Descriptive epidemiology

Epidemiology is the study of the patterns, causes, and control of disease in groups of people. In descriptive epidemiology, the three principal dimensions that are used to describe the occurrence of a disease are **time**, **place**, and **person** (see Table 1A.4).

Table 1A.2 Mortality indices

Index[a]	Calculation
Crude mortality rate	$\frac{\text{Number of deaths}}{\text{1000 population}}$ per year
Age-specific mortality rate	$\frac{\text{Number of deaths aged X}}{\text{1000 population aged X}}$ per year
Child mortality rate	$\frac{\text{Number of deaths aged} < 5 \text{ years}}{\text{1000 population aged} < 5 \text{ years}}$ per year
Infant mortality rate	$\frac{\text{Number of deaths aged} < 1 \text{ year}}{\text{1000 live births}}$ per year
Neonatal mortality rate	$\frac{\text{Number of deaths aged} < 28 \text{ days}}{\text{1000 live births}}$ per year
Post-neonatal mortality rate	$\frac{\text{Number of deaths aged 4 to 52 weeks}}{\text{1000 live births}}$ per year
Perinatal mortality rate	$\frac{\text{Number of stillbirths and deaths aged} < 7 \text{ days}}{\text{1000 births}}$ per year
Standardised mortality ratio	See Section 1A.5.

[a] The population in the denominator must be defined using the same period of time as that used to accumulate the numerator using the concept of **person-years at risk**. The population estimate used is typically the mid-year (July 1) population count estimate for the same year(s) and age(s) included in the numerator. Rates may also commonly be expressed per 100,000.

Table 1A.3 Fertility indices

Rate	Calculation	Notes
Crude birth rate	$\frac{\text{Number of live births}}{\text{1000 population}}$ per year	Poor indicator of fertility because the denominator includes men, children, and postmenopausal women.
General fertility rate	$\frac{\text{Number of live births}}{\text{1000 women aged 15 to 44}}$ per year	Denominator includes only women, typically of childbearing age (sometimes the age range 15 to 49 is used instead).
Age-specific fertility rate	$\frac{\text{Number of live births to women aged X}}{\text{1000 women aged X}}$ per year	More precise because it takes into account differences in fertility at different ages.
Total period fertility rate (TPFR)	Sum of the age-specific fertility rates	Indicates the average number of children that would be born to a woman during her lifetime, assuming that she experienced the current age-specific fertility rates and that she survived to the end of her reproductive life.

Table 1A.4 Dimensions of descriptive epidemiology

Dimension	Description
Time	Considers **when** the disease occurs and how it changes or has changed over time, including • Secular trends (i.e. trends over decades and centuries) • Seasonal variation (i.e. cyclical patterns in disease frequency, such as seasonal influenza) • Epidemic curves (i.e. acute increases in disease frequency) • Point events (i.e. the sudden emergence of disease at a particular time)
Place	Describes **where** the incidence is high or low and where the incidence is changing or has changed: • International (ecological comparisons may suggest hypotheses regarding causation) • National (compares urban–rural patterns and patterns related to deprivation) • Small areas (makes comparisons based on census data, IMDs, and town-centre data)
Person	Describes **who** is affected, based on characteristics such as • Age • Sex • Occupation or social class • Ethnicity • Behaviour and lifestyle

1A.2 Numerators, denominators, and populations at risk

In epidemiology, a **numerator** is a feature that has been counted (e.g. number of deaths); it forms the upper part of a fraction. A **denominator**, for epidemiological purposes, is usually the population from which the numerator was drawn. The denominator is the lower part of a fraction and it is often defined at a particular point in time.

The numerator and the denominator can be combined into a **ratio**, a **proportion**, or a **rate**, as described below. Some of the most frequent mistakes in applying epidemiological principles to real-world problems result from a failure to define the numerators and denominators accurately.

Ratio

$$\text{Ratio} = \frac{n_1}{n_2} = n_1 : n_2$$

where n_1 and n_2 are numbers.

For example,

$$\text{Ratio of males to females in a population} = \frac{\text{Number of males in the population}}{\text{Number of females in the population}}$$

A ratio is often expressed as the odds, which is a single number. For example, if a bag contains two white balls ($n_1 = 2$), three black balls ($n_2 = 3$), and five grey balls ($n_3 = 5$), then the ratio of black balls to white balls is 3:2 ('three to two'). This ratio can be simplified by dividing both the numerator and the denominator by the denominator to give 1.5:1 ('one and a half to one'). Expressed in odds, it is simply 1½.

Ratios are frequently used in epidemiology to compare the outcomes of two groups (e.g. odds ratio, risk ratio, rate ratio). See Section 1A.11.

Proportion

$$\text{Proportion} = \frac{n_1}{N}$$

where n_1 is a subpopulation of the whole study population, N.

If a bag contains two white balls ($n_1 = 2$), three black balls ($n_2 = 3$), and five grey balls ($n_3 = 5$), then $N = 10$, and the proportion of black balls is 3/10 or 0.3.

Disease risks and disease prevalence are proportions that are frequently used in epidemiology. For example, assuming all people in the population are either male or female, then

$$\text{Proportion of males in a population} = \frac{\text{Number of males in the population}}{\text{Number of males} + \text{Females in the population}}$$

Rate

$$\text{Proportion} = \frac{n_1}{N \times T}$$

where

- N is the numerator
- P is the number of people in the population
- T is a period of time, and $N \times T$ represents the quantity 'person-years at risk'

A rate is a measure of frequency with which a phenomenon occurs. The denominator reflects both the population and a timeframe and is often expressed in person-years.

Commonly used rates in epidemiology are incidence rates, mortality rates, and fertility rates.

For example,

$$\text{Incidence of epilepsy} = \frac{\text{Number of new cases of epilepsy}}{\text{Population} \times \text{Reporting period}}$$

Population at risk

Denominators should reflect the population from which the cases originated and should therefore only include those people who would have been counted as a case had they developed the disease. This is generally taken as the total number of people who were disease-free at the start of the study. The denominator should not include people who cannot possibly develop the disease. For example, people who have been immunised against a disease should not be included in studies examining the rate at which people acquire that disease, since these individuals cannot be considered at risk in the same way as people who have not been immunised. If such individuals were included in a study, then the true incidence would be underestimated.

1A.3 Time at risk

Time at risk describes the total amount of time that individuals within a study spend being at risk of developing the disease of interest. This concept is particularly important in the analysis of **cohort studies** because one of the difficulties with conducting cohort studies is that different subjects under study are typically at risk of the disease for different periods of time. For example,

- Some people may **join the study** after data collection has started.
- Other people may **develop the disease** of interest and thereby stop being at risk.
- Still other subjects may leave the at-risk population before the event of interest has occurred (e.g. if they are lost to follow-up or die from a cause other than that being investigated). This phenomenon is known as **right censoring**.
- Occasionally, some people may join the study after the event of interest has already occurred. This is known as **left censoring**; however, in most studies, theses subjects would be excluded at the time of enrolment.

To correct for the variation in different subjects' time at risk, the concept of **total person-time at risk** is used as the denominator in calculations of morbidity or mortality within many cohort studies. Person-time represents the sum of all the individual times at risk:

$$\text{Incidence rate} = \frac{\text{Number of new cases}}{\text{Total person-time at risk}}$$

Calculation of incidence rate using person-time at risk

Sometimes, participants are replaced by new people who are recruited into the study. For short-term studies or where relatively few individuals leave or join the at-risk population, it is reasonably accurate to use the number of individuals at the start of the study as the denominator when calculating the incidence.

However, where the study duration is longer or the likelihood of individuals leaving the at-risk population is greater, it is preferable to use a more accurate calculation of the incidence rate using **person-time at risk**. See Box 1A.3 for an illustration. As time progresses, the number of individuals at risk will fall as people die, become a case, or are lost to follow-up.

Box 1A.3 Cohort study illustrating the concept of time at risk

	Patient 1	Patient 2	Patient 3	Patient 4
Date of entry to study	1998	2000	1995	1997
Event	Death	Loss	Censored	Death
Date of event	2004	2003	2005	1999
Years at risk	6	3	10	2

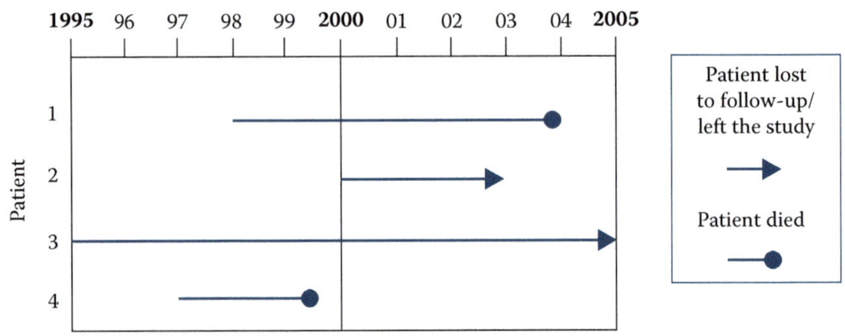

In this case, the event of interest is deaths; therefore, the mortality rate is calculated as:

$$\text{Mortality rate} = \frac{\text{Number of deaths in study period}}{\text{Person time at risk during study period}}$$

Mortality rate = 2/21

Mortality rate = 0.95 per person year or 95 per 1000 person years

1A.4 Methods for summarising data

See also Sections 1B.9 and 1B.10.

Data may be summarised **numerically** (using measures of location and measures of spread) or **graphically**. Different methods for summarising data are described in Sections 1B.9 and 1B.10, but the choice of method generally depends on the type of data in question (see Table 1A.5).

Discrete versus continuous data

Discrete data have a finite number of possible numerical values. Examples are the number of children with brown eyes in a class of 30 children or the number of times a person is admitted to the hospital over the course of their lifetime.

Table 1A.5 Types of data

Type of data	Description	Example
Nominal	Categorical data with no order	Country Blood group (A, B, AB, O)
Ordinal	Data do have an order, but it cannot be said with certainty that the interval between the first category and the second category is the same as the interval between the second category and the third.	Likert scale (strongly agree, agree, neutral, disagree, strongly disagree) Social class I, II, III, IV, V
Interval	These are quantitative data with meaningful intervals between the data; however, the ratios between the data are meaningless and the data do not have a true zero.	Temperature in degrees Celsius: In this example, zero is an arbitrary temperature, i.e. the temperature at which water freezes. Unlike the Kelvin scale, zero degrees Celsius does not imply that there is zero temperature. We also cannot say that 20°C is twice as hot as 10°C. However, we can say that the difference between 10°C and 30°C is twice the difference as between 10°C and 20°C.
Ratio	Ratio data have interval properties but also a true zero. Numbers on a ratio scale can be compared as multiples of one another.	Weight Height Kelvin temperature scale: In this case, 0 K is a true zero; 20 K is twice as hot as 10 K; and the difference between 10 K and 30 K is twice the difference as between 10 K and 20 K.

In contrast, **continuous data** include measurable quantities. Examples include length, volume, time, and many biological measurements. Continuous data frequently have an upper or lower limit (e.g. height cannot be less than zero).

Binary data

Binary data are a special type of discrete data that have only two possible values. Depending on how they are analysed, binary data may be considered to have properties of ordinal data, interval data, or ratio data. Binary data are very common in epidemiology, since they accurately describe a state of interest (e.g. whether a patient improved following a particular treatment or not; whether a case is alive or dead; or whether the case was in the treatment group or in the control group).

Binary data often take values such as true/false or male/female; however, for analysis, they are usually transformed into values of **zero** and **one**. Data of this type are often used in logistic regression (see Section 1B.14), where the values might represent the outcome variable itself or a binary coefficient reported as an odds ratio.

1A.5 Incidence, prevalence, and standardisation

Incidence and prevalence including direct and indirect standardisation.

Incidence and prevalence both measure the occurrence of a disease.

Incidence

The term incidence relates to the new occurrence of something, for example, a hip fracture, a diagnosis of carcinoma of the lung. There are two related measures of incidence, namely, the **incidence** and the **cumulative incidence** (see Table 1A.6). In contrast to the prevalence, the incidence of a disease is not affected by survival.

Prevalence

Prevalence relates to existing occurrences of a disease. The prevalence is also called the **point prevalence** (i.e. the proportion of a population with a disease). It is approximately equal to [incidence × duration] *provided* that the incidence and the death and recovery rates have been stable for the disease in question over time. The **period prevalence** relates to the proportion of the population with a disease during a specified period. See Table 1A.7.

Standardisation

This technique is required when making comparisons between populations of differing demographic structures, where crude mortality or morbidity rates would be misleading. Standardisation is, for example, the first step in addressing questions such as whether town A has a higher mortality rate than town B, or whether 10 new cancers in a workforce of 100 people over 10 years is more or less than we would expect. The technique is mostly used for comparing populations that differ in their age structure, but it may also be used when adjusting for other confounding variables such as differences in **gender**, **social class**, or **combinations** of these and other variables.

To standardise data, populations are divided into **strata** based on differences that might potentially influence the comparison that is being made. For example, to compare the number of deaths in a retirement community with the number of deaths in a town with a high proportion of young mothers, the mortality rates at different ages would need to be compared. One option is simply to present category-specific rates (i.e. age-specific mortality rates); however, this approach would involve presenting a large amount of data and would require the reader to make multiple different comparisons. Instead, standardisation combines category—the different specific rates into a **single summary rate** that has been adjusted to take account of the population's age structure.

Two forms of standardisation that are commonly used are **direct** and **indirect** standardisation.

Table 1A.6 Measures of incidence

Concept	Alternative name	Definition
Incidence	Incidence rate	Number of new events divided by the total person-time at risk during the follow-up period.
Cumulative incidence	Risk	Proportion of a population who *become* diseased in a defined time period. The cumulative incidence is a measure of the risk that an individual will become diseased during a defined time period (e.g. the **attack rate** during an epidemic).

Table 1A.7 Measures of prevalence

Concept	Definition
Point prevalence ('prevalence')	Proportion of a population with a disease *at* a particular point in time
Period prevalence	Proportion of a population who had the disease *during* a specified period

Direct standardisation

Direct standardisation may be used to compare two populations or the same population at two different periods of time. In direct standardisation, the age-specific (or stratum-specific) mortality rates of the **observed** population are known. These rates are then applied to a standard or reference population, such as the European standard population. To use this approach, data for a large number of subjects are generally required so that there are sufficient numbers in each stratum to be confident about the estimate.

Direct standardisation involves the following steps:

1. Identify a standard population (e.g. one of the populations being compared, their average, or an outside standard population).
2. For the populations being compared, take the age-specific mortality rate for each age band and multiply it by the size weighting of that age band from the standard population. This calculation gives the expected number of deaths in the standard population for each age band.
3. Sum all of these values to give the total expected number of deaths in the standard population.
4. Divide the number of deaths by the total standard population to give the **age-standardised rate**. (**Note:** This is an example of a **weighted average**.)
   a. The individual standardised rate has little meaning in its own right; however, it can be compared to the rate from another population that has been standardised in the same way as a **comparative mortality ratio** (see Box 1A.4).

Indirect standardisation

Indirect standardisation is used when age-specific rates are **unknown**, which is often the case with small populations. The technique relies on calculating the death rate that would have been **expected** in the study population had the rates from a standard population applied. This rate can then be compared with the deaths that were actually observed in order to give a standardised mortality ratio (SMR).

The following steps are involved in indirect standardised:

1. Identify a standard population with stratum-specific death rates (e.g. one of the populations being studied, or the European Standard Population).
2. Use these rates to calculate the expected number of deaths in each stratum of the study population.
3. Add up the expected number of deaths for each age band to give the total expected deaths.
4. Calculate the SMR based on the actual (observed) total number of deaths in the study population and the expected number of deaths that was calculated in step 3:

$$\text{SMR} = \frac{\text{Observed deaths}}{\text{Expected deaths}} \times 100\%$$

See Box 1A.4 for an example of indirect standardisation.

Two SMRs should be compared with caution because the number of expected cases in each group depends on the group's actual age/sex/ethnic composition.

When used to estimate the association between an **occupational exposure** and a disease, the SMR **underestimates** the true strength of the association because the general population contains both exposed and unexposed individuals. Therefore, in occupational mortality studies, comparisons are often made against two standard populations: (1) an unexposed population from the same type of occupation and (2) the general population.

Box 1A.4 Example of direct and indirect standardisation

Table B1A.4a shows the crude and age-stratified mortality ratios of two cities. The crude mortality ratio is higher for city A than city B, which is misleading given that the mortality rate is higher in city B in all age bands.

Table B1A.4a Distribution of deaths in city A and city B

	City A			City B		
Age group	No. deaths	Population	Rate per 1000 pyrs	No. deaths	Population	Rate per 1000 pyrs
0–29	4,000	5,000,000	0.8	2,000	2,000,000	1
30–59	15,000	4,000,000	3.75	4,000	1,000,000	4
60+	90,000	2,000,000	45	25,000	500,000	50
Total	109,000	11,000,000	9.909	31,000	3,500,000	8.857

Direct standardisation

A standard population is shown in Table B1A.4b.

Table B1A.4b Standard population

Age group	No. people
0–29	60,000
30–59	30,000
60+	10,000
Total	100,000

Table B1A.4c shows how the age-stratified death rates in city A, and city B from Table B1A.4a can be applied to the standard population in order to calculate their standardised mortality rates.

Table B1A.4c Calculation of age-standardised mortality rates for each city

	City A	City B
Age group	Expected deaths	Expected deaths
0–29	0.0008 × 60,000 = 48	0.001 × 60,000 = 60
30–59	0.00375 × 30,000 = 112.5	0.004 × 30,000 =120
60+	0.045 × 10,000 = 450	0.05 × 10,000 = 500
Total	610.5	680
Age-standardised rate per 100 pyrs	6.105	6.8

Box 1A.4 (*Continued*) Example of direct and indirect standardisation

The comparative mortality ratio can then be calculated as the ratio between the two age-standardised mortality rates:

$$\text{CMR} = \frac{6.8}{6.105} = 1.114$$

Therefore, after directly adjusting for age, the mortality in city B is 11.4% higher than in city A.

Indirect standardisation

Let us now assume that the age-specific mortality rates were unknown in city B but that the population distribution was known. In this situation, direct standardisation cannot be used; however, we can use indirect standardisation. This approach involves calculating the deaths that would be expected if a set of standard age-specific mortality rates were applied to the population, and then comparing this number to the observed deaths to generate an SMR. In this example, we will use the age-specific mortality rates from city A taken from Table B1A.4a as the standard. See Table B1A.4d.

Table B1A.4d Calculation of the SMR for city B

	City B
Age group	Expected deaths
0–29	0.0008 × 2,000,000 = 1,600
30–59	0.00375 × 1,000,000 = 3,750
60+	0.045 × 500,000 = 22,500
Total	27,850

The SMR can then be calculated using the observed deaths from Table B1A.4a and the expected deaths from Table B1A.4d:

$$\text{SMR} = \frac{O}{E} \times 100\%$$

$$\text{SMR} = \frac{31{,}000}{27{,}850} \times 100\% = 111.3\%$$

We can therefore conclude that the number of observed deaths in city B is 11.3% higher than would be expected if city B had the same pattern of mortality as city A.

1A.6 Years of life lost

One way to measure the impact of a health problem is to estimate how many years people might have lived had their lives not been curtailed by it. For example, deaths from road traffic collisions affect mostly young males who would otherwise have been expected to live into their 70s or 80s.

Years of life lost (YLL) is a measure of **premature mortality** and, as such, it explicitly places more importance on deaths that occur in young people than those in older people. YLL is therefore a **value-laden** statistic, which reflects the general wish of society to prevent avoidable causes of death in younger people and to avoid the loss to society of its investment in raising children and in supporting young adults.

To calculate YLL in its most simple form, an upper age limit (e.g. 75) is chosen. A person who dies at the age of 60 contributes 15 YLL (75 – 60 = 15) to the calculation, and a person who dies at age 15 contributes 60 YLL. Deaths occurring in people aged over 75 are not included in the calculation. Infant deaths may or may not be included.

For example, the total YLL in a population may be calculated as

$$\sum(\text{Deaths at each age 1 year} \times 74) + (\text{Deaths age 2 years} \times 73) + \ldots + (\text{Deaths age 74 years} \times 1)$$

In more complex calculations, an actuarial assessment is undertaken of the expectation of life for each person, where life expectancy is calculated using current life tables and age-specific mortality rates are applied to a hypothetical population (see Section 3B.6).

Note that YLL will underestimate the burden of disease due to chronic conditions, which typically have a low mortality in young people. To account for this phenomenon, **health-adjusted life expectancy** (**HALE**) may be used instead of the crude life expectancy, where

$$\text{HALE} = \sum(\text{Number of life years lived in each age group}) \times (\text{Mean health state score for that age group})$$

1A.7 Measures of disease burden

Measures of disease burden (event and time based) and population attributable risks (PARs), including identification of comparison groups appropriate to public health.

See Section 1A.10 for risks.

Various measures are used to assess the burden of disease affecting a community, including event-based and time-based measures. These metrics take into account both the **number** of events and the **impact** of these events on the population. The choice of measure often depends on what data are available for analysis.

Event-based measures of disease burden

These studies of **incidence** require data from routine sources:

- Death certificates (if the disease burden is in mortality rather than morbidity).
- Hospital episode data (if the disease results in hospital admissions).

- Disease registers (if a dedicated register for that particular disease exists).
- Statutory notifications (for certain infectious disease and for procedures such as terminations of pregnancy).
- Note that using health service data to assess disease burden may lead to an **underestimate** because the majority of care occurs outside the formal healthcare sector (i.e. self-care or other forms of informal care). See Section 4B.1 for more information.

Time-based measures of disease burden

Where there are no routine event-based data collected, a cross-sectional **prevalence survey** may be used.

Comparison groups used in public health

Comparison groups are often used as the control arm of a study (see Section 1A.19). At the population level, comparators are used in **needs assessment studies** and for assessing the quality of healthcare. Factors to consider when choosing comparison groups include the following:

- Size of population
- Area characteristics (rural/urban)
- Age structure
- Ethnicity
- Socio-economic characteristics (employment, education, income)
- Disease burden (mortality and morbidity)
- Health service usage
- Health service provision, funding, and organisation (especially for international comparisons)
- Provision of other relevant services (e.g. social care)

1A.8 Variation

Sources of variation, its measurement, and control.

When conducting causal epidemiological studies, researchers are generally interested in determining how an **outcome** (e.g. body weight) varies with respect to an **exposure** (e.g. physical activity). However, if the outcome is found to vary in the study population according to the exposure, this does not necessarily mean that the exposure caused the outcome nor does it even necessarily mean that the outcome was truly associated with the exposure. Other possible explanations must also be considered (see Table 1A.8).

In order to make conclusions about any observed association, other sources of variation should be limited as far as possible. If such factors cannot be eliminated, then efforts should be made to measure these sources of variation so that they can be taken into account when drawing conclusions. Only after other reasons for an association have been considered should the possibility of a causal relationship be considered (see Section 1A.13).

Sampling variability

Epidemiological studies are rarely conducted on a whole population; instead, a sample is usually studied. Even if large, unbiased, random samples are used, any estimates made on different samples will seldom be exactly the same as each other, and a sample value will rarely be the same as the true population value. For example, if several samples of 100 people were taken from a population of 1 million people, then the mean weight of one sample is not unlikely to be exactly the same as the mean weight of any other sample nor is it likely to be exactly the same as the mean weight of the whole population. In an unbiased study, the differences between the sample values and the population value occur due to chance. This difference is known as the **sampling error**, and it may be estimated as the **standard error** (see Section 1B.2). The standard error is the basis for calculating **p-values** and **confidence intervals** (see Sections 1B.3 and 1B.11).

Table 1A.8 Sources of variation

Source of variation	Description	Example	Further details
Chance (random error)	Random differences may occur between individuals in a population because of biological variation, measurement errors, or sampling variability.	Individual variation in the body size of individuals in a population leading to random differences in weight. Differences in weight due to technical limitations of the weighing scales.	1A.9
Bias (systematic error)	A bias exists when there are differences that are unrelated to the exposure of interest that cause some individuals to be systematically classified differently from others.	Interviewers probing certain people in greater detail about their level of physical activity than others.	1A.13
Confounding	Confounding exists when an apparent association between an exposure and a disease is, in fact, due to a third factor.	If people who drink are also more likely to smoke, then an observed association between alcohol intake and breast cancer might, in fact, be due to smoking.	1A.13, 1A.16
True causal association	Here, the exposure of interest directly causes the variation in the outcome.	Physical activity causes individuals to lose weight.	1A.12
Reverse causation	This phenomenon occurs when the outcome of interest causes variation in the exposure.	The association between physical activity and weight occurs because those people who are overweight are unable to mobilise easily, which therefore limits their physical activity.	1A.12

1A.9 Errors in epidemiological measurement

Common errors in epidemiological measurement, their effect on numerator and denominator data, and their avoidance.

See also Section 1B.10.

Measurement error can be defined as any mistake that occurs during the process of applying a standard set of values (i.e. a measurement scale) to a set of observations. In epidemiology, such errors can lead to the **misclassification** of cases and controls. It is important for researchers to acknowledge measurement error because doing so leads to more robust and defensible scientific results.

Measurement errors are either **random** (i.e. they occur due to chance) or **systematic** (i.e. they are persistent, non-random, differences that cause the observed measurement to differ from the true value). Random errors are **non-differential** (i.e. they affect all groups equally), whereas

Table 1A.9 Random and systematic errors in epidemiological measurement

	Random error	Systematic error
Cause	Occurs due to chance.	Occurs due to non-random factors.
Impact	Affects all groups equally (non-differential).	Affects some groups more than others (differential).
Exposure	Misclassification of exposures is *equal* for cases and controls (e.g. 20% of cases and 20% of controls are misclassified as being exposed).	Misclassification of exposures *differs* between cases and controls (e.g. 20% of cases misclassified as having been exposed but only 5% of controls misclassified).
Outcome	Misclassification of outcomes is *equal* for exposed and non-exposed (e.g. 30% of exposed and 30% of non-exposed are misclassified as having the disease).	Misclassification of outcomes *differs* between exposed and non-exposed (e.g. 19% of the exposed are misclassified as having the disease but only 7% of non-exposed are misclassified as having the disease).
Direction of bias	Bias is towards the null hypothesis (i.e. dilution of the study's findings).	Bias may be in any direction.
Threat to the study	Less threatening for a study than systematic error.	More threatening for a study than random error.
Example	A study of lung cancer in relation to proximity of residence to a coke oven classifies subjects (cases and controls) by distance of residence from the oven at the time of follow-up. Here, there is misclassification due to migration (not all people living near the oven at the time of follow-up will have lived there at the aetiologically relevant time); however, this error occurs randomly.	A study assessing the association between visual display unit (VDU) usage and spontaneous abortion. Here, cases are more likely to recall VDU usage compared with controls, particularly if there has been media interest in this hypothesis (recall bias). Therefore, the association measured is likely to be greater than the true association.

systematic errors are **differential** errors (i.e. they affect one group more than another). See Table 1A.9.

Effect of measurement errors

Measurement errors can affect

- **Dependent variables** (i.e. outcomes such as disease)
- **Independent variables** (i.e. risk factors such as exposures)
- **Confounding variables** (see Section 1A.13)
- **Effect modifiers** (see Section 1A.14)

Avoidance of measurement errors

Measurement error can be avoided or accounted for at various stages of a study (see Table 1A.10).

Table 1A.10 Avoiding and accounting for measurement error

Stage of study	Strategy for dealing with measurement error
Design	Set out to **measure reliability** using correlation coefficients (continuous variables) or Cohen's kappa (categorical variables). Ensure adequate blinding. Use standardised and validated measurement instruments. Use multiple sources of information (e.g. questionnaires, direct measurements, registries, and case records). Use multiple controls.
Data collection	Administer instruments equally to Cases and controls Exposed and unexposed persons
Data analysis	Conduct a **sensitivity analysis** to test the robustness of the findings (see Chapter 4D.5).
Reporting	Consider and describe the potential errors, both random and systematic.

1A.10 Concepts and measures of risk

See also Chapters 1A.5, 1A.7, and 2F.2.

Risk

Also called **cumulative incidence**.

Risk is the likelihood of some event. In an epidemiological sense, it is calculated as the proportion of individuals in a population initially free of the disease who develop the disease within the study period. Measures of risk may be **absolute** or **relative** (see Table 1A.11).

Attributable risk measures

All of the attributable risk (AR) measures described here assume that any observed association is causal. These measures can also all be calculated using risks or rates.

Table 1A.11 Absolute and relative risk measure

Type of risk measure	Description	Examples	Further details
Absolute	Public health effect that is attributable to a risk factor	• Attributable risk (AR) • AR fraction • Population attributable risk (PAR) • Population attributable fraction (PAF)	See the following text.
Relative	Ratio comparing the risk in one group to the risk in another group	• Odds ratio • Risk ratio • Rate ratio	Chapter 1A.11.

Attributable risk

Also called the **risk difference** or the **excess risk**, the **AR** is the difference in the risk or rate of disease between the exposed group and the unexposed group:

$$\text{AR} = R_e - R_0$$

where
R_e is the risk in the exposed group
R_0 is the risk in the unexposed group

Attributable fraction

Also called the **aetiological fraction** (or the **AR percent** when expressed as a percentage), this is the proportion of the disease among the exposed people that can be considered to be attributable to the exposure, after allowing for the risk of disease that would have occurred anyway:

$$\text{AF} = \frac{\text{AR}}{R_e} = \frac{R_e - R_0}{R_e}$$

The attributable fraction is a very useful epidemiological statistic, which is readily understood by non-epidemiologists. For example, in people who smoke, about 90% of lung cancers arise *because* of smoking.

Population attributable risk

The PAR is the excess rate of disease in the whole study population (of exposed and unexposed people) that is attributable to the exposure:

$$\text{PAR} = R_t - R_0$$

where
R_t is the risk in the whole population
R_0 is the risk in the unexposed group

Box 1A.5 Example: PAR of smoking in lung cancer

Mortality in whole population = 55 per 100,000
Mortality in non-smokers = 16 per 100,000
PAR = Rate in population − Rate in non-smokers
= 55 − 16
= 39 deaths per 100,000/year

See example in Box 1A.5.

When generalising for a broader population, the true prevalence of exposure in that broader population should be determined from an outside study; otherwise, it will have to be assumed that the broader population has the same exposure as the study population.

Population attributable fraction

This statistic estimates the proportion of disease in the study population that is attributable to the exposure (and thus the proportion of diseases that could be eliminated if the exposure were eliminated). Known also as the **preventable fraction** (or the **PAR percent** when expressed as a percentage), this is a key statistic for prioritising population interventions. It can be calculated in two ways:

$$\text{PAF} = \frac{\text{PAR}}{R_t} = \frac{R_t - R_0}{R_t}$$

$$\text{PAF} = \frac{\text{Prevalence in exposed population} \times (\text{RR} - 1)}{1 + \text{Prevalence in exposed population} \times (\text{RR} - 1)}$$

1A.11 Effect measures

Effect measures including odds ratios, rate ratios, and risk ratios (relative risk).

Effect measures are **relative risks** used to measure the strength of association between an exposure and an outcome (i.e. they are used to assess aetiological strength). The most commonly used such measures in epidemiology are the **risk ratio**, **rate ratio,** and **odds ratio**. Other relative risks include the **SMR** (see Section 1A.5) and the **hazard ratio** (see Section 1B.18). All of these measures reflect the increase in frequency of the outcome (e.g. disease) in one group (e.g. exposed) compared to another (e.g. unexposed).

Risk ratio

$$\text{Risk ratio} = \frac{\text{Risk of disease in exposed}}{\text{Risk of disease in unexposed}}$$

See Box 1A.6 for an example of how to calculate a risk ratio.

Rate ratio

$$\text{Rate ratio} = \frac{\text{Incidence rate in exposed}}{\text{Incidence rate in unexposed}}$$

Odds ratio

In a case–control study, the risk or rate cannot be calculated directly because subjects are selected on the basis of their diseases status, not on the basis of their exposure. The odds of either cases or controls having the exposure can, however, be calculated.

The odds ratio can be calculated based on the odds of exposure (in case–control studies) or, equivalently, the odds of disease (in any study design):

$$\text{Odds ratio} = \frac{\text{Odds of exposure in cases}}{\text{Odds of exposure in controls}}$$

$$= \frac{\text{Odds of disease in exposed}}{\text{Odds of disease in unexposed}}$$

Using a 2 × 2 table, this is calculated as

	Case	Control	
Exposed	a	b	a + b
Unexposed	c	d	c + d
	a + c	b + d	a + b + c + d

$$\text{OR} = \frac{a/c}{b/d} = \frac{a/b}{c/d}$$

If a case–control study is appropriately designed, and the disease is rare, then the odds ratio provides a good approximation of the risk ratio or the rate ratio.

Box 1A.6 Example: calculating the risk ratio

A consultant believes that hypertension is unusually common in patients in her clinic who have had a coronary bypass operation.

		Hypertension		
		Yes	No	
Coronary bypass	**Yes**	**15**	**467**	**482**
	No	**70**	**6364**	**6434**
		85	**6831**	

Risk ratio = (Risk of disease in exposed) ÷ (Risk of disease in unexposed)
= (15 ÷ 482) ÷ (70 ÷ 6434)
= 0.0311 ÷ 0.0109
= 2.86

In this clinic, patients who had had a coronary bypass operation were 2.86 times as likely to have hypertension as those who had not had a bypass.

1A.12 Association and causation

The concepts of association and causation are fundamental to the science of epidemiology. An association is a link between two variables. It is assessed by calculating a measure of effect (see Section 1A.12). However, as described in Section 1A.8, establishing an association does not necessarily mean that there is a **causal** link between the two variables. The association could also be due to **chance**, **bias**, **confounding,** or **reverse causation**.

Chance

Epidemiological studies make inferences regarding the wider population based on observations made on a sample. However, an association might be observed in the sample due to luck of the draw (i.e. where the sample does not truly reflect the wider population). The chance of observing such an unrepresentative association falls as the sample size increases.

The role of chance can be assessed using statistical hypothesis tests to calculate a **p-value** or by calculating **confidence intervals** (see Chapter 1B)

Bias

See Section 1A.13.

Confounding

See Section 1A.13.

Reverse causality

This phenomenon occurs where an association between an exposure and an outcome is in fact due to the outcome causing a change in the exposure. Examples of reverse causation are as follows:

- Some studies in developing countries have shown an association between the duration of breastfeeding and poor growth. However, the association is thought to be due to children with poor growth (due to low maternal dietary intake) being less likely to wean off breast milk [1].
- Studies have shown an association between sleep duration and health-related quality of life (HRQoL); however, it has been argued that poor HRQoL may lead to a greater risk of insomnia [2].
- The association between illicit drug use and psychological and social harm may, in part, occur because people suffering from psychological and social distress are more likely to take illicit drugs [3].

Note: A causal and reverse-causal association may occur simultaneously (likely to be the case in the latter two examples mentioned earlier).

Causality

Once all other potential reasons for an association have been considered, the likelihood of a causal association should be assessed. This is a judgement that should be made on the basis of valid study data *plus* a background of other evidence. The judgement of causality may be informed by the criteria listed in Table 1A.12, which were first proposed by **Bradford Hill** (1965).

Table 1A.12 Bradford Hill criteria for determining causality

Criterion	Description
Strength of association	The greater the magnitude of the risk observed (positive or negative), the less likely it is to be due to confounding. Associations of low magnitude do not necessarily mean that the finding is due to confounding.
Biological credibility/ plausibility	A finding is more credible if there is a known or postulated biological mechanism to explain it. However, an apparently implausible association might turn out to be a scientific discovery.
Consistency of findings	Most persuasive evidence comes from several studies with different methods showing similar results.
Temporal sequence	The exposure of interest should precede the outcome (this helps exclude reverse causation).
Dose–response	There may be a gradient of risk according to the amount of exposure. Note, however, that many biological phenomena demonstrate a threshold rather than a linear relationship. The relationship between alcohol and cardiovascular disease can show a 'J'-shaped curve, implying greater cardiovascular disease risk for people who drink no alcohol compared with people who drink small amounts.
Specificity	If the exposure is associated with one outcome or range of outcomes, this is evidence in favour of a causal effect relationship. However, there are few such one-to-one relationships, and many exposures cause several outcomes (e.g. smoking causes a plethora of diseases).
Coherence	The relationship should not conflict with the natural history of the disease.
Reversibility	If the risk of the disease decreases when the exposure is removed, then this is strong evidence of causality.
Analogy	Analogies with other well-established cause–effect relationships.

1A.13 Biases and confounding

Bias and confounding may lead to **spurious** associations being found between an exposure and an outcome. Both bias and confounding should be acknowledged and minimised in order to avoid incorrect conclusions being made about the causality of an association.

Bias

A bias is a **systematic error** that leads to a difference between the comparison groups with regard to how they are chosen, treated, measured, or interpreted. This error leads to an incorrect estimate of the association between the exposure and the risk of disease. Unlike confounding and the role of chance, the magnitude of a bias cannot be quantified.

Dozens of different types of bias have been described; however, these can be broadly categorised into two major types: **selection bias** and **information bias**.

Selection bias

Selection bias occurs when there are systematic differences between the following:

- Study participants and non-participants
- One group in the study (e.g. intervention group) and another (e.g. control group)

Examples of **selection bias** are shown in Table 1A.13.

Table 1A.13 Examples of selection bias

Type of selection bias	Description
Volunteer bias	This type of bias occurs because people who agree to participate in studies tend to be both healthier and more compliant than those who do not.
Control bias	Selection bias is a particular difficulty with case–control studies. Ideally, controls should represent the **same population** from which the cases were derived; however, this population is often difficult to define. For example, if cases are recruited from a hospital, then ideally controls should be a random sample of anybody who would have attended that hospital if they had developed the same disease. One option is to select other patients at the hospital who were admitted for a different disease; however, this approach often leads to an underestimation of any association because hospitalised patients tend to be more similar to one another with regard to the exposure than a member of the general population (e.g. if cases are patients with lung cancer, then a hospital-based control being treated for cardiovascular disease is more likely to smoke than a control drawn from the wider population). One method to reduce this type of selection bias is to conduct a **nested case–control study** (see Section 1B.17).
Healthy worker effect	This type of bias occurs in **occupational cohort studies**, which compare disease rates among individuals from a particular occupation with the general population. In general, employed people are healthier than the general population because the general population includes people who are too ill to work. To avoid this effect, the comparison group may be restricted to people employed at the same workplace but with a different job.
Follow-up bias	This phenomenon occurs when participants who are lost to follow-up differ systematically from those who remain contactable and where people who are lost to follow-up differ with respect to the exposure.

Information (measurement) bias

Information bias arises when errors occur in the way that the exposure or the outcome is assessed. Such errors may be **non-differential** or **differential** (see also Section 1A.9):

- With non-differential (random) misclassification, the classification errors are the same for both groups being compared (i.e. the misclassification is related neither to the exposure nor to the outcome). As a result, the two groups being assessed will appear to be more similar than they actually are, and therefore any observed association between exposure and outcome will be attenuated.
- With differential (systematic) misclassification, the classification errors occur differently depending on either the person's exposure or outcome status (i.e. the misclassification is related either to the exposure or to the outcome). This type of error can lead to the results being biased in either direction (i.e. overestimation or underestimation of the association). This type of error is therefore more problematic than non-differential misclassification because it can lead to spurious associations.

There are three main types of measurement bias: instrument bias, responder bias, and observer bias (see Table 1A.14).

Evaluating bias

Although bias **cannot be quantified**, attempts should always be made to contemplate the **direction** of the alleged bias and to use **internal validation**. For example, if some participants were incorrectly diagnosed initially, then, had there been no bias, we would expect these participants to have had the same exposures as the controls.

Table 1A.14 Types of measurement bias

<table>
<tr><th>Type of measurement bias</th><th>Description</th></tr>
<tr><td>Instrument bias</td><td>This type of bias occurs where there are systematic inaccuracies in a test or instrument.</td></tr>
<tr><td>Responder bias</td><td>Responder bias occurs where either the
• Information subjects provide about their exposure status differs according to the outcome or
• Information subjects provide about their outcome differs according to their exposure status
One example of this phenomenon is recall bias, where participants who develop a disease recall antecedent exposures differently from people without disease (which is particularly problematic in case–control studies).
Another example is the placebo effect, where people who receive an intervention are more likely to report favourable outcomes regardless of the physiological effects of the intervention.
Responder bias can be minimised by
• Blinding participants to the study hypothesis
• Using a placebo intervention for control groups
• Using objective exposure and outcome measures
• Collecting exposure data from past medical records</td></tr>
<tr><td>Observer bias</td><td>This bias occurs if there are systematic differences in the ways that the exposure or outcome data are collected between the two groups. For example, there may be inaccuracies or incompleteness in data collection that affects the groups to differing degrees.
Interviewer bias is a type of observer bias in which there is a systematic difference in the way that the investigator collects, probes for, or interprets data between groups. Observer bias can be minimised by blinding observers to participants' exposure and disease status and by using standardised protocols for data collection.</td></tr>
</table>

Minimising bias

Bias can be reduced in several ways (see Table 1A.15).

Bias in questionnaires can be reduced by

- Checking for known associations
- Seeking the **same information** in different ways
- Checking characteristics of **data collection** (time taken to complete the questionnaire)

Bias in intervention studies can be assessed by

- Self-reports
- Pill counts
- Measuring **biochemical** parameters
- Incorporating a safe **biochemical marker** in the placebo that can be detected in urine

Confounding

Confounding is a special form of bias that occurs when the association between an exposure is in fact the result of another variable. It occurs when an association is observed that is not due to the exposure being studied (i.e. there is a variable, called a **confounding factor**, which is associated with the exposure of interest and also with the outcome).

Table 1A.15 Methods for minimising bias

Method	Description
Randomisation	Randomisation with **true concealment** ensures that investigators are unable to predict or affect group allocation. Random allocation in intervention studies effectively removes selection bias.
Blinding	Blinding of **participants** avoids **respondent bias**. Blinding of **practitioners** who are treating study participants avoids **instrument bias**. Blinding of **observers** who collect measurements or analyse results avoids **observer bias**.
Irrelevant factors	Collect **irrelevant factors** to check for bias between groups and to mask the hypothesis under investigation.
Repeated measurement	Enhance the reliability and reproducibility of measurements by **repeating** measurements and assuring **inter-observer agreement** to reduce instrument bias.
Training	Study personnel should receive **standardised training** and have their performance monitored (e.g. time the duration of interviews to assess the degree of probing by interviewers).
Written protocol	Data should be collected according to a detailed written protocol using closed questions and direct observations.
Choice of controls	Choose **hospitalised controls** to increase comparability (they will have similar recall of events before admission). However, be aware that a hospital may have different catchment areas for different specialties.
Ease of follow-up	Choose cohorts that can **easily be followed up** long term (e.g. alumni groups).
High-risk cohorts	Choose cohorts with **above-average risk** of disease to shorten the follow-up period and thereby reduce losses to follow-up.
Duplication	Use **multiple sources** of data to assess exposure/disease status.

Note that a confounding factor must be associated with the outcome and must also be *independently* associated with the exposure of interest (i.e. a confounding factor cannot simply be an intermediate step in the causal chain). See Box 1A.7.

Confounding can be controlled either at the **measurement** stage or at the **analysis** stage (see Section 1A.16).

Mediating factors

Not every factor that is associated with both the exposure and the disease is a confounding variable. A variable that is associated with both the independent and dependent variables may alternatively be an intermediate step along the causal chain. This is called a **mediating factor** and it is not a confounding factor because it is not independently associated with the outcome. Longitudinal studies are required to determine whether a third variable is in fact a mediating factor. See Box 1A.8.

Direction of confounding

Confounding may be positive or negative:

- Positive confounding makes the association appear **more pronounced** (either in a positive or negative direction).
- Negative confounding makes the association appear **less pronounced** (i.e. diluted towards the null).

Box 1A.7 Example: Smoking as a confounding factor

Populations with high alcohol consumption tend to have high lung cancer rates, but this is simply because people who misuse alcohol are more likely to smoke than people who do not. Smoking, in turn, is causally associated with lung cancer. Smoking therefore confounds the apparent relationship between alcohol consumption and lung cancer.

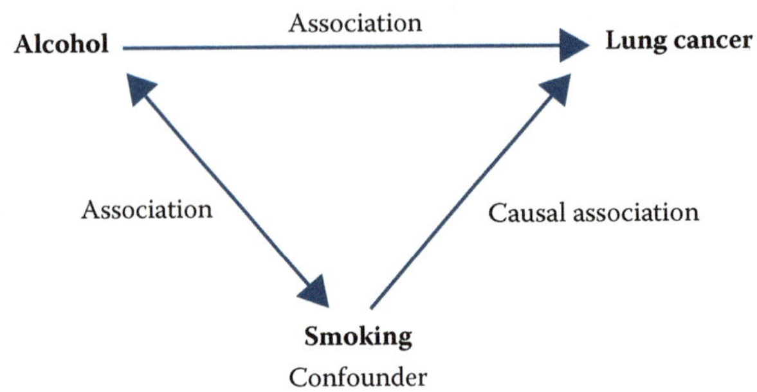

Box 1A.8 Example: Cholesterol as a mediating factor

There is a strong relationship between poor diet and the incidence of CHD. There is also a relationship between a poor diet and a high serum cholesterol level.

We know that a high serum cholesterol level is causally associated with a higher risk of a CHD event; however, serum cholesterol is not a confounding factor here. Since a high cholesterol level may be caused by a poor diet, it is in fact on the causal pathway of the relationship between diet and CHD. Accordingly, serum cholesterol is a mediating factor.

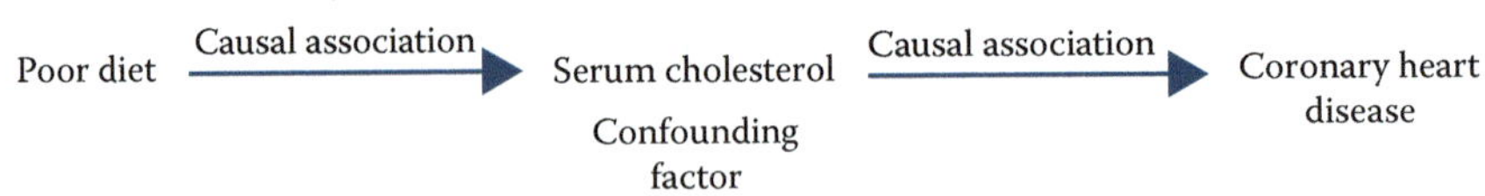

Residual confounding

Residual confounding occurs as a result of **unknown confounding factors** (i.e. confounders whose effects remain once all of the known confounding factors have been taken into account) or where confounding factors are **inaccurately measured**. The process of randomisation, which distributes both known and unknown confounding factors equally between groups, effectively eliminates residual confounding.

1A.14 Effect modification

Interactions, methods for assessment of effect modification.

Effect modification (also called **interaction**) occurs when the effect on the outcome of one causal factor varies according to the level of a third variable. This third variable is termed an **effect modifier**. For example, the effect of smoking on the risk of myocardial infarction is stronger in young people; therefore, age is an effect modifier in this case.

Assessment of effect modification

In order to assess whether an interaction exists, the association between an exposure and outcome should be assessed for different strata of the potential effect modifier. For example, where both smoking and age as risk factors for myocardial infarction, this process would involve examining the association between smoking and myocardial infarction for different age bands (see Table 1A.16).

Table 1A.16 Myocardial infarction in smoking

Age band	Odds of myocardial infarction, smokers compared to non-smokers (OR)
35–50	2.3
50–65	1.8
65+	1.4

Test for interaction

While examining the stratum-specific effects may provide a good indication of whether effect modification is occurring, stratum-specific estimates may vary in any case due to random variation, even if the true effect is the same for all strata.

The chi-squared test for interaction is used to test for heterogeneity between the stratum-specific estimates and provides a p-value as an indication of how likely it is that any observed heterogeneity is due to chance. However, this test has low power; therefore, the stratum-specific estimates should always be checked visually as well.

1A.15 Control of confounding

Strategies to allow/adjust for confounding in design and analysis.

Confounding can be countered at the **design** stage or it can be adjusted for at the **analysis** stage.

Design stage

At the design stage, confounding can be addressed through **restriction**, **matching**, and **randomisation** (see Table 1A.17).

Analysis stage

At the analysis stage, confounding can be corrected for by means of **stratification** or **multivariate analysis**. See Table 1A.18.

Table 1A.17 Techniques for dealing with confounding at the design stage

Technique	Method	Advantages	Disadvantages
Randomisation	Participants are allocated to groups at random.	If the sample is large enough, then randomisation removes both known and unknown confounding factors.	Not always possible.
Restriction	If sex and race are considered to be potential confounding factors, then consider only one particular group from across both factors (e.g. just black women).	Cheap.	Smaller pool of potential recruits; residual confounding factors if restriction is insufficiently narrow; cannot assess varying levels of a factor.
Matching	Nowadays only used for case–control studies (match for age, sex, ethnicity, smoking history, etc.).	Intuitive appeal; unique benefits of twin studies (see Section 1A.40); useful in small case series.	Difficult and expensive, especially where there are multiple controls for each case; cannot explore factors that have been matched; no control for factors that have not been matched.

Table 1A.18 Techniques for dealing with confounding at the analysis stage

Method	Details	Disadvantages
Stratification	Divide the confounding variables into strata and provide stratum-specific relative estimates (with confidence intervals) plus a weighted-average overall single estimate of the confounding effect (e.g. the **Mantel–Haenszel** method).	Unable to control simultaneously for more than a few confounding factors because the number of strata increases exponentially, so the number of individuals in each stratum falls.
Standardisation	See Section 1A.5.	See Section 1A.5.
Multivariate analysis	Mathematical models such as **multiple regression** and **logistic regression** (see Section 1B.14).	Sometimes viewed as a 'black box' (i.e. transparency is lost). However, this is a minor problem and multivariate analysis is usually the preferred method for dealing with confounding at the analysis stage.

1A.16 Descriptive and ecological studies

Design, applications, strengths, and weaknesses of descriptive studies and ecological studies.

Descriptive studies and ecological studies describe patterns of disease with regard to time, person, and place:

- Descriptive studies include **case reports** (a description of a one-off unusual finding) and **case series** (a description of several unusual findings that are linked in some way).
- **Ecological studies** are characterised by the unit of observation being a **group** (e.g. a population or community) rather than an individual.

Both types of study can use routinely collected data, and as a result they are relatively cheap and rapid to conduct. They are particularly useful for formulating research questions (see Table 1A.19).

Table 1A.19 Features of descriptive studies

Type	Descriptive studies (case reports/case series)	Ecological studies
Design	Astute clinician notices an unusual occurrence.	Describe a disease pattern for an entire population with regard to another parameter. Use group-level data: either **aggregate** (summaries of individual data), **environmental** (measurable at individual level but easier at group level), or **global** (attributes of a place that are not applicable at individual level, such as a district, or legislation). The correlation coefficient (r) can range from −1 to +1. Two main types: • Geographical studies • Time-series studies (see Section 1A.23)
Application	Case series are particularly useful in identifying the beginning of an epidemic. Hypothesis formulation.	International comparisons. Study of group-level effects (e.g. legislation). Hypothesis formulation.
Strengths	Rapid. Low cost.	Rapid. Low cost.
Weaknesses	Case report cannot be used to test for a valid statistical association (the observation may just be a coincidence). Case series are difficult to test because there is no appropriate comparison group. May not be generalisable Cannot assess disease burden.	Unable to control for unknown confounding factors. Only considers the average exposure (e.g. it would be unable to detect a J-shaped curve). Spatial autocorrelation (the analysis assumes that all areas are independent but they may not be). Leakage of exposures through migration. No information about individuals. Risk of the **ecological fallacy** (see in the following).

Box 1A.9 The ecological fallacy

The term ecological fallacy was first used in relation to an analysis of the 1930 US census. An analysis of the findings showed that the higher the proportion of new immigrants in a state, the higher its average literacy. Further analysis at the individual level showed, however, that new immigrants were less literate than citizens; however, they tended to settle in states where the native population was more literate. It would have been an ecological fallacy to conclude from the original analysis that new immigrants were more literate people than the citizens.

Ecological fallacy

An **ecological fallacy** is an error of logic that occurs when inferences are made regarding individuals, based on aggregate data from the population to which the individuals belong (see Box 1A.9).

1A.17 Analytical and intervention studies

Design applications, strengths, and weaknesses of cross-sectional, analytical, and intervention studies (including randomised controlled trials [RCTs]).

See Chapter 1B.9.

The choice of study design is key to conducting high-quality epidemiological research. There is rarely one single study design appropriate to answering an epidemiological question; more often, there are several potential designs that could be used. Practical concerns, such as costs and timescales, therefore guide which design should be used.

For all analytical studies, the first step is to articulate the research **hypothesis**, which involves stating the **exposure(s)** of interest, the **outcome(s)** of interest, and any possible **confounding factors**.

The main types of study design used in epidemiological research can be grouped into two overarching categories: observational and interventional (see Table 1A.20).

Table 1A.20 Epidemiological study designs

Design type	Description	Study designs
1. Observational	Individuals or communities are not allocated to specific groups (i.e. they are not allocated to receive an intervention).	• Cross-sectional • Case–control • Cohort
2. Interventional	Individuals or communities are allocated to specific groups (i.e. to receive an intervention). In **experimental** designs, participants are randomly assigned to groups. In **quasi-experimental** designs, the assignment is not random but is instead based on other factors.	• RCT • Non-randomised trial

Cross-sectional studies

In this type of study, all of the variables (i.e. exposures and outcomes) are measured at the same time. Cross-sectional studies can be descriptive or analytical. Ecological studies may also be cross sectional (see Box 1A.10).

See Table 1A.21 for the features of cross-sectional studies. An example of a cross-sectional ecological study is the study by Drain et al. [4] that compared HIV prevalence and rates of male circumcision in 118 developing countries and found that HIV prevalence was lower in countries where male circumcision was

Box 1A.10 Types of cross-sectional studies

Type of cross-sectional study	Description
Descriptive	Description of the point prevalence of a disease or an exposure in a population (but not both). Used to assess the burden or distribution of diseases or risk factors.
Analytical	Comparison of different exposures with occurrences of the outcome of interest to investigate associations.
Ecological[a]	Neither the exposure nor the outcome is measured at the individual level.

[a] Note that ecological studies need not necessarily be cross-sectional: they can also be longitudinal.

Table 1A.21 Features of cross-sectional studies

Feature	Description
Design	Determines the **simultaneous** prevalence of exposure and disease. Measures the prevalence of diseases, characteristics, and healthcare usage and make comparisons between these.
Sampling	Sampling needs to be representative of the population under study. A random sample is preferable and the sample needs to be sufficiently large.
Application	Hypothesis formulation. Analytical cross-sectional studies can be used to test hypotheses.
Analysis	Disease **frequency**: Odds or prevalence Measure of **effect**: Prevalence ratio, prevalence difference, odds ratio.
Strengths	Can study multiple exposures and outcomes. Rapid and cheap. Useful for rare diseases. Useful for detecting disease burden.
Weaknesses	Because cross-sectional studies measure prevalence, not incidence, the findings cannot differentiate between the determinants of aetiology and survival. Difficult to determine if an outcome or an exposure came first, because both were assessed simultaneously (i.e. risk of reverse causation). May be subject to recall bias if inquiring about past exposures.

commoner. They cautioned that the interpretation of this study should to take account of the ecological fallacy (see Section 1A.16) and the potential for confounding (e.g. religious practice may be associated with higher circumcision rates *and* with lower prevalence of high-risk sexual behaviours).

Case–control studies

In this type of study, a group of individuals with the outcome of interest (**cases**) are compared to a group of individuals who do not have the outcome of interest (**controls**). See Table 1A.22 for the features for case–control studies. For example, in a study of sudden infant death syndrome (SIDS), characteristics such as sleeping position and type of mattress were compared in a group of children who had died from SIDS and a matched group of children who had not.

Nested case–control studies

Sometimes, a case–control study is enclosed ('nested') within a cohort study. In this instance, both the cases and the controls are taken from within the population of a cohort study. Nested case–control studies can be useful when it would be **too expensive** or otherwise unfeasible to perform laboratory tests on the entire cohort.

Some advantages of nested studies are that they

- Avoid selection bias by drawing cases and controls from the same cohort
- Are cost-effective
- Can avoid recall bias by using data collected before the onset of disease

Cohort studies

In a cohort study, a group of individuals is selected who do ***not*** initially have the outcome of interest. A range of exposures is quantified for cohort members. At the end of the study, those people who have developed the outcome of interest are compared with those who have not developed the outcome of interest, according to the exposure of interest. Cohort studies can be **prospective** or **retrospective** (where the exposures and outcomes have already occurred and recorded in past records).

The **Framingham study** is an example of a prospective cohort study, which followed residents of a town in Massachusetts. The outcomes of interest were cardiovascular endpoints (e.g. myocardial infarction) and the exposures of interest included serum cholesterol and blood pressure. See Table 1A.23 for the features of cohort studies.

Intervention studies (including randomised controlled trials)

In an intervention study, the epidemiologist is able to allocate the exposure of interest across the study population (see Table 1A.24). For example, in the 4S Study [5], a group of Scandinavian volunteers was randomised to receive either 20 mg of simvastatin daily or placebo. The intervention and control groups were compared according to the numbers of deaths and numbers of major cardiovascular events in each group.

Variations of the randomised control trial

There are several important variations of the randomised control trial to note, including **crossover trials, factorial trials**, and **cluster randomised trials** (see Table 1A.25).

Table 1A.22 Features of case–control studies

Feature	Description
Design	In the hypothesis, state the exposure(s) and outcome of interest. Choose subjects who do and do not have the **disease** of interest and compare them with respect to the exposure of interest. The selection of controls is the most critical issue (see Section 1A.24). The ideal ratio of cases to controls is 1:1, but if cases are limited, then it is possible to increase number of controls disproportionately up to 1:4 (beyond this ratio, there is little additional gain in power).
Sampling	**Selection of cases** Selection is usually either **population based** (all cases within a defined population in a given time) or **hospital based** (all cases attending a named hospital). The population approach is generally preferable because the patients attending a hospital may not be representative of the whole population. In all case–control studies, a precise **case definition** is required. **Selection of controls** Controls should be selected from the same population as the cases and may be matched for certain characteristics that are *not* being tested. This approach is easier in population-based studies and is more complicated in hospital-based studies (see Section 1A.24). The selection of cases and controls must be independent of their exposure to the putative risk factors of interest.
Application	Case–control studies can be **retrospective** (all cases of disease have been diagnosed before the study starts) or **prospective** (new cases are identified during the lifetime of the study).
Analysis	First, compare the cases and controls for baseline differences. **Disease frequency**: cannot be determined using this study design (because the cases were chosen precisely because they had the disease). **Measure of effect**: odds ratio.
Strengths	Rapid and cheap. Ideal for **rare diseases/outcomes**. Useful for diseases with long latent periods. Can simultaneously examine a large number of potential exposures.
Weaknesses	Selection bias (exposure and disease have already occurred). Temporal relationships may be difficult to establish. Recall bias (of information on exposure and disease). Poor for rare exposures (unless high AR percentage). Cannot compare incidence rates (unless population based). Misclassification of exposure/disease status (random → null; non-random → any direction). Temptation of data fishing (if multiple hypotheses are tested, then, on average, 1 in 20 will be significant at the $p < 0.05$ level simply because of chance; see Section 1B.11).

Table 1A.23 Features of cohort studies

Feature	Description
Design	In the hypothesis, state the exposure and outcome(s) of interest. Choose subjects on basis of their **exposure** (all subjects should be disease-free at the start). Follow the cohort to study **temporal relationships**; therefore, consider the ease of follow-up when selecting a prospective cohort (e.g. alumni).
Sampling	For common exposures, a population-based sample is usually chosen to limit selection bias. For rare exposures, the cohort may be chosen on the basis of exposure (e.g. workers exposed to asbestos). **Note:** If a workplace cohort is chosen, then cohort members are likely to be healthier than the general population (the **healthy worker effect**). See Section 1A.13.
Application	Able to measure incidence directly in both groups.
Analysis	**Disease frequency**: rate, risk, odds, mean, or median **Measure of effect** • Relative: Rate/risk/odds ratio • Absolute: Rate/risk/odds difference • Other: Vaccine efficacy, difference in mean/median Must also **compare** groups to ensure **similarity** of potential confounding factors. Can estimate effect of loss to follow-up by comparing the two extreme situations (i.e. that all of the people lost to follow-up developed the disease, and then that none of them did). Survival analysis can also be conducted (see Section 1B.18).
Strengths	Able to follow **temporal** relationships. Well suited to **rare exposures**. **Multiple effects** of a single exposure. Minimises selection bias (prospective cohort studies). Useful for diseases with **long latency** periods (retrospective cohort studies).
Weaknesses	Time-consuming. Expensive. Risk of loss to follow-up (→ poor validity [power and bias], especially if loss to follow-up >30% or if loss to follow-up is disproportionate between two groups). Inefficient for rare diseases. Records may be inadequate for ascertainment (retrospective cohort studies). Healthy worker effect (see Section 1A.14).

Table 1A.24 Features of intervention studies

<table>
<tr><th>Feature</th><th>Description</th></tr>
<tr><td>Design</td><td>These studies are epidemiological experiments in which the investigators allocate the exposure. The intervention is generally allocated at random (an RCT) in order to control for confounders (see Section 1A.25); but an alternative is to use systematic allocation.

Stopping rules<ul><li>An independent group must monitor the interim results to ensure the welfare of participants.</li><li>If there is extreme benefit or extreme harm, the trial should be stopped early but only if this is definitely not a temporary or random fluctuation in the results.</li><li>Procedures are also needed for immediate unblinding in the event of an isolated serious complication.</li><li>An extremely high significance (i.e. extremely low p-value) is needed to justify early termination of trial.</li><li>It is controversial whether different stringencies in significance are needed to stop a trial early because of beneficial and harmful effects.</li></ul>Compliance
Non-compliance → Two groups more similar → Result tends towards the null → Trial less able to detect a true effect.
Can improve compliance by using run-in period before randomisation, during which all potential participants receive treatment/placebo to determine their acceptability to patients.</td></tr>
<tr><td>Sampling</td><td>The study population needs to be representative of the reference population (i.e. the population to which the results of the trial will be extrapolated).
Individuals are then randomised to either the intervention or the control group (see Section 1A.25).</td></tr>
<tr><td>Application</td><td>Can investigate therapeutic or preventive interventions, at the level of either the individual or the population (e.g. fluoridation).</td></tr>
<tr><td>Analysis</td><td>Disease frequency: rate, risk, odds, mean, or median.
Measure of effect<ul><li>Relative: Rate/risk/odds ratio</li><li>Absolute: Rate/risk/odds difference</li><li>Other: Vaccine efficacy, difference in mean/median</li></ul>Start with a table comparing the two groups for their baseline characteristics.
Consider the placebo effect.
Analyse by intention to treat (see Section 1A.20).</td></tr>
<tr><td>Strengths</td><td>The evidence generated can be of extremely high quality.
If the sample is large enough, then the validity can be guaranteed.
Blinding minimises observation bias (where blinding is impossible, independent examiners should assess the endpoints).</td></tr>
</table>

(continued)

Table 1A.24 (*Continued*) Features of intervention studies

Feature	Description
Weaknesses	Generalisability. Is the **study population** similar enough to the reference population for the results to be applicable? If inclusion/exclusion criteria are too strict, then it may not be. Is the **intervention** comparable to the treatment that would be received outside a trial (with regard to clinicians' interest and attentiveness)? **Efficacy** is the effect under ideal conditions; **effectiveness** is the real-life effect. Ethical issues: There must be sufficient doubt (**equipoise**) about the alternatives: • Study will be not be feasible if the treatment under investigation is already too widely accepted. • Study will be unethical if the existing evidence suggests harm from giving or withholding the treatment. Potential to be extremely high **cost**. Potential **biases** from • Loss to follow-up of many subjects (more likely with long follow-up periods). • Unequal follow-up (in terms of accuracy or completeness) between the two groups. • Observation bias (unlikely with mortality but more likely with cause of death; can be minimised by double blinding). • Placebo effect (response to any therapy regardless of physiological effect). The true effect of intervention is the percentage effect in the treatment group minus the percentage effect due to placebo.

Table 1A.25 Variations of RCTs

Type	Details
Crossover	Each participant acts as their own control by receiving two or more treatments at different times in the trial. The order in which participants receive the treatments is determined by random allocation. This design is only suitable for interventions with long-term outcomes.
Factorial design	Two or more interventions are compared singly and in combination against a comparison group (i.e. there may be four groups: intervention A, intervention B, interventions A and B, and control). This design allows the investigator to study two interventions and how they interact; however, it requires large numbers of study participants.
Cluster	In this design, groups of participants are randomised, rather than randomising them individually. See Section 1A.21.

1A.18 Small-area analysis

Analysis of health and disease in small areas.

The prevalence of a particular disease at a small area level may be markedly different from its prevalence at a regional or national level. Therefore, analysing data at these larger geographical areas might mask pockets of high risk.

Similarly, it may not be valid to extrapolate health survey data (such as the *Health Survey for England*) down to a local level. There is, therefore, a case for high-quality research to be commissioned at a local level, although often the cost implications may be prohibitive. See Section 3A for details of small area boundaries in the United Kingdom.

One of the most notable examples of small-area analysis is the Dartmouth Atlas (see Box 1A.11).

Difficulties with small-area analysis

There are several difficulties inherent to conducting small-area studies:

- There may be **little variation** in exposure by area (making analytical studies difficult).
- Data errors and **chance** variation may have a greater effect on the results.
- The data available at a small area may often be limited. For example, accurate population data may not be available, meaning that no appropriate denominator is available.

Box 1A.11 Small areas analysis

Dartmouth Atlas of Health Care

First published in 1996, this project analyses Medicare data to describe how medical resources are distributed and used across the United States. Healthcare may be classified as being either

- **Effective and necessary**
- **Preference sensitive** (some better-informed patients would choose other options)
- **Supply sensitive** (driven by how many hospitals and doctors a region has)

The atlas highlights areas of unwarranted variation in supply-sensitive care.

In the United Kingdom, the NHS Atlas of Variation in Healthcare showed almost a 30-fold variation in the percentage of patients in PCT areas who received all nine key care processes recommended for people with diabetes.

Sources: www.dartmouthatlas.org; www.rightcare.nhs.uk/atlas; Wennberg, J., *Tracking Medicine: A Researcher's Quest to Understand Healthcare*, 2010, by permission of Oxford University Press.

1A.19 Validity, reliability, and generalisability

Validity

Validity is the degree to which an instrument **measures what it purports to measure**. It is important that all variables are measured accurately, including exposures, outcomes, and potential confounders. There are various different ways of describing the validity of a test or measurement instrument, including the **criterion validity, face validity, content validity,** and **construct validity** (see Table 1A.26).

Measuring validity

It is possible to assess the degree of criterion validity against a gold standard by measuring the correlation between the two measures. For continuous measures, the **correlation coefficient** is used (see Section 1B.16), whereas for binary outcome measures, the validity can be assessed by calculating the sensitivity and specificity (see Section 2C.2).

Improving validity

Validity may be evaluated and improved by

- **Testing/measuring** it against a gold standard or against expert opinion
- **Triangulation** using multiple research methods
- Addressing **measurement bias** (e.g. by using blinding and standardised protocols)

Reliability

Reliability, also known as **repeatability** or **reproducibility**, is a measure of the consistence of an instrument's performance. A test is 100% reliable if it always produces the same result when measuring the same thing.

Types of reliability

There are several methods for assessing the reliability of an instrument, including **intra-observer reliability**, **inter-observer reliability**, **equivalence**, and **internal consistency** (see Table 1A.27).

Measuring reliability

Intra- and inter-observer reliability can be measured using the **correlation coefficient** or the **kappa statistic**.

Correlation coefficient

For continuous measures, the correlation between measures on two different occasions can be

Table 1A.26 Types of validity

Type of validity	Description
Criterion	There are two types of criterion validity: • **Concurrent validity** (how well the instrument compares to another 'gold standard' measure) • **Predictive validity** (how well the instrument predicts what it aims to predict, such as the likelihood of having a disease)
Face	How well the instrument corresponds to expert opinion, in terms of how it measures the variable of interest
Content	How representative is the instrument of the concept that it is measuring? For example, does a questionnaire on depression cover all the relevant symptoms?
Construct	How well the instrument measures what it should theoretically be measuring rather than some other concept. For example, does a questionnaire on leadership accurately assess whether somebody is a good leader or a good manager?

Table 1A.27 Types of reliability

Type	Description
Intra-observer reliability	Also known as **intra-measurement reliability** or **test-retest reliability**, this type of reliability describes the consistency of results when the instrument is used by the **same observer on the same subject** on two or more occasions.
Inter-observer reliability	The consistency of the results when the instrument is used on the **same subject by two or more observers**.
Equivalence	The consistency between **two instruments** that are meant to measure the same thing (e.g. a questionnaire in two different languages). Equivalence is calculated as the **equivalence reliability coefficient**.
Internal consistency	The consistency of different parts of an instrument (e.g. different questions within a questionnaire). This is only relevant in some circumstances and is measured using **Cronbach's alpha**.

assessed using the correlation coefficient (see Section 1B.16). A measure with a correlation coefficient >0.70 is generally considered to be reliable.

Kappa statistic

The kappa statistic indicates how closely two different measurements (binary or nominal) are aligned. Table 1A.28 is a contingency table for the kappa statistic.

The agreement due to chance varies according to the proportion of results that are reported as positive or negative. The kappa value is interpreted as shown in Table 1A.29.

Kappa has some limitations:

- Using kappa to assess agreement assumes that the raters are independent.
- It tells the reader nothing about the reasons for any variation.

An example of the use of the kappa statistic is shown in Box 1A.12.

Table 1A.28 Contingency table for kappa statistic

		Observer 1		
		No	Yes	Total
Observer 2	No	*a*	*b*	***a* + *b***
	Yes	*c*	*d*	***c* + *d***
Total		***a* + *c***	***b* + *d***	***a* + *b* + *c* + *d***

Generalisability

Generalisability, also known as **external validity**, is the extent to which a study's findings are applicable to other populations or situations. The degree of generalisability is a judgement, which should consider

Table 1A.29 Interpretation of the kappa statistic

Kappa value	Degree of agreement beyond chance
0	None
0–0.2	Slight
0.2–0.4	Fair
0.4–0.6	Moderate
0.6–0.8	Substantial
0.8–1.0	Almost perfect

Box 1A.12 Example: kappa statistic

Two doctors reported the results of 29 patients. They agreed with each other in 22 cases (75.9%), From the following table, we can see that the resultant kappa statistic is 0.542, representing moderate agreement.

$I_o = 0.759$

$I_e = 0.473$

kappa = 0.542

all aspects of the study and the context of the other population in question. Relevant factors include

- Eligibility criteria
- Characteristics of participants
- Location and other aspects of the setting
- Interventions
- Exposures
- Measurement of outcomes

For a study to be generalisable, it must also have good internal validity.

1A.20 Intention-to-treat analysis

It may seem intuitive to compare the groups in an intervention study according to the actual interventions received by the participants. This is known as an **analysis by treatment received**.

It is generally preferable, however, to perform the analysis on the *a priori* group to which each participant was originally assigned. In other words, the analysis should be conducted without consideration of whether each participant actually received or adhered to the treatment they were offered, or whether or not they were lost to follow-up. This approach is known as an **intention-to-treat analysis** and it has a number of advantages.

Advantages of intention-to-treat analysis

The advantages of intention-to-treat analysis over analysis by treatment received are as follows:

- The **actual research question** being asked concerns the effect of *offering* the treatment to patients in the real world, as opposed to the actual physiological effect of their receiving it.
- The **balance of unknown confounding factors** achieved at randomisation is impossible to recreate once non-compliers are removed from the two groups (hence the maxim *'once randomised, always analyzed'*).
- People who switched from their allotted groups may **differ systematically** from those who remained (e.g. patients who were too sick to cope with side effects may have tended to transfer to the placebo group).

Participants lost to follow-up

Strictly speaking, in an intention-to-treat analysis, participants lost to follow-up should be kept in the analysis. This can be achieved either by seeking the outcomes of people who were lost to follow-up or by imputing their outcomes (see below). An alternative approach is to exclude people lost to follow-up from the main analysis but to conduct a **sensitivity analysis** using imputed results.

Imputing results

There are four principal strategies for imputing the results of people lost to follow-up (see Table 1A.30).

Strategies 3 and 4 put bounds on the possible results and may therefore be used in a sensitivity analysis.

Table 1A.30 Strategies for imputing results

Imputation strategy	Description
1. Assume the best.	Assume that all the people that are missing were free of the disease.
2. Assume the worst.	Assume that all the people that are missing developed the disease.
3. Best-case scenario for the intervention.	Assume that all people missing from the intervention group were free of the disease but that all those missing from the control group developed the disease.
4. Worst-case scenario for the intervention.	Assume that all the people missing for the intervention group developed the disease but that all those missing from the control were disease-free.

1A.21 Clustered data

Clustered data—effect on sample size and approaches to analysis.

Clustered data are not fully independent of each other. Rather, they are linked according to a particular characteristic (e.g. time, place, or person). Standard statistical techniques depend on the assumption that observations are independent of each other. This assumption is not true when the data are clustered since observations in the same cluster will be more similar to each other than if they were independent. See Box 1A.13 for an example of a clustered study.

Clustered data

Common types of clustered data include

- Multiple observations on the same subject at the same time
- Repeated observations on the same subject over time
- Cluster randomised trials
- Clustered sampling surveys

Cluster randomised control studies

In some studies, it is more appropriate to randomise groups (clusters) of people rather than individuals. For example,

- If the intervention is provided at a community level (e.g. water fluoridation, mosquito spraying)
- If individual randomisation would result in considerable contamination (e.g. individuals receiving a sexual health education programme might discuss what they learned with individuals in the control group and thereby influence their outcomes)

Statistical considerations for clustered data

In each of these circumstances, the effect of clustering must be taken into account at the statistical analysis stage; otherwise, associations that do not truly exist are more likely to be reported as significant.

Sample size

Clustered trials and surveys require an increased sample size to compensate for the tendency of individuals within each cluster to be more similar to each other than to individuals in other clusters.

The amount by which the sample size needs to be increased is called the **design effect** and this depends on the number of individuals per cluster and the **intra-class correlation** coefficient (i.e. the ratio of inter-cluster variance to total variance).

Analysis

At the analysis stage, there are several ways of accounting for the effect of clustering, such as by

- Calculating **summary statistics** for each cluster and then analysing these using standard techniques
- Calculating **robust standard errors** that account for clustering
- Using more sophisticated techniques, such as generalised estimating equations and multilevel models

Random and fixed effects

Random and fixed effects are statistical models that can be employed within analysis of variance (ANOVA)* or a multilevel regression analyses of clustered data:

- **Random-effects** models explicitly model the similarities between individuals in the same cluster (i.e. a random sample of all possible values of that variable).
- In contrast, a **fixed-effects** model refers to assumptions about the independent variable (e.g. that it can only take the values high, medium, or low). With a fixed-effects model, the conclusions will be restricted to these three values.

---

* ANOVA is a collection of statistical procedures that compares means by dividing the overall observed variance into different parts. See Box 1B.12.5.

Box 1A.13 Example: Accounting for clustering in studies

The ten towns' study started in 1990, and compared ten towns in England and Wales. Five of the towns had high levels of cardiovascular disease and five had low levels. In one study within the project, researchers surveyed school children to determine *'Whether markers of nutrition, cardiovascular health and type 2 diabetes differ between school pupils who eat school dinners and those whose school day meal is provided from home'.*

In order to take account of clustering, the researchers assigned the town of residence as a **fixed effect** and assigned the school attended as a **random effect**. Because the analysis used both fixed and random effects, it is termed a 'mixed model'.

Source: Adapted from Whincup et al., 2005; *Ten Towns Heart Health Study*, www.tentowns.ac.uk.

1A.22 Numbers needed to treat

Numbers needed to treat—calculation, interpretation, advantages, and disadvantages.

The numbers needed to treat (NNT) is a useful statistic that indicates how many patients would need to be treated with a particular intervention for one patient to benefit with respect to the defined outcome. It is the **reciprocal of the absolute risk reduction** and is particularly

Box 1A.14 Number needed to treat (NNT)

Calculation	$\text{NNT} = \dfrac{1}{\text{Absolute risk reduction}}$
Interpretation	The NNT answers the question *'How many patients would I need to treat in order for one extra patient to benefit?'* An analogous measure in screening studies is called the **number needed to screen**. If the treatment or exposure is harmful (i.e. the result is a negative number), then the minus sign is omitted and the measure is renamed the **number needed to harm**.
Advantages	A more intuitive expression of the absolute risk.
Disadvantages	The NNT depends on the baseline risk of the disease in the study sample; therefore, it is not generalisable to populations where the baseline risk of disease differs. It is tempting to compare NNTs for different therapies but this is only justified when the baseline risks of the disease are similar. A drug that reduced mortality from 90% to 80% has the same NNT as a drug that reduces mortality from 40% to 30% but the latter would have a greater relative impact. Caution is needed when calculating the NNT from meta-analyses.

Box 1A.15 Example: Number needed to treat

In the 4S Study, during a 5.4-year period, 256 of 2223 patients (11.5%) in the placebo group died, compared with 182 of 2221 patients (8.2%) in the group who were treated with simvastatin.

Absolute risk reduction = 0.115 − 0.082 = 0.033

$$\text{NNT} = \frac{1}{0.033} = 30 \text{ patients}$$

useful since it takes into account the frequency of the outcome and thus reflects the public health impact of the intervention (e.g. the impact of offering low-dose aspirin in preventing cardiovascular disease).

Analogous measures can be used to compare screening programmes (number needed to screen) and harmful exposures (number needed to harm). See Box 1A.14.

See Box 1A.15 for an example of how NNT is calculated.

1A.23 Time trend analysis, time-series designs

A **time-series analysis** considers the situation where both the exposure and the outcome are measured over time. If there are secular increases or decreases, or seasonal variations, in both variables, then the variables will be correlated with time. This phenomenon is known as **serial correlation**, and time will therefore be a confounding factor in the analysis.

For example, both rainfall and hospital admissions are higher in winter. In answering the question whether high rainfall is associated with increased hospital admissions, this seasonal correlation would first need to be accounted for.

Note: The unit of analysis in time-series studies is often at a population level; such analyses are therefore examples of ecological studies.

Applications

Examples of applications of time-series studies are

- Descriptive study of change in the pattern of a disease or risk factor over time
- Assessment of the correlation between an exposure and an outcome over time (e.g. between temperature and cases of meningococcal disease)
- Evaluating the impact of an intervention using an interrupted time-series analysis (e.g. the effect of a smoking ban on smoking rates)
- Analysing the effect of an unplanned event (see Box 1A.16)
- Making future projections to aid health service planning

Time-series designs

Figure 1A.1 shows four different interrupted time-series designs. In each of the four graphs, the horizontal axis represents time and the vertical axis represents the magnitude of the observed effect.

Analysis to estimate effect size

Approaches for estimating effect size in time-series studies include

- Smoothing out the noise in curves (i.e. peaks and troughs) by using **moving averages** (e.g. autoregressive integrated moving average [ARIMA] modelling)
- **Segmented regression analysis** of each separate part of an interrupted time series

Difficulties with time-series designs

Table 1A.31 describes some of the challenges associated with time-series studies.

Box 1A.16 Example: Effect of the financial crisis on suicides

An **interrupted time-series analysis** was conducted to study of the effect of the 2008 financial crisis on suicides rates in Spain (i.e. an unplanned event).

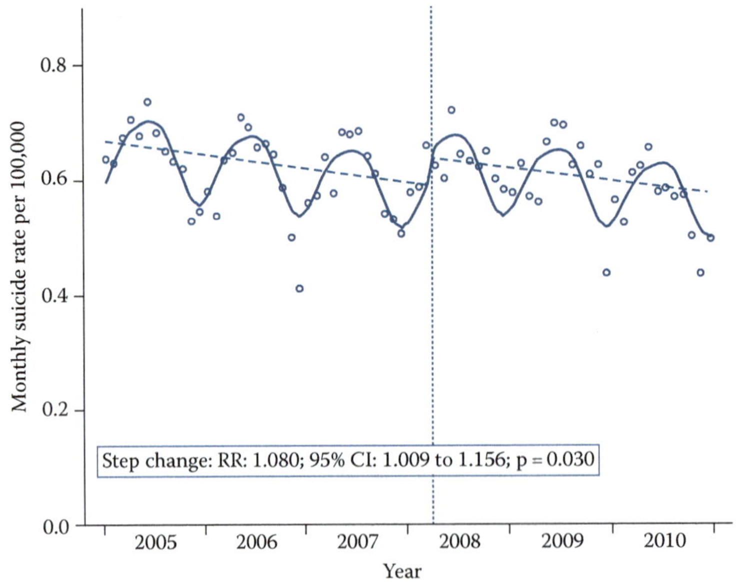

Seasonally adjusted. Circles = observed rates; solid line = modeled rates fitted to the data; dashed line = deseasonalised trend. Vertical dotted line = onset of the financial crisis

This analysis demonstrates a rate ratio of 1.080 after adjustment for seasonal effects, suggesting that the financial crisis was associated with an 8% increase in suicides.

Source: Lopez Bernal, J.A. *et al. Eur. J. Publ. Health,* 2013.

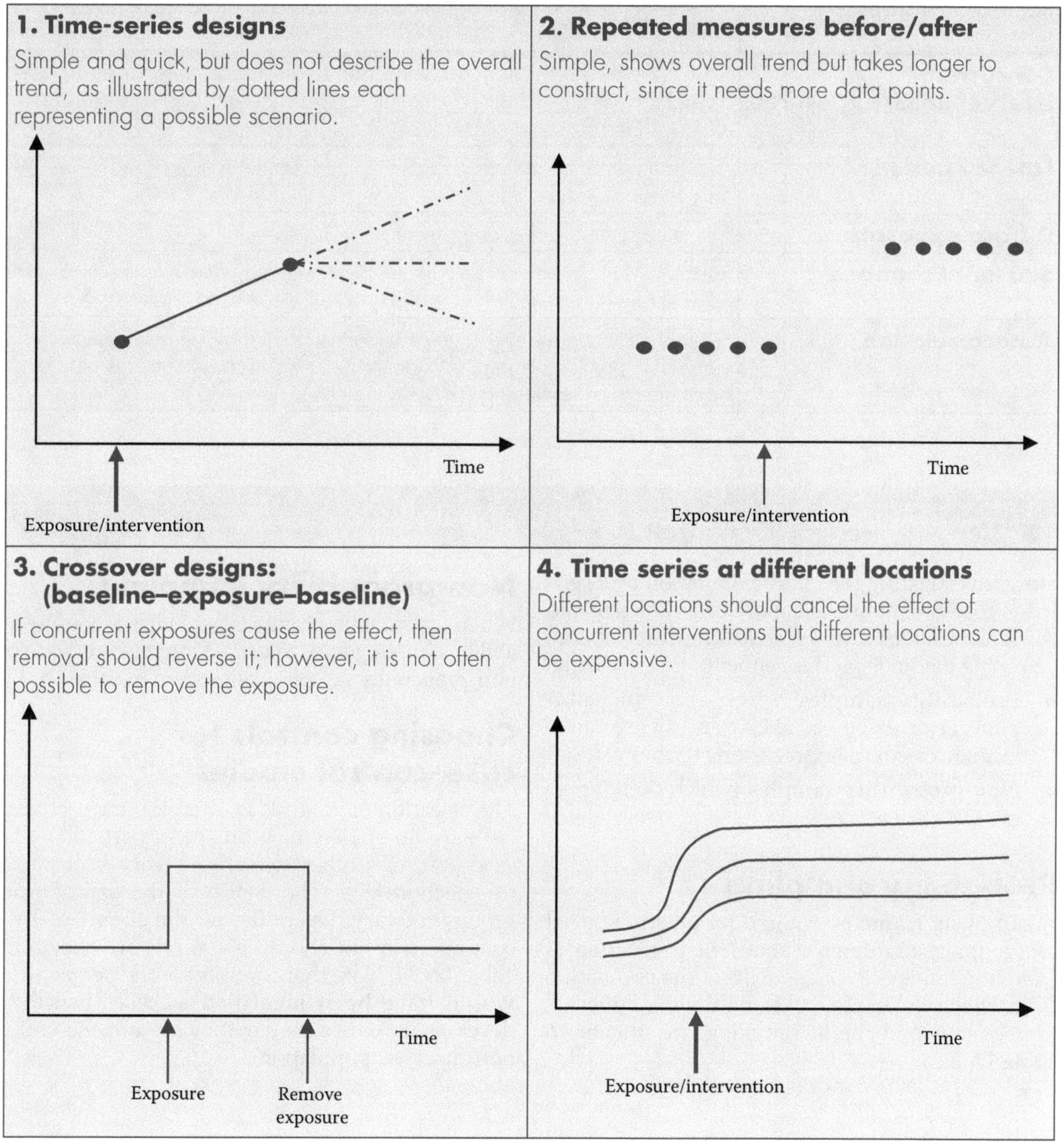

Figure 1A.1 Study designs for time series.

Table 1A.31 Challenges associated with time-series analyses

Challenge	Description
Secular changes	For example, changes in age structure, classifications of disease, or diagnostic techniques.
Concurrent interventions/exposures	For example, a reduction in deaths from heart disease might be observed at a time of falling smoking prevalence and increasing use of effective therapies such as statins.
Latency period	A long time period between exposure and manifestation of its effect (e.g. smoking and cancer).
Diffuse exposure	Exposure spread out over many months or years.
Seasonal changes	Fluctuations in patterns of the outcome over time may confound the observed associations (this phenomenon can be adjusted for in the analysis).
Autocorrelation	For many outcomes, the value at one time point may be affected by the value in a previous time point. Techniques exist to adjust for this type of autocorrelation, including ARIMA modelling.

1A.24 Methods of sampling from a population

Since investigating the entire population by a census is costly, sampling is a more cost-effective and convenient alternative for collecting information. Sampling methods produce either of the following:

- **Probability samples** (which allow the sampling error to be calculated and hence allow inferences to be made regarding the population)
- **Non-probability samples** (which do not permit such inferences)

Probability sampling

A **sampling frame** is required for all studies that aim to make an inference about the population. A sampling frame is a complete list of the population from which the sample is to be drawn. Different methods of probability sampling are shown in Table 1A.32.

Non-probability sampling

When the sampling frame is not known, non-probability sampling may be used. Different methods of non-probability sampling are shown in Table 1A.33.

Choosing controls for case–control studies

The selection of controls is often the most critical issue for an epidemiological study, particularly in case–control studies, which are very vulnerable to selection bias. The choice of the comparison group will vary depending on the situation. Two common ways of choosing controls are shown in Table 1A.34. Note that controls are the people who **would have been identified** as cases had they developed the disease (i.e. they are **not** the entire non-diseased population).

Table 1A.32 Methods of probability sampling

Method	Description	Advantages	Disadvantages
Random	Start with a sampling frame. Sampling frames include postcode address files, the electoral register, or a GP practice list. Draw a random sample from the sampling frame.	Purest form of probability sampling. Allows the sampling error to be calculated.	Relatively inconvenient in practice. Inefficient for rare outcomes. A sample frame is not always available.
Systematic	Start with a sampling frame Calculate a sampling interval (n) : $\frac{\text{(Number in population)}}{\text{(Number in sample)}}$ n = Draw every nth person from the sampling frame.	More convenient than random sampling. Allows the sampling error to be calculated.	Potential for bias if there are underlying patterns in the sampling frame.
Stratified	Assign members of the population into relatively homogeneous subgroups ('strata') before sampling. Draw a random sample of subjects from each stratum.	Improves the accuracy of estimation. Efficient. Allows the sampling error to be calculated.	Requires accurate information about the population. Choice of relevant stratification variables can be difficult. Not useful if there are no homogeneous subgroups.
Cluster	Used when there are 'natural' clusters in the population (e.g. GP practices within a borough). A random sampling technique is used to choose which clusters to include in the study. In single-stage cluster sampling, all the elements from each of the selected clusters are used (e.g. all patients in selected practices). In two-stage cluster sampling, elements from each of the selected clusters are selected at random (i.e. a sample of patients from within the selected practices).	Convenient for fieldwork. Cost-efficient. Allows calculation of the sampling error.	Increased sampling error.

Table 1A.33 Methods of non-probability sampling

Method	Description	Advantages	Disadvantages
Convenience	Subjects are chosen on the basis of being readily available.	Useful for preliminary research because it is extremely efficient.	Sampling error cannot be calculated. Volunteer bias.
Purposive	Subjects are chosen purposively on the basis of a judgement that they have particular features (e.g. used for selecting controls required for epidemiological studies).	Useful for rare characteristics. Useful for qualitative research.	Sampling error cannot be calculated. Volunteer bias.
Quota	Begin by determining the demographic characteristics of interest (e.g. age, sex, ethnicity). Select subjects to represent the proportional distribution of these characteristics within the population.	Representative with regard to the known characteristics.	Sampling error cannot be calculated. Potentially unrepresentative in terms of other characteristics. Volunteer bias.
Snowball	Ask subjects to recommend acquaintances who meet the sample criteria.	Very cost-efficient. Useful where no sample frame exists. Enables the researcher to reach groups that are otherwise hard to reach.	Sampling error cannot be calculated. Volunteer bias.

Table 1A.34 Choice of controls in case–control studies

Type of control	Sampling strategy	Advantages	Disadvantages
Controls within the healthcare system	Purposive (through registers, hospital records, referral data)	Easily identified. By being in hospital, the controls, like the diseased cases, are more aware of antecedent events (i.e. more similar to diseased cases, therefore less recall bias). Same hospital, therefore same influences on choosing that hospital. More cooperative than healthy people.	Ill, therefore different from the healthy population (e.g. more likely to smoke and drink heavily). A given hospital may have secondary and tertiary activities, so patient selection differs. Different specialties within the same hospital may have different catchment areas.
Population controls	Random sampling or purposive sampling (friends, relatives, and neighbours of cases may be more motivated to participate)	Healthy population.	General public does not recall antecedent events as well as patients who are ill. Less motivated to participate. Healthier people are less likely to be at home during the daytime. Costly and time-consuming.

1A.25 Methods of allocation in intervention studies

Interventional studies differ from observational studies in that the epidemiologist allocates the intervention of interest. The process of allocation is therefore of pivotal importance. Ideally, subjects will be allocated in such a way that the two groups are identical, meaning that the only difference between the two groups will be the intervention under investigation.

In order to minimise allocation bias, subjects should be allocated to their groups only *after* ensuring that they are **eligible**, have **consented** to participate, and have been fully **enrolled**.

Allocation may be **systematic**, **volunteered**, or at **random**.

Systematic allocation

Here, allocation is determined in advance (e.g. it is decided that recruits will be allocated alternately into groups or that all recruits presenting on alternate days will be allocated to the same alternate group). There is much potential for **selection bias** because

- The order is predictable and so the recruiter may be tempted to interfere with the order of recruits
- There may be underlying patterns to the order in which recruits present

Volunteer allocation

Allocation is determined on the basis of which recruits volunteer to participate. This is highly unsatisfactory because of extreme **selection bias**.

Randomisation

The unique advantage of random allocation is that if the groups are large enough then, on average, they will be similar with respect to all variables. This similarity includes all confounding factors, both known and unknown. Randomisation also eliminates intervention selection bias.

There are several types of randomisation that may be used for allocating recruits. See Table 1A.35.

Allocation concealment

The person recruiting a participant should not know to which arm of the study the participant will be allocated. This concealment avoids selection bias. Methods of allocation concealment include using opaque sealed envelopes, computer randomisation, and telephone randomisation.

Note the difference between allocation concealment and blinding/masking: it is not always possible to **mask** the intervention from participants or assessors (e.g. surgery versus drugs), but it should always be possible for the allocation method to be **concealed**.

Table 1A.35 Types of randomisation

Type of randomisation	Description
Simple	Known also as **unrestricted randomisation**, participants are allocated purely on the basis of chance (e.g. using a computer generated random number or a coin toss). Potential for **unequal group sizes** (not an issue with large studies).
Blocked	This is a technique for obtaining equal group sizes. First, the ratio of participants between the allocation groups is set (e.g. 1:1). A block size is then chosen (e.g. four). All permutations of assignments that meet the ratio are then listed for that block size (with these examples, the blocks would be AABB, BBAA, ABAB, BABA, ABBA and BAAB). Finally, the allocation sequence is generated by randomly selecting blocks from this list. The block size can be varied periodically to make prediction of the allocation sequence even more difficult.
Stratified	This approach may be used in smaller trials to ensure that potentially confounding variables are evenly distributed between the groups. Recruits are subdivided into strata (e.g. according to ethnicity or gender) and individuals within each stratum are randomised.
Cluster	Groups, rather than individuals, are randomised to receive the different interventions. This design needs to be fully taken into consideration at the design stage to ensure a sufficiently large sample size is used (see Section 1A.21).
Matched pair	Individuals or groups are first matched according to baseline data, by matching them on as many variables as possible. The intervention is then randomly allocated to one member of the pair, with the other member of the pair receiving the control.
Stepped wedge	The population is divided into groups and then the intervention is progressively introduced, in random order, across the groups until every group is receiving it. This approach is used when other allocation methods would be unfeasible because of a widespread belief that the intervention will be beneficial.

1A.26 Surveys

Design of documentation for recording survey data, construction of valid questionnaires, and methods for validating observational techniques.

A survey is a standardised method for collecting the same information from each study participant. Often this method involves the use of a questionnaire. Either the **participant** or the **researcher** can record survey data.

Survey documentation

The design of the survey documentation should ensure that the data recorded are

- Complete
- Accurate
- Understandable and legible
- Stored in a format suitable for analysis
- Secure, to protect respondents' **confidentiality**

Documentation of data can be

- **Hard copy**: Questionnaires for postal surveys for participants to complete (or questionnaires plus prompts for researchers to complete during face-to-face or telephone surveys)
- **Online**: Allows documentation to be tailored to responses; if required, can provide prompts when invalid/incomplete/no responses are received

Investigators who will be recording survey data need to know

- **Where** to record information
- What **type** of answer is required
- **Directions** for completing the survey (if items are not relevant, respondents need to know which question to answer next, such as 'NO → move to question 5')

Researchers recording survey data from participants also need prompts/clarifications with information on

- **Screening**: to ensure that appropriate participants are interviewed
- Directions if there is **no response** to a particular item

Documentation layout can help by providing

- **Appropriately sized** spaces to indicate where responses are needed and in what form
- **Clear navigation** to guide participants through the survey

Construction of valid questionnaires

Validity is the extent to which a tool explores what it is purported to measure (see Section 1A.19). A questionnaire's validity will depend on the range of factors listed in Table 1A.36.

Other ways to maximise validity are to

- Use an **existing tool** if an appropriate one exists
- Increasing the **sample size**
- **Triangulate** with other sources of evidence (e.g. observation)

Validating observational techniques

For further detail on validity, see Section 1A.19.

Enhancing validity

Methods for enhancing validity are listed in Table 1A.37.

Table 1A.36 Characteristics of valid questionnaires

Characteristic	Implications	Technique to maximise validity
Sample selected	Unrepresentative sample may lead to bias.	Obtain a *sampling frame* (exhaustive list of all possible experimental units). Random selection of sample. Stratification of sample.
Response rate achieved	Uneven or very low response rate is potentially subject to bias.	Advance warning letters. Incentives for responding. Data method: Face to face or telephone better than postal (though more costly).
Content of questionnaire (content validity and construct validity)[a]	Questions should be chosen carefully to ensure that the questionnaire addresses the research question. For psychometric questionnaires, conceptual model needed first to define dimensions of the construct to be measured.	Researching content through Existing tools Literature review Qualitative interviews Expert opinion
Quality of the questions asked	Participants need to understand what the questions asked require and be prepared to give this information honestly.	Generate clear and non-judgemental questions: pilot and test on potential participants and revise. Data collection to suit the subject: face to face better to explain questions; postal or computer-assisted survey designs may be better for privacy.

[a] Note the difference between psychometric questionnaires (analysed by a summative score) and survey tools (analysed by the individual question).

Table 1A.37 Methods for enhancing the validity of observational studies

Consideration	Methods
Sampling strategy	Ensure appropriate selection of participants, and appropriate settings for making observations.
Reflexivity	Consider the observers' effect on what they are observing.
Recording	Record observations using observers trained comprehensively and systematically. Use a checklist to record observations.
Cross-checking	Cross-check observational data by means of • **Repeated observations** by the same, or other, observers in the same setting • Recorded observations (e.g. **videotape**) • **Triangulation** with other research methods

1A.27 Studies of disease prognosis

The prognosis is the expected course and outcome of a disease. Studies of prognosis estimate the frequency with which different outcomes can be expected to occur. **Cohort studies** are used for analysing prognostic factors (e.g. the Framingham study [11] investigated cardiovascular prognostic factors). **Disease registers** (e.g. regional cancer skin cancer register) can also be used to analyse prognosis.

Prognostic factors

Prognostic factors are patient characteristics that guide the prediction of outcomes. These factors are similar to risk factors but they occur after the onset of disease and they predict disease outcome, whereas risk factors occur before the disease has occurred and predict disease onset.

Prognostic factors may include

- Demographic characteristics (e.g. age, sex)
- Clinical features (e.g. tumour stage, co-morbidities, genetics)
- Behaviours (e.g. smoking, diet)

Prognostic studies

Prognostic studies are typically cohort studies that start with a cohort of patients who already have the disease and which analyse disease outcomes as they occur. Often, **survival analytical** techniques are used (see Section 1B.18); these techniques analyse the time to an event, which may be **negative** (e.g. death) or **positive** (e.g. remission). Different exposures can also be compared (such as the prognostic factors described earlier).

1A.28 Epidemiological research ethics

Ethics and etiquette of epidemiological research.

Ethics is the philosophical discipline concerned with understanding how human beings should act, what is good, and what kind of life is best. In 1979, Beauchamp and Childress [12] identified four principles associated with ethical medical practice: see Box 1A.17.

In public health, beneficence implies acting in the best interests of the population or society as a whole [13]. Public health specialists should always act in a just way, ensuring the fair distribution across the population of both benefits and risks. At a population level, there is sometimes a tension between these principles, because of the conflicting aims associated with benefiting an individual and of providing optimal conditions for the well-being of the community as a whole (see Box 1A.18).

Box 1A.17 Principles of medical ethics

Principle	Concepts
Autonomy	Human rights, dignity, freedom
Non-malfeasance	Do no harm
Beneficence	Do good
Justice	Equity, fairness

Box 1A.18 Examples of conflicts between ethical principles in public health

- Fluoridation of the water supply does not permit individual informed consent. It may occur despite the opposition of many people.
- If healthcare resources are redistributed with the aim of providing equitable services, this redistribution may harm people from whom resources are removed.

While there are many ethical issues relating health research, it would also be unethical not to undertake research where knowledge is lacking or uncertainty exists.

Declaration of Helsinki

The principles first set out by the World Medical Association in the 1964 Declaration of Helsinki are regarded as the foundation of modern research ethical guidance. They have since undergone several revisions. The principles cover

- The safeguarding of research subjects
- Informed consent
- Reducing risk
- Adhering to approved research plans/protocols

Informed consent

Truly informed consent requires all of the features listed in Box 1A.19.

Confidentiality

Research may involve the collection of private or sensitive information. Such confidential information should not be shared with anyone without consent except when there is a clear **ethical justification** (e.g. approval by a human subjects research review panel) or a **legal requirement** (e.g. regulations to protect children).

The use of identifiable data in research without consent requires demonstrating

- The **importance** of the research
- The **minimal risk** to the people whose information is used
- The promise of **benefit** to society
- An obligation to maintain the **confidentiality** of the information

Scot Ethics committees

In research studies, ethical principles are protected by the requirements of local or national research ethics committees (RECs). Proof of ethical approval is often a prerequisite of journals for considering a study for publication.

ENG + SCOT In England and Scotland, any research conducted in the NHS must receive approval from an ethics committee before commencing. An REC will consider issues such as whether the study has the potential to benefit society/participants, how participants are recruited, how participants' confidentiality will be protected, as well as any possible effects of the study on health or well-being and the processes for obtaining informed consent.

WA Any research requires the approval of a local ethics committee. It will subsequently be subject to local research governance arrangements that

Box 1A.19 Features of informed consent in clinical research

Feature	Description
Competence	Do subjects understand what is involved? Children over a certain age can assent to take part but may lack full capacity for providing truly informed consent.
Voluntariness	Are participants free to leave a trial at any point? Have they been put under excessive pressure to enrol in a research project? Patients need to be confident that their standard of care will not be affected by their decision to take part in a study.
Understanding	Understanding the **risks, burdens,** and **benefits** of the study.
Documentation	Written consent is required in trial settings. In cluster randomised trials, communities may be asked to give consent but it is not always clear who, if anyone, can provide consent on behalf of a community.

seek to ensure that the research is conducted in a manner consistent with the approval given by the ethics committee. Where the research setting is in primary care, the researcher is required to seek local management approval from the local health board, which may decline approval if it believes that the research poses a risk either to patients or to the delivery of NHS services.

ENG + WA In England, the National Research Ethics Service (NRES) provides guidance, training, and support on research ethics.

IRE The Irish Council for Bioethics Guidance (2004) stipulates that all research involving or impacting on human participants requires ethics review by an REC. Procedures vary for obtaining permission to undertake research in a hospital setting. Usually, an application must be submitted to the hospital's REC, but national committee approval may be accepted as sufficient by some hospitals, and regional approval may be accepted by smaller hospitals in the regional network. For community-based research, protocols may be submitted to the REC under the joint auspices of the Faculties of Occupational Health and of Public Health Medicine of the Royal College of Physicians of Ireland.

SA In South Africa, there is a national process controlled by the *Ethics in Health Research: Principles, Structures and Processes Research Ethics Guidelines* (2004). Biomedical RECs at the various universities must be registered and structured according to these guidelines.

AUS Ethical approval comes from a formally constituted Human Research Ethics Committee (HREC). The National Health and Medical Research Council publishes guidelines for the establishment and accreditation of RECs. Ethics committee approval must be obtained before research on humans can begin.

NZ In New Zealand, all health and disability research that involves human subjects must be sent for ethical review. This requirement covers observational research (e.g. descriptive studies using already collected personal information or information obtained by questionnaires and interviews) as well as experimental research (e.g. clinical trials). The only exceptions are certain types of audit and related activities (e.g. quality assurance and programme evaluation), public health investigations (e.g. outbreak investigations and surveillance), and where a statutory exclusion applies (e.g. official statistics).

The main system for ethical review is the set of health and disability ethics committees (HDECs). There are six regional committees and a multiregional committee for research carried out nationally or in more than one region. Research may be reviewed by an accredited institutional ethics committee (IEC) established by universities and private companies, but in most circumstances it will also need to be reviewed by a HDEC. Additional review is required in some specific areas, notably clinical trials of a pre-registration medicine, research involving assisted human reproduction, and research involving the manipulation of human genetic material (e.g. gene therapy).

1A.29 Life-table analysis

Appropriate use of statistical methods in the analysis and interpretation of epidemiological studies, including life-table analysis.

Statistical tests are covered in greater detail in Section 1B. Life tables are covered in Chapters 1B.18 and 3A.7.

Choice of statistical method

Questions to consider include the following:

- What is the **hypothesis** being tested?
- Are the data **independent**? Or are they matched, clustered, or correlated?
- What are the **input** variables (e.g. intervention or control)?
- What are the **output** variables (e.g. measure of morbidity)?

Hypothesis testing

The null hypothesis (H_0) states that there is **no association between exposure and disease**.

Assuming that the null hypothesis is true, the *p*-value is the probability due to chance alone of obtaining a result at least as extreme as the observed result.

Usually, a **two-sided** *p*-value is used (i.e. the probability of observing such a large difference, without specifying the direction of the difference). A **one-sided** *p*-value is used to increase the precision of an estimate where there is a strong prior belief. For example, when comparing radical mastectomy against lumpectomy, there is a strong prior belief that the more radical procedure will be at least as curative as the limited procedure, so the question is simply whether lumpectomy is as effective as mastectomy.

Choice of outcome measure

The choice of statistical method and outcome measure will depend on the nature of the study (see Table 1A.38).

Choice of statistical test

See Section 1B.

Table 1A.38 Outcome measures

Study type	Outcome measure	Details
Correlation study	Correlation coefficient (*r*)	See Section 1B.14 (linear regression and correlation coefficients).
Case–control study	Odds ratio	$\text{Odds ratio} = \frac{\text{Odds (cases)}}{\text{Odds (controls)}}$ where $\text{Odds} = \frac{\text{Proportion exposed}}{\text{Proportion unexposed}}$ Confidence intervals can be constructed using the natural log of standard error of the odds ratio (lnOR). Note that the confidence interval is not symmetrical around the odds ratio. If the confidence interval includes 1, then there is no significant difference between the groups.
Cohort study	Risk ratio	$\text{Risk ratio} = \frac{\text{Risk (exposed)}}{\text{Risk (unexposed)}}$ where $\text{Risk} = \frac{\text{Number of cases}}{\text{Number at risk to start}}$
	Rate ratio	$\text{Rate ratio} = \frac{\text{Rate (exposed)}}{\text{Rate (unexposed)}}$ where $\text{Rate} = \frac{\text{Number of cases}}{\text{Number of person – years}}$
	SMR	$\text{SMR} = \frac{\text{Observed deaths}}{\text{Expected deaths}}$
Intervention study	Risk ratio, rate ratio, AR, or PAR	
Life-table analysis (see Sections 1B.15 and 1B.16)	Survival probability	Cumulative chance of death in a given time period.
	Confidence intervals	95% confidence intervals may be calculated using a formula by Kalbfleisch and Prentice.
	Life expectancy	In the UK calculated as the average time someone is expected to live
	Proportional hazards	A statistical method for comparing survival rates in different groups. If there is no difference between groups, then the ratio of hazards between the groups is constant over time (even though the underlying hazards will change) and the logged cumulative hazard curves will be parallel.

1A.30 Epidemic theory and analysis of infectious disease data

Epidemic theory (effective and basic reproduction numbers, epidemic thresholds) and techniques for analysis of infectious disease data (construction and use of epidemic curves, generation numbers, exceptional reporting, and identification of significant clusters).

An epidemic is the occurrence of a number of cases of a disease that exceeds the number of cases normally expected for that disease in that area at that time.

Techniques for analysing infectious disease data include

- Construction and use of epidemic curves, generation of numbers
- Exceptional reporting
- Identification of significant clusters

Reproduction numbers

Reproduction numbers are used to describe the spread of an epidemic and include the **effective reproduction number** and the **basic reproduction number**.

Effective reproduction number

The effective reproduction number (R) is the average number of secondary cases of an infectious disease per primary case observed in a population:

- If the disease is endemic $R \approx 1$
- At the start of an epidemic $R > 1$
- In order to control an infectious disease and lead to a decrease in cases $R < 1$

Basic reproduction number

The basic reproduction number (R_0) is defined as the average number of secondary infections produced when one infected individual is introduced into a host population where **everyone is susceptible** (i.e. the situation where R would be at its maximum). This number gives a measure of the infectiousness of the organism independent of how many immune people there are in the population.

An infection will take hold in a population only if $R_0 > 1$.

Secondary attack rate

The secondary attack rate is the **risk** of **secondary cases** among **all those people exposed** to a primary case. It is often difficult to establish everyone who has been exposed to a primary case; therefore, this calculation is normally conducted in a defined exposure setting, such as a household:

$$\text{Household secondary attack rate} = \frac{\text{Number of secondary cases in affected households}}{\text{Total number of household contacts of a primary case}}$$

The household secondary attack rate is used to estimate the spread of the infection in a household setting and can give an indication of the infectivity of the organism and the effect of control measures.

Population thresholds

Important population thresholds for an infectious disease include the **critical population size**, the **epidemic threshold**, and the **herd immunity threshold** (see Table 1A.39).

Generation numbers

Cases may be described according to when they were identified and when they developed the infection (see Table 1A.40).

Serial interval

The serial interval, also called the **generation interval**, is the time interval between the onset of

Table 1A.39 Important population thresholds

Threshold	Description
Critical population size	The minimum number of people required for a given infectious agent to remain endemic. Varies depending on the structure and distribution of the population, hygiene measures, preventative measures, etc.
Epidemic threshold	The fraction of the population who must be susceptible for an epidemic to occur. Below this value, an epidemic outbreak will not occur.
Herd immunity threshold	The proportion of people in a population who must be immune for the incidence of infectious disease to decrease: $\text{Herd immunity threshold} = \frac{R_0 - 1}{R_0}$

Table 1A.40 Types of case in an outbreak

Type of case	Description
Index case	The first recognised case in an outbreak
Primary case	The original case in an outbreak (may only be recognised in retrospect and may not necessarily be the index case)
Secondary case	A case that acquired their infection from a primary case
Tertiary case	A case that acquired their infection from a secondary case

a given set of clinical symptoms or signs in two successive cases (e.g. between a primary case and a secondary case). This time interval depends on a combination of the incubation period, the latent period, and the duration of infectiousness (see Chapter 2G.1).

Note: The serial interval can sometimes be shorter than the incubation period if there is a long duration of infectiousness before symptoms start (i.e. the latent period is shorter than the incubation period). Sometimes, a secondary case may even develop symptoms before the primary case if the secondary case happened to have a shorter incubation period.

Epidemic curves

Epidemic curves are graphic representations of the number of new cases by date of onset. They are used to display the magnitude and time trend of an outbreak. The features of an epidemic curve are listed in Table 1A.41 with examples provided in Box 1A.20.

Some of the uses of an epidemic curve are

- Determining the **current position** in the course of the epidemic and possibly **projecting** its future course
- Estimating the probable **time of exposure** (if the disease and its usual incubation period are known) so that the investigation can be focused on that specific time period
- Identifying **outliers** (all of whom are worthy of investigation since their unusual exposure may provide clues about the source)
- Drawing inferences about the epidemic **pattern** (e.g. whether it is an outbreak resulting from a common source exposure, from person-to-person spread, or from both)

Table 1A.41 Features of an epidemic curve

Feature on epidemic curve	Phenomenon or phenomena
Sudden rise in the number of cases	Common source
Steep rise then a gradual fall	Single source (or 'point source') epidemic, with all cases occurring within a single incubation period
Plateau (rather than a peak)	Prolonged exposure period ('continuous common source epidemic')
Series of progressively taller peaks one incubation period apart	Person-to-person spread (a 'propagated' epidemic)
Early outlier	Background (unrelated) case Or a source of the epidemic Or a person who was exposed earlier than most of the other affected people
Late outlier	Unrelated to the outbreak Or a case with a long incubation period Or a person who was exposed later than most of the other affected people Or secondary cases (i.e. the person may have become ill after being exposed to someone who was part of the initial outbreak)

Source: Reproduced from the National Center for Chronic Disease Prevention and Health Promotion, 2006.

Geographical patterns

The assessment of an outbreak by **place** provides information about the geographical extent of a problem and may also reveal clusters or patterns that provide clues to the identity and origins of the problem (see Table 1A.42). A simple and useful technique for looking at geographical patterns is to plot a 'spot map' of the area showing where the affected people live or work or where else they may have been exposed.

Exception reporting

Surveillance involves the systematic collection and analysis of data and the communication of results. Early warning procedures aim to detect any divergence from the usual frequency of disease or symptoms as soon as possible.

UK In the United Kingdom, this work was previously coordinated by the Health Protection Agency (HPA) now part of Public Health England (see Figure 1A.2).

Significant clusters

A cluster is a collection of events in space and/or time that is believed to be greater than would be expected by chance. If the population density varies between suspect areas, then a spot map will be misleading. To correct for this, the **attack rate** in each area should be calculated.

Box 1A.20 Examples of the main types of epidemic curves

(a) Point source

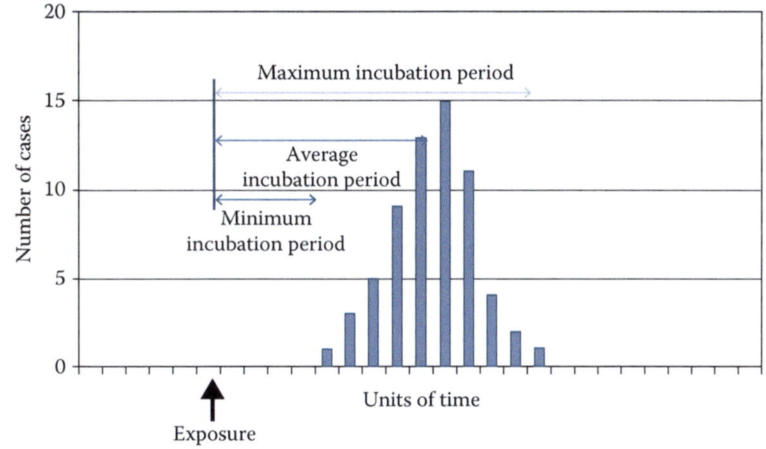

(b) Continuous source

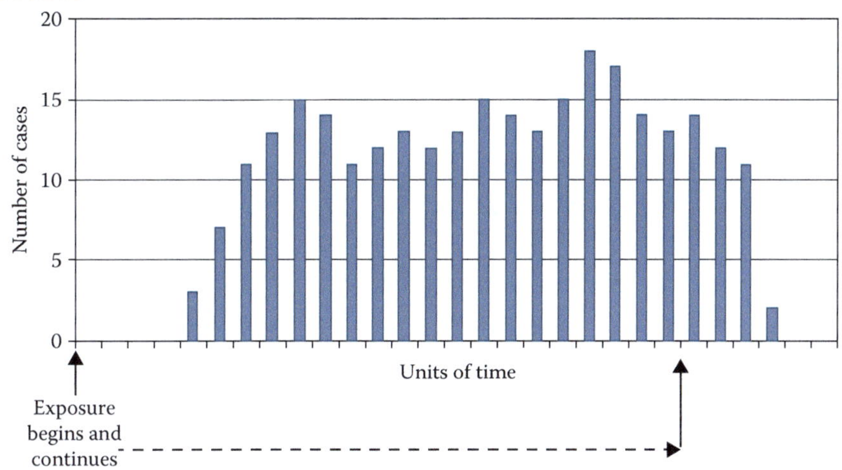

(c) Propagated source

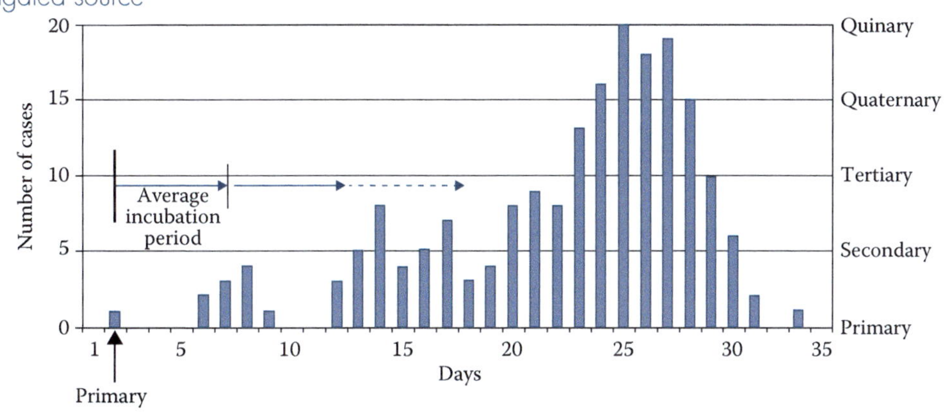

Table 1A.42 Geographical patterns in epidemiology

Setting	Clusters
Community	Water supply Wind currents Proximity to a restaurant or shop
Hospital ward	Focal source (person-to-person spread) Scattered common source (e.g. catering company)
Surgical infection	Operating room Recovery room Ward

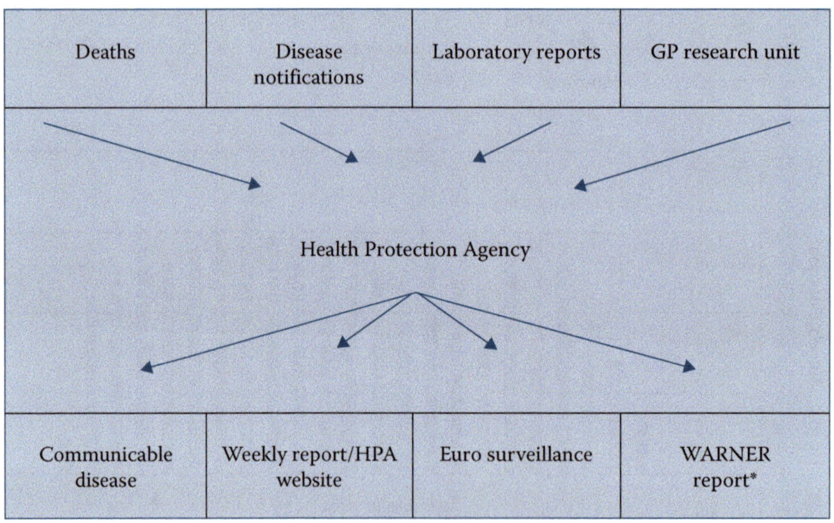

Figure 1A.2 Coordination of infectious disease information prior to April 2013. * Weekly analysis report of notifications above expected rates.

1A.31 Combining studies

Systematic reviews, methods for combining data from several studies, and meta-analyses.

The process of combining the results from several studies offers a number of advantages, which are listed in Box 1A.21.

Systematic reviews

A systematic review is defined by the Cochrane Collaboration as *'A review of a clearly formulated question that uses systematic and explicit methods to identify, select and critically appraise relevant research, and to collect and analyze data from the studies that are included in the review'.*

Systematic reviews are essential for decision-makers who need access to reliable information, such as healthcare providers, policymakers, and

Box 1A.21 Advantages of combining studies

Advantage	Explanation
Increased power and precision	A large single trial is preferable to a combination of small studies, but many underpowered studies may be published, all showing a similar effect size but lacking in significance.
Greater generalisability	Results taken from several studies may be relevant to a wider patient population.
Efficiency and cost	It is quicker and cheaper to perform a systematic review than to embark on a new study.

Table 1A.43 Steps involved in conducting a systematic review

Step	Description
1. Literature search	A thorough, systematic search of the published and grey literature (see Section 1A.34).
2. Critical appraisal	Review of the studies found to determine which are relevant and valid.
3. Amalgamation	Merger of the valid studies. When this is done quantitatively (i.e. to produce a single summary estimate of an effect), it is termed a **meta-analysis**.

researchers. There is a vast quantity of evidence available on most healthcare subjects, making it almost impossible for a non-specialist to keep up to date. Therefore, decision-makers need unbiased scientific reviews that appraise and summarise the information for them in order to provide a reliable basis for their decisions.

The systematic review process involves three main steps (see Table 1A.43).

Two organisations that undertake high-quality systematic reviews are the Cochrane Collaboration and the Campbell Collaboration (see Box 1A.22).

Meta-analyses

The process of combining trials relies on the quality of the constituent studies and on their being similar with regard to exposures and outcomes. If there are enough studies with sufficiently similar characteristics that their results can be combined, then a meta-analysis may be possible. Since the patients in one trial are likely to differ in a systematic way from those in another, it is wrong to compare individual trials. However, since the individual studies are internally randomised, their effect sizes can be synthesised.

Methods

When results are combined in a meta-analysis, a summary estimate is calculated. This value is a weighted average of the treatment effects of all of the eligible studies. Each study is assigned a weight, which determines the relative importance of that study in the meta-analysis and is based largely on the sample size. The estimate for each study is then multiplied by its weight in order to calculate the weighted average:

$$\text{Weighted average, } e = \frac{\sum (w_i \times e_i)}{\sum w_i}$$

where

e is an estimate (e.g. the OR)

e_i is the value of the estimate for each study i

w_i is the weighting for each study

Box 1A.22 Examples: Systematic reviews

Cochrane collaboration: collection of systematic reviews of medical and public health interventions. See Section 1A.38.

www.cochranecollaboration.org

Campbell collaboration: collection of systematic reviews of social and educational policies, including some health-related outcomes.

www.campbellcollaboration.org

There are various ways of weighting the studies, including

- The inverse variance method (where the weight of a study is the inverse of the variance of the measure of effect in that study)
- The Mantel–Haenszel weights

Forest plots

The findings of a meta-analysis can be displayed using a forest plot, which provides a visual representation of the results of the individual studies and of the summary estimate. Figure 1A.3 shows a forest plot of four studies.

Approaches to meta-analysis

There are two main approaches to meta-analysis: **fixed-effect** meta-analysis and **random-effects** meta-analysis (Table 1A.44).

The issue of heterogeneity and problems with using the random-effects methods are described in greater detail in Chapter 1B.19.

Bias in meta-analysis

Bias in meta-analyses may result from **poor trial quality** (e.g. inadequate concealment) exaggerating the treatment effect or from **publication bias**. The existence of publication bias means that studies showing an effect are more likely to be published than those that do not. Publication bias can be detected using **funnel plots** that display the effect size versus the study size (the funnel would be expected to be symmetrical if no publication bias existed).

See Chapter 1B.20.

Meta-analyses of observational studies

Meta-analysis is often described with reference to RCTs. However, it is also possible to conduct meta-analyses of observational studies, which may be useful when it is not possible to collect data from RCTs, for example, where the intervention is already in common usage. However, meta-analyses of observational studies are subject to other types of bias, and the impact of confounding factors is hard to control.

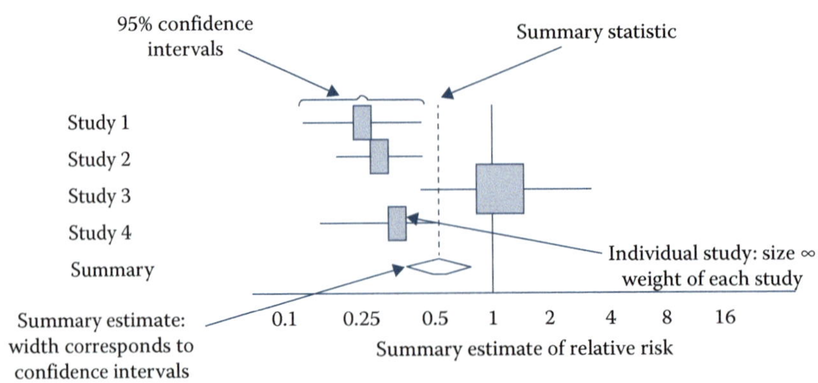

Figure 1A.3 Forest plot showing the estimates of relative risk for four studies.

Table 1A.44 Fixed- and random-effects in meta-analysis

Characteristic	Fixed-effect meta-analysis	Random-effects meta-analysis
Appropriate uses	Only used if there is no evidence of heterogeneity.	May be used if there is heterogeneity between studies (although it may be argued that calculating a summary measure is inappropriate if there is considerable heterogeneity).
Assumptions	Assumes that the underlying treatment effect is the same in all of the constituent studies and that the observed variation between studies is entirely due to sampling variation.	Aims to allow for heterogeneity by assuming that the treatment effect follows a distribution whose mean is the overall effect.
Summary estimate	Summary estimate is calculated as a weighted average.	Summary estimate is calculated as a weighted average but the formula for weighting is different.
Weighting	Weighting is largely determined by each study's size.	Weights are smaller and more similar to each other than in fixed effects, causing smaller studies to be given increased weight.
Confidence interval	Narrower confidence interval and smaller *p*-value for the summary estimate.	Wider confidence interval and larger *p*-value for the summary estimate.

1A.32 Electronic bibliographical databases

Electronic bibliographical databases and their limitations.

The health literature is colossal: there are currently over 30,000 medical journals, some of which have been in print for over 100 years. Bibliographic databases allow researchers to search these publications using Boolean operators such as AND, OR, and NOT. Certain databases (e.g. PubMed) contain journal material only; others (e.g. Popline and Google Scholar) include other forms of literature, such as reports and books.

Databases such as PubMed can be searched either using free text words in the title or abstract ('keyword') or by using a thesaurus term that has been grouped hierarchically. Using thesaurus terms such as the Medical Subject Headings (MeSH) terms has a number of advantages and disadvantages (see Box 1A.23).

Search strategy

The following steps should be followed when conducting a search of the literature [15]:

1. Define the research question.
2. Choose which databases to search (see the following).
3. Define limits (e.g. time period).
4. List the individual terms that constitute the research question.
5. Choose either keyword or thesaurus search strategy or a combination of the two.

Box 1A.23 Thesaurus terms

Advantages	Automatically include all synonyms for a particular term, including American and British spellings Plural and singular
Disadvantages	Prolonged time delays between publication and indexing mean that thesaurus terms may not keep pace with new areas of research.

6. If keyword, then list all similar terms, spellings, etc., by using a wildcard term denoted by typing an asterisk (e.g. diabet* will search for diabetes, diabetology, diabetologist, and diabetic).
7. If thesaurus, then identify thesaurus terms within the hierarchy.
8. Search for individual terms.
9. Combine individual terms (use AND to narrow the search and OR to broaden the search).
10. Set further limits (e.g. restrict by language or just review papers).
11. Save the papers identified.
12. Scan the titles for additional related terms to include in the search strategy.
13. Save the refined research strategy for future use.

Limitations of databases

No single database has access to all forms of publication, and no one library will have access to all databases. There is a tendency in public health to concentrate on health databases; however, being a multidisciplinary specialty, other databases should also be searched (e.g. economics, anthropology). There is also often a bias towards English language publications.

Databases have a limited span of years and research that predates a database is sometimes wrongly ignored. There is often a time delay between the publication of a study and its appearance in the database. Using the Internet can sometimes overcome this delay. However, using the Internet as a database is risky because there are no quality controls. It does, however, offer access to the grey literature and to full-text information.

1A.33 Grey literature

Grey literature is defined as written material issued by a body with a primary activity that is not publishing. As such, the grey literature is not readily available through traditional publication channels such as books and journals. Some advantages and disadvantages of using the grey literature are shown in Box 1A.24.

Box 1A.25 gives some examples of materials from the grey literature.

Box 1A.24 Advantages and disadvantages of using grey literature

Advantages	The Internet makes this easier to access. Presents less orthodox views. Provides perspective to published material.
Disadvantages	Traditionally difficult to access—especially older publications published in paper form only and stored only in specialist libraries (e.g. King's Fund). Little or no quality control: The onus is on the reader to assess a publication's quality and credibility.

Box 1A.25 Grey literature

- Technical and scientific reports
- Conference papers
- Internal reports from government and non-governmental organisations
- Government documents
- Theses
- Fact sheets
- Unpublished reports

1A.34 Publication bias

Publication bias is a tendency for journals to report positive results (where something was found to happen) rather than negative results (where something was found not to happen) and especially neutral results (no conclusive finding). This type of bias exists because researchers are less likely to submit, and publishers are less likely to publish, negative and neutral results. Publication bias is important because it distorts meta-analyses (see Chapter 1A.31).

The non-reporting of RCTs is increasingly regarded as a form of scientific and ethical misconduct. In an effort to address the problem, registers such as the meta Register of Controlled Trials have been established, where researchers must define the trial's primary outcome at the outset of the study. Many medical journals have agreed to publish only registered RCTs.

Other options for detecting or reducing publication bias are

- Active discouragement of studies that do not have sufficient power to detect effects
- Publication of study protocols
- Examining effects in meta-analyses using funnel plots

1A.35 Evidence-based medicine and policy

The term 'evidence-based medicine' (EBM) first appeared in 1992, and it relates to the **explicit** use of the current best evidence for decision-making at the level of the **individual patient**. In addition to clinical skills, a practitioner of EBM requires expertise in

- Retrieving, ranking, and interpreting the evidence
- Communicating evidence to patients
- Applying evidence to clinical decisions

Some advantages and disadvantages of EBM are shown in Box 1A.26.

Evidence-based policy

Since the late 1990s, there have been calls for more explicit use of evidence when making public policy decisions (i.e. a move towards engineered policies rather than policies of conviction). The

Box 1A.26 Evidence-based medicine (EBM)

Advantages	Explicit use of best evidence. Opinion of 'medical expert' demoted to the least valid form of evidence.
Disadvantages	Publication bias (failure to publish negative results). Retrieval bias (limitations of databases). Lack of evidence does not imply a lack of benefit. There is often a lack of robust evidence for non-drug treatments. Evidence typically applies to populations, not necessarily to individuals. Diminishes the value of clinical nous.

theory of evidence-based policy is that decisions should be shaped using processes such as those illustrated in Box 1A.27.

In the real world, there are very few examples of evidence-based policy occurring in this way. Instead, decision-makers tend to absorb the evidence, which then appears unexpectedly in the future as policy. This phenomenon is known as the **enlightenment** model [16].

Box 1A.27 Evidence-based policy

Problem identified by policymakers → Problem solved by researchers → Solution adopted as policy

Or

New knowledge → Knowledge adopted into policy

1A.36 Hierarchy of research evidence

Hierarchy of research evidence—from well-conducted meta-analyses down to small case series.

The traditional hierarchy of evidence ranked study designs in the following order:

1. Systematic reviews and meta-analyses
2. RCTs
3. Cohort studies
4. Case–control studies
5. Cross-sectional surveys
6. Case series and case reports

However, this list is now seen as being too simplistic since the most appropriate study design typically depends on the research question being asked. Many alternative systems have since been described to rank studies. One widely used example is the Levels of Evidence scheme published by the Oxford Centre for Evidence-Based Medicine (see Box 1A.28). Another system is the Grades of Recommendation, Assessment, Development, and Evaluation (GRADE) Working Group system, which is used by the Cochrane Collaboration and the World Health Organization (WHO), see Table 1A.45.

Box 1A.28 Oxford Centre for Evidence-Based Medicine levels of evidence [17]

Question	Step 1 (Level 1[a])	Step 2 (Level 2[a])	Step 3 (Level 3[a])	Step 4 (Level 4[a])	Step 5 (Level 5)
How common is the problem?	Local and current random sample surveys (or censuses)	Systematic review of surveys that allow matching to local circumstances[b]	Local non-random sample[b]	Case-series[b]	n/a
Is this diagnostic or monitoring test accurate? (diagnosis)	Systematic review of cross sectional studies with consistently applied reference standard and blinding	Individual cross sectional studies with consistently applied reference standard and blinding	Nonconsecutive studies, or studies without consistently applied reference standards[b]	Case-control studies, or poor or non-independent reference standard[b]	Mechanism-based reasoning
What will happen if we do not add a therapy? (prognosis)	Systematic review of inception cohort studies	Inception cohort studies	Cohort study or control arm of randomised trial[a]	Case-series or case–control studies, or poor quality prognostic cohort study[b]	n/a
Does this intervention help? (treatment benefits)	Systematic review of randomised trials or *n*-of-1 trials	Randomised trial or observational study with dramatic effect	Non-randomised controlled cohort/follow-up study[b]	Case–series, case–control studies, or historically controlled studies[b]	Mechanism-based reasoning
What are the COMMON harms? (treatment harms)	Systematic review of randomised trials, systematic review of nested case-control studies, *n*-of-1 trial with the patient you are raising the question about, or observational study with dramatic effect	Individual randomised trial or (exceptionally) observational study with dramatic effect	Non-randomised controlled cohort/follow-up study (post-marketing surveillance) provided there are sufficient numbers to rule out a common harm. (For long-term harms the duration of follow-up must be sufficient.)[b]	Case-series, case-control, or historically controlled studies[b]	Mechanism-based reasoning

(continued)

Box 1A.28 (*Continued*) Oxford Centre for Evidence-Based Medicine levels of evidence [17]

Question	Step 1 (Level 1[a])	Step 2 (Level 2[a])	Step 3 (Level 3[a])	Step 4 (Level 4[a])	Step 5 (Level 5)
What are the RARE harms? (Treatment Harms)	Systematic review of randomised trials or *n*-of-1 trial	Randomised trial or (exceptionally) observational study with dramatic effect			
Is this (early detection) test worthwhile? (Screening)	Systematic review of randomised trials	Randomised trial	Non-randomised controlled cohort/follow-up study[b]	Case–series, case–control, or historically controlled studies[b]	Mechanism-based reasoning

[a] Level may be graded down on the basis of study quality, imprecision, indirectness (study PICO does not match questions PICO), because of inconsistency between studies, or because the absolute effect size is very small; Level may be graded up if there is a large or very large effect size.

[b] As always, a systematic review is generally better than an individual study.

Table 1A.45 Hierarchy of the GRADE system of ranking the quality of evidence

Study design	Quality of evidence	Lower if	Higher if
Randomised trial →	High	Risk of bias −1 Serious −2 Very serious	Large effect +1 Large +2 Very large
	Moderate	Inconsistency −1 Serious −2 Very serious	Dose response +1 Evidence of a gradient
Observational study →	Low	Indirectness −1 Serious −2 Very serious	All plausible confounding +1 Would reduce a demonstrated effect or
	Very low	Imprecision −1 Serious −2 Very serious	+1 Would suggest a spurious effect when results show no effect
		Publication bias −1 Likely −2 Very likely	

1A.37 Cochrane collaboration

The Cochrane Collaboration was established in 1993 and named after the British epidemiologist **Archie Cochrane** (1909–1988). Cochrane was a notable contributor to the development of epidemiology as a science. Between 1960 and 1974, he was director of the Medical Research Council Epidemiology Research Unit in Cardiff.

The Cochrane Collaboration is an international, non-profit, independent organisation. It produces and disseminates systematic reviews of healthcare interventions and promotes the search for evidence in the form of clinical trials and other studies of the effects of interventions. As of 2012, there were over 26,000 people working within the Cochrane Collaboration in over 100 countries.

A key function of the collaboration is to produce systematic reviews (meta-analyses) of RCTs (see Section 1A.32). Cochrane Reviews are systematic assessments of the evidence of the effects of healthcare interventions, which are intended to help people make informed decisions about healthcare. They are published as part of the quarterly Cochrane Library and in the **Cochrane Database of Systematic Reviews**. Other components of the library include the Cochrane Methodology Register and the Health Technology Assessment Database.

1A.38 Genetic epidemiology

Understanding of basic issues and terminology in the design, conduct, analysis, and interpretation of population-based genetic association studies, including twin studies, linkage, and association studies.

See Chapter 2D for details of public health genetics.

The principles of genetic epidemiological studies [18] are summarised in Table 1A.46 and described in the following text.

Family studies

Family studies are performed in order to determine whether there is a genetic component to a particular disorder. They aim to detect whether there is a higher risk of disease in family members of an affected person than in the general population.

Table 1A.46 Genetic studies

Study question	Appropriate study designs	Unit of analysis/results obtained
Is there a genetic component to the disorder?	Family studies	FRR Relative recurrence risk
What is the contribution of genetics as opposed to environment/other sources to the trait?	Family—twin, adoption	Percentage concordance, discordance
What is the model of transmission of the genetic trait?	Family—segregation	Multigeneration family trees, preferably with more than one affected member
What is the location of the disease gene(s)?	Family—linkage	LOD score Recombination fraction

This tendency can be measured by calculating the **familial relative risk (FRR)** (or relative recurrence risk [RRR]) for a particular type of relative), for example,

$$\text{Sibling FRR} = \frac{\text{Risk of disease in siblings}}{\text{Risk of dieases in the general population}}$$

A higher FRR is a necessary, though not sufficient, attribute to decide that there is a heritable component to a disorder.

Twin studies

Twin studies explore the relative contributions of genes and the environment by comparing identical (monozygotic) and non-identical (dizygotic) twins to explore the relative contributions of genes and environment to health and disease. They are often used to examine the effects of genes on behaviours.

Identical twins can be considered to share their genes and their environment. Non-identical twins act as a control in that they share the same environmental factors but are only as genetically alike as any other siblings.

Genetic disorders are expected to have a higher correlation (known as **concordance**) among identical twins compared to non-identical twins. The strength of this genetic predisposition is expressed as the **heritability** (e.g. asthma has a heritability of 60%). Note that heritability is a population-based statistic (i.e. a measure of variance within a population), not a measure of the relative contribution of genes in an individual nor a measure of their risk. Furthermore, the heritability of a condition is unrelated to the number of genes that influence it.

Concordance may be **pairwise** or **probandwise**:

- **Pairwise** concordance is the percentage of concordant pairs (i.e. both twins affected) in a group of twins where at least one member of each pair is affected.
- **Probandwise** concordance is the percentage of twins whose twin becomes affected during the study, in a group of twins where just one member of each pair is affected.

Limitations of twin studies

There are several important limitations associated with twin studies. For example,

- Identical twins may not have identical gene expression
- The intrauterine environment of identical twins may not be exactly the same (e.g. often one twin receives a greater proportion of the placental blood supply)
- Twins may differ in certain ways from the general population; therefore, results may not be generalisable

Linkage studies

Linkage studies are based on the principle that if a disease 'runs in a family', then genetic markers that 'run in the family' in the same pattern are likely to be close in the genome to the gene that causes the disease. This proximity can be assumed because genes that are located close together are more likely to be inherited together. Linkage studies aim to find the broad region on the genome at which the gene is located.

Linkage disequilibrium occurs when a genetic marker shares the same inheritance pattern as the disease of interest more commonly than would be expected by chance. Linkage may be quantified using the **LOD score**, which is the logarithm of the odds of linkage. Traditionally, a LOD score >+3 is considered to be significant, which corresponds to a one-sided p-value of 10^{-4}. By studying the linkages between many genes, it is possible to create of a genetic map called a **linkage map**.

Limitations of linkage studies

- These studies only indicate the broad region of the gene.
- Strong linkage patterns only tend to occur with rare, highly penetrant, recessive diseases.

Association studies

Association studies measure the relative frequency with which a particular polymorphism occurs together with the disease of interest in a population (i.e. the extent to which the polymorphism is associated with the disease). This assessment is analogous to the way in which traditional epidemiological studies investigate associations between environmental risk factors and disease. Association studies are normally conducted using a **case–control design**. If the odds of having a particular allele are greater among cases than controls, then the allele may either have a causal role or it may be correlated with the causal allele.

Association studies frequently follow linkage studies: the linkage study identifies the broad region of the gene and then specific genes in this region can be investigated using association studies.

Another type of association study is a **family-based association study**. Here, families are identified that contain both affected and unaffected individuals. The transmission of alleles from parents to their affected and unaffected offspring is compared using statistical methods.

Limitations of association studies

- Many different mutations in a gene may lead to the disease; therefore, the effect of any single mutation may be attenuated by the presence of other genes, leading to no association being found.

1B

Statistics

Public health specialists need an understanding of statistical principles both for several different parts of the Membership of the Faculty of Public Health (MFPH) examination and for public health practice.

To aid with revision, the order of this chapter, like the rest of the book, closely follows the order of the 2014 Faculty of Public Health MFPH Part A syllabus. However, since certain earlier sections of this chapter require prior knowledge of some later sections, Table 1B.1 suggests an alternative order for reading this chapter. In addition, Chapter 6D lists the statistical formulae that candidates must memorise for the examination.

Table 1B.1 More logical order for reading Chapter 1B

Topic	Syllabus points
Probability theory	1B.1 Elementary probability theory 1B.4 Independence of events 1B.5 Conditional probability
Measures of location and dispersion	1B.9 Measures of location and dispersion and their appropriate uses
Displaying data	1B.10 Graphical methods in statistics
Sampling distributions and inference	1B.6 Standard statistical distributions 1B.7 Sampling distributions 1B.8 Principles of making inferences from a sample to a population
Quantification of uncertainty	1B.2 Methods for the quantification of uncertainty 1B.3 Estimation of confidence intervals
Hypothesis tests and their interpretation	1B.11 Hypothesis testing 1B.12 Type 1 and type 2 errors 1B.13 Problems of multiple comparisons
Sample size and power	1B.15 Sample size and statistical power
Tests comparing two groups	1B.14 Tests for comparing two or more groups
Regression	1B.16 Regression and correlation 1B.17 Regression techniques
Survival analysis	1B.18 Comparison of survival rates
Statistics for meta-analysis	1B.19 Heterogeneity 1B.20 Funnel plots
Bayesian statistics	1B.21 Role of Bayes' theorem

1B.1 Elementary probability theory

Probability is a measure of the likelihood that an event will occur. It is expressed as a positive number between 0 (event never occurs) and 1 (event is certain to occur). There are several approaches to calculating the probability of an event (see Table 1B.2).

Rules of probability

Two rules determine how two or more probabilities may be combined: the **addition rule** and the **multiplication rule**. An example of their application is shown in Box 1B.1.

Addition rule ('OR')

This rule is used to find the probability P that **at least one event** will occur out of two or more possible events.

For non-mutually exclusive events,

$$P(\text{A or B}) = P(\text{A}) + P(\text{B}) - P(\text{A and B})$$

otherwise expressed as

$$P(\text{A or B}) = 1 - P(\text{neither A nor B})$$

For mutually exclusive events, *if* A and B are mutually exclusive then, by definition, they cannot occur together. Therefore, $P(\text{A and B}) = 0$. Based on the first formula earlier, we can see that the probability that at least one mutually exclusive event will occur is

$$P(\text{A or B}) = P(\text{A}) + P(\text{B})$$

Note: $P(\text{A})$ is the probability that event A will occur; $P(\text{A or B})$ is the probability that at least one of event A *or B will occur;* $P(\text{A and B})$ *is the probability that both event A and event B will occur; etc.*

Multiplication rule ('AND')

This rule is used to calculate the probability of the **joint occurrence** of two or more events. The general rule is

$$P(\text{A and B}) = P(\text{A}) \times P(\text{B}|\text{A})$$

where $P(\text{B}|\text{A})$ is the probability that event B will occur given that event A has already occurred (i.e. the 'conditional probability'; see Section 1B.5).

Note: The vertical bar | is pronounced 'given'.

Independent events:

For independent events, event B is not affected by event A. Here, $P(\text{B}|\text{A}) = P(\text{B})$ and therefore, the multiplicative rule can be simplified to

$$P(\text{A and B}) = P(\text{A}) \times P(\text{B})$$

Please see Sections 1B.4 and 1B.5 (recommended).

Table 1B.2 Approaches to calculating the probability of events

Approach	Method for defining probability
Subjective	Personal degree of belief that an event will occur, such as a doctor's opinion for clinical decision-making. This is based on a priori beliefs and is the approach used in Bayesian statistics (see Section 1B.21).
Frequentist	Proportion of times an event would occur in a large number of similar repeated trials, e.g. number of 'heads' in coin tossed 100 times.

Box 1B.1 Application of the rules of probability

A smoking cessation programme has a probability of 0.4 that any individual completing the programme will quit smoking. If two random individuals (Adam and Ben) who never meet complete the programme, what is the probability that

1. At least one of them quits smoking
2. Both of them quit smoking

		Adam	
		Quits (0.4) P(A)	Does not quit (0.6) 1 − P(A)
Ben	Quits (0.4) P(B)	Both men quit (0.16)	Only Ben quits (0.24)
	Does not quit (0.6) 1 − P(B)	Only Adam quits (0.24)	Neither man quits (0.36)

1. From the table earlier, we can see that at least one of them quits smoking in all but the bottom right quadrant. Using the addition rule,

$$P(\text{A or B}) = 1 - P(\text{neither A nor B})$$

$$P(\text{A or B}) = 1 - 0.36$$

$$P(\text{A or B}) = 0.64$$

Alternatively,

$$P(\text{A or B}) = P(\text{A}) + P(\text{B}) - P(\text{A and B})$$

$$P(\text{A or B}) = 0.4 + 0.4 - 0.16$$

$$P(\text{A or B}) = 0.64$$

Note: The result is not simply the probability that Adam quits (0.4) + the probability that Ben quits (0.4) as this would include the probability of them both quitting twice.

2. As Adam and Ben never meet, the probability of both of them quitting smoking are independent events; therefore, it can be calculated as

$$P(\text{A and B}) = P(\text{A}) \times P(\text{B})$$

If Adam and Ben were friends, then their smoking habits might influence each other's (see Sections 1B4. [independence of events] and Section 1B.5 [conditional probability]):

$$P(\text{A and B}) = 0.4 \times 0.4$$

$$P(\text{A and B}) = 0.16$$

as already shown in the top left quadrant of the table earlier.

1B.2 Methods for the quantification of uncertainty

As described in Sections 1B.7 and 1B.8, most epidemiological studies rely on making observations on random sample of a population, rather than the whole population. Observations made on a sample are unlikely to be exactly the same as those in the population as a whole; therefore, they are subject to some degree of uncertainty. This uncertainty, caused by observing a sample rather than the whole population, is known as the **sampling error**. In general, the larger the sample, the smaller the sampling error. The most common method for measuring the likely sampling error is to determine the **standard error**.

Note: Sampling error is not the only reason why the observations in a sample may differ from those in the whole population. See Section 1A.13, which explains how ***bias*** *may also lead to such differences.*

Standard error

The standard error (se) estimates how precisely a population parameter (e.g. mean, difference between means, proportion) is estimated by the equivalent statistic in a sample. The **standard error is the standard deviation of the sampling distribution** of the statistic. The method of calculating the standard error therefore depends on type of statistic in question (see Table 1B.3).

The calculations of **confidence intervals** (see Section 1B.3) and **hypothesis testing** (see Section 1B.11) are both based on standard errors.

We advise reading Section 1B.3 on confidence intervals.

Table 1B.3 Calculation of standard error for different statistics

Type of outcome variable	Statistic	Calculation of the standard error
Continuous	Mean	$se = \frac{\sigma}{\sqrt{n}} \approx \frac{s}{\sqrt{n}}$ The population standard deviation (σ) is rarely known; therefore, the sample standard deviation (s) is used instead:
	Difference between means (large sample)	$se \approx \sqrt{\frac{s_1^2}{n_1} + \frac{s_0^2}{n_0}}$
	Difference between means (small sample)	$se \approx s_p\sqrt{\frac{1}{n_1} + \frac{1}{n_0}}$ where $s_p = \sqrt{\frac{(n_1 - 1)s_1^2 + (n_0 - 1)s_0^2}{(n_1 + n_0 - 1)}}$ σ = Population standard deviation, s = Sample standard deviation, n = Number in the sample
Binary	Proportion (or risk)	$se = \sqrt{\frac{\pi(1-\pi)}{n}} \approx \sqrt{\frac{p(1-p)}{n}}$ The probability or risk in the population (π) is rarely known; therefore, the sample proportion (p) is used instead:
	Difference between proportions	$se \approx \sqrt{\frac{p_1(1-p_1)}{n_1} + \frac{p_0(1-p_0)}{n_0}}$ π = Population probability or risk, p = Sample proportion or risk, n = Number in the sample
Binary over time	Count	$se \approx \sqrt{\lambda}$
	Rate	$se \approx \frac{\sqrt{\lambda}}{T}$ λ = Mean count in the sample, T = Total person-years of observations

1B.3 Estimation of confidence intervals

Confidence intervals are a way of gauging how accurately a **sample statistic** estimates a **population parameter**. They provide an **interval estimation** rather than a point estimation.

Calculation of confidence intervals

As seen in Sections 1B.6 and 1B.7, the sampling distribution of a mean is a normal distribution. Furthermore, the sampling distributions of other statistics (e.g. proportions and rates) can usually be approximated by the normal distribution. 95% of the values in a normal distribution lie within 1.96 standard deviations above or below the mean value (see Figure 1B.1). In a sampling distribution, the mean value is equivalent to the true population parameter and the standard deviation is equivalent to the standard error of the sample statistic. Therefore, 95% of sample statistics (from unbiased random samples) would lie within 1.96 standard errors above or below the

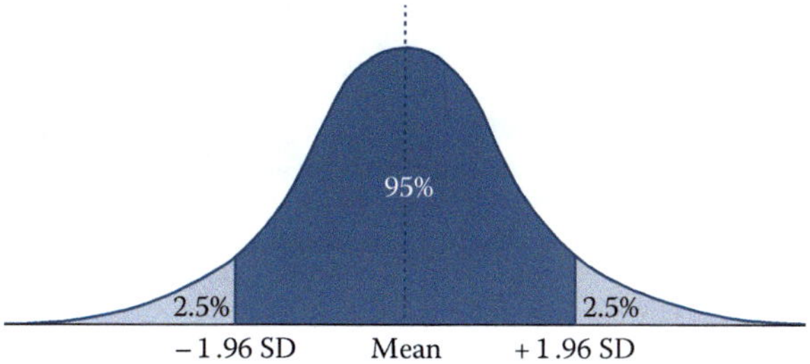

Figure 1B.1 The normal distribution.

Box 1B.2 Example: Calculating the confidence interval of a mean

The mean pO_2 arterial blood test for a sample of 56 patients with COPD was 8.9 mol/L, with a standard deviation of 0.8 mmol/L. What is the 95% confidence interval for the mean pO_2 of the population of all COPD patients?

Standard error	$\frac{0.8}{\sqrt{56}}$ $= 0.11$
95% confidence interval	= 8.9 +/− (1.96 × 0.11) = Between 8.7 mmol/L and 9.2 mmol/L

true population parameter. From this, we can also infer that there is a 95% probability that the true population parameter lies within 1.96 standard errors above or below any sample statistic. The interval between 1.96 standard errors above or below a sample statistic is therefore known as the **95% confidence interval**:

$$95\%CI = Sample\ statistic \pm (1.96 \times se)$$

This relationship is true whether the sample statistic is a mean, a difference between means, a proportion, a regression coefficient, etc.—only the method for calculating the standard error changes (see Section 1B.2). The only exceptions are for very small samples, where the 95% confidence interval may be calculated using other distributions (e.g. using the t-distribution for means in a small sample).

To calculate other confidence intervals, we use different multiples of the standard error (e.g. for a 99% confidence interval, we use 2.58 times the standard error):

$$99\%CI = Sample\ statistic \pm (2.58 \times se)$$

Boxes 1B.2 and 1B.3 give two examples 95% confidence interval calculations.

Box 1B.3 Example: Calculating the confidence interval for two proportions

57% of the 864 patients at a stop-smoking clinic had quit smoking by the end of the programme, compared with 42% of 795 patients at a neighbouring clinic. What was the difference in quit rates between the two clinics?

$$\text{Standard error (difference in proportions)} = \sqrt{\frac{0.57(1-0.57)}{864} + \frac{0.42(1-0.42)}{795}}$$

$$= 0.0243$$

$$\text{95\% confidence interval for the difference} = \text{Sample value} +/- (1.96 \times \text{Standard error})$$

$$= (0.57 - 0.42) +/- (1.96 \times 0.024)$$

$$= \text{Between } 0.102 \text{ and } 0.198$$

$$= \text{Between } 10.2\% \text{ and } 19.8\% \text{ difference}$$

Box 1B.4 Overlap of confidence intervals

Degree of overlap	Interpretation
95% confidence intervals do not overlap.	Significant difference* at the 5% significance level (i.e. strong evidence of a true difference).
95% confidence intervals overlap but the point estimates are outside the confidence intervals of the other.	Unclear: Requires calculation of a significance test.
Point estimate of one sample falls within the 95% confidence intervals of the other.	No significant difference at the 5% significance level (i.e. no strong evidence of a true difference).

Note: Most epidemiologists now avoid dichotomising between significant and non-significant differences. Instead, they quote the confidence interval and/or *p*-value and then describe the strength of evidence that this provides (e.g. weak, modest, strong, very strong evidence).

Interpretation of confidence intervals

A confidence interval is a **range of values** indicating the **precision** with which the sample estimate is likely to represent the population from which the sample was drawn. For a 95% confidence interval, the true value for the population will lie within this range on 19 occasions out of 20. For a 99% confidence interval (which will be a wider range), the true value will lie within the range expressed 99 times out of 100.

For measures of **absolute risk**, where a 95% confidence interval includes **zero**, there is no evidence at the $p = 0.05$ level that there is a true difference.

For measures of **relative risk**, where a 95% confidence interval includes **one**, there is no evidence at the $p = 0.05$ level that there is a true difference.

In any diagram showing two or more point estimates and their associated confidence intervals, there are three possibilities regarding the overlap of the points and intervals. These may be interpreted as shown in Box 1B.4.

Section 1B.11 follows on from here and covers confidence intervals.

1B.4 Independence of events

The application of probability theory to independent events is covered in Section 1B.1.

Much of the science of epidemiology relates to establishing whether events are independent or not. If they are not independent, then they are said to be **associated**. For example, smokers have a greater risk of developing lung cancer; therefore, smoking is not independent of developing lung cancer—rather, the two phenomena are associated.

Epidemiologists estimate the likelihood that two events are associated by calculating measures of effect such as an **odds ratio** (see Section 1A.11) or a **regression coefficient** (see Sections 1B.16 and 1B.17). The *p*-values and confidence intervals can then be calculated to give an indication of how likely it is that any observed association was due to chance (see Sections 1B.2 and 1B.3).

1B.5 Conditional probability

As we saw in Section 1B.1, the probability that an event (B) will occur given that another event (A) has already occurred is a conditional probability and is denoted by $P(B|A)$.

The formula for calculating a conditional probability can be derived from the multiplication rule described in Section 1B.1:

$$P(\text{A and B}) = P(\text{A}) \times P(\text{B}|\text{A})$$

$$P(\text{A}) \times P(\text{B}|\text{A}) = P(\text{A and B})$$

$$P(\text{B}|\text{A}) = \frac{P(\text{A and B})}{P(\text{A})}$$

Conditional probability allows epidemiologists to evaluate how different treatments or exposures influence the probability that outcomes, such as disease or mortality, will occur. It also provides a useful way to evaluate diagnostic tests. See Box 1B.5.

Section 1B.9 follows on from here and covers measures of location and dispersion.

Box 1B.5 Breastfeeding Example: conditional probabilities

In a study of feeding modalities, preterm infants were randomised into two groups. The treatment group was fed by nasogastric (NG) tube, and the control group was bottle-fed. The purpose of the study was to test whether, compared to bottle-feeding, NG feeding would increase the likelihood that the infant was being breastfed at the time of discharge from hospital.

In the below table, the rows represent the treatment group (NG tube versus bottle), and the columns represent the feeding status at the time of discharge from hospital (i.e. exclusive breastfeeding versus partial/no breastfeeding).

	Exclusive breastfeeding at discharge		
	No	Yes	Row total
Bottle-fed	27	20	47
NG tube fed	10	32	42
Column total	37	52	89

In order to calculate the conditional probability of breastfeeding given that NG feeding has occurred, we can use the conditional probability formula:

$$P(\mathrm{B} \mid \mathrm{A}) = \frac{P(\mathrm{A\ and\ B})}{P(\mathrm{A})}$$

$$P(\text{breastfeeding} \mid \text{NG fed}) = \frac{P(\text{NG fed and breastfeeding})}{P(\text{NG fed})}$$

From the table earlier, we can see that

$$P(\text{NG fed and breastfeeding}) = \frac{32}{89} = 0.360$$

$$P(\text{NG fed}) = \frac{42}{89} = 0.472$$

Therefore,

$$P(\text{breastfeeding} \mid \text{NG fed}) = \frac{0.360}{0.472} = 0.76$$

Note: This is the same as the 'risk' of breastfeeding among the NG fed group, and we would obtain the same result if we calculated risk from a 2 × 2 table in the usual way,

i.e.

$$\text{'Risk' of breastfeeding among NG fed} = \frac{\text{Number NG fed who were breastfeeding at discharge}}{\text{Total number NG fed}} = \frac{32}{42} = 0.76$$

Source: Reproduced from Fleiss, J.L., *Statistical Methods for Rates and Proportions*, 3rd edn., New York: John Wiley & Sons, p. 77, 1981. With permission.

1B.6 Standard statistical distributions

A statistical distribution is an arrangement of the values of a variable that shows how frequently each value is observed or is expected theoretically to occur.

Normal distribution

The normal (or **Gaussian**) distribution is a bell-shaped, symmetrical curve that is described by two parameters:

Mean (μ)

Variance (σ^2)

The normal distribution is important for several reasons:

- It provides a good description of the frequency distribution of **many variables in biology** (e.g. height, systolic blood pressure, birthweight) (see Section 1B.10).
- It describes the **sampling distribution of a mean** (i.e. if many samples were taken, their means would be normally distributed around the true population mean). Known as the **central limit theorem**, this phenomenon means that the normal distribution is the basis of many statistical tests used when making inferences from a population (see Section 1B.7), including hypothesis testing (see Section 1B.11) and the calculation of confidence intervals (see Section 1B.3).
- Other distributions **approximate to the normal distribution** when the sample size is **sufficiently large**. This convergence means that statistical tests for proportions, rates, and means may be based on approximations to the normal distribution.

The standard normal distribution has a **mean of 0** and **variance of 1**. Any normally distributed variable can be converted to a standard normal distribution by subtracting the mean from each observation and dividing by the standard deviation:

$$\text{Standard normal distribution, } z = \frac{x - \mu}{\sigma}$$

In the normal distribution,

68% of the area under the curve is within 1 standard deviation of the mean.

95% of the area is within 1.96 standard deviations.

99% of the area is within 2.58 standard deviations (see Figure 1B.2).

Note: The area under the curve of a normal distribution beyond a given z-value is used to calculate p-values (see Section 1B.11).

Binomial distribution

The binomial distribution shows the frequency of events that have two possible outcomes. It is constructed from two parameters: n (sample size) and π (true probability). When the sample size is large, the binomial distribution approximates to the normal distribution (see Figure 1B.3).

This distribution is used for discrete data with two outcomes (e.g. success or failure) and also the sampling distribution for proportions. **Note:** Since a proportion or a probability cannot be negative, the binomial distribution has no negative values.

Poisson distribution

The Poisson distribution shows the frequency of events **over time** in which the **events occur independently** of each other. An example is the rate of deaths due to myocardial infarction. The Poisson distribution is used in the analysis of **rates** (e.g. incident rates of disease). Since it leads to a prediction of randomly occurring events, it allows a determination to be made as to whether observed events are occurring randomly or not.

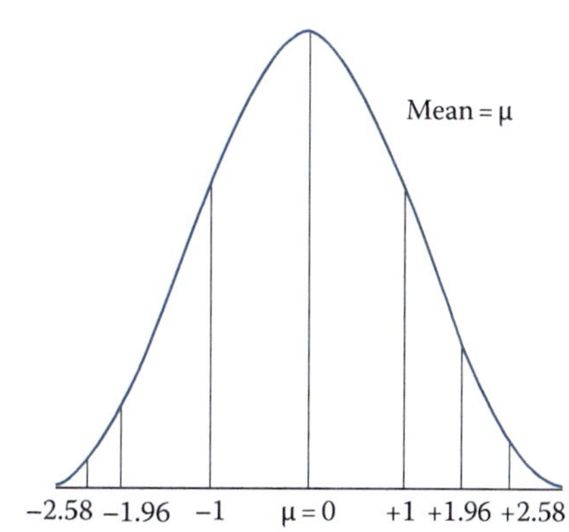

Figure 1B.2 The standard normal distribution.

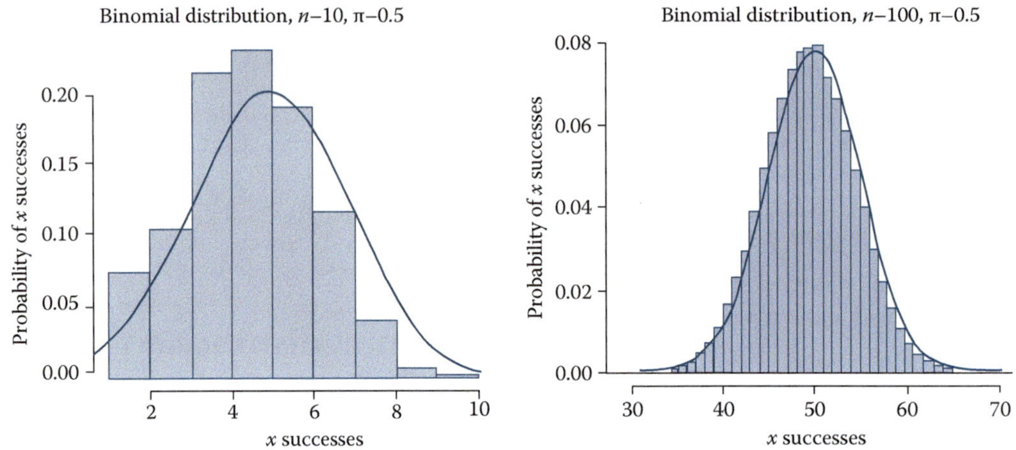

Figure 1B.3 Graph of binomial distribution approximating normal distribution as sample size increases, where *n* is the sample size, π is the probability, and *x* represents the number of successes obtained.

The Poisson distribution assumes that the data are **discrete**, that they occur at **random**, and that they are **independent** of each other. In the Poisson distribution, the parameter is the **variance, which is equal to the mean**, and therefore the standard deviation is equal to the square root of the mean. As a result, small samples give asymmetrical distributions, and large samples approximate the normal distribution (see Figure 1B.4).

The horizontal axis shows *x*, which is the **number** of occurrences of an event within a particular time period. The vertical axis shows the **probability** of obtaining *x* events during that period.

Like the binomial distribution, the Poisson distribution has no negative values, since a count or a rate cannot be negative.

Other distributions

Table 1B.4 lists the features and applications of some other distributions of continuous variables.

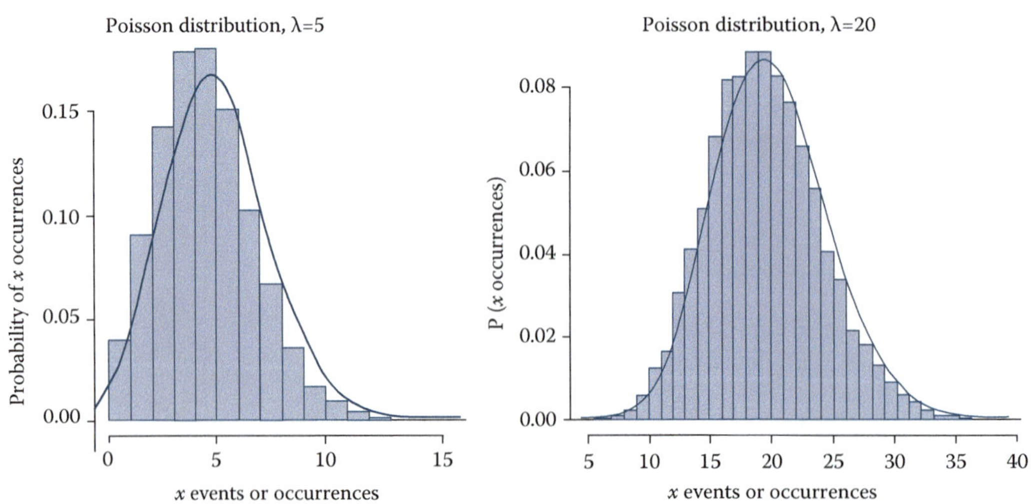

Figure 1B.4 Approximation of Poisson distribution to normal distribution as λ (the mean or expected value) increases.

Table 1B.4 Probability distributions of continuous variables

Distribution	Parameter(s)	Features	Uses and assumptions
t-distribution (also called '*Student's t-distribution*')	Degrees of freedom.	The shape is similar to the normal distribution but the tails are more spread out. As the degrees of freedom increases, the *t*-distribution approaches the normal distribution.	**Uses** Estimating the mean of a normally distributed population when the sample size is small. Testing hypotheses with a single mean (small sample). Testing hypotheses with two means (small samples). Confidence intervals.
Chi-squared	Degrees of freedom.	The shape is right-skewed, taking positive values. With increasing degrees of freedom, it approximates the normal distribution.	**Uses** Analysing categorical data, e.g. significance test for two categorical variables (comparison of observed and expected events). **Assumptions** If n is >40, then all x are >1 If n is >20 but <40, all x should be >5; otherwise, use **Fisher's exact test**.
f-distribution	It is defined by a ratio of two parameters: degree of freedom of the numerator and denominator of the ratio.	It is skewed to the right. Values are positive.	**Uses** Useful for comparing two variances and more than two means using ANOVA.

1B.7 Sampling distributions

Studies can rarely be conducted on a whole population. However, it is possible to make reliable inferences about the population by drawing a random sample and making observations on this sample (e.g. systolic blood pressure or the presence of a disease). Such measurements are used to generate a **statistic** for the sample (e.g. mean, proportion, or rate).

Using mean systolic blood pressure as an example, if many different samples, all of the same size, were taken from the same population, then the frequency distribution of these sample means is known as the **sampling distribution**. The mean systolic blood pressure in each sample would not always be the same; neither would it always be the same as the true population mean systolic blood pressure. However, the mean of this frequency distribution will be almost the same as the true population mean.

Of course, in reality, only one sample is usually taken in a study; therefore, the sampling distribution is theoretical. The shape of the sampling distribution depends on the type of statistic (see Table 1B.5).

Epidemiological studies are generally interested in how one variable (the outcome) differs with respect to another variable (the exposure). Therefore, epidemiologists are often interested in **differences** in means or difference in proportions

Table 1B.5 Shape of sampling distribution for different statistics

Type of outcome variable	Statistic	Shape of sampling distribution
Continuous	Mean	Normal
Binary	Proportion (or risk)	Binomial[a]
Binary over time	Rate	Poisson[a]

[a] As described in Section 1B.6, when the sample is large, the binomial and Poisson distributions approximate to the normal distribution.

(e.g. the difference in mean systolic blood pressure in men compared to women). These differences also have a sampling distribution, and the difference between means itself has a normal sampling distribution providing that each of the means is normally distributed. The sampling distribution of a difference between proportions can also be reasonably approximated by a normal distribution under most circumstances.

Sampling distributions are the basis for making inferences from a sample to a population (see Section 1B.8)

1B.8 Principles of making inferences from a sample to a population

In epidemiological studies, observations in a sample are rarely of interest in their own right but rather for what they tell us about the population from which the sample was taken. The process of making conclusions about a population based on observations in a sample is known as **inference**. Inferences are only valid if the sample correctly represents the population (e.g. an unbiased random sample).

Using a sample to make inferences is more efficient in terms of time and resources than obtaining details on the entire population, which may often be impossible. However, the process of sampling introduces a degree of error. The **standard error** measures how precisely a population parameter (such as the mean, difference in means, or proportion) is estimated by the equivalent sample statistic (see Section 1B.2).

There are two main methods of statistical inference: **estimation** and **hypothesis testing**, both of which are derived from standard errors.

Estimation

An **estimate** is a measurement made from a sample. This normally includes

- A **point estimate** (e.g. mean, difference in means, proportion)
- An **interval estimation**, which expresses the uncertainty associated with the point estimate (e.g. a **confidence interval**; see Section 1B.3)

Hypothesis testing

This is a way of assessing how unlikely it is that a particular finding in a sample was due to chance or, in other words, the likelihood that the finding observed in the sample was a true finding within the population (see Section 1B.11).

Section 1B.2 follows on from here and covers standard errors.

1B.9 Measures of location and dispersion and their appropriate uses

Data may be summarised according to two parameters:

- **Location**, which typically describes an **average value** or **central tendency** of the data
- **Dispersion**, which describes the **spread** of the data

Measures of location

The measures of central tendency that are most widely used in statistics are described in Table 1B.6.

Measures of dispersion

The principal measures of dispersion are shown in Table 1B.7.

Table 1B.6 Measures of location

Measure	Definition	Calculation	Advantages	Disadvantages
Arithmetic mean	The average value based on the **sum** of a set of numbers. For a **sample**, the mean is denoted by $\bar{x}$ (pronounced 'x-bar'). For a **population**, the mean is denoted by the Greek letter μ (pronounced 'mu').	$\bar{x} = \frac{\sum x_i}{n}$ $\mu = \frac{\sum x_i}{n}$	Amenable to statistical analysis.	Sensitive to outliers. Poor for asymmetrical distributions.
Geometric mean	An average based on the **product** (rather than the sum) of a set of numbers. The nth root of the product of n numbers; also, the arithmetic mean of the logarithm of the values exponentiated.	$G = \sqrt[n]{x_1 \times x_1 \times \cdots x_n}$ For log transformed values where $u = \log(x)$, $G = \exp(\bar{u}) = e^{\bar{u}}$	More appropriate for positively skewed distributions.	Cannot be used if any values are zero or negative.
Median	Value at the centre of the distribution.	If all observations are arranged in ascending order of value, then the median is the middle value (i.e. half the observations lie above and half below).	Unaffected by extreme outliers. Good for skewed distributions.	Value determined solely by rank, so carries no information about any other values.
Mode	Most commonly occurring value or values.	Value(s) that occur(s) with the highest frequency.	Not greatly affected by extreme values. Can provide extra insights (e.g. suicide is bimodal, affecting young and old adults).	Not amenable to statistical analysis. Sometimes no mode exists. Data containing more than one mode may be difficult to interpret.
Percentiles	Values are ranked and divided into 100 groups where the 100th percentile is the largest value. The *n*th percentile will have *n*% values below it and (100 – *n*)% values above it. **Note:** The 50th percentile is the **median**, the 25th percentile is the **lower quartile**, and the 75th percentile is the **upper quartile**.	Useful for comparing measurements (e.g. BMI in groups of similar age and sex).	Comparisons made at extreme ends of the distribution are often less informative than those at the centre.	

Table 1B.7 Principal measures of dispersion

Measure	Definition and calculation	Units	Advantages	Disadvantages
Range	Difference between maximum and minimum sample values.	Units are the same as data.	Intuitive. Simple—only depends on two observations.	Sensitive to the size of the sample.
Interquartile range (IQR)	Middle 50% of the sample. Calculated as the upper quartile (the value below which 75% of the data lie) minus the lower quartile (the value below which 25% of the data lie).	Units are the same as data.	More stable than the range as the sample size increases.	Unstable for small samples. Does not allow further mathematical manipulation.
Variance	Average squared deviation of each number from its mean $(x - \bar{x})$ Variance in a sample: $s^2 = \frac{\sum(x_i - \bar{x})}{(n-1)}$ **Note:** $(n-1)$ = *the degrees of freedom* Population variance: $\sigma = \frac{\sum(x_i - \mu)}{n}$	Units are the squared units of the data.	Takes into account all values. Useful for making inferences about the population.	Units are different from the units of the data.
Standard deviation	The square route of the variance: $s = \sqrt{\frac{\sum(x_i - \bar{x})}{(n-1)}}$	Units are the same as data.	Most commonly used. Units are the same as the data. Useful for making inferences about the population.	Sensitive to some extent to extreme values. Will vary depending on the units of observation.
Coefficient of variation	Ratio of the standard deviation to the mean to give an idea of the size of the variation relative to the size of the observation: $c_v = \frac{s}{\bar{x}}$	No units as long as the mean and standard deviation are converted to the same units. May be expressed as a percentage: $c_v = \frac{s}{\bar{x}} \times 100$	Allows comparison of the variation of populations that have significantly different mean values.	Where the mean value is near zero, the coefficient of variation is highly sensitive to changes in the standard deviation.

1B.10 Graphical methods in statistics

Graphics can be a highly effective means of conveying statistical information. Different types of data are better suited to different types of data (see the following).

In the MFPH Part A examination, you may be asked to describe a graph. The key features that should be described are

1. The type of graph
2. The axes or equivalent
3. The type of data plotted (e.g. mortality)
4. The units of analysis
5. Any obvious findings
6. What interpretation, if any, can be made from the findings (NB: you will not normally be able to interpret a *causal* relationship from a graph)

Categorical data

The type of chart used should be chosen carefully based on the **nature** of the data, the **analysis** conducted, and the **message** to be conveyed.

Bar charts

These charts use bars to represent the frequencies, or relative frequencies, of the observations, such that the height of each bar equates to the frequency or relative frequency of its category (see Figure 1B.5):

Frequencies: Counts

Relative frequencies: Percentage

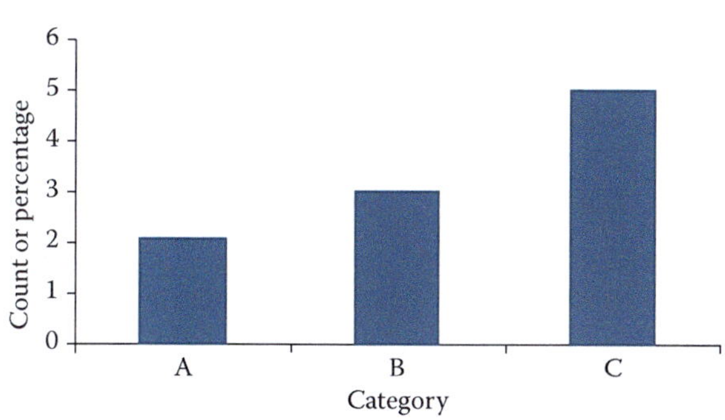

Figure 1B.5 Schematic of a bar chart.

Pie charts

The pie is a circle divided into a number of slices, each representing a different category. The size of each slice is proportional to the relative frequency of that category. Starting at the 12 O'clock position, the categories should be ordered clockwise in descending order according to their size. An example is shown in Figure 1B.6.

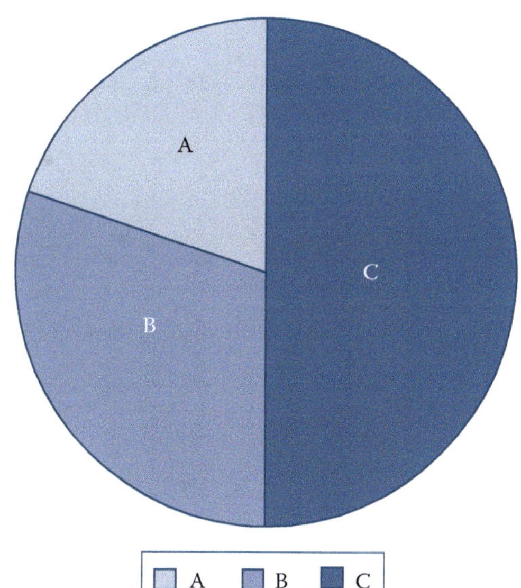

Figure 1B.6 Schematic of a pie chart.

Continuous data

Stem-and-leaf display

This is a quick technique for displaying numerical data graphically. A vertical stem is drawn, consisting of the first few significant figures. Any digit after the stem is called the leaf (i.e. the leaf is the last digit of the data value). An example is shown in Figure 1B.7. A **back-to-back** stem-and-leaf plot can be used to display data from two groups. Table 1B.8 lists the advantages and disadvantages of stem-and-leaf display.

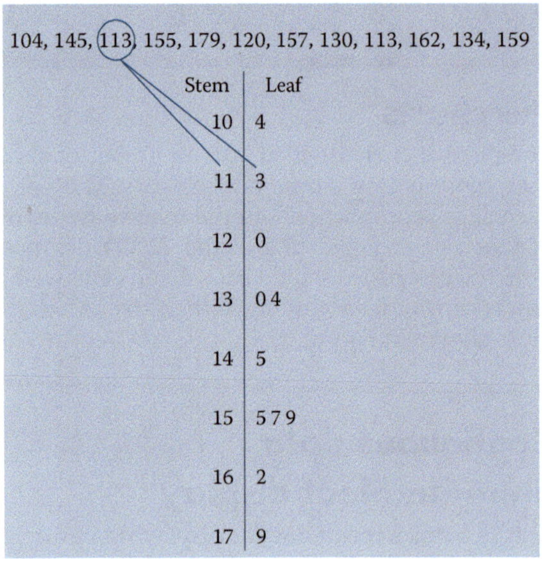

Figure 1B.7 Example of stem-and-leaf display constructed from 12 data points.

Table 1B.8 Advantages and disadvantages of stem-and-leaf display

Advantages	Disadvantages
Quick and easy to construct. Actual values are retained.	Cumbersome for large datasets.

Boxplots

Also known as a **box-and-whiskers** plot, a boxplot shows

- A measure of **central location** (the median)
- Two measures of **dispersion** (the range and interquartile range)
- The **skewness** (from the orientation of the median relative to the quartiles)
- Potential **outliers** (marked individually)

An example is shown in Figure 1B.8, and the advantages and disadvantages of boxplots are listed in Table 1B.9.

Histograms

Histograms divide the sample's values into many intervals, which are called **bins**. The area of a bar is proportional to the number of observations falling within its bin (i.e. the bin's frequency). Examples are shown in Figure 1B.9. Note that in contrast to bar charts, there should be **no gaps** between the bars of a histogram. This is important because it reflects the fact that the data are continuous. Table 1B.10 lists the advantages and disadvantages of histograms.

Frequency polygons

This is drawn by joining the midpoints of the tops of the bars in a histogram (see Figure 1B.9).

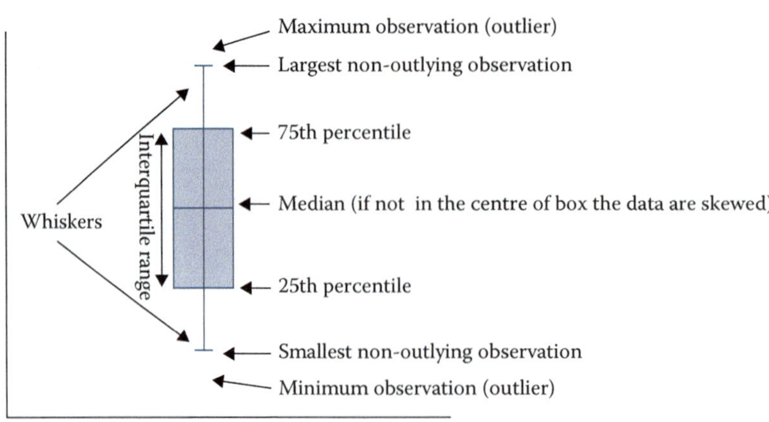

Figure 1B.8 Schematic of a Boxplot.

Table 1B.9 Advantages and disadvantages of boxplots

Advantages	Disadvantages
The spacing between the different parts of the box a large amount of information. Boxplots are especially useful when comparing two or more sets of data.	Exact values are not retained.

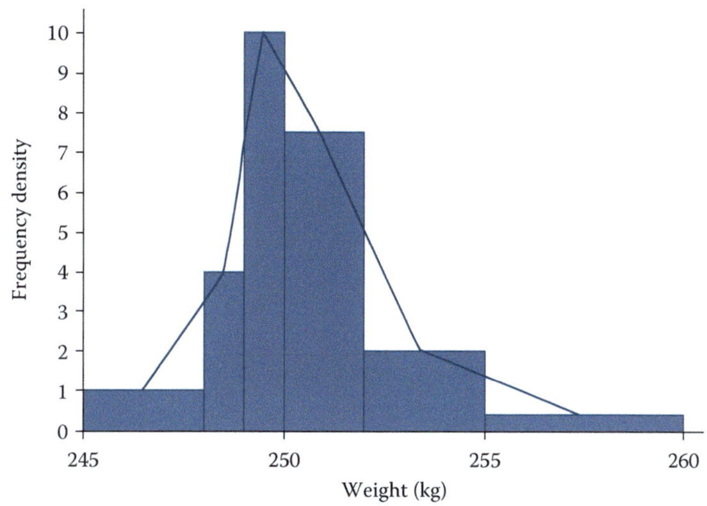

Figure 1B.9 Schematic of a histogram with a frequency polygon (blue line) overlaid.

Table 1B.10 Advantages and disadvantages of histograms

Advantages	Disadvantages
Demonstrates central tendency (mean, mode, median) Demonstrates the shape of the frequency distribution (e.g. symmetrical or skewed, unimodal, bimodal, or multimodal)	Cannot read exact values because the data are grouped into categories More difficult to compare two datasets Can only be used with continuous data

Frequency distributions

These charts are essentially the frequency polygon that would be drawn for a very large sample divided into a very large number of bins, which leads to a smooth line. Examples of some important frequency distributions are shown in Figure 1B.10.

Cumulative frequency distribution

A **running count** starting with the lowest value and displaying how the number and % of observations accumulate (Figure 1B.11).

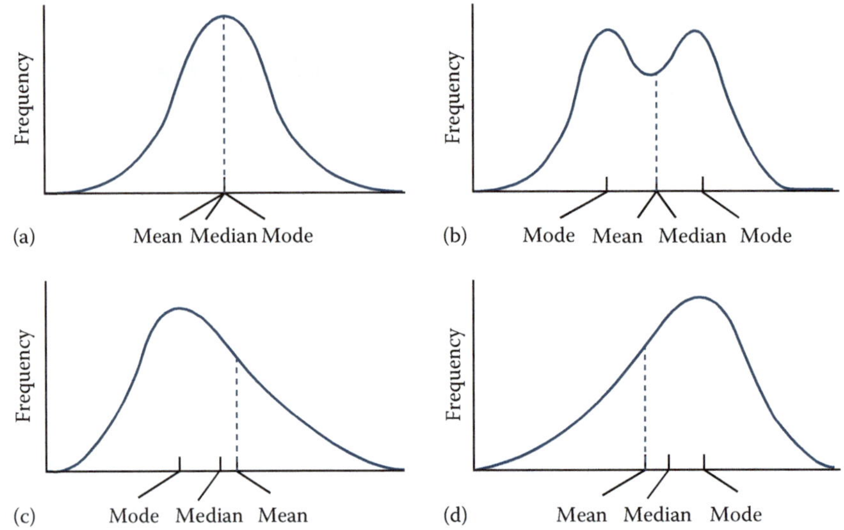

Figure 1B.10 Frequency distributions: (a) normal distribution, (b) bimodal distribution, (c) positively (right) skewed distribution, (d) negatively (left) skewed distribution.

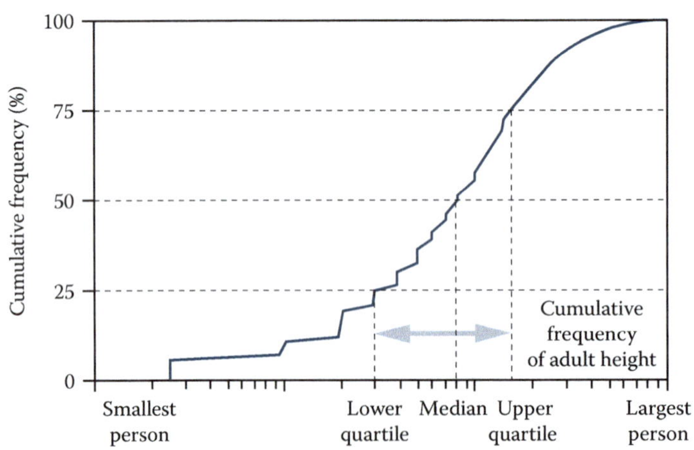

Figure 1B.11 Cumulative frequency distribution.

Association between two variables

Bivariate data are best displayed using **scatter plots**.

Scatter plot

Here, the data from two variables are plotted one against the other, in order to explore the association between them. A trend line is drawn to illustrate whether any correlation is

Positive, negative, or non-existent
Linear or nonlinear
Strong, moderate, or weak

The strength of any correlation is determined by observing the spread of the points about the line. Examples of scatter plots are shown in Figure 1B.12, and the advantages and disadvantages are listed in Table 1B.11.

Section 1B.6 follows on from here and covers standard statistical distributions.

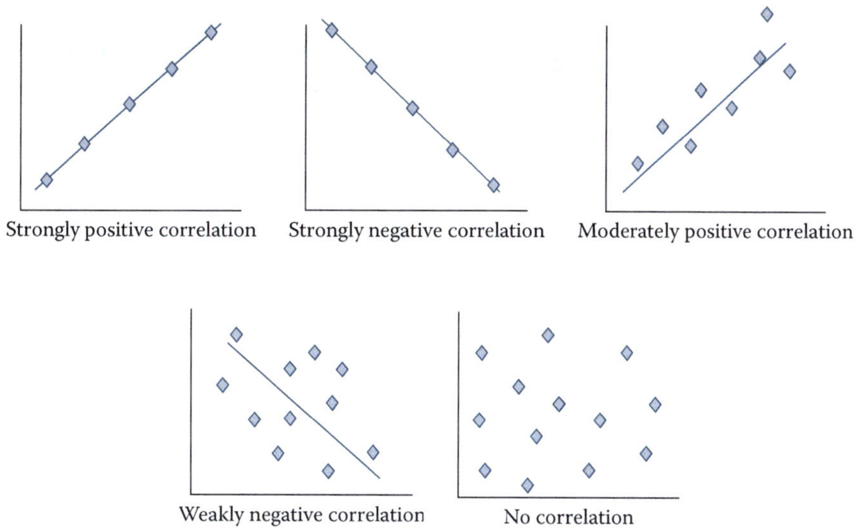

Figure 1B.12 Example scatter plots, each displaying the correlation between two variables.

Table 1B.11 Advantages and disadvantages of scatter plots

Advantages	Disadvantages
Shows a trend in the data relationship.	Hard to visualise results in large datasets.
Retains exact data values and sample size.	Flat trend line gives inconclusive results.
Shows minimum, maximum, and outliers.	Data on both axes must be continuous.

1B.11 Hypothesis testing

In the earlier parts of this chapter, we mostly focused on data for a single group or sample. However, epidemiological studies are often interested in comparing the outcomes of two or more exposure groups or assessing the association between an outcome and an exposure variable.

In order to investigate the association between two variables, the following process is generally used:

1. Calculate a measure of the **magnitude of the difference** in the outcome between exposure groups in the sample. This may be a difference between two means, an odds ratio, a regression coefficient, etc.
2. Calculate a **confidence interval** for the difference (see Section 1B.3).
3. Conduct a **hypothesis test** to derive a p-value.

The latter two steps assist in making inferences about whether any association found in the sample is likely to be a true association in the population or was simply due to chance (see Section 1B.8).

A hypothesis test assumes the **null hypothesis**, that is, there is no association between the exposure and the outcome in the population. The outcome of the test is expressed as a p-value.

Steps in hypothesis testing

Step 1

To answer a statistical question, a **hypothesis** is first formulated. For example, in an RCT, the hypothesis may be that the intervention group will have a lower incidence of disease than the control group.

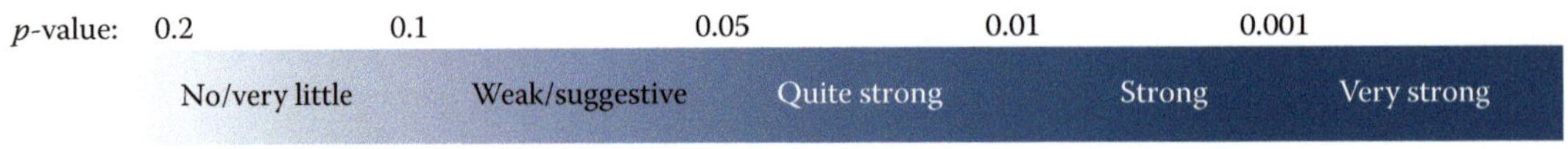

Figure 1B.13 Strength of evidence against the null hypothesis at different *p*-values.

Step 2
Define a **null hypothesis** (H_0). This is a statement that assumes there is no difference (or no relationship) between the variables being tested. For every null hypothesis, there is an **alternative hypothesis** (H_A), which assumes that a difference or relationship does exist. Both the null hypothesis and the alternative hypothesis are true/false statements, which are answered according to the significance level chosen (e.g. $p = 0.05$). For example,

H_0 = The incidence of the disease is the same in the intervention group and the control group

H_A = The incidence of the disease differs between the intervention group and the control group

Step 3
Collect the data.

Step 4
Calculate a **test statistic** using a statistical test. Numerous tests exist (e.g. *z*-test, χ^2 test, linear regression), and these are described in more detail in Sections 1B.14 and 1B.17.

Step 5
Derive the ***p*-value** for the test statistic from a known probability distribution found in statistical tables (note that these tables are not currently provided to candidates in the UK MFPH Part A examination).

Step 6
Interpret the *p*-value in terms of the strength of the evidence to **accept** or **reject** the null hypothesis.

Interpreting the *p*-value

A *p*-value provides an estimate of the probability of recording an association at least as large as the association found in the sample if there was no true association in the population.

For example, if $p = 0.001$, there is 0.1% likelihood that, if the null hypothesis were true, this result would be obtained by chance alone. In the past, *p*-values <0.05 were frequently reported as being 'statistically significant' and *p*-values >0.05 as 'not statistically significant'. However, this is an arbitrary cut-off, and it is now considered preferable to present actual *p*-values and to interpret the strength of evidence against the null hypothesis as a gradient (see Figure 1B.13).

Note: In the MFPH Part A examination, it is unlikely that candidates will be provided with a lookup table for test statistic distributions, so it is acceptable to memorise the $p = 0.05$ that corresponds to certain distributions to comment on their significance at the 5% level.

It is important to remember that a very small *p*-value (e.g. 0.001) does not signify a large effect. Rather, it signifies that the observed effect—whatever its size—is highly unlikely to be due to chance. For example, a very small *p*-value may arise when an effect is small but the sample size is very large. Conversely, a larger *p*-value may arise when the effect is large but the sample size is small.

1B.12 Type 1 and Type 2 errors

The findings from a study may lead to the acceptance or rejection of the null hypothesis. However, the findings of the study sample may or may not reflect the 'true' situation in the population at large, as illustrated in the contingency table shown in Table 1B.12, where the null hypothesis is that A = B.

The magnitudes of type 1 (α) and type 2 (β) error rates are generally set in advance as part of a

Table 1B.12 Contingency table displaying Type 1 and Type 2 errors

		'True' finding	
		A = B	A ≠ B
Results from study	A = B	Correct	Type 2 error (β)
	A ≠ B	Type 1 error (α)	Correct

Table 1B.13 Differences between Type 1 and Type 2 errors

	Type 1 error	Type 2 error
Symbol	α.	β.
Definition	False positive.	False negative.
Description	Null hypothesis was wrongly rejected. Study shows an effect which in reality does not exist.	Null hypothesis was not rejected when it should have been. Study does not detect an effect that existed in reality.
Relationship with power and significance	Significance level = α.	Power = $1 - \beta$.
Typical value	0.05 or 0.001.	0.8.
Aide memoire	Type 1 error = *p*-value.	Type 2 (*two*) error = sample size too small.

power calculation used to determine the appropriate sample size of the study (see Section 1B.15). Table 1B.13 summarises the differences between type 1 and type 2 errors.

Type 2 errors are generally considered to be **less serious** than type 1 errors because a type 2 error is only an error in the sense that an opportunity to reject the null hypothesis was missed.

Note that there is a **trade-off** between type 1 and type 2 errors: the more the study restricts type 1 errors by setting a low level of α, the greater the chance that a type 2 error will occur.

1B.13 Problems of multiple comparisons

The hypothesis to be tested should always be stated **before** a study begins, together with the list of variables that will be analysed. The reason for prespecifying the hypothesis is that once the results have been collected, there may be a temptation to search for associations using additional variables. This practice is known as **data mining** or **data fishing**. As more and more such tests are performed, the likelihood of a type 1 error increases (i.e. the chance of falsely concluding that an association is significant). Indeed, at the $p = 0.05$ level of significance, 1 in 20 tests will appear significant simply due to chance alone.

If multiple comparisons are going to be made, a method should be used to adjust the acceptable *p*-value for the number of tests performed, such as the **Bonferroni correction**.

Using this correction, an investigator testing n outcomes should divide the original α by n:

$$\text{Adjusted } \alpha = \frac{\text{Original } \alpha}{n}$$

See Box 1B.6.

Section 1B.15 follows on from here.

Box 1B.6 Example: Bonferroni correction

Suppose we were investigating the association between salt intake and 15 different types of cancer. Instead of testing at the $p = 0.05$ level for a single cancer, we would test at the $p = 0.0033$.

Adjusted $\alpha = 0.05 \div 15 = 0.0033$ level.

Using this threshold would ensure that the overall chance of making a type 1 error was kept at <1 in 20.

1B.14 Tests for comparing two or more groups

Parametric and non-parametric tests for comparing two or more groups.

In order to test for associations between an exposure and an outcome, we can either use a **statistical test** or some form of **regression**. The type of **exposure variable** determines whether we use a statistical test or regression (see Table 1B.14). As can be seen, some form of regression can generally be used in any situation (see Sections 1B.16 and 1B.17).

The specific statistical test or type of regression to be used will depend on the **outcome variable**, specifically whether it is numerical, binary, categorical, or a rate or count. Other factors may also influence the choice of test, such as the **sample size** or the **distribution** in the population. For example, if the distribution is markedly non-normal, then non-parametric tests may be appropriate. Tables 1B.15 through 1B.17 list the common statistical tests and the circumstances in which they are used.

If the outcome is a count or a rate, then the **Poisson regression** or **Cox regression** is generally used. There are also statistical tests used with these methods, including ***z*-tests** ('Wald tests') of rate

Table 1B.14 When to use statistical tests or regression

Type of exposure variable	Statistical test or regression
Binary (two groups)	Statistical test (e.g. *z*-test) Regression
Unordered categorical (>2 groups)	Statistical test (e.g. ANOVA) Regression
Ordered categorical	Regression Rarely—statistical tests (e.g. χ^2 test for trend)
Numerical	Regression
Multiple exposure variables	Regression Some statistical tests (e.g. 2-way ANOVA or Mantel–Haenszel)

Table 1B.15 Tests for numerical outcome variables

Exposure variable	Type of data		Parametric test	Non-parametric test
Binary	Unpaired	Large sample	*z*-test	
		Small sample	*t*-test	Mann–Whitney *U*-test or Wilcoxon rank sum test
	Paired	Large sample	Paired *z*-test	
		Small sample	Paired *t*-test	Wilcoxon signed rank test
Unordered categorical			One-way ANOVA	Kruskal–Wallis test

Table 1B.16 Tests for binary outcome variables

Exposure variable	Type of data		Parametric test
Binary	Difference between proportions		z-test
	2 × 2 table (OR)	Large sample	χ^2 test
		Small sample	Fisher's exact test
	Paired/matched 2 × 2 table (OR)		McNemar's χ^2 test
Unordered categorical	r × 2 table		χ^2 test
	Paired/matched 2 × 2 table		McNemar's χ^2 test
Ordered categorical	r × 2 table		χ^2 test for trend

Table 1B.17 Tests for categorical outcome variables

Exposure variable	Type of data	Parametric test
Binary	2 × c table	χ^2 test
Unordered categorical	r × c table	χ^2 test
Ordered categorical	r × c table	χ^2 test for trend

ratios and the **log-rank test** for hazard ratios (see Sections 1B.17 and 1B.18).

Parametric tests

The z-test and t-test are parametric tests. They are used for comparing percentages, proportions, and means of groups. The z-test is used for large samples and the t-test for samples <60.

z-Test

The z-test is used for testing the difference between the means or proportions of two groups. This test is based on the standard normal distribution and it gives a z-score ('standard normal deviate') that indicates by how many standard deviations the observed difference differs from the null hypothesis.

A z-score of 1.96 is equivalent to a two-tailed p-value of 0.05; therefore, a z-score >1.96 can be considered statistically significant at the 5% level (i.e. provides strong evidence against the null hypothesis).

The formula for the z-test is

- Difference in means

$$z = \frac{\bar{x}_1 - \bar{x}_0}{se(diff)}$$

where
$\bar{x}_1$ is the mean in exposed (or intervention) group
$\bar{x}_0$ is the mean in unexposed (or control) group
$se(diff)$ is the standard error of the difference in the means (see Section 1B.2).

- Difference in proportions

$$z = \frac{p_1 - p_0}{se(diff)}$$

where
p_1 is the proportion in exposed (or intervention) group
p_0 is the proportion in unexposed (or control) group
$se(diff)$ is the standard error of the difference in the proportions

Note that this error is calculated in a slightly different way from the calculation of confidence intervals described in Section 1B.2. Instead, the following formula is used:

$$se \approx \sqrt{\frac{\bar{p}(1-\bar{p})}{n_1} + \frac{\bar{p}(1-\bar{p})}{n_0}}$$

where $\bar{p}$ is the average proportion for the two groups.

For paired data (e.g. two readings from the same person at different times or matched case–control study pairs), the pairing should be taken into account in the analysis. In order to do this, the difference between the observations for each pair is calculated and then these differences are then treated as a single observation. The following formula (**paired z-test**) can then be used based on the mean and the standard error of these differences:

$$z = \frac{\bar{x}}{se(\bar{x})}$$

t-Test

When the sample is small (usually fewer than 60 observations), methods based on the t-distribution are used instead of the normal distribution. This test is calculated in the same way as the z-test but it also takes into account the degrees of freedom, and the results should be looked up on a t-distribution table rather than a z-distribution table in order to determine the p-value (one or two-tailed). **Note:** These tables are not currently provided in the MFPH Part A examination.

Unpaired t-test:

$$t = \frac{\bar{x}_1 - \bar{x}_0}{se(diff)}, \quad \text{degrees of freedom} = n_0 + n_1 - 2$$

Paired t-test:

$$t = \frac{\bar{x}}{se(\bar{x})}, \quad \text{degrees of freedom} = n - 1$$

where n is the number of pairs.

Chi-squared test

The chi-squared (χ^2) test is used for comparing the counts of categorical responses between two or more independent groups. As such, it can only be used for **actual** numbers (i.e. counts, not proportions or percentages). In order to perform the χ^2 test, the data should be placed in an ***r* × *c* contingency table** where r is the number of exposure groups in the rows and c is the number of possible outcomes in the columns. Proceed as follows:

1. For each observed number, calculate the **expected** number.
2. Subtract the expected number from the observed number $(O - E)$.
3. Square the result and divide the result by the expected number $(O - E)^2 \div E$.
4. X^2 is the total of these results for all cells (i.e. the sum of [3]).
5. Look up X^2 using (degrees of freedom = [rows – 1] × [columns – 1]) to find the p-value.
   - In summary, the formula for the χ^2 statistic is

$$\chi^2 = \sum \frac{(O-E)^2}{E}, \quad d.f. = (r-1) \times (c-1)$$

Note that MFPH Part A examination candidates are not currently provided with the distribution tables. It is, therefore, important to remember that for a 2 × 2 table,

χ^2 of $1.96^2 = 3.84$ corresponds to $p = 0.05$.

Therefore, $\chi^2 > 3.84$ corresponds to $p < 0.05$ (i.e. it is 'statistically significant at the 5% level' or 'provides strong evidence against the null hypothesis').

An example is shown in Box 1B.7.

McNemar's χ^2 test

For paired binary data (such as an individually matched case–control study or repeated measures of the same variable in each participant), it would be inappropriate to present the data in a normal 2 × 2 contingency table or to use the χ^2 test, since this would not take into account the fact that the data were paired. Instead, the data should be presented in pairs in a way that shows the agreement or discordance between the pairs. For example, in a matched case–control study, if the case and the control were both exposed, then this is **agreement**, whereas if the case was exposed but the control was not, or vice versa, this is **discordance** (see Box 1B.8).

The data of interest are the discordant pairs (i.e. cells r and s in the lower table in Box 1B.8). These cells are used to calculate the odds ratio (OR):

$$OR = \frac{r}{s}$$

and the p-value using McNemar's test:

$$\text{McNemar's } \chi^2 = \frac{(r-s)^2}{r+s}, \quad (d.f. = 1)$$

Box 1B.7 Chi-squared test: Example

The paté at a restaurant is implicated in an outbreak of listeriosis.

Here are the **observed** numbers of guests that ate paté, and the numbers who were ill with listeriosis:

Observed number of cases

		Listeriosis		
		Yes	No	
Ate paté	**Yes**	**12**	**24**	36
	No	**42**	**48**	90
	Total	54	72	126

First, calculate the row and column totals. Now calculate the **expected** number for each cell assuming paté was **not** linked to listeriosis as follows:

Expected number of cases in cell yes/yes = 36 × 54 ÷ 126 = 15.43. Calculate the **expected number of cases** by subtracting from the row and column totals:

Expected number of cases

		Listeriosis		
		Yes	No	
Ate paté	**Yes**	15.43	20.57	36
	No	38.57	51.43	90
	Total	54	72	126

Now calculate $\frac{(O-E)^2}{E}$ for each cell

		Listeriosis	
		Yes	No
Ate paté	**Yes**	0.76	0.57
	No	0.31	0.23

Now calculate $X^2 = \sum \frac{(O-E)^2}{E} = 0.76 + 0.57 + 0.31 + 0.23$

$X^2 = 1.87$

Therefore, we can conclude that eating paté was not significantly associated with listeriosis at the $p < 0.05$ level.

Box 1B.8 Presenting data for analysis in case–control studies

For an unmatched study (e.g. unmatched case–control study), the data may be displayed as follows:

	Case	Control	
Exposed	a	b	a + b
Unexposed	c	d	c + d
	a + c	b + d	a + b + c + d

However, for a matched study, the data should instead be presented in pairs, with the cases in the rows and the controls in the columns:

		Controls		
		Exposed	Unexposed	
Cases	Exposed	q	r	q + r
	Unexposed	s	t	s + t
		q + s	r +t	q + r + s + t

Note: q, both exposed; r, case exposed control unexposed; s, case unexposed control exposed; t, both unexposed.

Here, each cell represents a set of matched pairs rather than individuals. As a result, the total (q + r + s + t) should be half the sample size.

As with χ^2, McNemar's $\chi^2 > 3.84$ corresponds to $p < 0.05$ (i.e. it is 'statistically significant at the 5% level'). See Box 1B.9.

Chi-squared test for trend

The chi-squared (χ^2) test for trend is another type of χ^2 test used for **ordered categorical** exposure variables. It tests the null hypothesis that there is no linear increase in the log odds per exposure group.

ANOVA

The same principles as the *t*-test (and *z*-test) are used in the ANOVA, which is used when there is a numerical outcome and more than two groups need to be compared. In this situation, an *f*-test is used and the null hypothesis is that the means of all the groups of observations are equal:

$$f = \frac{\text{Between-groups mean squares}}{\text{Within-groups mean squares}},$$

$$d.f. = \text{No.groups-1, no.observations-no.groups}$$

ANOVA is a **one-way** ANOVA. For example, if three groups of human volunteers were treated separately with drug 1, drug 2, and saline solution (control) to assess whether there were any differences in renal function, then the 'factor' concerned here is the treatment received, and this is a 'one-way' or 'one-factor' ANOVA.

Two factors can also be tested, using two-way ANOVA. Drugs may affect male volunteers to a

Box 1B.9 Example: McNemar's Chi-squared test

A matched case–control study is conducted to assess the association between maternal smoking and childhood asthma. The results of the study are presented in the following table:

		Controls		
		Maternal smoking	Maternal non-smoker	
Cases	Maternal smoking	15	30	45
	Maternal non-smoker	9	70	79
		24	100	124

To test whether there was any association between maternal smoking and asthma, perform the following:

1. Calculate the odds ratio:

$$OR = \frac{r}{s} = \frac{30}{9} = 3.33$$

2. Conduct a hypothesis test:

$$\text{McNemar's } \chi^2 = \frac{(r-s)^2}{r+s}, \quad (d.f. = 1)$$

$$\text{McNemar's } \chi^2 = \frac{(30-9)^2}{30+9} = 11.31$$

This is strong evidence to reject the null hypothesis of no association between maternal smoking and childhood asthma.

greater or lesser extent than females. By selecting samples of females and samples of males for each treatment, sex then becomes 'factor 2'. Comparisons could then be made between the different treatments and between the different sexes to test for interaction.

A second extension of one-way ANOVA is made when comparing two dependent variables simultaneously across two or more groups. This extension is called multivariate analysis of variance (**MANOVA**). For example, the means of dependent variables (reading, writing, IQ, mathematics) may be tested across two groups (males, females).

Note that ANOVA is a special type of regression analysis, and most datasets for which ANOVA is appropriate can be analysed by regression yielding the same results. With two groups, one-way ANOVA is exactly equivalent to the usual two-sample t-test, and we have $f = t^2$.

Tests for multiple exposure variables

Testing for multiple exposure variables usually involves either multiple regression (see Section 1B.17) or standardisation (see Section 1A.5); however, there are also statistical tests that can sometimes be used, including

- Two-way ANOVA or MANOVA for numerical outcomes
- The Mantel–Haenszel method for binary outcomes or rates

Non-parametric tests

Samples that are normally distributed can be described by two parameters: the mean and the standard deviation. A difference between samples, or between a sample and the population, may be measured by examining differences in their means. These differences can be tested using **parametric** tests, such as the ***z*-test** or the ***t*-test**.

Where a population is not normally distributed, its shape cannot be described using the mean and standard deviation alone. Instead, any differences between two groups should be tested using a **non-parametric** test. These tests focus on the **rank ordering** of the data rather than on their actual values. Non-parametric tests are generally only used for **small** samples; if the samples are large, then the lack of normality is not problematic and parametric tests can be used.

Non-parametric tests are used in the following situations:

- The data are definitely **not normally distributed** (although in these situations it is often preferable to **transform** the data, e.g. using log transformation).
- The outcomes are **ordered categorically but have no scale** (e.g. 'completely disagree', 'mostly disagree', 'neither agree nor disagree,' 'mostly agree', 'completely disagree'). In other words, the data have **ordinal but not interval** properties.
- To deal with **outliers**.

Non-parametric tests have a number of disadvantages, including the following:

- Low power (type 2 errors are more likely).
- Calculating confidence intervals is more difficult.
- Can only generally be used for simple **bivariate analysis** (i.e. unable to adjust for confounding or test for interaction).

Wilcoxon rank sum test

This test is used for **paired** data whose differences, when plotted, look roughly symmetrical. Proceed as follows:

1. Find differences between individual pairs.
2. Omit zero values.
3. Ignoring the signs (+ or –) for the moment, rank the differences in order, placing identical values halfway between the ranks that they would have occupied if they were unique.
4. Reapply the signs (+ or –).
5. Find the sum of the positive ranks and the sum of the negative ranks (these are called the 'rank totals').
6. Ignoring the signs again, take the smaller 'rank total' from [5].
7. Look up this 'rank total' in the Wilcoxon table (either the 1% or the 5% section) according to the number of pairs in the sample.
8. If the 'rank total' is larger than the number in the table, then the result is insignificant at that *p*-value.

Mann–Whitney U-test

This is used for **unpaired** data where the data, when plotted, do not appear symmetrical. Proceed as follows:

1. Rank the results from both groups in a single list (typing each in a different colour).
2. Add up the ranks for the two samples separately (by reading off the different colours): these are the 'rank totals'.
3. Use the smaller of the 'rank totals'.
4. Look up in the Mann–Whitney table (either the 1% or the 5% section) using n_1 as the number of observations in one group and n_2 as the number of observations in the other.
5. If the number from [3] is larger than the number found in [4], then the result is insignificant at this *p*-value.

Section 1B.16 follows on from here.

1B.15 Sample size and statistical power

Sample size and power calculations are important components of the design phase of an experiment. They allow the researcher to determine

- How large a sample is needed to obtain accurate and reliable results
- How likely it is that the statistical test to be used will detect effects of a given size in a particular situation

Sample size

Sample size calculations are a crucial part of the study design because they help ensure that studies have sufficient participants to answer the study question, but not so many participants to be wasteful. In general, there are four factors to consider when calculating the required sample size: the size of the difference, the significance level, the power, and the exposure in the baseline population (see Table 1B.18).

Power

The power of a study is the probability that it will be able to detect a difference if it truly exists in the population. The power of a study to detect a true effect is generally set at 80% or more. If the power of an experiment is low, then there is a high probability that the experiment will be inconclusive. Note that power can be increased at the expense of significance. In case–control studies, power can be increased for a limited number of cases by increasing the ratio of controls to cases.

The power should always be calculated in advance, so that an appropriately sized sample is recruited. Different methods are used for estimating power for different study designs. It is generally considered **unethical** to undertake an underpowered study involving human participants. However, for logistical or financial reasons, this may not always be possible. In the case of very rare conditions, for example, the sample size may be fixed. In these situations, the fixed sample size can be used to calculate the power of the study (i.e. to assess the likelihood that it will detect a statistically significant effect).

Meta-analyses can be conducted to pool the results from several studies and thereby increase the power of detecting a finding if one exists (see Section 1A.33).

Other factors to consider

Table 1B.19 describes a number of situations where the sample size will need to be increased or decreased.

Table 1B.18 Factors in sample size calculations

Factor	Details	Effect on sample size
Size of difference	Effect size needed for result to be clinically or experimentally meaningful.	Smaller effect size requires larger sample.
Significance level	*p*-value (i.e. the type 1 error rate). Usually, a significance level of 0.05 is used.	Smaller *p* requires larger sample.
Power	Probability that the study will be able to detect a difference if it truly exists. This is 1 minus the type 2 error $(1 - \beta)$. Usually, a power of ≥80% is used.	Higher power requires larger sample.
Exposure in baseline population	For case–control studies, this is the prevalence of the exposure in controls. For cohort and intervention studies, this is the prevalence of outcome in unexposed individuals (e.g. disease rate in the population).	Smaller prevalence requires larger sample.

Table 1B.19 Circumstances where the sample size will need to be adjusted

Adjustment needed to the sample size	Situation
Sample size should be **increased**.	High loss to follow-up
	Low response rate
	Cluster sampling (see Section 1A.21)
	Confounding
	Interaction
Sample size can be **decreased**.	Matched case controls

Note that increasing the sample size can only reduce the likelihood of errors caused by chance: it cannot compensate for bias.

Section 1B.14 follows on from here and covers tests for comparing two groups.

1B.16 Regression and correlation

Regression and correlation are related statistical techniques. Both examine the relationships between two or more variables, but they do so in different ways. In this section, we focus on linear regression; other types of regression are discussed in Sections 1B.17 and 1B.18.

Linear regression

As seen in Section 1B.10, in order to examine the association between two numerical variables, a scatter plot is usually drawn. If the relationship appears to be linear on the scatter plot, then we can draw a best-fitting straight line and calculate the equation for this line. Note that the scatter plot should always be examined prior to calculating the equation because a straight line may not be the best way of describing the data. For example, if the association is U-shaped or exponential, then linear regression would not be appropriate unless the data were first transformed (e.g. using log transformation).

Regression is the process of deriving an equation for the best-fitting line through the points on the scatter plot. This line can be found by minimising the squared distances between points and the line, which is known as the **least squares technique** (see Figure 1B.14). Regression analysis is conducted using statistical computer packages such as SAS™, SPSS™, or Stata™.

The regression equation can be used to determine by how much one variable (y) changes when another variable (x) changes by a certain amount. For a straight line, the line has the following equation:

$$y = a + bx$$

where a is the intercept with the y-axis and b is the gradient.

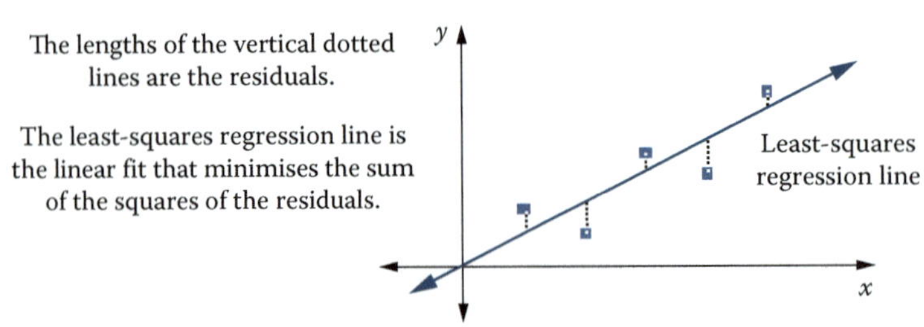

Figure 1B.14 Least squares regression line.

The gradient of the line (*b*) is known as the **regression coefficient** (or β coefficient). If there was no association between the two variables, then the gradient of the slope would be zero. Therefore, linear regression tests the null hypothesis that the regression coefficient = 0. Accordingly, if the confidence interval does not cross zero, there *is* evidence of an association.

Correlation

Correlation estimates the **strength** of any linear association between two variables. The strength of the association can be represented by **Pearson's correlation coefficient (*r*)** which reflects how closely to the regression line the data lie (see Figure 1B.11).

The value of *r* can vary from –1 through 0 to +1 (see Box 1B.10).

The association can be tested using a form of the *t*-test (based on *r* and *n*) at degrees of freedom = $n - 2$, where

r^2 measures how much of the variation in the *y* variable is accounted for by the linear relationship in the *x* variable. For example, if $r^2 = 64$, then the regression model explains 64% of the variation in the *y* variable (other variables may explain the remaining 26%).

Box 1B.10 Interpretation of *r*

Value of *r*	Interpretation
+1	Perfect positive correlation.
Positive values	When one value increases, the other variable increases.
0	No correlation.
Negative values	When one value increases, the other variable decreases.
–1	Perfect negative correlation.

Pearson's correlation coefficient is a parametric statistic. Non-parametric correlation methods, such as **Spearman's ρ** (rho), are used when distributions are not normal.

1B.17 Regression techniques

Appropriate use, objectives and value of multiple linear regression, multiple logistic regression, principles of life tables, and Cox's regression.

Uses of regression

Regression analysis is used for estimating the relationships among variables. It is particularly useful for assessing the effect on the outcome variable of changing one of the exposure variables while all of the other exposure variables are kept fixed.

Testing for associations between two variables

This technique is known as simple (or univariate) regression. It tests the association between one exposure variable (independent variable) and one outcome variable (dependent variable). It is primarily used for the univariate analysis of **continuous exposure variables** (because other statistical tests cannot be used in these circumstances; see Section 1B.14) or **ordered categorical variables** (because other statistical tests often cannot be used). However, univariate regression can also be used with any other type of exposure variable as an alternative to the statistical tests described in Section 1B.14.

Multiple regression

Regression techniques are also available that allow multiple exposure variables to be assessed simultaneously. Known as **multiple regression**, this technique can be used to adjust for confounding by including potentially confounding variables in the regression model. Interaction terms (i.e. where the simultaneous influence of two or more variables is

Table 1B.20 Types of regression and their uses

Type of regression	Outcome variable	Measure of effect	Type of model
Linear	Numerical	Difference in means	Additive (linear)
Logistic	Binary	Odds ratio	Multiplicative (log scale)
Poisson	Time to binary event (count)	Rate ratio	Multiplicative (log scale)
Cox	Time to binary event (count)	Hazard ratio	Multiplicative (log scale)

not additive) can also be included in regression models to test for **effect modification** (where the effect of an exposure on the outcome variable depends on the level of exposure to a confounding variable).

Predictive modelling

As well as testing for associations between an outcome and an exposure (causal modelling), regression can be used to predict what the outcome may be for a given set of exposures. For example, a predictive model may be used to estimate a person's blood pressure based on their age, height, and gender. Note that predictive modelling should only be performed within the limits of the data available, since any extrapolation beyond this range may be inaccurate.

Types of regression

There are four main types of regression. As with the statistical tests described in Section 1B.14, the choice of regression method depends on the type of **outcome variable** (see Table 1B.20).

Logistic, Poisson, and Cox regressions are all **multiplicative models** and the results of the regression output are expressed on a log scale. These results therefore need to be exponentiated in order to give the measure of effect.

The Poisson regression and Cox regression can both be used with counts of binary events; in general, the Poisson regression is used for **rates**, whereas the Cox regression is used for **survival times**.

1B.18 Comparison of survival rates

Poisson regression, used in the analysis of binary events (e.g. deaths from a given disease), assumes that the event rates are constant throughout the study period. This assumption may, however, not be valid, particularly in longitudinal studies where a cohort of individuals is followed over time. For example, the rate of death from various diseases will increase as the cohort ages. Equally, if the cohort is being followed after a particular event (e.g. cancer surgery), then the rate of deaths may be very high initially, then decrease, and then gradually increase again. Methods used in analyses of survival must therefore not assume that such rates are constant.

Two key statistics used in survival analysis are

- The **survival function** $S_{(t)}$—The probability of not experiencing the event of interest, at least to time *t* (this can be illustrated in a survival curve)
- The **hazard function** $h_{(t)}$—The conditional probability of experiencing the event of interest at time t having survived to that time (i.e. the rate at the specific moment in time *t*)

Note: Despite the name 'survival analysis', the event of interest does not necessarily have to be death. For example, it could be recurrence of a tumour, readmission to hospital, or even a positive event such as quitting smoking.

Two methods can be used to generate survival functions and survival curves, namely, **life tables** and the **Kaplan–Meier** method.

Life tables

See also Section 3A.6 for the application of life tables to demographics rather than survival analysis.

Life tables are generally used to display patterns of survival in a cohort of individuals when we do not know the exact survival time of each individual but we do know the number of survivors at specific intervals of time. There are two types of life tables:

- **Cohort life tables**—These show the actual survival of a group of individuals through time. This is the main life-table method used in survival analysis.
- **Period (or current) life tables**—These use current age-specific death rates (or rates of another event) applied to a hypothetical population in order to calculate expected survival times. This is used more often in demographics (see Chapter 3A.6).

In a cohort life-table analysis, at specific time intervals (t) (e.g. days, months, or years), the following data are collected:

- The **number of individuals alive** at the beginning of each time interval (a_t)
- The **number of deaths** (or other events if the event of interest is not death) during each time interval (d_t)
- The number of individuals **censored** during each interval (i.e. lost to follow-up, died from another cause, or reached the end of the study period) (c_t)

From these data, it is possible to calculate the following:

- The **number of persons at risk** during each interval (n_t). This is the total number of people alive at the beginning of the interval adjusted for any people who are censored:

$$n_t = a_t - \frac{c_t}{2}$$

where c_t is divided by 2 on the assumption that on average censorship occurs half way through the time period.

- The **risk of dying** during the time interval (r_t):

$$r_t = \frac{d_t}{n_t}$$

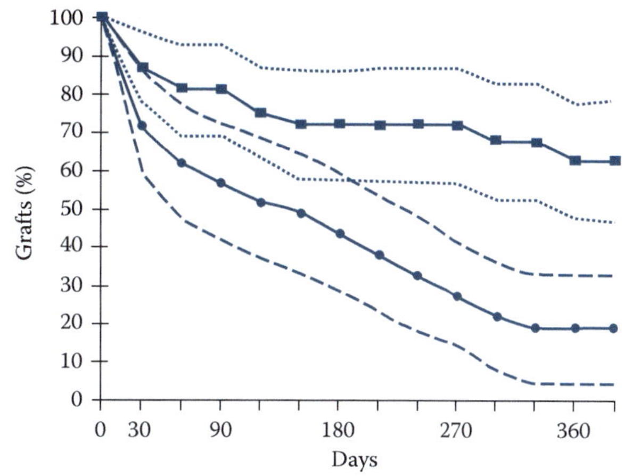

Figure 1B.15 Example of life-table survival curves showing survival of hemodialysis access grafts in two different groups and their associated 95% confidence intervals. (From Constantinos T. Sofocleous, et al. *J. Vasc. Intervent. Radiol.*, JVIR 1, 13(8), 775, August 2002. DOI: 10.1016/S1051-0443(07)61985-X.)

- The **chance of surviving** during the time interval (s_t):

$$s_t = 1 - r_t$$

- The cumulative chance of surviving up to that time period from the start of the cohort, known as the **survival function** ($S_{(t)}$):

$$S_{(t)} = S_{(t-1)} \times s_t$$

A 95% confidence interval about $S_{(t)}$ can be calculated at each time interval. A **survival curve** can then be constructed from the survival function (see Figure 1B.15).

Kaplan–Meier method

The Kaplan–Meier method is similar to the life-table method but it calculates the survival function **each time an event occurs** rather than at given time intervals. Often, in cohort studies, the exact day an event occurs is known (particularly if the event is death); therefore, it is preferable to use this information rather than the fact that it occurs at some point during a given time period.

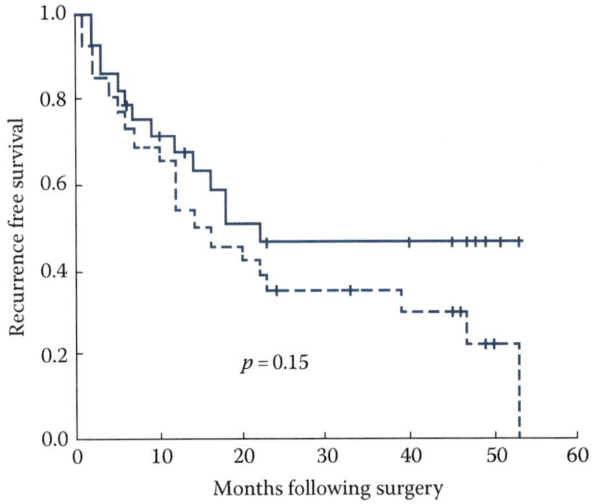

Figure 1B.16 Example of a Kaplan–Meier curve showing survival following surgery in two different groups of patients.

Each time (t) that either the event of interest occurs or a person is censored, the risk of the event (r_t) is calculated by dividing the number of events at that time (d_t) (which is usually 1) by the number of people at risk at that time (n_t). In the same way as for the life-table method, this can then be used to calculate the probability of surviving at time t (s_t) and thus the survival function ($S_{(t)}$). These values can then be used to draw a survival curve as a **step function** with a step at each occurrence of an event or a censorship (see Figure 1B.16).

Comparing survival curves in two groups

Differences in survival rates between two groups may be visually apparent from survival curves, but quantifying the differences requires statistical methods.

Log-rank test

The comparison of survival curves can be assessed quantitatively using the log-rank test. This is a special application of the Mantel–Haenszel chi-squared procedure and is carried out by constructing a separate 2 × 2 table for each interval of the life tables (or each interval to an event if using the Kaplan–Meier method), in order to compare the proportions between the groups who died during each interval. For each such time interval, the observed number of deaths in each group is calculated, together with the number of deaths that would be expected if there were no difference between the groups.

The log-rank test is used to test the null hypothesis that there is no difference between the populations in the probability of an event (e.g. death) occurring at any time point.

The log-rank test is most likely to detect a difference between groups when the risk of an event is consistently greater for one group than another. It is unlikely to detect a difference when survival curves cross, as can happen, for example, when comparing a medical with a surgical intervention. When analysing survival data, the survival curves should therefore always be plotted to check for this phenomenon.

Because the log-rank test is purely a **test of significance**, it cannot provide an estimate of the size of the difference between the groups nor a confidence interval. To calculate these parameters, some assumptions must be made about the data. Common methods used are the hazard ratio, including the Cox proportional hazards model.

Cox regression

Also known as **proportional hazards regression**, this form of regression is based on the proportional hazards assumption, which states that the ratio of hazards (i.e. the instantaneous risk of dying at time t) remains the same in both groups. For example, if the risk of dying in one group at a particular point in time is twice that of the other group, then at any other time, it will still be twice that of the other group. Cox regression analyses the effect of exposure variables on survival. The output is the **log hazards ratio**, which can then be exponentiated into a hazard ratio.

Hazard ratio is interpreted in a similar way to a relative risk (i.e. a value of 1 indicates no difference; values >1 indicate a raised hazard; values <1 a decreased hazard). As with other forms of regression, multiple exposure variables can be included in order to adjust for confounding.

1B.19 Heterogeneity

Heterogeneity refers to differences between observations, populations, or studies. It is particularly an issue in systematic reviews and meta-analyses, since these aim to arrive at a conclusion based on the results of various studies that may have been conducted in slightly different ways (see Section 1A.33). Heterogeneity may preclude pooling the data from different studies.

There are three main types of heterogeneity that may lead to variation between the results of individual studies, namely, **statistical**, **methodological**, and **clinical**. See Table 1B.21.

Statistical heterogeneity can be tested for to assess whether the observed variability in study results (i.e. the effect sizes) is greater than would be expected due to chance.

Testing for statistical heterogeneity

There are several ways of testing for statistical heterogeneity. The most commonly used are **Cochran's** Q statistic and the I^2 **statistic**.

Cochran's Q statistic

Known also as the χ^2 test for heterogeneity, this approach tests the null hypothesis that the true effects in the studies are the same (i.e. a low p-value suggests strong evidence of heterogeneity). The test has low power when there are few studies; therefore, a significance level of 10% is often used (i.e. $p < 0.10$ suggests that heterogeneity is present).

I^2 statistic

This was developed because Q has low power (although the I^2 test may also have relatively low power). It provides a measure of the degree of inconsistency in the studies' results by describing the percentage of total variation across studies that is due to heterogeneity rather than chance. The formula is:

$$I^2 = 100\% \times \frac{(Q - d.f.)}{Q}$$

I^2 scores heterogeneity between 0% and 100%. As a rule of thumb, 25% = low heterogeneity, 50% = moderate heterogeneity, and 75% = high heterogeneity.

Random-effects meta-analysis and meta regression

As discussed in Section 1A.31, if there is evidence of heterogeneity between studies in a meta-analysis,

Table 1B.21 Types of heterogeneity

Type of heterogeneity	Description
Statistical	Also known as 'study heterogeneity', this relates to differences in the reported effects between studies. It may be explained by methodological or clinical heterogeneity.
Methodological	This is due to differences in study design and presents comparability problems for meta-analysis.
Clinical	This relates to differences between studies relating to • characteristics of the patient population • interventions • outcome measures As with methodological heterogeneity, clinical heterogeneity may preclude the pooling data from these studies.

Source: Kirkwood, B.R. and Sterne, J.A.C. *Essential Medical Statistics*, 2nd ed., Blackwell Science Oxford, UK, 2003.

then random-effects approach to meta-analysis may be used. In contrast to the fixed-effects approach, the random-effects approach aims to allow for such heterogeneity.

There is, however, disagreement over whether it is appropriate to use random-effects models to combine studies in the presence of heterogeneity because the heterogeneity may be due to another important factor. For example, studies conducted in different countries might show differing associations between a dietary substance and diabetes. These observed differences may reflect the fact that the dietary substance only occurs in populations with a certain genetic factor. Clearly, it is important to take account of such a phenomenon in a meta-analysis. For example, if another variable is found to explain the observed heterogeneity, then it may be possible to incorporate this variable into a **weighted regression estimate** using a method known as **meta-regression**.

1B.20 Funnel plots

The funnel plot (Figure 1B.17) is a type of scatter plot that is commonly used to visualise potential **publication bias** in meta-analyses [22] (see Section 1A.33). It is also increasingly being used in other situations, such as comparing performance between several organisations or clinical teams (see Figure 1B.18 for a funnel plot comparing outcomes in fertility clinics for women aged under 35).

For a meta-analysis, the estimated **treatment effect** values from the component studies are plotted against a measure of their **precision** (e.g. study size or standard error). Appropriate confidence intervals are then added. As the sample sizes of the component studies increase, the precision of their estimated treatment effect increases. This gives the graph its funnel shape. So, in the absence of bias, the results from small studies should scatter widely at one end of the graph, with the spread narrowing among the larger studies.

Interpreting funnel plots

Meta-analysis

If the funnel plot is asymmetrical at the bottom, this indicates a **small study effect** (i.e. the phenomenon of small trials tending to report larger treatment benefits than larger trials). If a small study effect exists, the summary effect measure of the meta-analysis will overestimate the treatment effect.

A small study effect is often due to **publication bias**; however, there may be other reasons. For example, studies targeting particularly high-risk patients tend to be smaller as there are fewer very high-risk patients to sample from, but the intervention may be more likely to produce a greater effect in these patients.

Formal tests exist to test for funnel plot asymmetry (e.g. Egger's regression, which tests whether small studies have larger effect sizes than would be expected).

Funnel plots of performance

In a plot of **performance** (e.g. surgical complication rates), those institutions plotted outside the confidence interval envelopes are revealed as outliers that may warrant further investigation.

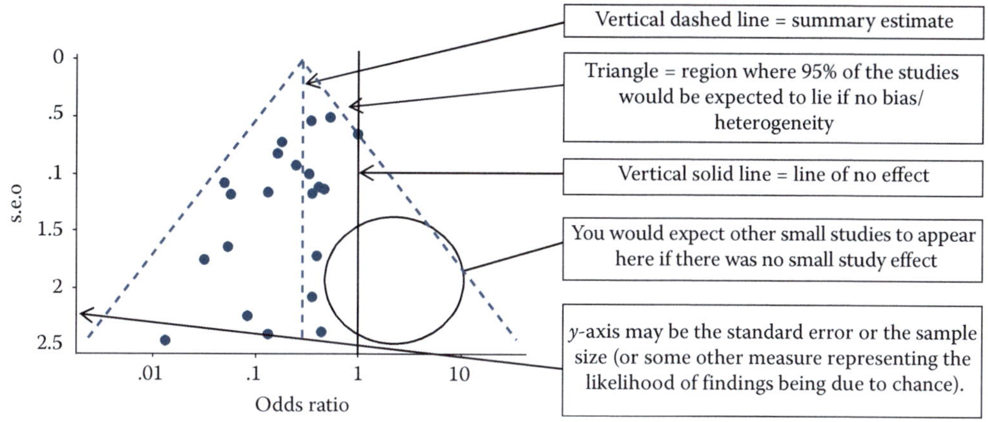

Figure 1B.17 Funnel plot of studies in a meta-analysis.

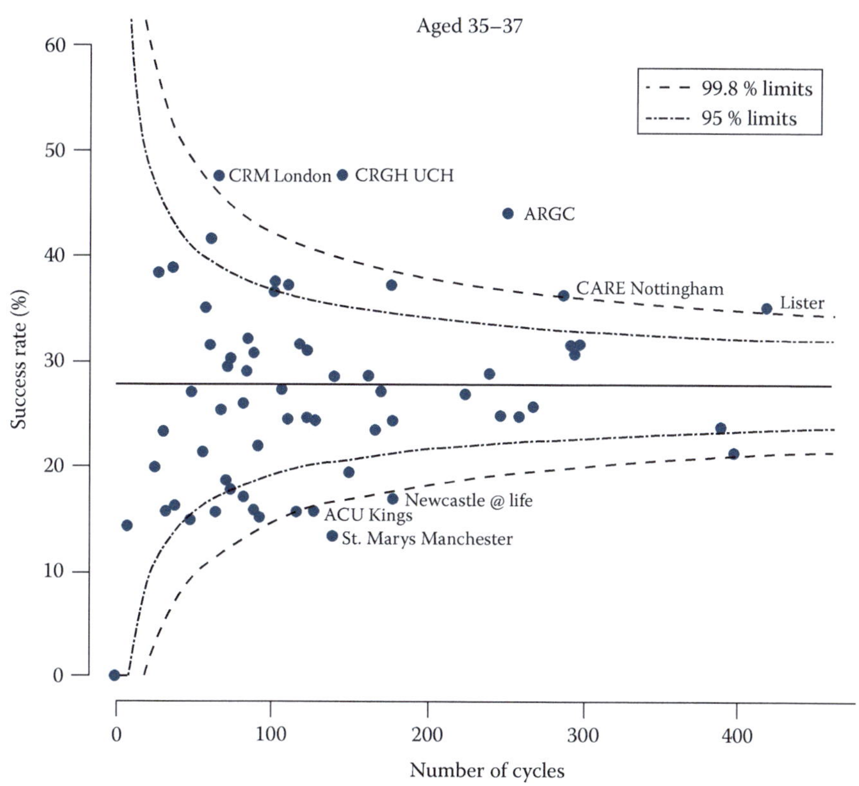

Figure 1B.18 Funnel plot comparing outcomes in fertility clinics.

1B.21 Role of Bayes' theorem

Bayesian methods incorporate **prior beliefs** into calculations of probability. In real clinical situations, for example, existing knowledge about a particular patient will affect how much credence clinicians place on a laboratory test performed on that patient. Bayesian methods incorporate this prior knowledge into the probability calculations.

According to Bayes' theorem, the probability of A occurring, given B, depends on three factors: the probability of A, the probability of B, and the probability of B given A (see Table 1B.22).

Using these three measures, the probability of A occurring given that B occurred is computed as

$$P(A|B) = \frac{P(B|A) \times P(A)}{P(B)}$$

This is Bayes' formula for relating conditional probabilities.

Advantages and disadvantages of Bayesian statistics compared with classical statistics are listed in Box 1B.11.

An application of Bayesian statistics to screening tests is discussed in Chapter 2C.5.

Diagnostic test in a Bayesian framework

Posterior odds of disease = prior odds × likelihood ratio of a positive test result

$$\text{Prior odds} = \frac{\text{Prior probability}}{1-\text{Prior probability}}$$

$$\text{Likelihood ratio} = \frac{\text{Sensitivity}}{1-\text{Specifictiy}}$$

$$\text{Posterior probability} = \frac{\text{Posterior odds}}{1+\text{Posterior odds}}$$

Table 1B.22 Bayesian probability

Factor	Alternative name	Symbol	Description
Probability of A	Prior	$P(A)$	Probability of A occurring on its own, irrespective of B
Probability of B	Normalising constant	$P(B)$	Probability of B occurring on its own, regardless of A
Probability of B, given A	Likelihood	$P(B|A)$	Probability of B occurring given that A occurred

Box 1B.11 Bayes' theorem

Advantages	More flexible Makes use of all available knowledge, therefore possibly more **ethical**. Mathematics is **not** controversial.
Disadvantages	Different users will obtain **different conclusions** if they choose different priors. Prior beliefs can be difficult to quantify.

Example

The likelihood ratio (LR) for a positive cytomegalovirus (CMV) test = 13.3
The prevalence of CMV infection after bone marrow transplantation ~33%
The prior probability of severe disease = 0.33

$$\text{Prior odds} = \frac{\text{Prior probability}}{1-\text{Prior probability}} = \frac{0.33}{0.67} = 0.493$$

$$\text{Posterior odds} = 0.493 \times \text{Likelihood ratio} = 0.493 \times 13.3 = 6.557$$

$$\text{Posterior probability} = \frac{6.557}{1+6.557} = 0.868$$

Therefore, there is an 87% chance of developing severe disease with CMV after transplantation, which is greater than the pretest probability, indicating the usefulness of the test.

Source: Petrie, A. and Sabin, C., *Medical Statistics at a Glance*, 2nd edn, Oxford, UK: Blackwell Publishing, 2005.

1C

Assessment and Evaluation

Approaches to the assessment of healthcare needs, utilisation and outcomes, and the evaluation of health and healthcare.

The fact that a particular health service is currently provided does not necessarily mean that it is effective or that it is necessarily appropriate for the population served. Public health specialists have an important role in assessing the need for a service and the quality and appropriateness of what is currently provided. These tasks require a sound knowledge of research methods coupled with a range of practical skills in order to

- Measure patients' health, illness, and quality of life
- Study the quality, safety, access, and cost-effectiveness of health services
- Involve relevant stakeholders, such as clinicians, patients, and communities, in making assessments and implementing improvements

1C.1 Need for health services

Uses of epidemiology and other methods in defining health service needs and in policy development.

In public health, the generic term **need** is used to indicate a number of concepts relating either to the illnesses that people experience (i.e. need for **health**) or to their treatment (i.e. need for **healthcare**). Bradshaw [24] described four specific types of need (see Box 1C.1).

The need for health services is sometimes implicitly equated to ill health. However, authors such as Culyer and Wagstaff [25] equate the need for interventions with the **potential to benefit** from them. Therefore, even if a person is unwell, if an intervention offers them no clinical benefit, then there is no need for the intervention. In contrast, if a person is healthy, but would have a greater chance of staying healthy if they received a preventive service, there is a need for that service.

A key role of public health specialists is to assess the health needs of a given population. When conducted systematically, this process is known as a **health needs assessment** (HNA). The findings of an HNA should be used to guide the allocation of resources to improve the health of the population and reduce health inequalities. Conducting an HNA offers an opportunity to

- Consult the population
- Establish or maintain cross-sectoral partnerships
- Ensure that healthcare provision is evidence based (by withdrawing non-evidence-based interventions and introducing evidence-based interventions not currently offered locally)

ENG Since the introduction of the Local Government and Public Involvement in Health Act (2007), health service commissioners and local authorities have been required to produce **joint strategic needs assessments (JSNAs)** detailing the health and wellbeing of their local community. These assessments follow the principles of a generic HNA but, in addition, they explicitly consider the social care needs of the population, and they involve non-health agencies in their assessment process.

Corporate needs assessment

In this type of HNA, public health specialists consider the **views** of interested parties, aiming to tailor the provision of healthcare to accord with these opinions. See Box 1C.2.

Comparative needs assessment

This process uses data from surveys or hospital activity data. It compares the findings **observed** locally with those that would be **expected** from a reference population (e.g. regional or national data). For the comparisons to be valid, adjustments to the reference population are required to reflect the characteristics of the local population (e.g. adjustment for age, ethnicity, smoking rates). Note that the local prevalence of a particular condition may not always be known (e.g. many cases of chlamydia infection are undetected).

Box 1C.1 Bradshaw's four types of need

Type of need	Description
Normative	Needs as deemed by a clinician
Felt	Requirement of patients to feel better
Expressed	Demand (e.g. visits to a GP)
Comparative	Need in one area compared with that in another

Box 1C.2 Advantages and disadvantages of corporate needs assessments

Advantages	Disadvantages
Being an **incremental** process, it allows services to be altered a little at a time, guided by feedback from interested parties. Can be conducted relatively **quickly**. No need to collect large amounts of data. **Responsive** to interested parties.	Can be driven by **power** rather than by need. Can be **disproportionately influenced** by the reaction of participants to certain events, (e.g. to newspaper headlines). An incremental process may be inappropriate where **large-scale** or **radical reform** is required.

Evidence-based needs assessment

Evidence from the literature—ideally in the form of guidelines or consensus statements—should be used to shape the local provision of healthcare. Such provision should be adjusted to take account of local circumstances including the prevalence of the disease in the local population and the findings of patient surveys. Note that high-quality literature for a particular condition may not exist or the messages from the literature may be conflicting.

Conducting a needs assessment

The Health Development Agency (now part of NICE) outlined a five-step approach to conduct an HNA (see Table 1C.1).

Data sources for conducting a needs assessment

The NHS Information Centre for Health and Social Care and the Association of Public Health Observatories in England [26] produced a **core dataset** outlining the data sources that should

Table 1C.1 Steps involved in a needs assessment

Step	Description
Scope	Identify the following: • Population to be considered • Aims of the HNA • Stakeholders • Resources needed to conduct the HNA • Risks involved
Identification of potential priorities	Gather various data to **describe the population**, then interpret these data through discussion with stakeholders (see data sources section).
Selection of a priority	Choose a disease according to its **health burden**. Select interventions that are **effective** and **acceptable**.
Change	Specify the aims of the intervention. Use **change management** techniques (e.g. action planning, monitoring, risk management).
Review	**Learn** from the project by measuring impact, then disseminate the findings and identify the next priority.

Source: Adapted from Cavanagh, S. and Chadwick, K., *Health Needs Assessment: A Practical Guide*, London, UK: National Institute for Clinical Excellence, Available online at www.nice.org.uk/page.aspx?o=513203, 2005.

Table 1C.2 Data for a needs assessment

Type of data	Description and examples of data sources
Socio-demographics	Age, sex, ethnicity, socio-economic circumstances
Social and environmental context	Employment rate, overcrowding
Lifestyle/risk factors	Modelled or surveyed smoking prevalence
Burden of ill health	Service activity (e.g. hospital admissions from HES for cancer) Epidemiology (e.g. from cancer registry data)
Services	Service mapping to understanding the volume and characteristics of the services currently provided Useful data sources may include • Waiting times data (e.g. proportion of people seeking sexual health advice offered who were offered a GUM appointment in 48 h) • Offers of service (e.g. proportion of eligible women who were offered cervical screening) • Patient views (e.g. local results of the national patient survey programme)

be used for conducting a needs assessment (see Table 1C.2).

The data should be discussed with stakeholders (see Section 1C.2) to help interpret them appropriately as measures of need. For example, the perceived burden of ill health may be different when assessed using activity data as opposed to epidemiological data and discussing the data with stakeholders can provide different perspectives.

Routinely collected activity data often **underestimate** needs, since they generally do not include

- Unmet need (e.g. when a patient is unable to access a service)
- People who self-care (see Chapter 4B.1)
- People pay for private treatment

In contrast, existing local epidemiological data often **overestimate** need because some of the people with the condition

- Do not need treatment (e.g. patients with arthritic hips who are unfit to undergo surgery)
- Do not want treatment
- Have already had treatment

Note that need is not a binary concept. While some conditions (e.g. diabetes) are diagnosed using a cut-off point, levels of need typically vary among people above the cut-off; moreover, being below the cut-off does not necessarily mean that a patient has no need for the service. For example, patients with an HbA1c levels above 48 mmol/mol (6.5%) have diabetes. However, patients with an HbA1c of 42–47 mmol/mol are at high risk of diabetes and need lifestyle advice and annual retesting.

1C.2 Participatory needs assessment

If a needs assessments is conducted solely by the commissioner of health services or by third parties, then the local population may be reluctant to accept the findings and conclusions. In order to improve engagement, the local community should participate in the process which requires the following:

- Clear objectives (so the population are aware of the purpose of the exercise and the extent to which different elements are up for consultation)

- Use of accepted methods and data sources
- Support from appropriate experts
- Effective communication techniques
- Views of groups of people whose voices are rarely heard but which should be taken into account (e.g. ethnic minorities, older people, children, young mothers, and transient populations)
- Involvement of the community in all steps of the process

This type of HNA often produces **qualitative** rather than quantitative information, based on data collected during

- Key informant interviews
- Group workshops
- Focus groups
- Visual methods (e.g. mapping or 'transect walks' where groups are given low-cost cameras, or encouraged to use their mobile phone cameras, to take pictures that illustrate their needs)

If done well, the participatory process sheds light on the raw quantitative data collected and identifies potential needs that service providers may not otherwise have recognised.

ENG Various ways of involving patients, or members of the local community, in planning services are covered in

- 5e (public and patient involvement in health service planning)
- 2i (involvement of the general public in health programmes and their effects on healthcare)
- 4c (user and carer involvement in service planning)

1C.3 Service utilisation and performance

Formulation and interpretation of measures of utilisation and performance.

With such a high proportion of most countries' GDP being spent on healthcare, it is incumbent on health services to account for how this money is spent and the extent to which health services are meeting their stated aims.

In many developed counties, health service utilisation data are routinely collected and collated for every episode of care. Such information is used both for **paying** health service providers and for secondary purposes such as **commissioning** and **research**. The range of routine data sources used in the NHS is described in more detail in Chapter 3B.2. Here, we describe how activity data may be used to measure performance and some of the issues that need to be considered in the interpretation.

Health systems will typically ensure that the requisite information on each episode of care is entered correctly by defining a **minimum dataset**. Typical requirements for each episode of care will vary depending on the service but are likely to include many of the items listed in Table 1C.3.

Such datasets are typically collated at different aggregate levels so that performance may be measured according to clinical team, organisational, or national goals. Furthermore, by analysing several episodes of care for the same patient, it becomes possible to monitor performance across a clinical pathway (see Chapter 5C). For example, the NHS has national goals for access for certain conditions (e.g. to investigate suspected cancer, there is a maximum 2-week wait from the general practitioner (GP) referral to secondary care appointment). Some examples are given in Table 1C.4.

As shown in Table 1C.4, there are typically several possible interpretations of any utilisation measure; therefore, additional contextual information is needed if utilisation data are to be

Table 1C.3 Activity data typically required for each episode of health service use

Domain	Description
Patient characteristics	Socio-demographics and contact details (e.g. name, age, sex, address) **Note:** In some situations, it may be appropriate for these fields to be removed (e.g. name) or changed (e.g. date of birth to year of birth, address to lower super output area [SOA]).
Clinical information	Diagnosis Procedures Prescriptions
Pathway/service use	Referred by and/or where referred on to Duration of stay Referral date Appointment/admission date
Provider details	Clinical team Consultant or lead clinician
Specific/bespoke data	PROMs Satisfaction measures (e.g. friends and family test) Research data

used appropriately for monitoring performance. In particular, the following factors should be considered:

- **Patient factors**: patients with co-morbidities are likely to require more complex care and may have poorer outcomes; therefore, a consideration of the **case mix** is essential.
- **System factors**: the intensity and duration of service utilisation may be greater if other services are unavailable. For example, patients with alcohol dependence arriving in A&E on a Friday may stay in hospital for the weekend if community detoxification placements are not available at weekends.

Table 1C.4 Examples of how activity data may be used

Data	Measure	Interpretation
Referral and appointment dates	Waiting times	Indicator of barriers to **access**, due to • Insufficient resources (e.g. need to employ more staff) • Suboptimal care pathways • Lack of effective preventive interventions
Duration of stay	Total bed days	Indicator of • **Morbidity** (fewer bed days may indicate that patients being admitted to hospital were less sick on arrival) • **Efficiency** (fewer bed days for the same procedure may indicate a more efficient service) • **Effectiveness** (fewer bed days after an operation may indicate that perioperative care was better)
Episodes and patient/clinical characteristics	Number of admissions/ procedures or patient group	Indicator of • **Volumes** of care provided • **Appropriateness** of care (e.g. high hospitalisation rates for ambulatory care-sensitive conditions such as diabetes or COPD may indicate suboptimal primary care)
Date of admission previous admission data	Readmission rates	Indicator of • **Morbidity** (admitted patients might have been sicker on arrival) • **Effectiveness** (readmission within 30 days of an index admission may indicate suboptimal discharge planning during the index admission)
A&E attendances or unscheduled admissions	Unplanned care	Indicator of barriers to **access**, due to • Inadequate care pathways • Lack of effective preventive interventions

1C.4 Measures of supply and demand

See Chapter 4D.1.

1C.5 Study design to assess health services

Study design for assessing effectiveness, efficiency, and acceptability of services, including measures of structure, process, service quality, and outcome of healthcare.

In health services, it is incumbent on those providing, commissioning, and responsible for performance management to assess whether current services are effective, efficient, and acceptable or to institute improvements and new services to improve these characteristics.

Studies to assess health services can range in scale and formality from multi-centre RCTs conducted with academic partners over several occasions to a survey of patients visiting a clinic on a single day to inform the design of a new clinic form.

For a fuller description of different study designs, see the following:

Chapter	Research question	Study designs
Section 1A.19	Acceptability Effectiveness (when experimental or quasi-experimental not possible)	Epidemiological research (observational studies such as cross-sectional, case–control, cohort studies)
	Effectiveness (when no evidence base exists)	Experimental and quasi-experimental studies (e.g. RCTs)
Section 1A.33	Effectiveness (when an evidence base does exist)	Combining the results of several studies (e.g. systematic reviews and meta-analyses)
Chapter 4D.5	Efficiency	Economic evaluations (e.g. cost-benefit, cost-utility, cost-effectiveness, and cost-minimisation analyses)
Chapter 5C.2	Implementation Quality	Quality improvement tools (e.g. plan–do–study–act)

Different study designs may be more or less appropriate depending on both the research question and the context. A prime example is the RCT. While RCTs are generally considered the gold standard for many research questions, they have specific limitations relating to their use in health services research at a local level (see Table 1C.5).

To decide the most appropriate design, consider the aim and purpose of the study, as well as the nature of the new service and the existing evidence base (see Table 1C.6).

For studies of health service quality, it is important to consider which dimensions of quality are most important. Chapter 1C.6 describes some frameworks for defining the quality of healthcare, including **Donabedian's** structure and **Maxwell's** seven dimensions of quality.

Table 1C.5 Limitations of using RCT in a local health services research context

Limitation	Description
Resources	The funding, expertise, and time needed for a well-run RCT are usually unavailable in these settings.
Timescales	An intervention's impact on health may not manifest itself for decades, and the cost of the requisite long-term RCT follow-up is often prohibitively expensive.
Changes in policy	Changes in national policy may require rapid alterations in local health service provision, which an RCT may hinder.
Multi-site studies	Differences in the ways that health services are delivered across the country may preclude multi-site RCTs.
Organisational research questions	In health services, the intervention is often at an organisational level (e.g. evaluation of a service reconfiguration). It is generally impracticable to reconfigure only half a service at random. While cluster designs may address some of these problems, they are not always feasible due to small numbers.

Table 1C.6 Factors influencing the choice of study design in health services research

Factor	Issues to consider
The **aim** of the study	If the study seeks to assess the acceptability of a service, a descriptive cross-sectional survey is the best approach. If the study is seeking to assess the effectiveness of a new intervention, a trial is more suitable.
Whether the study is for **summative or formative** purposes	In health services research, it is often desirable to refine and improve an intervention as it is implemented (using the quality improvement techniques such as PDSA). In experimental designs with a predefined control group, there is little scope to amend an intervention once the trial has started.
Available **resources**	Not only financial resources but also expertise and time.
Whether this is an **existing** or a **new** or **proposed** service?	For existing services that are available universally, there is unlikely to be a suitable group against which to compare the effects of the intervention; therefore, a descriptive study (e.g. cross-sectional survey) may be most appropriate. However, it may still be possible to compare data from before and after the service started. For a new service, it is desirable to implement the service in some areas but not other comparable areas, preferably chosen at random. This allows comparisons of health status and patient satisfaction to be made between the implementation and control areas.
What is the **existing evidence base?**	If several studies have already been undertaken in this area, a review of the literature could be all that is needed to decide which services to commission and how they should be implemented. For a particularly novel intervention, with little existing evidence, an in-depth case study of a pilot or pilots may be helpful prior to rollout.

1C.6 Structure, process, and outcomes

Measures of structure, process, service quality, and outcome of healthcare.

Donabedian [28] proposed the framework of **structure, process,** and **outcome** to assess the quality of care. An additional category, **output**, is often added or combined with outcome (see Box 1C.3).

Box 1C.3 Donabedian's framework

Donabedian's framework
Structure
Process
Output
(Outcome)

Structure

The structure of a health service considers of all of the **inputs** to the activity, including

- Staff
- Budgets

Table 1C.7 Using structure as a measure of quality

Advantage	Disadvantage
Resource information is relatively **easy** to measure.	Structural data **may not be comparable** between systems. For example, with regard to staffing, all nurses may not be working at the same level of responsibility or may not have received the same level of training.

- Buildings
- Beds

An advantage and disadvantage of using structure as an indicator of quality are shown in Table 1C.7.

Process

These are the **activities** that constitute the intervention and may be considered as follows:

- Strategies, plans, and procedures
- Referral patterns
- Prescription practices
- Consultations (duration, number)
- Bed occupancy
- Waiting times

Some advantages and disadvantages of using this domain are shown in Table 1C.8.

Outputs

These are the **products** of the activity. Examples are

- Numbers of operations conducted
- Length of stay (an indicator of effectiveness)
- Waiting times (an indicator of access)

Outcomes

These are changes in **health status** that are attributable to the activity. Examples are

- Death (mortality rates)
- Disability (and quality of life)
- Discharge (and complications such as emergency readmissions)

Some advantages and disadvantages of using outcomes as a measure of quality are shown in Table 1C.9. The challenges of using outcomes to evaluate health services are illustrated with respect to smoking cessation in Box 1C.4.

Table 1C.8 Advantages and disadvantages of using process as a measure of quality

Advantages	Disadvantages
Relatively **easy** to obtain in centralised healthcare systems such as the NHS. Some processes are **directly related to outcomes** (e.g. immunisation coverage).	Processes do not necessarily predict health outcomes.

Table 1C.9 Advantages and disadvantages of output and outcome as a measure of quality

Advantages	Disadvantages
Ultimately, the **aim** of health service interventions is to improve outcomes.	Not necessarily related to performance since it is affected by **case mix** (i.e. by patient characteristics).
Surrogate endpoints can indicate health outcomes (e.g. CD4 counts in an HIV/AIDS drug trial).	Outcomes are often relatively **long term**, so they may be difficult or impossible to measure in short-term trials.
	Often costly to collect, or incomplete. An exception is mortality data, but these may be difficult to link to interventions.

Box 1C.4 UK Example: Stop-smoking services

Structure	Number of staff employed as stop-smoking advisors. Budget for nicotine replacement therapy and other smoking cessation aids.
Process	Number of prescriptions of NRT or smoking cessation aids. Advisors' training. Number of clients setting quit dates.
Output	Number of 4-week quitters (ideally verified using exhaled carbon monoxide readings).
Outcome	Ideally the morbidity and mortality from smoking-related diseases. However, outcomes have to be attributable to the intervention, and the effects of stop-smoking services on lung cancer deaths may not be apparent for 20 years. Surrogate endpoints could be used instead and include length of stay in hospital for ex-smokers undergoing surgery.

1C.7 Measuring health

Measures of health status, quality of life, and healthcare.

Given the broad definition of health used in public health, more specific definitions are required for describing individual health status. At an aggregate level, a variety of health indicators is required to describe a population's health, including health status and quality of life.

Health status

The WHO's *International Classification of Functioning, Disability and Health* (ICF) is a universal system for measuring health and disability. It classifies health from the perspectives of the body, the individual, and society. The ICF is used in national and international surveys to **measure health**, including the prevalence and degree of disability. It is also used in clinical settings for **assessment** purposes, for informing **treatment decisions**, and for measuring the **impacts of care**.

This system was updated in 2000. Previously, the classification focused on the three concepts of **impairment**, **disability,** and **handicap**, but the categories in the current version are **body structure/function**, **activities**, **participation**, and **environment** (see Table 1C.10).

Health-related quality of life

In clinical trials, increasing importance is being placed on measuring HRQoL. The reason is that for many potentially **fatal conditions** (e.g. lung cancer) and for many **long-term conditions** (e.g. epilepsy), treatments may not affect life expectancy but can still have a profound impact on the quality of life. Studying HRQoL may reveal whether and why a particular treatment is acceptable or not to patients. For example, a trial of cancer chemotherapy might reveal that small treatment benefits, such as a few weeks' extra life expectancy, were outweighed by intractable nausea and vomiting.

There are several theoretical models for measuring quality of life, which take into account the factors listed in Box 1C.5 to different degrees.

HRQoL scales contain several items that build up a composite picture of health status. Except in exceptional circumstances, such as people with dementia or very young children, HRQoL scales should be **completed by the patient** rather than by a carer or clinician.

Some examples of HRQoL scales are listed in Box 1C.6.

Table 1C.10 WHO ICF (2000)

	Body structure/Function	Activities	Participation	Environment
Description	Pathology and clinical measures.	Symptoms and health status.	Effect of disability on life.	Barriers or facilitators to function and participation in the environment.
Measurement	Usually observed by clinicians or measured using instruments.	Self-reported measure of what the person can do.	Usually self-reported. This is the extent to which the condition affects the person's normal life.	Self-reported or observed.
Examples of measures	Blood pressure, temperature, tumour size as assessed on CT.	Beck Depression Inventory Activities of daily living scales.	HRQoL.	ICF checklist for clinicians.
Example 1 (prostate)	Examination: enlarged prostate. Test: increased prostate-specific antigen levels in serum.	Self-report: trips to the toilet per day.	Self-report: person cannot go to cinema because they need the toilet too often.	Observation: workplace has only one toilet (barrier). Self-report: family and friends supportive (can discuss problem openly).
Example 2 (hip)	Clinical examination: reduced joint mobility. Investigation: joint degeneration seen on radiograph.	Self-report: pain or distance that patient can walk.	Self-report: isolation—cannot walk to the park.	Observation: route to park requires walking up several steps but there is no stair rail (barrier).

Box 1C.5 Components of quality of life

Factor	Description
Expectations	Differences between a person's present experience and his or her hopes and expectations. For example, a professional pianist would be more affected by the loss of the use of a finger than would a window cleaner.
Needs	Ability or capacity of a person to satisfy basic human functions (e.g. eating, sleeping, enjoying music).
Normal living	Ability of the person to do what he or she wants to do (rather than being free of disease or symptoms).

Box 1C.6 Examples of QoL scales

Type	Example scales
Generic	Short Form 36 (SF36) Nottingham Health Profile (NHP) EQ5D (EuroQoL)
Disease related	Functional Assessment of Cancer Therapy
Specific aspects of quality of life	Hospital Anxiety and Depression Scale Multidimensional Fatigue Scale

A fuller description of generic quality of life scales also given in Chapter 4D.5, with their application to economic evaluations.

Measures of healthcare

There are many ways to measure the quality of healthcare. These include the methods described in Chapter 5E.2; financial accountability, described in Chapter 5F; as well as adherence to standards and compliance with best-practice guidelines.

Frameworks to assess quality

Two standard frameworks used for measuring the quality of healthcare are those of Donabedian (see Chapter 1C.6) and Maxwell. Maxwell's framework [29] consists of six dimensions of quality, namely, access, relevance, equity, efficiency, effectiveness, and acceptability. See Table 1C.11.

Patient/service user views

The opinions of patients and service users should be collected and acted upon wherever possible (see Box 1C.7). Such information may be used to guide the following:

- **Patients** in their choice of care. For example, if there is a choice of hospital or care environment, then patient views may be useful for informing this decision.
- Commissioners in their decisions regarding the awarding of contracts to healthcare providers.

Considerations for assessing acceptability

Tables 1C.12 and 1C.13 describe some factors that should be considered when using surveys to assess the acceptability of health services.

ENG Patient-reported outcome measures (PROMs) collect information on patient's perceptions of the effectiveness of a healthcare service (see Box 1C.8).

See also Section 1C.10 for methods of evaluating healthcare.

Table 1C.11 Maxwell's dimensions of quality

Dimension	Description
Access	Whether patients can see a clinician when they wish. Whether there are any tangible or intangible barriers to access. Barriers reflect how uninviting or unsuited the service is to particular groups and may be tangible or intangible: **Tangible barriers** • Geography (services near to home or public transport) • Finance (user charges, costs attached to attending services, e.g. lost income, childminding fees) • Opening hours, waiting times **Intangible barriers** • Languages used • Female doctors available to see female patients
Relevance	Whether the services provided are **appropriate** to patients' needs.
Equity	Whether services are provided **fairly** (not necessarily equally; see Section 1C.10).
Efficiency	Whether the **costs** of providing interventions are justified by the **benefits**. Economic evaluations (Section 4) are used to address this question.
Effectiveness	Whether the outcomes of the interventions are reflected in **improvements** in health (see Section 1C.6).
Acceptability	Whether the patient (and, in some cases, the practitioner) is **satisfied** by the care provided. Considerations of acceptability may include • The degree to which patients are treated with **respect** • Whether or not the service is offered in an **appropriate setting** (clean, sufficient privacy) • Whether the service is appropriate for **client group** (e.g. toys available for children) • Whether patients are fully informed about their care (e.g. translation services provided, lay terminology used to describe the treatment options and procedures

Box 1C.7 ENG Patient/service user views

Source of patient opinion	Uses
Complaints and compliments	• Informal comments and complaints (e.g. through conversations with staff and on social media) • Formal complaints made directly to services • Ombudsman's reports • Complaints reported to a third party
Surveys	• National patient and staff surveys • General practice surveys • Local bespoke surveys • PROMs (see Box 1C.8)
Social media	Sentiment analysis of social media feeds, such as Twitter

Table 1C.12 Surveys for assessing the acceptability of health services

Consideration	Details
Who is surveyed?	Sample selection is important: it should be considered carefully and recorded. Should people who have already complained be asked their opinions, or all patients? Different degrees of satisfaction are seen among different sections of the population, with key determinants being age, socio-economic status, and ethnicity.
When is the survey taken?	During care or after? There is a trade-off between patients' capacity to remember care accurately versus asking someone when they are still in the vulnerable position of still receiving care.
Where is the survey performed?	Satisfaction results are generally higher if answered within healthcare setting compared with outside, (e.g. the patient's home).

Table 1C.13 Factors affecting responses to surveys of health services

Factor	Details
Individual	Every person has different values, tolerances, and ideas of what is acceptable.
Patient group	Old versus young and long-term versus day-case patients have different requirements for appropriate services.
Service	Inpatient versus community clinics have different dimensions and different requirements for humane and accessible care.
Priorities	There may be a trade-off between accessibility and humanity (e.g. the need to see a GP promptly may take priority for some over seeing the same GP on each visit).

Box 1C.8 PROMs

ENG PROMs seek to assess the quality of care from a patient's perspective. NHS Trusts in England have been collecting standardised PROMs since for four health conditions: hip replacements, knee replacements, hernia, and varicose veins. PROMs are recorded using short, self-completed questionnaires that ask out about patients' health or quality of life at different points in time before and after the procedure.

The NHS Information Centre for Health and Social Care published PROM results for the first time in 2012. Most patients reported an improvement after hip and knee replacements but the proportion varied markedly between hospital providers.

Source: Health and Social Care Information Centre, Patient survey suggests benefit from common procedures varies markedly by NHS provider, http://www.ic.nhs.uk/proms, 2012.

1C.8 Population health outcome indicators

Population health indicators reflect—at a population level—the effect of healthcare and public health policies and activities (Box 1C.9). They can be used to

- Prompt the assessment of local health outcomes, particularly in relation to national targets
- Monitor variation in healthcare (particularly using small-area analysis; see Section 1A.18)
- Monitor trends in healthcare, to answer questions such as 'Is effectiveness of healthcare improving?' [31]
- Monitor of quality of life as part of a population needs assessment (see Sections 1C.1–1C.2)

Box 1C.9 Public Health Outcomes Indicators for England 2013–2016

In England, the public health outcomes framework is centred on two overarching measures:

1. **Healthy life expectancy** (i.e. it takes account of health quality as well as the length of life)
2. **Health inequalities** (i.e. differences in life expectancy and in healthy life expectancy, between different communities)

The indicators are used to promote greater improvements in healthy life expectancy in more disadvantaged communities. There are **four domains** that contribute to achieving these goals (see table) plus premature mortality.

Domain	Examples indicators
1. Wider determinants of health	16–18 year olds not in education, employment, or training (NEET) People with mental illness or disability living in settled accommodation
2. Health improvement	Low birthweight of term babies Breastfeeding
3. Health protection	Air pollution Population vaccination coverage
4. Healthcare public health and preventing	Tooth decay in children aged 5
Premature mortality	Mortality from causes that are considered preventable

Source: Part 1: A public health outcomes framework for England, 2013–2016, Department of Health. www.dh.gov.uk

Table 1C.14 Characteristics of useful population health indicators

Characteristic	Description
Validity	The indicator should be valid and precise.
Consistency	It should be collected consistently and regularly over time. If the definitions or the data collection method changes, it will be problematic to monitor trends and detect improvements or deteriorations.
Availability	The indicator should be available at appropriate geographical levels (e.g. common conditions should be available at small area levels, and vice versa).
Suitability	The indicator should be suitable for making comparisons between population subgroups. For example, if an indicator is to be used for monitoring inequalities, it must be possible to link to data on deprivation, age, ethnicity, or gender.

Parrish [33] proposed that population health outcomes metrics should cover the following three elements:

1. **Life expectancy from birth** (or age-adjusted mortality rate)
2. **Condition-specific changes in life expectancy** (or condition-specific or age-specific mortality rates)
3. **Self-reported level of health** (including functional status and experiential status)

The choice of specific indicators will depend in part on the data available and on relative priorities in each setting; however, useful indicators will meet the criteria in Table 1C.14.

1C.9 Deprivation measures

Deprivation measures are used to describe a population according to social and economic disadvantage. Public health specialists use them to identify people or areas with high levels of disadvantage and deprivation, in order to offer them targeted programmes and resources. Deprivation may be measured at the **individual** or **area** levels.

Individual indicators

UK In the United Kingdom, the most commonly used indicator of deprivation at the individual or household level is the **National Statistics Socio-economic Classification** (NSSEC). The former system of social class (I–V), which was based on occupation, has been replaced by a classification based on occupation and economic group. The Office of National Statistics now uses this system in all official statistics and surveys. Using the scale shown in Table 1C.15, a person or household is assigned to a category according to the current or former occupation of the **household reference person** (i.e. the person responsible for owning or renting the household's accommodation).

Other individual indicators

Alternative markers of socio-economic status that are sometimes used in public health include

- Income
- Occupation
- Years of education
- Housing (e.g. owner/renter or occupancy per room)
- Commodities (e.g. ownership of a car, television)

Table 1C.15 National statistics socio-economic classification

NSSEC category		Definition
1		Higher managerial and professional occupations
	1.1	Large employers and higher managerial occupations
	1.2	Higher professional occupations
2		Lower managerial and professional occupations
3		Intermediate occupations
4		Small employers and own account workers
5		Lower supervisory and technical occupations
6		Semi-routine occupations
7		Routine occupations
8		Never worked and long-term unemployed

Source: The Office for National Statistics, The National Statistics Socio-economic Classification, http://www.ons.gov.uk, 2007.

Area indicators

Different countries have adopted various area-level indicators of socio-economic deprivation according to national circumstances and the availability of data. In the United Kingdom, the indices of multiple deprivation (IMDs) are used to score and to rank small areas. The focus is on deprivation rather than affluence because the prime purpose of these indicators is for **directing state resources** to areas of need. They are also used for setting **targets**, **monitoring** social and health inequalities, and sometimes as a proxy for individual socio-economic circumstances where no individual-level indicator is available (e.g. in health records).

The IMDs are comprised of seven domains (except in Wales, which has separate domains for housing and services):

1. Income
2. Employment
3. Education and skills, training
4. Health deprivation and disability
5. Housing and services
6. Living environment
7. Crime and disorder (called community safety in Wales)

Each domain is built from local indicators, which are mainly based on administrative data (e.g. from taxation and benefits systems). The score and rank for each domain can be used on its own but then the domains are **weighted** and **combined** into a single IMD. In England and Northern Ireland, indices have also been created for specific population groups (e.g. children and older people). Distinct features of these systems by country are in Table 1C.16.

IRE Two indices of area-level deprivation are in use in Ireland, based on information derived from the census:

1. The **Small Area Health Research Unit** [35] index incorporates the following area-based parameters:
   A. Proportion of population unemployed or seeking a first job
   B. Proportion of population in social class 5 (semi-skilled manual occupations, including farmers on < 30 acres of land) or class 6 (unskilled manual occupations)
   C. Proportion of households with no car
   D. Proportion of households in accommodation rented from the local authority
2. The **Pobal Haase–Pratschke Deprivation Index** (HP Index) [36] was developed by consultants Trutz Haase and Jonathan Pratschke and funded by the not-for-profit organisation Pobal, which manages programmes on behalf of the Irish Government and the European Union (EU). The HP Index includes indicators of deprivation relevant to rural as well as to urban areas.

Table 1C.16 Indices of deprivation in the United Kingdom

Country, index	Government department or agency	Local areas	Population of local area	Number of local areas
Northern Ireland Multiple Deprivation Measure[a]	Northern Ireland Statistics and Research Agency	SOA	2000	890
Scottish Index of Multiple Deprivation (SIMD, 2009, 2012)	National Statistics, Scottish Government	Data zones	500–1000	6,505
English Indices of Multiple Deprivation (IMD)	Communities and Local government	Lower-layer super output areas (LSOA)	1500	32,842
Welsh Index of Multiple Deprivation ('Welsh Townsend')[b]	Welsh Assembly Government	LSOA	1500	1,896

[a] http://www.nisra.gov.uk/deprivation/nimdm_2010.htm.
[b] http://www.wales.gov.uk/topics/statistics/theme/wimd/?lang=en.

Analyses are based on small areas (mean size 100 households, 18,488 areas in total). Three dimensions of affluence/disadvantage are included:

1. Demographic profile
2. Social class composition
3. Labour market situation

AUS The Australian Bureau of Statistics [39] provides summary indices at the individual, family, household, and area levels. These indices incorporate measures of demographics, education, employment, and income. In contrast to the United Kingdom, the Australian indices consider both **advantage** and **disadvantage**. Some of the more commonly used indices are

1. Four Socio-Economic Indexes for Areas (SEIFA), which summarise disadvantage and advantage
2. Accessibility/Remoteness Index of Australia (ARIA), indicating access to services
3. Community Socio-Educational Advantage (ICSEA), which describes school populations
4. Socio-economic position, based on education, income and employment

HK In Hong Kong, there is a growing awareness of the links between deprivation, poverty, and health. Although there are no formal population indicators, information about use of hospital services and socio-economic status can be derived from studies such as the Thematic Household Survey [THS] as well as from the data systems in the hospital authority.

SA The **South African Indices of Multiple Deprivation 2007** (SAIMD 2007) were developed by the Centre for the Analysis of South African Social Policy from Oxford University, using principles similar to those in the UK Indices of Deprivation. The most recent indices are available at data zone level (small geographical units). In contrast to the UK Indices of Deprivation, the SAIMD 2007 comprises just four domains of deprivation, in Table 1C.17.

Jarman

UK The Jarman score is based on factors that affect patients' demand for primary care but is sometimes used as a proxy for deprivation. It is a measure of **GP practice workload** and is used to calculate additional payments to practices. Factors are determined from the **census** and include

- Elderly living alone
- One-parent families
- Children under 5 years old
- Unemployed (as percentage of economically active population)
- Overcrowded households
- Moved house within the last year
- Born in the New Commonwealth or Pakistan

ENG *Reproduced from* Guyatt et al. [43].

Table 1C.17 Domains of the South African Indices of multiple deprivation 2007 and the National Prevalence of Deprivation

Domain	Description	National Population in Deprivation (%)
Income and material deprivation	Living in a low-income household or one without a fridge, TV, or radio	72%
Employment deprivation	Working age population unemployed or unable to work due to sickness or disability	38%
Education deprivation	No secondary schooling.	27%
Living environment deprivation	Households with no running water, toilets or electricity. Or overcrowded dwellings or shacks	67%

Townsend

A census-based measure of comparative deprivation, which is measured at **ward level** and is defined by the **proportion of households** that

- Have more than one person per habitable room
- Have no car
- Are not owner occupied
- Include a person who is unemployed

Carstairs [41]

The Carstairs index is similar to the Townsend index but it is based on an **unweighted** combination of four census variables for the **residents** living in an area:

1. Residents living in households headed by an unskilled person
2. Unemployed males
3. Overcrowding
4. Residents with no car

Note that the currencies of Jarman, Townsend, and Carstairs are limited by the currency of census data (i.e. in 2012, the information used to form the indices was 10 years old).

Reproduced from Carstairs [42] and Morgan [43].

1C.10 Evaluation

Principles of evaluation, including quality assessment and quality assurance.

The terms evaluation, assessment, monitoring, and appraisal are sometimes used interchangeably as approaches to examining health services. Evaluation usually involves a combination of the other three elements and its prime purpose of evaluation is to inform decisions, often about the following:

1. New or proposed services
   A. Should we introduce a proposed service or intervention?
   B. What is the best way to address an identified health need?
2. Existing services
   A. Should we discontinue an existing service?
   B. How well is a current service addressing an identified health need? (quality assessment)
   C. Is the current service meeting required levels of delivery? (quality assurance)
   D. What aspects of the service require improvement or changing?

Good evaluations are characterised by the features listed in Table 1C.18.

It is important to ensure that the goals of an evaluation are of relevance to commissioners, providers, and patients or service users. The evaluation's recommendations will have a greater likelihood of leading to service

Table 1C.18 Features of a good evaluation

Feature	Details
Clear purpose	The design of the evaluation and the terms of reference should be agreed **at the start** of the process.
Clear goals	In particular, it is important to distinguish between • **Formative evaluations** (for an ongoing programme, to provide feedback leading to iterative improvements) • **Summative evaluations** (once a programme has finished or reached a particular point, to decide how well the programme met its aims)
Clear objectives	It should be clear what the service is intended to do and what indicators are to be used as markers of meeting these objectives.
Robust processes	Data should be valid and reliable but collection need not be burdensome for the service. In many circumstances, it may be possible to conduct evaluations without data collection using available evidence and routinely collected data.
Sufficient resources	Sufficient resources should be available to conduct the evaluation, including time, expertise, and funding.
Flexibility	The evaluation should have sufficient flexibility to adapt to changes in health services and in the local or national context.
Stakeholder engagement	The support and engagement of stakeholders is needed at all stages of the evaluation.

improvements if stakeholders are involved in generating recommendations.

A range of methods can be used for evaluation, depending on the evaluation's **goals**, the existing **evidence** base, and the available **resources**. However, the steps listed in Box 1C.10 are usually applicable.

In their influential book, Pawson and Tilley [44] call for more 'realistic' evaluations. See Box 1C.11.

Quality assessment and quality assurance

In public health, the terms **quality assessment** and **quality assurance** are often used interchangeably with the term **evaluation**. Note, however, that in other fields, the term quality assurance may relate to the process of ensuring that a service **meets a defined standard**.

Box 1C.10 Steps in conducting evaluations

Describe (the intervention or service)

Identify (the issues for the evaluation to address)

Design (the study, data collection required)

Collect and analyse (the data: compare with other areas, identify strengths and limitations, distinguish what is amenable to change)

Recommend

Disseminate (to funders, providers, and service users)

Use (to change services)

Source: WHO, Evaluation in health promotion. Principles and perspectives, WHO Regional Publications, European Series, no. 92, 2001.

Box 1C.11 Pawson and Tilley paradigm for evaluating services

Realistic evaluation

Pawson and Tilley describe a new **paradigm** for evaluating services, which the argue will lead to greater validity and utility from the evaluation findings. The authors argue that *'scientific evaluation requires a careful blend of theory and method, quality and quantity, ambition and realism'* and that interventions are assumed to have the following characteristics.

Interventions:

1. Are **theories** (i.e. they are based on a hypothesis such as if we do **x**, then we expect *y*)
2. Are **active** (i.e. they 'work' or not, regardless of volition; however, in reality, the reasoning and reaction of stakeholders is critical to success)
3. Are **chains of theory** (i.e. success of the programme depends on each stakeholder in the chain sustaining the assumptions and decisions of earlier stakeholders)
4. Exist within open, **multiple systems** (therefore, we should ***expect*** variation in delivery of the 'same' intervention)
5. Are **leaky** and prone to be borrowed (we should ***expect*** interventions to evolve as elements from one programme are integrated into another)
6. Change the conditions that make them work (as programmes mature, we should expect to see familiarisation, bringing about habituation, which can either be self-defeating or affirming)

Source: Pawson, R., Chapter 2: Realist methodology, in *Evidence-Based Policy*, Sage Publications, London, UK, 2006, pp. 17–37.

1C.11 Equity in healthcare

Equity and equality are distinct concepts (see Box 1C.12).

As with the concept of fairness, there are different viewpoints as to what constitutes equity, including **vertical** and **horizontal** equity.

Vertical equity

Vertical equity requires **unequal healthcare for unequal need**. For example, in a system that is vertically equitable, sicker people on a waiting list would be prioritised above patients who were less sick but had been waiting longer on the same list. Similarly, a progressive taxation system (where the rich face a disproportionately large tax burden) is vertically equitable.

Horizontal equity

Horizontal equity requires **equal healthcare for equal need**. It can be considered in the four ways outlined in Table 1C.19; however, it is recognised that equity of access and equity of use are overlapping concepts.

In his seminal paper, Julian Tudor Hart (1971) described inequities resulting from the introduction of market forces in the NHS. He coined the phrase the **inverse care law**, to describe this phenomenon, namely, that

> *'the availability of good medical care tends to vary inversely with the need of the population served'.*

Tudor Hart's evidence of the inverse care law came from a study of GPs in South Wales; but in subsequent years, empirical evidence of the inverse care law has been found in numerous settings.

In 2000, Victora and colleagues [47] proposed the **inverse equity hypothesis** to explain how health inequalities can widen as new public health

Box 1C.12 Equity and equality

	Equity	Equality
Definition	Fairness Distributive justice	Sameness
Issue	Differences in health due to avoidable inequalities (e.g. distance from home to a general practice surgery)	Avoidable and unavoidable differences (e.g. differences in healthcare use as a result of genetic diseases versus as a result of an informed choice not to have treatment)

Table 1C.19 Types of horizontal equity

Type	Definition	Advantages	Disadvantages
Equal spending for equal need	Budgets are allocated according to health need. For example, resources might be targeted according to SMRs and area-level deprivation indicators (see 4D.3).	Simple to measure because spending can be clearly identified.	Healthcare for a particular condition will cost varying amounts in different settings (e.g. the cost of a visit from a district nurse may be greater in rural than urban areas because of the greater distances involved).
Equal access for equal need	Access can be considered in terms of removing the barriers to service use. These barriers could be **geographical** (distance to the service), **financial** (cost to the user), or related to **time** (whether services are open only during office hours).	A defining principle of healthcare systems such as the NHS. Important for providers to consider whether their supply of services is equitable.	Barriers to access are often **intangible** (e.g. cultural) and therefore difficult to identify.
Equal use for equal need	This concept assumes that people should have the same healthcare demands for the same symptoms, so that any differences seen reflect barriers to access. One example often quoted is that of coronary bypass rates in areas of different SMR for CHD. Note that many studies that purport to measure access in fact measure healthcare use.	Overcomes the problem of intangible barriers to access.	Assumes that people with the same symptoms have the same demand for healthcare.
Equal health for equal need	This is clearly the ultimate aim for equity in health services.	Gold standard.	Subject to factors outside the control of healthcare, which may be **unavoidable** (e.g. genetics) or **avoidable** (e.g. poverty).

interventions are introduced. Typically, a new intervention will reach people in higher socio-economic circumstances first and only later affect the poor. The authors demonstrated the hypothesis held for Brazil Child Health, where absolute morbidity and mortality had fallen but inequity ratios had grown. Their hypothesis has been tested subsequently in relation to other changes in the profile of disease (e.g. the shift in HIV treatment in sub-Saharan Africa from higher socio-economic groups at the start of the epidemic to lower socio-economic groups in the late 2000s) [48].

1C.12 Clinical audit

A clinical audit is a **systematic review** of care, as measured against **explicit criteria**. It is a central component of **clinical governance**, which is a local system for assuring the quality of patient care and for making ongoing improvements. Audit and research require similar methods and can set out to answer similar questions. The distinction between audit and research relates to whether the learning is generalisable outside its setting (see Box 1C.13).

Audit cycle

In order for lessons to be learnt from an audit exercise, the process should always be seen as an **ongoing cycle** rather than a one-off event (see Figure 1C.1). The steps involved in conducting an audit are described in Table 1C.20.

Box 1C.13 Distinction between audit and research

Concept	Description
Research	Results can be generalised outside the setting of the study
Audit	Results are pertinent only to the setting under study

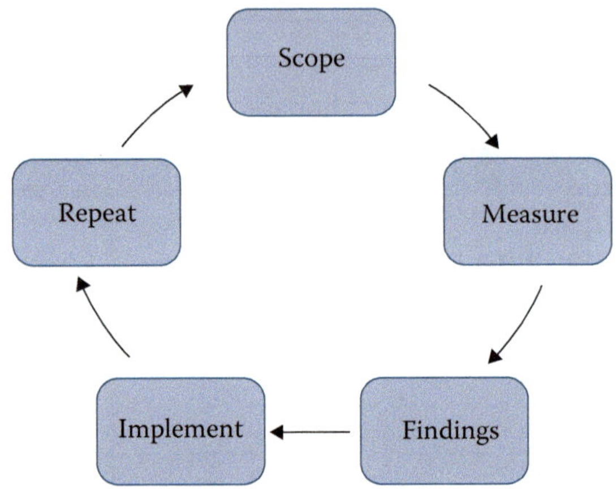

Figure 1C.1 The steps involved in conducting an audit.

Successful audit

Table 1C.21 lists the factors that may influence the success of an audit, based on the work of Baker and colleagues [49] and Johnston and colleagues [50].

UK In England and Wales, the **Healthcare Quality Improvement Partnership** (HQIP) was established to increase the impact of clinical audit on healthcare quality. HQIP funds the **National Clinical Audit and Patient Outcomes Programme** on a range of topics, including acute services, cancer, cardiac, mental health, and women and children.

Table 1C.20 The audit process

Scope	Begin by selecting criteria against which to audit. Useful sources of criteria include national standards (e.g. NICE quality standards) and national guidelines (e.g. NICE Health Technology appraisals). The **criteria** should be • Explicit statements that define what is being measured • Elements of care that can be measured objectively The **scope** of the audit can then be determined by deciding • Which patients should be included • Over what time period they should be audited • Which aspects of care should be considered An appropriate **sample** should be chosen by using a strategy such as the following: • **Interval sampling**, such as all patients visiting a clinic in a given period of time (e.g. January to March). • **Two-stage sampling**, where a small sample is selected first. If unequivocal conclusions can be drawn, then no more data are collected; however, if the results are ambiguous, then a larger sample is selected.
Measure	Measure observed performance against the selected criteria. Data sources include • **Registers**—to identify patients • **Patient records**—to examine aspects of care • **Electronic systems**—for rapid retrieval of information • **Teams** delivering the care—to find out if information is collected and the extent to which this information is suitable
Findings	Use the findings to identify areas for change. Ensure that the findings are shared with those who need to know, including • Teams working in the area of the audit • Area service directors • Boards Produce short summaries of findings that are readily understandable.
Implement	Implement the findings of the audit by making improvements to the service. Consider adopting **change management** approaches (see Section 5C).
Repeat	Check that these improvements are in place and are making a difference by repeating the audit cycle.

Table 1C.21 Drivers and barriers to success in audit

	Drivers of success	Barriers to success
Time	Ensure that protected time available to conduct audits.	Lack of time is the main reason for failure and incompleteness.
Strategy	Incorporate the requirement for audit into job descriptions and structured programmes.	Lack of an overall plan for audits.
Skills	Training for clinical staff. Availability of specialist audit staff.	Lack of expertise or advice in project design and analysis.
Resources	Modern medical records and IT systems. Dedicated audit staff. Funding to conduct the audit and implement changes.	Incomplete or inaccessible notes or patient records limit the robustness and comprehensiveness of audits and therefore weaken their influence on improving service quality.
Organisational culture	Dialogue between purchasers and providers. Whole team participates in the audit and in the implementation of change. Supportive learning environment with a no-blame culture.	Lack of trust between staff conducting the audit and staff being audited, which can hamper full disclosure and reduce opportunities for honest reflection.

1C.13 Confidential inquiry processes

Confidential inquiries are national investigations into serious untoward incidents. They are an example of a national investigation of serious concerns. Confidential inquiries conducted in England are described in Box 1C.14. Other examples of national investigations with implications for health are

- Clinical Standards Advisory Group (1991–2000)
- Bichard Inquiry into the Soham murders (2004), which made recommendations regarding child protection procedures following the murder of two young girls
- The Francis Inquiry (2013) into serious service failures at Mid Staffordshire Hospital NHS Foundation Trust that resulted in over 200 excess deaths (the main review findings and implications are covered in Chapter 5E.2)

Box 1C.14 Confidential inquiries in the United Kingdom

- National Confidential Inquiry into Suicide and Homicide in Mental Health Services (www.national-confidential-inquiry.ac.uk)
- The National maternal, newborn, and infant clinical outcomes review programme, run by MBRRACE-UK (Mothers and Babies—Reducing Risk through Audits and Confidential Enquiries across the UK), which collects data on maternal deaths, perinatal, neonatal and infant mortality and causes of stillbirth (www.npeu.ox.ac.uk/mbrrace-uk)
- National Confidential Enquiry into Patient Outcome and Death (NCEPOD) (www.ncepod.org.uk)
- Confidential Inquiry into premature deaths of people with learning disabilities (http://www.bris.ac.uk/cipold/)

The purpose of all such investigations is to identify what went wrong and to draw general lessons that can be shared and acted upon.

A **case–control** study design is often employed in this type of inquiry and is used to detect risk factors that predispose to unexpected deaths or other untoward incidents. Both quantitative and qualitative data may be used, including

- Routinely collected data (e.g. hospital episode statistics [HES])
- Hospital records
- Confidential surveys of individuals (including hospital staff, HM Coroner, families, GPs, patients' friends)

Confidential inquiries produce **reports** that are circulated widely and make **recommendations** for health services on how to minimise the risk of similar events happening again. The reports sometimes include **self-audit tools** that health services may use to assess their own risk.

1C.14 Delphi methods

This is an iterative technique for **generating consensus** about a particular issue **without face-to-face meetings**. The process works as shown in Box 1C.15.

The Delphi technique was originally used for making technology forecasts, but it has also proved useful in public health—especially in fields where **data are lacking** or as a way of **engaging people** who would not otherwise be involved. Its advantages and limitations are shown in Box 1C.16. An example of how the Delphi method is used in practice is given Box 1C.17.

Box 1C.15 Steps in the Delphi technique

Steps	Description
Step 1	A group of experts is contacted and surveyed.
Step 2	Views of the group are shared anonymously among the same group, highlighting areas of disagreement.
Step 3	Respondents are asked if they wish to change their views in light of step 2.
Step 4	Steps 2–3 are repeated several times until consensus is reached.

Box 1C.16 Advantages and limitations of the Delphi method

Advantages	Limitations
Anonymity and written process avoids some of the pitfalls of face-to-face discussion (e.g. each contribution is valued equally, with reduced potential for personality to influence responses).	Written survey format may be more suitable for some respondents than others.
Time-efficient since it does not rely on bringing together disparate, busy groups.	Open to manipulation from the administrators of the process.
Encourages open critique and admission of errors by encouraging contributors to revise earlier judgements.	Does not always produce useful results. Sometimes, future developments are more accurately predicted by unconventional thinking than by iterative consensus from accepted experts.

Box 1C.17 Example: Dephi technique

In an attempt to describe different service models that were used in Community Mental Health Practice, investigators used a Delphi method to generate a *'valid and reliable set of categories to describe the clinical work practices of intensive case managers'*. Eight case managers took part in the process, which involved a combination of

(a) The Delphi method to generate a list of categories to describe their working practices
(b) Face-to-face discussions to refine this list

The authors described the Delphi method as being'... an effective, straightforward, and time-efficient way of obtaining a workable consensus'.

Source: Reproduced from Fiander, M. and Burns, T., *Psych. Serv.*, 51, 656, 2000.

1C.15 Economic evaluation

Economic evaluation is a core component on health service evaluation. In order to make decisions about healthcare provision, it is important to have considered the relative costs and benefits of different interventions.

See Chapter 4D.5 for a full description economic evaluation.

1C.16 Epidemiological basis for preventive strategies

The epidemiology of a disease can act as a guide for its prevention. Factors that are found to be associated with the disease, and which meet the criteria for causation, can provide useful targets for preventive strategies (see Section 1A.13).

Levels of prevention

Preventive interventions are considered at three levels: primary, secondary, and tertiary (see Table 1C.22).

Note that primary prevention is not the same as screening (which seeks to identify the

Table 1C.22 Levels of prevention

Level of prevention	Definition	Example
Primary prevention	Aims to prevent or delay the onset of the disease in people who are at risk but who do not currently have the disease	Low-dose aspirin given to people at sufficient risk of developing ischemic heart disease
Secondary prevention	Aims to prevent or delay further progression or complications in people known to have the disease	An exercise programme offered to patients who have had a myocardial infarction
Tertiary prevention	Aims to reduce long-term disability that would otherwise result from the disease	Removing allergens from the environment of a patient with asthma

Table 1C.23 Population and high-risk approaches to prevention

Strategy	Description	Example
Population approach	The whole population receives health promotion and disease prevention interventions, which seeks to reduce risk across the population because everybody is at risk.	Legislation for wearing seat belts in cars.
High-risk approach	Health promotion and disease prevention is targeted at groups or individuals identified from epidemiological studies as being most at risk.	Chlamydia screening targeted at people aged 15–24 (who have the highest prevalence of the disease in the population).

members of a population who are at sufficient risk of the disease to warrant further action or investigation).

Preventive strategies

There are two main approaches to preventive medicine: the **population approach** and the **high-risk** approach (see Table 1C.23).

Epidemiological strategies to identify high-risk groups include

- Ecological studies to identify groups with highest incidence of disease (see Section 1A.17)
- Analytical studies to link risk factors and diseases (e.g. blood pressure, diabetes, and coronary heart disease [CHD])
- Genetic studies to identify families and individuals with genetic risk factors (e.g. gene for hypercholesterolemia; see Section 2D.9)
- Population screening to identify individuals who have known risk factors (e.g. diabetes for heart disease, age profile for chlamydia infection)

The epidemiologist **Geoffrey Rose** (1992) outlined the rationale for a population-based preventive approach in his seminal work, *The Strategy of Preventive Medicine*. This approach is useful for tackling common conditions that are distributed normally and which have a widespread cause. The classic example is deaths from CHD due to hypertension (see Figure 1C.2 and Box 1C.18).

However, the **prevention paradox** (see Section 2H.4) significantly limits the appropriateness of the population approach. Current thinking therefore emphasises the need for a combination of both the population and the targeted approaches to prevention [52].

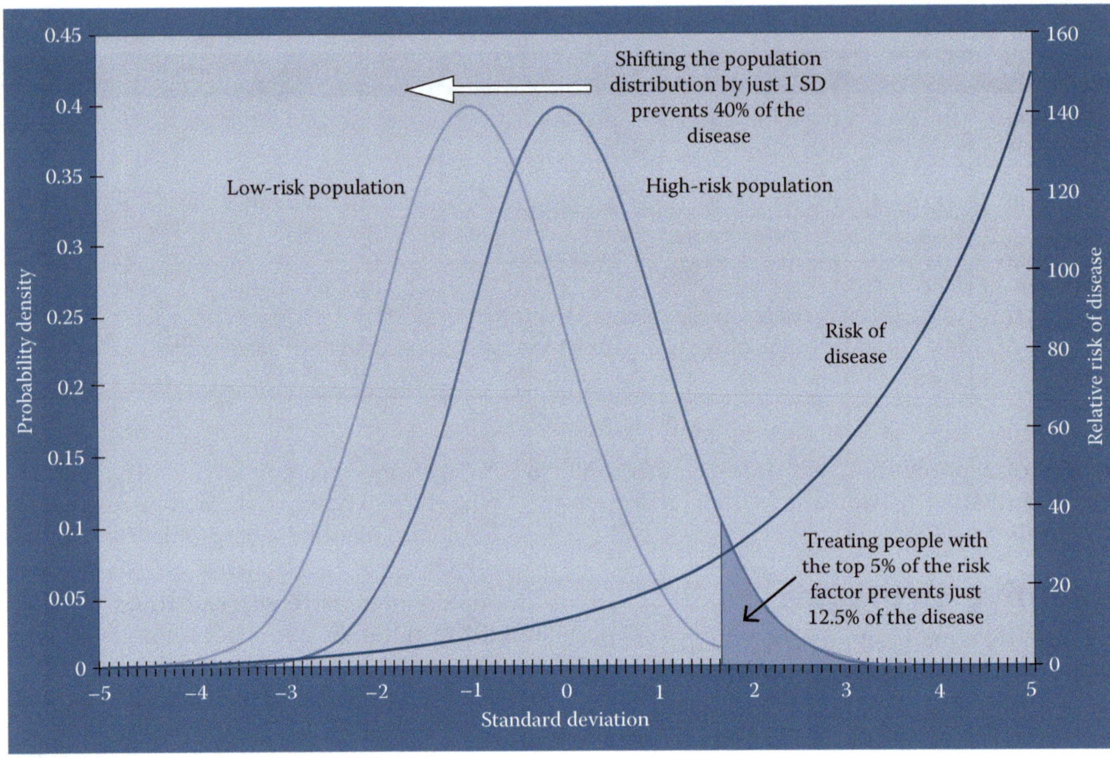

Figure 1C.2 Effects of a population-based versus a high-risk-based approach to preventing heart disease. (From Jackson, R., *BMJ*, 332, 617, 2006.)

Box 1C.18 Example: Controlling risk factors for heart disease

The blood pressure of the population is normally distributed; therefore, a minority of people have very high blood pressures. In Figure 1C.2, the top 5% of the population with the highest blood pressures are represented by the white triangular area. These people are at high risk of CHD.

However, since the number of such high-risk people is small, their burden of disease on the overall population is modest. In this example, these 5% of people represent 12.5% of the burden of disease. Therefore, many more cases of CHD occur in people with lower blood pressure (i.e. to individuals who fall outside the dark blue triangular area). Targeting only the top 5% of the population with very high levels could at best reduce disease by 12.5%.

An approach that slightly reduced blood pressure across the whole population would, in contrast, have a considerably larger impact, in this example reducing disease by 40%.

Sources: Rose, G., *The Strategy of Preventive Medicine*, Oxford: Oxford University Press, 1992.

1C.17 Health and environmental impact assessments

The potential effects of **transport**, **employment**, and **economic** policy decisions on health are often profound (both good and bad). However, it is rare to know in advance what the environmental and public health impacts of a policy will be. Therefore, in order to gauge which options will produce the most beneficial (or least harmful) effects, an **environmental impact assessment (EIA)** and a **health impact assessment (HIA)** should be undertaken. These exercises use systematic processes to consider and estimate the likely impact of a policy decision.

All member states of the EU are legally required to conduct an EIA for any major civil engineering project. Some EIAs consider health as a criterion against which to assess the proposal. Even then, health is typically covered only superficially, so the WHO **Ottawa Charter** for Health Promotion [55] proposed an analogous process of HIAs. These assessments concentrate solely on the potential effects of a proposed policy on the health of the population (see Box 1C.19).

Box 1C.19 Examples of policies that might require an Impact Assessment

Type of policy	Example
Transport strategies	London Heathrow Airport Terminal 5
Civil engineering	New landfill site
Urban regeneration	Olympics regeneration in East London
Lobbying	Manchester Airport second runway expansion
Developing countries	Donor aid project appraisals

Steps in undertaking a health impact assessment [56]

There are five key steps to an HIA: screening, scoping, appraisal, reporting, and monitoring (see Box 1C.20). Throughout the HIA process, it is important to engage in a dialogue with relevant stakeholders, including the general public.

Challenges

Challenges to conducting an HIA may include a lack of evidence, time and resources, as well as barriers to implementation.

Evidence

A crucial point to consider is whether there is any existing evidence on which to base recommendations. For new projects, the health impacts may not previously have been considered, observed, or measured. Quantifiable evidence often proves to be more influential than qualitative evidence, but it may be not be feasible to collect.

The evidence for an HIA may originate from several sources, often coming from stakeholders with conflicting perspectives. HIAs may therefore require the appraisal and synthesis of contradictory information.

Time and resources

Some HIAs demand rapid results despite being allocated few resources. In these circumstances, it may not be possible to conduct the HIAs with the same degree of rigour as a longer-term or better-funded study. This trade-off needs to be acknowledged explicitly during the scoping and reporting stages of an HIA.

Action

A final, but pivotal, challenge is to ensure that the findings and recommendations of the HIA are actually implemented. For this to happen, the decision-makers responsible for the programme need to be actively engaged in the HIA during the reporting stage.

Box 1C.20 Steps in undertaking an HIA

HIA steps	Details
1. Screening	Establish whether there is any **health relevance** to a policy, programme, or other development.
2. Scoping	For proposals with health relevance, decide the **questions** that the HIA should address, together with the **reporting arrangements**. A decision should be made as to whether the HIA will consider determinants at the • Individual level (e.g. genetics, lifestyles) • Environmental level (e.g. air, water quality) • Institutional level (e.g. availability of services) • A combination of the three
3. Appraisal	Assess the potential health impacts either through **rapid appraisal** (over a few days or weeks) or through **in-depth assessment** (weeks or months), depending on results of the scoping exercise. Information considered in the HIA will include • An analysis of secondary data sources • Interviews with key informants • Field observations • A review of the peer-reviewed and grey literature
4. Reporting	**Conclusions** are written, together with **recommendations** to minimise the negative impacts and maximise the positive impacts of the development.
5. Monitoring	Actual impacts are **monitored** to enhance the evidence base for future HIAs and to assess the extent to which the HIA's recommendations were acted upon.

1D

Principles of Qualitative Methods

Many types of scientific studies generate quantitative data about an issue. For example, a study might measure the proportion of people affected by a condition who have a particular risk factor. Sometimes, however, the information required to answer a question pertains more to the character of an issue, rather than to any numerical value. Qualitative methods aim to explore this second type of inquiry (i.e. those that relate to the **kind** or the **quality** of things). These methods are used for answering **how, what,** or **why** questions. For example, qualitative research questions in public health include the following:

- What influences parents' decisions to vaccinate their children?
- How do different patients view their illnesses?
- Why would some patients decline information about their condition?

Many public health specialists will be involved in conducting qualitative research to inform service development; others will be involved in commissioning or appraising such research. Therefore, whether or not they engage in such research themselves, all public health specialists require some knowledge of qualitative methods and their appropriate use in an applied health context.

1D.1 Overview of methods of data collection

Semi-structured, narrative and in-depth interviewing, focus groups, action research, participant observation.

Four of the most widely methods for collecting qualitative data are the following:

1. One-to-one interviews, which may be
   a. Semi-structured
   b. In-depth
   c. Narrative format
   d. A combination of the earlier
2. Focus groups
3. Action research
4. Participant (or non-participant) observation
   a. These methods are described in Table 1D.1.

The robustness of qualitative research is often judged according to the same criteria as are used to evaluate quantitative research, including

- **Reliability**—the degree to which the collection of data in a study was consistent and **repeatable**
- **Validity**—how well a study's findings represent the **'true'** state of affairs
- **Generalisability**—the extent to which the findings from one setting can be **applied** to another

Table 1D.1 Four methods of qualitative data collection

	Semi-structured and in-depth interviewing	Focus groups	Action research	Participant (or non-participant) observation
What is done?	The interviewer uses a topic guide, rather than a rigid set of questions. Issues should arise naturally in the conversation. In-depth interviews can be conducted over several hours. Researchers may also conduct several interviews at different stages with the same individuals.	A facilitator leads a small number of people (usually 5–10) in a structured conversation. The focus is not on the responses to the facilitator but more on the reactions of participants to each other.	The people under study (e.g. service users) are actively involved as researchers. Action research enables researchers to make changes to projects during the course of the research, not simply at the end.	Researchers actively take part in a setting as they collect their data, either as a member of the community (e.g. a nurse in a hospital). Observation can also be achieved as a non-participant (e.g. attending team meetings but not responsible for contributing to any agenda items).
How is this used?	**Uses** Generating new concepts and ideas about an issue.	**Uses** Understand target audiences. Exploring subjects that are difficult to discuss individually (e.g. sexual beliefs and behaviours).	**Uses** Involving people who would otherwise not normally take part in research. Community development.	**Uses** Immersing the researcher in the experiences of the people under study. Gaining insight into subcultures that are not usually open to study or observation.

Note that the concepts of validity and reliability are underpinned by a **positivist perspective** on research (i.e. that there is one true answer and that a well-designed study would be able to reproduce the same findings if conducted by different people at different times). Many qualitative researchers follow a **constructivist** tradition (i.e. research will not yield one 'true' view of an issue but could yield several valid perspectives depending on who is conducting the research and when the research was conducted).

See Chapter 4A for a discussion of positivism, constructivism, and other theoretical concepts that underlie qualitative research.

For both traditions, the quality of qualitative data collection may be enhanced using the methods described in Table 1D.2.

Table 1D.2 Methods for improving the quality of data collection in qualitative research

Method	Description
Data collection tool	Using the **same data collection tool** (interview schedule, observation, or topic guide) for each interview, group, or observation.
Single researcher	Using **one researcher** (interviewer, facilitator, or observer) for all interviews/groups/observations, or agreeing a common approach or goal with all researchers.
Standardised training	Providing the same **training** and **written guidance** to researchers to keep discussions on topic but still enabling enough flexibility for participants to express their views.
Record keeping	Producing an **accurate record** of the discussion, interview, or observations through electronic recording of interviews (audio or video) rather than note-taking, not only because it ensures an **accurate record,** but also because it enables the researcher to **listen fully** and take part in the discussion. However, recording may not be appropriate or feasible in all situations, and it may dissuade some subjects from participating. Explicit consent must always be obtained for recording data collection. Noting/recording observations as soon as possible afterwards to ensure that they are recalled correctly.

1D.2 Contribution of qualitative methods to public health research and policy

Qualitative research has an important role in influencing public health research and policy. Its principal contributions fall into three areas: policy formulation, development, and evaluation (see Table 1D.3). Note that qualitative research has two distinct roles in evaluation: explaining the outcomes and revealing unintended consequences and changes in perceptions.

Table 1D.3 Principal contributions of qualitative research to public health policy

Area	Contribution	Description
Formulation	Research questions or policy problems.	Defining the boundaries of an issue, creating a contextual understanding (e.g. how a problem developed and why, which people are central to addressing it).
Development	Methods or tools.	What questions to ask, how they are understood by potential respondents, how to interpret their responses (see Box 1D.1).
Evaluation	Explain the outcomes found.	A quantitative evaluation may measure effects, but the intervention itself remains a 'black box'. Qualitative methods can help unpick what worked and why, providing insight for refining or modifying the intervention.
	Reveal unintended consequences and perceptions.	Quantitative evaluations also measure the extent to which an intervention achieved predetermined effects. By asking open questions, qualitative studies can uncover outcomes that were not anticipated at the start.

Box 1D.1 How qualitative methods can be used to decide which questions to ask [57]

The National Survey of Sexual Attitudes and Lifestyles (NATSAL) [58] is a large cross-sectional survey that provides data on sexual health, lifestyles, and attitudes. In the 2010 survey, it was decided for the first time to collect data on sexual function and dysfunction. However, this area was previously ill defined. Being a private and sensitive topic, carefully crafted questions were required that could obtain useful information without alienating participants.

Qualitative research on a comparatively small sample of people was undertaken to decide what questions should be part of a sexual function questionnaire and how the questions should be asked. The research team began by conducting 32 semi-structured interviews with a purposive sample (some interviewees were members of the public, some were selected from GP practices, some had a higher risk of problems by virtue of their diagnosis (e.g. diabetes), while others had sought clinical advice for a sexual function problem).

The researchers developed a conceptual framework setting out four dimensions that emerged as being central to this issue, namely, psychophysiological aspects, severity (if a difficulty was present), relationships, and overall self-rating.

Once the tool was developed, the researchers piloted its use with 12 general practice patients to understand how people might interpret the questions and how the questions might be rephrased in ways that would encourage more honest responses. This tool was subsequently validated on over 1000 people.

Source: Mitchell, K.R. and Wellings, K., *J. Sex Res.*, 50(1), 17, 2013.

1D.3 Appropriate use, analysis, and presentation of qualitative data

The uses, analysis, and presentation of qualitative data are quite distinct from those of quantitative data.

Appropriate use

Table 1D.4 sets out the principal applications of the different types of qualitative data collection methods.

Analysis

Qualitative data are analysed in different ways depending to a degree on the method of data collection used but more importantly according to the goals of the research. Some analytical methods involve an extremely detailed interrogation of the data. For example,

- **Interpretative phenomenological analysis** (IPA) focuses on individuals' experiences of a particular phenomenon
- **Discourse analysis** focuses on the linguistic attributes of the data (i.e. the style and syntax of the language used, not simply the content)

The principal methods of qualitative analysis used most frequently in public health are **thematic content** analysis, **grounded theory**, and **framework analysis** (see Box 1D.2).

There are several ways of enhancing the validity and the credibility of qualitative analysis, which are summarised in Table 1D.5.

- In addition, **reflexivity** is an important dimension that should be considered in any qualitative analysis (see also Chapter 4A). The concept of reflexivity recognises that the researcher affects the environment and the people whom he or she is researching.

Presentation

As with quantitative research, many peer-reviewed journals require authors to complete checklists to ensure the comprehensive and transparent reporting of qualitative research (e.g. the COREQ checklist, 2007).

Such checklists typically require researchers to meet the requirements listed in Table 1D.6.

From interviews and focus groups, short quotes should be selected (i.e. in the participants' own words)

Table 1D.4 Applications of qualitative investigation

Semi-structured and in-depth interviewing	Focus groups	Action research	Participant observation
Exploring people's accounts of experiences and beliefs	Exploring shared experiences and beliefs Generating large amounts of data in a relatively short time Exploring *how or whether* people come to a consensus or viewpoint	Aims to change practice as well as study it Cyclical research design where data gathering, planning, observing, and reflecting all feed into the next planning cycle. Participants are therefore also the researchers Particularly useful for • Evaluation • Assessing health needs Can use innovative research methods (e.g. drama, charts, creative arts)	Exploring what people actually do, not just what they say they do Capturing information on familiar and routine areas of life that enables views or perceptions that are tacitly understood to become explicit

Box 1D.2 Types of qualitative analysis

Method	Description
Thematic content	The simplest form of analysis, this usually involves reporting interviewees' comments in a structured form. Useful for areas where not much is known and as a starting point for other types of analysis. (**Note:** Thematic content analysis is distinct from **thematic analysis**, which is a broad term for a range of qualitative analytic approaches).
Grounded theory	Used for developing theories rather than testing theories that have already been generated. Data collection takes place in a cyclical process: themes that are identified from the analysis are fed back into the topics to be discussed during subsequent interviews, and new data are used to refine the analysis on an ongoing basis. The analysis involves organising content into codes and continually refining these codes. Data collection ends when **saturation** is reached (i.e. interviews where no new codes start to appear).
Framework	Used for developing practical strategies as a result of research. Analytical themes can be chosen before the analysis (or indeed sometimes even before data collection begins); however, the themes are refined on analysis.

that best encapsulate the findings or which convey the themes in memorable ways. For each quote, include the setting and the speaker. From observations, quotes or short extracts of dialogue should be selected, and contextual information should be provided (e.g. this was at *x* meeting when *y* was being discussed).

The ways in which qualitative data are presented should be tailored to the audience. For example, the website www.healthtalkonline.org presents patient stories to patients in the form of online video clips. Sometimes, qualitative data may be presented in graphical or pictorial form (e.g. a study of a local area may include research participants' hand-drawn maps).

Table 1D.5 Methods for enhancing the validity and credibility of qualitative analysis

Method	Description
Deviant data	Identification of **disconfirming** cases or **deviant data**, then accounting for these (i.e. not solely quoting supportive data).
Coding	Developing a **coding structure** with other researchers.
Feedback	**Presenting back** to interviewees to check that the material accurately represents what they thought.
Counting responses	**Counting responses** in themes to give an indication of how common a particular response was heard (e.g. 'seven participants said x' or 'most participants said y').
Transparency	Being as **transparent** as possible in the presentation of the findings and including raw data if possible (e.g. quotes).
Description	Providing a detailed description of the **process** of analysis.
Comparing methods	**Comparing** the findings using other study methods (e.g. questionnaires) to explore the **effect of the interviewer/facilitator** on findings. For example, a health service employee may hear only positive comments about the health service.
Comparing findings	**Comparing** and **contrasting** the findings with the findings from other studies and with attitudes expressed at beginning of the study or with other data collected in the current study.

Table 1D.6 Typical requirements in presenting qualitative data

Study aspect	Requirement
Context	Provide context to the data (i.e. introduce the study **background** and **rationale**; report the methods used to **collect** and **analyse** the data).
Themes	Summarise the data in themes. Within each theme, include **examples** as articulated by participants in the form of select quotes or short extracts of dialogue (noting the requirement to anonymise; see Section 1D.3).
Reflexivity	Comment on reflexivity (i.e. what effect did the study team have on the findings generated?) and how these data fit with what is already known.

1D.4 Ethical issues

All research involves risks. In general, qualitative research raises fewer ethical concerns than studies requiring invasive procedures (e.g. drug trials). However, there are still significant ethical implications that should be considered and the risk of harm to participants should always be minimised (see Table 1D.7).

Potential strategies for managing such ethical issues are listed in Table 1D.8.

Table 1D.7 Ethical considerations

Ethical issue	Description
1. Costs	Participants often need to give their **time and energy** to take part in research.
2. Psychological harm	Participants are put at risk of psychological harm to participants through • Disclosure of confidential or sensitive information • Reaction from others In interviews and focus groups, participants are generally **aware** of what they are sharing; however, in observation studies, disclosure may be **unwitting**. Participants may receive **negative responses** to the information or views that they disclose, either during data collection (from other participants) or after reporting (from readers).

Table 1D.8 Strategies for managing ethical issues in qualitative research

Stage of research	Strategy	Details
Before data collection	Risk assessment	Ensure that the **likely benefits** of the research outweigh the likely costs (i.e. the anticipated new insights or information are worth the risks involved).
	Literature review	Search for **published studies** to explore whether similar research has been conducted before.
	Clarity of purpose	Be **clear to participants** as early as possible about the aims of the research and their role as a participant (assuming that sharing this information does not conflict with the goals of the study).
	Informed consent	Seek **informed consent**. Provide information before the study and allow time for reflection. Enable participants to withdraw at any time. For vulnerable adults and children, the consent of a responsible adult may be required.
	Ground rules	In focus groups, explain and seek agreement of the **ground rules** for behaviour towards each other (i.e. respecting other participants' opinions and not sharing what was heard in the focus group with others outside).
After data collection	Anonymisation	In reporting, **anonymise participants** (i.e. remove names and do not provide positions or settings if such information would allow someone to guess the respondent's identity).
	Data protections	Ensure that any personal data held about participants is stored securely in line with **information governance** and **data protection** principles.
	Contact details	Provide **contact details** so that participants can report any concerns they may have about the research.

1D.5 Common errors and their avoidance

Qualitative research should not be undertaken lightly. On the surface, qualitative research can seem deceptively easy. For example, data collection may appear to involve chats or discussion, and analysis using quotes and narratives may seem more accessible to some readers than statistical data. However, major problems can arise with qualitative research, which may limit the extent to which qualitative studies are of value in public health. Some of these problems occur due to methodological errors, whereas others are legitimate challenges that researchers may encounter during the course of a study. See Table 1D.9.

Table 1D.9 Problems that may be encountered in qualitative research and mitigation strategies

Issue	Possible error or reason	Strategies to manage the situation
Inadequate sample	Too few participants, or participants lack the profile or experience needed to address the research question.	Allow sufficient preparation time to engage potential participants (may require several meetings). Engage decision-makers early in the research process.
	Logistical barriers to attendance.	Remove barriers to participation by • Providing travel expenses, crèche facilities, refreshments, etc. • Conducting the research near to participants' homes or workplaces
		Consider other data collection methods (one-to-one interviews are often easier to coordinate than focus groups).
Data lack credibility	**Interviews**: interviewees feel constrained from saying what they actually think.	Make interviewees comfortable through • Sensitive choice of location for the interview and the arrangement of room • The conduct of the interviewer (e.g. assurances of confidentiality, dress, and manner suited to the interviewee) In the analysis, reflect explicitly on whether only socially acceptable views were expressed and what the interviewee perceived as being acceptable.
	Groups: Individuals may feel constrained from saying what they actually think by the supposed or voiced opinions of other members of the group. There is a risk of **false consensus** because of pressure to be agreeable with each other.	As with interviews, make members of the group comfortable through by choosing the location and arrangement the room sensitively. Emphasise at start that there are 'no wrong answers' and that 'all comments are valid'. Reflect explicitly in the analysis **why** socially acceptable were views expressed and **how** members constrained or enabled the free expression of opinion (e.g. by laughing, expressing surprise).
	Observation: Participants behave differently when the observer is present.	Avoid drawing attention to observation (e.g. no conspicuous note-taking). Observe over long periods because behaviour may eventually revert to 'normal'. In the analysis, explicitly reflect on how behaviour changed and why.
	Analysis: Insufficient or too superficial.	Allow sufficient time and resources to conduct high-quality analysis in keeping with aims of the study. Be transparent about the methods used at all stages.

(continued)

Table 1D.9 (*Continued*) Problems that may be encountered in qualitative research and mitigation strategies

Issue	Possible error or reason	Strategies to manage the situation
Findings sidelined	**Time lag**: Study concludes too late to inform decisions.	Set realistic timescales at the start of the study. Ensure that the research plan is commensurate with time available.
	Study findings are **at odds with decision-makers' agenda**.	Understand policymakers' agenda at the start of the and throughout the project. Consider tailoring the ways in which findings are conveyed without changing the findings themselves.
	Findings **not well known**.	Plan the dissemination strategy at the start of the research, including which communication methods will be used for relevant audiences (e.g. peer-reviewed article for scientific audiences, executive summary for the management team, a short video for a public meeting).

1D.6 Strengths and weaknesses of qualitative research

As with all research, the strengths and weaknesses of qualitative research are determined by whether

- The **method was appropriate** to answer the research question
- The data were collected and **analysed appropriately**
- Sufficient resources were available to ensure that all stages of the research could be conducted properly

Qualitative research tends to produce in-depth information from a small number of people or settings. This attribute can both be a strength or a weakness, depending on the **perspective** of the person using the research.

Qualitative research typically has a lower profile in health journals than quantitative research. Although the volume of qualitative research being published is increasing, quantitative research still dominates mainstream journals. For example, fewer than 10% of *BMJ* publications are qualitative in nature. One reason may be that qualitative studies do not fit neatly into **hierarchies of evidence**; therefore, it can be problematic to compare the value of the qualitative evidence compared with the value of quantitative studies.

The features outlined in Table 1D.10 are less inherent strengths or weaknesses of qualitative research but rather some factors that may enhance or limit a qualitative study's potential to be well received and to influence policymakers.

Table 1D.10 Factors affecting the potential of qualitative research to influence policy

Facilitators	Barriers
Depth of data: Qualitative research often examines issues in great detail.	**Generalisability**: Qualitative research may be sidelined if it is not seen as being readily generalisable to other settings.
Flexibility: Not restricted to predetermined, narrowly focused questions. Instead, allows open research questions to be addressed. Iterative analytical approaches mean that unexpected or novel insights often emerge.	**Reliability**: The extent to which the individual researcher can shape the findings may be viewed as a weakness of qualitative research.
Memorable and compelling stories produced: Narratives of human experience produced from qualitative studies can be evocative.	**Acceptability** findings may not fit with policymakers' existing agendas.
Qualitative research has the capacity to reveal **subtleties** and **complexities**.	**Perceived credibility**: Rigour is more difficult to demonstrate than in quantitative research.
Potential to **engage communities** and other **stakeholders** in the data-gathering process.	**Volume of data**: Time intensive to collect and analyse well (and observers may need to be in place for years to collect data).

References

1. Marquis, G.S., Habicht, J.P., Lanata, C.F., Black, R.K., and Rasmussen, K.M. (1997) Association of breastfeeding and stunting in Peruvian toddlers: An example of reverse causality. *Int J Epidemiol* 26(2), 349–356. doi:10.1093/ije/26.2.349.
2. Faubel, R., Lopez-Garcia, E., Guallar-Castillón, P., Balboa-Castillo, T., Gutiérrez-Fisac, J.L., Banegas, J.R., and Rodríguez-Artalejo, F. (August 2009) Sleep duration and health-related quality of life among older adults: A population-based cohort in Spain. *Sleep* 32(8), 1059–1068.
3. Macleod, J., Oakes, R., Oppenkowski, T., Stokes-lampard, H., Copello, A., Crome, I., Davey Smith, G., Egger, M., Hickman, M., and Judd, A. (2004) How strong is the evidence that illicit drug use by young people is an important cause of psychological or social harm? Methodological and policy implications of a systematic review of longitudinal, general population studies. *Drugs Educ Prev Policy* 11(4), 281–297.
4. Drain, P.K., Halperin, D.T., Hughes, J.P., Klausner, J.D., and Bailey, R.C. (2006) Male circumcision, religion, and infectious diseases: An ecologic analysis of 118 developing countries. *BMC Infect Dis* 6, 172, doi:10.1186/1471-2334-6-172.
5. 4S Study. (1994) Randomised trial of cholesterol lowering in 4444 patients with coronary heart disease: The Scandinavian Simvastatin Survival Study (4S). *Lancet* 344, 1383–1389.
6. www.dartmouthatlas.org.
7. www.rightcare.nhs.uk/atlas.
8. Wennberg, J. (2010) *Tracking Medicine: A Researcher's Quest to Understand Healthcare*. New York: Oxford University Press.
9. Whincup et al. (2005) Ten Towns Heart Health Study. www.tentowns.ac.uk.
10. Lopez Bernal, J.A. Gasparrini, A., Artundo, C., and McKee, M. (2013) The effect of the late 2000s financial crisis on suicides in Spain: An interrupted time-series analysis. *Eur J Publ Health*.
11. Framingham Heart Study website www.framinghamheartstudy.org.

12. Beauchamp, T.L. and Childress, J.F. (2001) *Principles of Biomedical Ethics* (5th ed.). Oxford, UK: Oxford University Press.
13. McKeown, R.E. and Weed, D.L. (2002) Ethics in epidemiology and public health II. Applied terms. *J Epidemiol Commun Health* 56, 739–741.
14. National Center for Chronic Disease Prevention and Health Promotion. (2006) Steps of an Outbreak Investigation—www.cdc.gov/excite/classroom/outbreak/steps.htm.
15. Eyers, J.E. (1998) How to do (or not to do)—Searching bibliographic databases effectively. *Health Policy Plan* 13, 339–342.
16. Buse, K., Mays, N., and Walt, G. (2005) *Making Health Policy*. Maidenhead, UK: Open University Press.
17. Oxford Centre for Evidence-Based Medicine Levels of Evidence. (2011).
18. Dorak, M.T. (2007) Genetic epidemiology. www.dorak.info/epi/genetepi.html.
19. Fleiss, J.L. (1981) *Statistical Methods for Rates and Proportions* (3rd ed.). New York: John Wiley & Sons, p. 77.
20. Sofocleous, C.T., Hinrichs, C.R., Weiss, S.H., Contractor, D., Barone, A., Bahramipour, P., Brountzos, E., and Kelekis, D. (August 2002). Alteplase for hemodialysis access graft thrombolysis. *J Vasc Intervent Radiol JVIR 1*, 13(8), 775. DOI: 10.1016/S1051-0443(07)61985-X.
21. Kirkwood, B.R. and Sterne, J.A.C. (2003) *Essential Medical Statistics* (2nd edn.). Oxford, UK: Blackwell Science.
22. Egger, M., Davey Smith, G., Schneider, M., and Minder, C. (1997) Bias in meta-analysis detected by a simple, graphical test. *BMJ* 315, 629–634.
23. Petrie, A. and Sabin, C. (2005) *Medical Statistics at a Glance* (2nd ed.). Oxford, UK: Blackwell Publishing.
24. Bradshaw, J.R. (1972) The taxonomy of social need. In: McLachlan G (ed) *Problems and Progress in Medical Care*. Oxford, UK: Oxford University Press, pp. 69–82.
25. Culyer, J. and Wagstaff, A. (1991) *Need, Equality and Social Justice*.New York: Centre for Health Economics, University of York. Accessed online (17/7/2014) at: http://www.york.ac.uk/media/che/documents/papers/discussionpapers/CHE%20Discussion%20Paper%2090.pdf.
26. The NHS Information Centre for Health and Social Care and the Association of Public Health Observatories in England. (2008).
27. Cavanagh, S. and Chadwick, K. (2005) *Health Needs Assessment: A Practical Guide*. London, UK: National Institute for Clinical Excellence. Available online at: www.nice.org.uk/page.aspx?o=513203.
28. Donabedian, A. (1966) Evaluating the quality of medical care. *Millbank Memorial Fund Quarter* 44, 166–206.
29. Maxwell, R.J. (1984) Quality assessment in health. *BMJ* 288, 1470–1472.
30. Health and Social Care Information Centre (2012). Patient survey suggests benefit from common procedures varies markedly by NHS provider. Accessed online (17/7/2014) at: http://www.ic.nhs.uk/proms.
31. Lakhani, A., Coles, J., Eayres, D. et al. (2005) Creative use of existing clinical and health outcomes data to assess NHS performance in England: Part 1—Performance indicators closely linked to clinical care. *BMJ* 330, 1426–1431.
32. Department of Health. Part 1: A public health outcomes framework for England, 2013–2016. www.dh.gov.uk.
33. Parrish, R.G. (2010) Measuring population health outcomes. *Prev Chronic Dis* 7(4), A71. Accessed online (17/7/2014) at: http://www.cdc.gov/pcd/issues/2010/jul/10_0005.htm.
34. The Office for National Statistics. (2007) The National Statistics Socio-economic Classification, http://www.ons.gov.uk.
35. Small Area Health Research Unit. (2011) SAHRU Deprivation index. Accessed online (17/7/2014) at: http://www.sahru.tcd.ie/.
36. Trutz Haase. (undated) Key features of the pobal HP deprivation index. Accessed online (17/7/2014) at: http://trutzhaase.eu/deprivation-index/the-2011-pobal-hpdeprivation-index-for-small-areas/.
37. The Scottish Government. (2009) Scottish index of multiple deprivation: Guidance. The Scottish Government Publications. Available from http://www.scotland.gov.uk/Resource/Doc/288642/0088311.pdf.
38. The Scottish Government. (2012) Scottish index of multiple deprivation. The Scottish Government Publications. Available from http://www.scotland.gov.uk/Topics/Statistics/SIMD.
39. The Australian Bureau of Statistics. (2012) Information paper: Measures of Socioeconomic Status 1244.0.55.001 Canberra. Available from: http://www.abs.gov.au/AUSSTATS/abs@.nsf/DetailsPage/1244.0.55.001New%20Issue%20for%20June%202011 (accessed October, 2013.)

40. Guyatt, G., Oxman, A.D., and Akl, E.A. (2011) GRADE guidelines: 1. Introduction—GRADE evidence profiles and summary of findings tables. *J Clin Epidemiol* 64, 383–394. Accessed online (17/7/2014) at: http://www.jclinepi.com/article/S0895-4356%2810%2900330-6/fulltext"\l"sec5"http://www.jclinepi.com/article/S0895-4356%2810%2900330-6/fulltext#sec5.

41. Carstairs, V. and Morris, R. (1989) Deprivation, mortality and resource allocation. *Commun Med* 11, 364–372.

42. Carstairs' Deprivation Index for Scottish Postcode Sectors, 1991 and 2001. www.datalib.ed.ac.uk/EUDL/carstairs.html. (1989).

43. Morgan, O. and Baker, A. (2006) Measuring deprivation in England and Wales using 2001 Carstairs scores. *Health Statist Quarter* 31, 28–33. Available online at: www.statistics.gov.uk/articles/hsq/HSQ31deprivation_using_carstairs.pdf.

44. Pawson, R. and Tilley, N. (1997). *Realistic Evaluation*. London, UK: Sage Publications.

45. WHO. (2001) Evaluation in health promotion. Principles and perspectives. WHO Regional Publications, European Series, no. 92.

46. Pawson, R. (2006) Realist methodology. In *Evidence-Based Policy*. London, UK: Sage Publications, pp. 17–37.

47. Victora, C.G., Vaughan, J.P., Barros, F.C., Silva, A.C., and Tomasi, E. (2000) Available from http://www.thelancet.com/journals/lancet/article/PIIS0140-6736(00)02741-0/abstract.

48. Hargreaves, J.R., Calum Davey, C., and White, R.G. (2012) Does the "inverse equity hypothesis" explain how both poverty and wealth can be associated with HIV prevalence in sub-Saharan Africa? *J Epidemiol Community Health*. doi:10.1136/jech-2012-201876. Accessed online (17/7/2014) at: http://jech.bmj.com/content/early/2012/12/11/jech-2012-201876.extract.

49. Baker, R., Robertson, N., and Farooqi, A. (1995) Audit in general practice: Factors influencing participation. *BMJ* 311, 31–34.

50. Johnston, G., Crombie, I.K., Davies, H.T.O. et al. (2000) Reviewing audit: barriers and facilitating factors for effective clinical audit. *Qual Health Care* 9, 23–26.

51. Fiander, M. and Burns, T. (2000) A Delphi approach to describing service models of community mental health practice. *Psychiatry Services* 51, 656–658.

52. Manuel, D.G., Lim, J., Tanuseputro, P. et al. (2006) Revisting rose: Strategies for reducing coronary heart disease. *BMJ* 332, 659–662.

53. Jackson, R. (2006) Preventing coronary heart disease: Does Rose's population prevention axiom still apply in the 21st century? *BMJ* 332, 617.

54. Rose, G., *The Strategy of Preventive Medicine*. Oxford: Oxford University Press, 1992.

55. WHO. (1986) Ottawa Charter for Health Promotion. First International Conference on Health Promotion, Ottawa, Ontario, Canada, November 21, 1986. WHO/HPR/HEP/95.1. Geneva, Switzerland: WHO. Available online at: www.who.int/hpr/NPH/docs/ottawa_charter_hp.pdf.

56. International Association for Impact Assessment. (2006) Health impact assessment: International best practice principles. Accessed online (17/7/2014) at: http://www.iaia.org/publicdocuments/special-publications/SP5.pdf.

57. Mitchell, K.R. and Wellings, K. (2013) Measuring sexual function in community surveys: Development of a conceptual framework. *J Sex Res* 50(1), 17–28. Accessed online (17/7/2014) at: http://www.ncbi.nlm.nih.gov/pubmed/22047590.

58. Mitchell, K.R., Ploubidis, G.B., Datta, J., and Wellings, K. (2012) The Natsal-SF: A validated measure of sexual function for use in community surveys. *Eur J Epidemiol* 27(6), 409–418. Accessed online (17/7/2014) at: http://www.ncbi.nlm.nih.gov/pmc/articles/PMC3382648/ doi: 10.1080/00224499.2011.621038. Epub 2011 Nov 2.

59. Anderson, C. (October 11, 2010) Presenting and evaluating qualitative research. *Am J Pharm Educ* 74(8), 141. PMCID: PMC2987281 Presenting and Available from: http://www.ncbi.nlm.nih.gov/pmc/articles/PMC2987281 Evaluating Qualitative Research.

60. Noble, M., Dibben, C., and Wright, G. (2010) *The South African Index of Multiple Deprivation 2007 at Datazone Level (modelled)*. Pretoria, South Africa: Department of Social Development.

61. OCEBM Levels of Evidence Working Group. The Oxford 2011 Levels of Evidence. Oxford Centre for Evidence- Based Medicine. Available from: http://www.cebm.net/index.aspx?o=5653.

62. Department of Health (2013) Patient Reported Outcome Measures (PROMs): Update on data collection. Accessed online (17/7/2014) at: http: //www.dh.gov.uk/health/2013/01/proms-data-collection/.

63. Rist, R.C. (1994) Influencing the policy process with qualitative research. In N. Denzin and Y. Lincoln (eds.) *Handbook of Qualitative Research*. Thousand Oaks, CA: Sage Publications, Inc., pp. 545–557.

64. Maxwell, R.J. (1992) Dimensions of quality revisited: From thought to action. *Qual Health Care* 1(3): 171–177. Accessed online (17/7/2014) at: http://www.ncbi.nlm.nih.gov/pmc/articles/PMC1055007/?page=1

Section 2

DISEASE CAUSATION AND THE DIAGNOSTIC PROCESS IN RELATION TO PUBLIC HEALTH

Prevention and Health Promotion

In order to improve the health of a population, practitioners need a broad understanding of what affects the health of an individual and the evidence base behind approaches to improve it.

Section 2 covers a wide range of subjects, starting with an introduction to different ways of conceptualising the study of disease in **epidemiological paradigms**. The fundamentals of how disease is caused and where threats to health originate are covered in the sections on the **epidemiology** of specific diseases, the environment, genetic factors, communicable diseases, and **health and social behaviour**. Finally, the theory and practice of protecting and improving health is covered in the sections on **diagnosis and screening**, **health promotion,** and **disease prevention**.

2A

Epidemiological Paradigms

There exist a wide range of epidemiological paradigms that propose different explanations for variations in health experiences and the prevalence of disease. Public health practitioners need an awareness of these different paradigms in order to understand when and how diseases develop, as well as where best to target public health actions.

Three common paradigms for explaining how risk factors at different stages in life may lead to ill health are the following:

1. Programming approach
2. Adult risk factor approach
3. Life-course approach

2A.1 Programming, life-course, and adult risk factor approaches

Each of the following three paradigms can be used as a way of considering the epidemiological influences on an individual during the life course.

Programming

This epidemiological paradigm considers the **long-term effects of environmental exposures** during **critical periods** of growth, including in utero development and early life. Programming is also known as the 'critical period model' because it assumes that there are specific periods during which certain exposures will have lasting effects on the structure or function of body organs.

The classic example of this is the **Barker hypothesis,** which states that an effect of in utero malnutrition is an increased risk of coronary heart disease (CHD) in adulthood. This hypothesis has since been extended to a wide range of chronic diseases, such as type 2 diabetes and hypertension.

Adult risk factor

The *adult risk factor approach,* in use since the 1950s, considers the impact of **lifestyle** and **behaviours** on the onset and progression of diseases, including smoking, diet, exercise, and alcohol consumption. One disease may have multiple risk factors; and one behaviour may be a risk factor for multiple diseases. The relative contributory effects of different risk factors can be assessed using multiple regression analysis.

Life course

The life-course model combines elements of the **programming** and the **adult risk factor** paradigms. It considers how various biological and social factors throughout gestation and life affect health and disease in adult life independently, cumulatively, and interactively. For example, one model proposes that different risk factors may accumulate throughout life, that they exhibit a dose–response effect, and that they have long-term consequences.

A limitation of this paradigm is that few researchers will have access to a sufficiently wide range of biological and social data on large, longitudinal cohorts of subjects in order to assess the outcomes of interest.

2B

Epidemiology of Specific Diseases

Epidemiology of specific diseases (and their risk factors) of public health significance.

This section covers the occurrence and distribution of certain key diseases within the population. Clearly, it is impossible for anyone to have an encyclopaedic knowledge of all diseases. However, it is important that public health specialists have an overview of the epidemiology of those diseases that are of particular public health concern in order to guide them in prioritising, organising, and allocating resources.

The key public health diseases are either

- Frequent causes of **premature death** (e.g. cardiovascular disease, cancers, trauma)
- Common causes of **morbidity** or the high use of healthcare resources (e.g. diabetes, asthma and chronic obstructive pulmonary disease (COPD), depression, schizophrenia, Alzheimer's disease)
- Sharply **changing** in their **incidence or prevalence** in a particular area of the world (e.g. obesity in developed countries)
- Often **preventable** (e.g. lung cancer)

2B.1 'Important' diseases

Knowledge of the defining clinical features, distribution, causes, behavioural features, and determinants of diseases that currently make a significant impact on the health of local populations, with particular reference to those that are potentially preventable; require the planned provision of health services at individual, community, and structural levels; or are otherwise of particular public concern, for example, mental health.

The World Health Organisation's (WHO) **global burden of disease** project provides an estimate of the relative importance of all communicable and non-communicable diseases, together with 'intentional harms' such as suicide and war. The global burden of disease does not account for the degree to which illnesses are preventable or can be treated. Instead, it provides a useful guide to which illnesses have the greatest impact on morbidity and mortality in the world—and thus their public health importance.

EUR As Figure 2B.1 shows, neurological, cancer, cardiovascular disease, musculoskeletal disorders, and mental and behavioural disorders account for most of the burden of disease in Western Europe. The burden of a particular disease depends very much on the setting: communicable disease and maternal, perinatal, and nutritional conditions are responsible for most of the mortality in Africa. In Europe, by contrast, non-communicable disease accounts for over 80% of mortality.

Similarly, the burden of different diseases varies across the age groups. Although there is some variation in the age at which the major non-communicable diseases have the highest incidence, the burden is consistently highest in people aged over 70 as exemplified by mortality from cardiovascular and circulatory diseases (see Figure 2B.2).

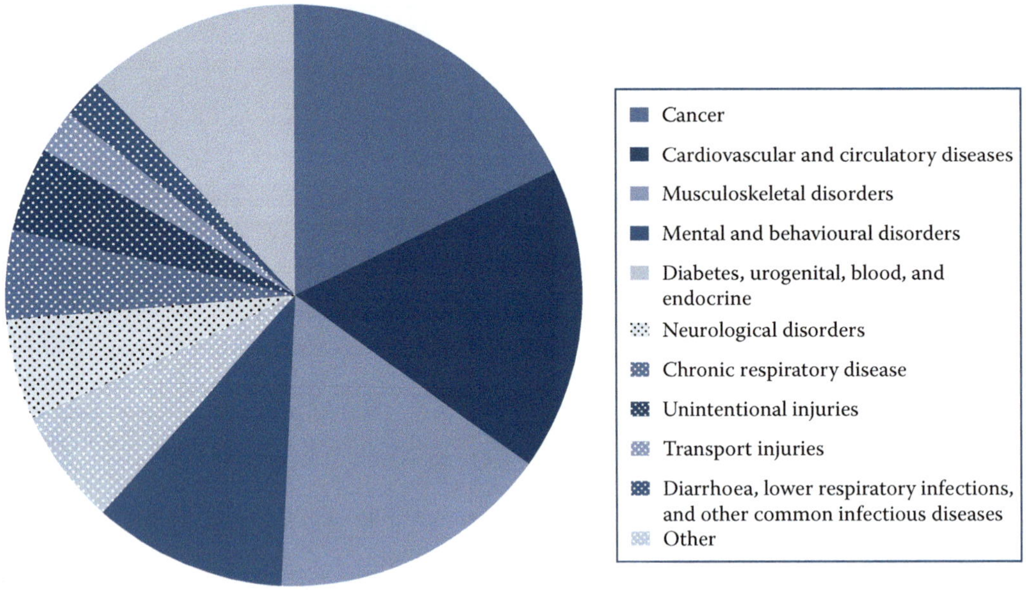

Figure 2B.1 Disability adjusted life years (DALYs) by cause, Western Europe (2010). (From *Global Burden of Disease study 2010*; http://www.healthmetricsandevaluation.org/gbd/visualizations/gbd-2010-patterns-broad-cause-group?unit=pc&sex=B&metric=daly&stackBy=region&year=5.)

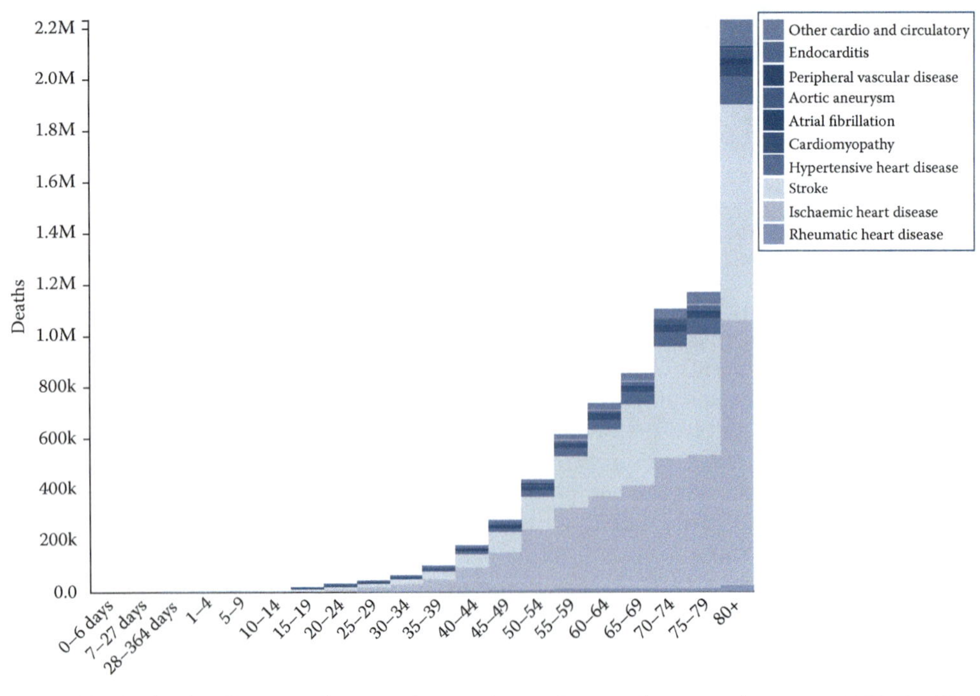

Figure 2B.2 Global deaths from cardiovascular and circulatory diseases by age (2010). (From *Global Burden of Disease study 2010*; http://www.healthmetricsandevaluation.org/gbd/visualizations/gbd-2010-patterns-broad-cause-group?unit=pc&sex=B&metric=daly&stackBy=region&year=5.)

Public health disease knowledge

The descriptive aspects of disease that are most important to public health specialists are

- Incidence and prevalence
- Morbidity and mortality
- **Burden** (e.g. population attributable risk (PAR) fraction of a risk factor such as hypertension or the number of disability-adjusted life years (DALYs) caused by a disease)
- **Time** (trends—whether the incidence is rising or falling)
- **Place** (whether there are areas where the disease is particularly common or rare)
- **Person** (the type of person who is most at risk, with regard to demographics, lifestyle, health circumstances, and workplace)
- **Prevention** (primary, secondary [early detection through tests/screening], and tertiary)

Tables 2B.1 through 2B.12 cover the aspects of non-communicable diseases that have a notable impact on the burden of disease in developed countries or are otherwise of considerable public health importance.

Neuropsychiatric conditions

Table 2B.1 Depression

Feature	Description
Clinical characteristics	Depression is a mood disorder characterised by low mood that (1) exceeds normal sadness or grief in intensity or duration and (2) is accompanied by functional disabilities. Symptoms include negative thoughts, low mood, lack of positive emotions ('anhedonia'), and changes in bodily functions such as disturbed appetite, early-morning wakening, and reduced libido. Other mood disorders include *major depression* (which may be psychotic or non-psychotic) and bipolar disorder (characterised by pronounced mood swings).
Known causes/ aetiological mechanisms	The causes are debated. Depression involves neurochemical abnormalities, hormonal risk factors, and genetic characteristics and may be triggered by adverse life events or social conditions.
Public health relevance	Commonest psychological disorder. The 2nd highest cause of disability globally as measured by years lost due to disability (YLDs) in 2010. The 11th leading contributor to the global burden of disease (DALYs) in 2010. Can mostly be diagnosed and treated in primary care.
Prevalence in the United Kingdom	Half of all women and a quarter of all men will have a depressive episode in their lifetime.
Time	Increasing incidence worldwide.
Place	People living in deprived industrial areas are more likely to be treated for depression than people living in other areas.
Person	**Gender**: women > men. **Age**: increasing incidence with increasing age. **Ethnicity**: sometimes seen as a Western construct; there may be under-detection in some cultures.

(*continued*)

Table 2B.1 *(Continued)* Depression

Feature	Description
	Socio-economic circumstances: unemployed people are twice as likely to have depression than those in employment. **Life events**: depression can follow adverse life events (e.g. divorce, bereavement, redundancy). **Disease**: may follow chronic or serious disease or occur during or after pregnancy. **Family**: increased risk in people with a family history of depression.
Prevention	**Secondary**: effective treatment to prevent long-term sickness and reduce the risk of suicide.

Table 2B.2 Suicide and parasuicide

Feature	Description
Clinical characteristics	Suicide is the act of intentionally causing one's own death, whereas parasuicide is an unsuccessful suicide attempt. Over half the people who complete suicide have a history of parasuicide. In the United Kingdom, as in many countries, the determination of suicide as a cause of death is based on a coroner's verdict and not on medical opinion. It has been suggested that when monitoring suicide prevalence, unexplained deaths should also be reported, since many of these may be suicides [3].
Public health relevance	A leading cause of death among young adults. Recent increases associated with the global financial crisis.
Prevalence in the United Kingdom	Suicide rate ~8 per 100,000 per year.
Time	Strong decline in the 1960s attributed to the switch from coal gas to safer natural gas.
Place	Between 2008 and 2010, the United Kingdom saw an increase in suicides thought to be associated with the financial crisis [4]. Within the United Kingdom, suicide rates are higher than average in London. In Europe, Sweden and Hungary have some of the highest rates, while Catholic countries tend to have lower recorded rates.
Person	**Gender**: men > women. **Age**: rates are higher in people aged over 50. **Socio-economic circumstances**: highest among low-income groups, especially in unemployed and homeless people. **Disease**: associated with mental illness including depression and schizophrenia; however, there is frequently no history of mental illness. **Family**: higher rates among single, widowed, or divorced people.
Prevention	Primary: addresses risk factors (e.g. through active labour market programmes, family support programmes, and debt relief programmes). Secondary: through management of mental illness and people with a history of parasuicide.

Table 2B.3 Dementia

Clinical characteristics	Dementia is a neurodegenerative syndrome involving memory loss, confusion, and problems with speech and understanding. The two principal types are **Alzheimer's disease** and **vascular dementia**. Other forms include dementia with Lewy bodies, excessive alcohol use, and the Creutzfeldt–Jakob disease (CJD).
Known causes/ aetiological mechanisms	Loss of acetylcholine receptors and neurons in the brain occurs in Alzheimer's disease. Vascular dementia includes single-infarct dementia following a stroke and multi-infarct dementia following multiple very small strokes.
Public health relevance	Dementia is growing in prevalence and importance as the population ages. There are no cures for most forms of dementia. Acetylcholinesterase inhibitors are currently recommended by NICE for treating mild to moderate disease but have only modest efficacy. Dementia is extremely costly in terms of the burden it places on unpaid carers. It is also extremely costly in terms of healthcare and social care services. The UK government is committed to increasing the funding for dementia from £26.6 m in 2010 to £66 m in 2015. Plans have been proposed to include dementia screening in the NHS.
Prevalence in the United Kingdom	One person in 20 aged over 65 years and one person in 5 over 80 years of age develops dementia.
Time	Prevalence steadily rising, as proportion of older people in the population increases.
Place	Prevalence higher in countries with older populations (e.g. Western Europe has a higher prevalence than South Asia or Africa).
Person	**Gender**: risk slightly greater for women than men. **Age**: risk increases with age (see prevalence). **Lifestyle**: risks include smoking; sedentary lifestyle; high-fat, high-salt diet that increases risk of vascular dementia; and excessive alcohol (Korsakoff's syndrome). **Disease/disability**: associated with hypertension, hypercholesterolaemia, obesity, and Down's syndrome. **Family**: genetic risk of early-onset forms of Alzheimer's disease with the apolipoprotein E4 (*APOE4*) allele. **Other**: protective factors include exercise, healthy diet, and undertaking memory and cognition exercises (e.g. doing crosswords); head injury may increase risk.
Prevention	**Secondary**: people with mild memory loss are encouraged to use their memory and cognitive skills to preserve them

Table 2B.4 Schizophrenia

Clinical characteristics	A chronic, often lifelong, psychotic condition or group of conditions characterised by three types of symptom: • **Positive**: third-person auditory hallucinations, delusions • **Negative**: flat affect, low mood, withdrawal from social life, lack of motivation • **Cognitive**: memory, concentration problems Symptoms develop gradually: before diagnosis, a patient's behaviour and mood may have been deteriorating for some several years. Treatment can control many of the symptoms but may also lead to severe side effects such as drowsiness and blurred vision (short term) or (with older drugs) movement disorders such as *tardive dyskinesia* (long term).
Known causes/ aetiological mechanisms	Unknown. Studies have investigated neuroanatomical and neurochemical abnormalities, including larger ventricles and an imbalance in serotonin and dopamine transmission. Twin studies and other family studies indicate a genetic element. Injury and infection during pregnancy or early in life have also been investigated.
Public health relevance	High burden of disease since it is a chronic illness. Associated with a higher risk of mortality from physical illness, injury, and suicide. Diagnosis/definition and treatment may be controversial. Often requires treatment under a section of the Mental Health Act. Stigmatised condition.
Prevalence in the United Kingdom	1% lifetime prevalence.
Time	Health service data suggest falling incidence in the United Kingdom since the 1960s but lack of good corroborating evidence.
Place	Commoner in urban areas than in rural. Worldwide incidence fairly similar.
Person	**Gender**: men > women. **Age**: onset usually late adolescence. Rarely presents below age 10 or above age 40. **Ethnicity**: high rates of diagnosis in African–Caribbean people but could be an artefact, possibly due to over diagnosis. **Socio-economic circumstances**: commoner in low-income groups, especially homeless people, and in prisoners—but note the *social drift* caused by schizophrenia. **Lifestyle**: associated with cannabis. **Disease**: associated with other forms of psychosis (e.g. post-pregnancy, drug-induced psychosis). **Family**: higher risk if a family member is affected. **Other**: symptoms appear after stressful life events.
Prevention	**Secondary**: symptom control with antipsychotics and psychosocial therapies (e.g. CBT) **Early intervention**: to promote early detection of psychosis and treatment.

Table 2B.5 Parkinson's disease

Clinical characteristics	Progressive neurodegenerative condition leading to loss of dopamine-containing cells in the *substantia nigra*. Symptoms include disordered movements, such as walking, swallowing, and writing.
Known causes/ aetiological mechanisms	Unknown. Most cases are idiopathic. Genetic studies have identified several candidate genes (e.g. *parkin*).
Public health relevance	Parkinson's disease is a common cause of falls, fractures, and hospital admissions and is a costly disease, especially in the later stages, due to its social care burden. Diagnosis can be difficult in the early stages—there are no laboratory tests—since symptoms develop gradually and may be mistaken for normal ageing.
Prevalence in the United Kingdom	Approximately 200 per 100,000 although misdiagnosis and undiagnosed cases are common.
Time	No marked geographical variation. Prevalence stable, but mortality for patients aged under 75 years is decreasing with better treatment.
Person	**Gender**: men slightly more than women. **Age**: prevalence rises with age (up to 2% of the population aged 80 and over affected). Around 1 in 7 cases is diagnosed below the age of 60 years (1 in 10 cases below age 40). **Family**: mostly sporadic. **Others**: Older antipsychotic drugs can induce symptoms of parkinsonism, as does the recreational drug MPTP. Head trauma (e.g. through boxing) can increase risk of Parkinson's disease. Environmental exposures, such as herbicides, are possibly linked.

Cardiovascular diseases

Table 2B.6 CHD

Clinical characteristics	Angina, which may be *stable* (chest discomfort on exertion or under emotional stress) or *unstable* (chest discomfort at rest). Myocardial infarction (MI) ('heart attack')—ischaemia of the myocardium, leading to chest/arm discomfort, sweating, shortness of breath, nausea. Heart failure—ineffective pumping by the heart, resulting in breathlessness, oedema, tiredness. Stroke—see Table 2B.7. Peripheral artery disease—leading to claudication and ischaemia. Cardiac arrest—abrupt cessation of pumping by the heart, which may be *shockable* or *non-shockable*. Cardiovascular disease is the commonest cause of cardiac arrest.
Known causes/ aetiological mechanisms	Atherosclerosis (narrowing of the coronary arteries due to a build-up of fat) leads to vessel stenosis. Ischaemia occurs if the artery becomes occluded. Heart failure results from cardiac ischaemia.
Public health relevance	Leading individual cause of death in England (65,000 deaths in 2010[5]). Potentially preventable. Source of health inequalities: disproportionately affects people in deprived areas.
Incidence in the United Kingdom	200 cases of MI per 100,000 population per year.
Time	Mortality rates fell by about 70% in the United Kingdom between 1980 and 2010.
Place	Geographical inequalities: Scotland has a higher mortality than England; deprived areas have higher prevalence than affluent areas.
Person	**Gender**: men > women (but risk for women increases after the menopause). **Age**: risk increases with age. **Ethnicity**: mortality greater for South Asian population in the United Kingdom, low prevalence in Chinese and African–Caribbean populations. **Socio-economic circumstances**: higher mortality in people on lower incomes age <75. **Lifestyle**: smoking, sedentary lifestyle, high-fat/high-salt diet; heavy drinking (light drinking may be protective), stress. **Disease**: diabetes, hypertension, hypercholesterolaemia, obesity. **Family**: family history is a risk factor. Some rare genetic risk factors (e.g. familial hypercholesterolaemia).
Prevention	**Primary**: lifestyle measures to reduce smoking, encourage physical activity, balanced diet. **Secondary**: providing treatment for high-risk people (e.g. people who have already had an MI and people with diabetes or hypertension).

Table 2B.7 Stroke

Clinical characteristics	Stroke is a form of cardiovascular disease affecting the brain (i.e. it is a form of cerebrovascular disease). Two major types of stroke: • **Ischaemic stroke** (most strokes) is caused by thrombosis or embolism causing an occlusion of a cerebral blood vessel, leading to cerebral ischaemia. • **Haemorrhagic strokes** are caused by burst blood vessels. **Transient ischaemic attacks** (TIAs) occur when blood supply to the brain is interrupted for a short time. They are similar to strokes but the symptoms resolve within 24 h. Common signs of stroke include weakness or paralysis on one side of the body (apraxia), slurred speech (dysarthria) or difficulty finding words (aphasia), loss of sight/blurred vision, and confusion or unsteadiness. Longer-term effects depend on the affected part of the brain, the severity of the stroke, and the general health of the patient.
Public health relevance	Third commonest cause of death in the United Kingdom and commonest cause of disability. Potentially preventable with lifestyle changes and medication. High burden on unpaid carers and social care services.
Incidence in the United Kingdom	Approximately 200 people per 100,000 population per year.
Time	Age-adjusted incidence declining in Western Europe but overall incidence increasing due to ageing population.
Person	**Gender**: men > women (though risk for women increases after menopause). **Age**: risk increases with age. **Ethnicity**: higher risk for South Asian, African, African–Caribbean. **Socio-economic circumstances**: higher mortality (in under 75s) in people on lower incomes. **Lifestyle**: smoking, sedentary lifestyle, high-salt/high-fat diet, heavy drinking (via hypertension). **Disease**: hypertension, coronary artery disease, obesity, diabetes, hypercholesterolaemia, previous stroke, or TIA. **Family**: higher risk if a family member has had a stroke.
Prevention	**Primary**: lifestyle modification to increase exercise, eat a healthy diet, and reduce alcohol intake; hypertension screening and treatment; cholesterol screening and treatment; anticoagulation for people with atrial fibrillation (or another risk factor) to risk of emboli. **Secondary** (after a stroke): multidisciplinary care on a stroke unit, lifestyle modification, anticoagulation, hypertension monitoring and treatment, peer support, awareness campaigns and reconfiguration of services to promote earlier recognition of stroke, and faster care to improve outcomes (e.g. *FAST* campaign—face, arms, speech, time [6].)

Common western forms of cancer in Western Europe

Table 2B.8 Common cancers

Cancer type	Breast	Lung	Colorectal/ bowel	Prostate	Cervical
Public health relevance	Major cause of mortality in women, rare in men. Better prognosis with early detection and treatment. Controversy over benefits of screening.	High case fatality rate, which has barely decreased. Large proportion of cases preventable.	Known risk factors. Better prognosis with early detection and treatment.	Relatively high incidence in older men. Controversy over benefits of screening.	Common cause of cancer in women. Early detection improves prognosis. Risk factors linked to social exclusion (social deprivation, STIs, etc.).
Incidence in the United Kingdom [7] (2010) (per 100,000 per year)	80	67	66	66	5
5-year survival (%)	85	8	55	80	65
Time/place	Survival improving in the United Kingdom.	Survival *not* improving.	Survival rate improving; higher in countries with Western-style diet.	Survival rate improving; more men die *with* it than *from* it.	Second most common cancer in women aged <35; higher in countries with high prevalence of HPV.
Person	**Gender**: women > men **Age**: greater proportion of cases in older women. **Deprivation**: higher incidence in more affluent communities	**Gender**: men > women but increasing number of women affected **Age**: 95% occur in over 50s. **Deprivation**: death rates higher in more deprived communities	**Gender**: men ≥ women (12:10) **Age**: 90% occur in over 50s. **Health**: bowel polyp, previous bowel cancer; obesity, inflammatory bowel disease, familial adenomatous polyposis	**Gender**: men only **Age**: rare under 50 years. **Ethnicity**: most common in men of African descent, least common in Asian men **Genetics**: rare but links to *BRCA-2*.	**Gender**: women only **Age**: median age at diagnosis is 48. **Deprivation**: higher incidence in deprived than affluent women

Table 2B.8 *(Continued)* Common cancers

Cancer type	Breast	Lung	Colorectal/ bowel	Prostate	Cervical
	Ethnicity: less common in groups that start families early (e.g. Bangladeshi). **Genetics**: ~5% of cancers due to genetic factors, mainly *BRCA-1* or *BRCA-2*. **Lifestyle**: exercise and breastfeeding are protective.	**Exposure**: asbestos, radon. **Lifestyle**: smoking (9/10 cases), passive smoking; diet high in fruit and vegetables may lower risk.	**Lifestyle**: diet high in meat and fat, low in fibre. Lack of exercise and high waist circumference increase risk. **Genetic**: increased risk if first-degree relative affected. Rare genetic risk factors: polyposis coli, HNPCC.	**Exposure**: radiation.	**Health**: HPV infection strong risk factor; vaccine introduced in England for girls; immunosuppression due to smoking and HIV. Poor diet increases risk. **Lifestyle**: many sexual partners/ sex at an early age increases risk.
Prevention	**Secondary**: Screening programme via mammogram for women aged 50–70.	**Primary**: Reduce smoking prevalence, exposure to carcinogens (e.g. asbestos) **Secondary**: None available but trials ongoing	**Primary**: Diet (cut meat, add fibre), reduce central obesity. **Secondary**: Screening programme: faecal occult blood test age 60–74.	No evidence based prevention strategies. Screening via prostate specific antigen (PSA) not recommended in England.	**Primary**: Safer sex, HPV vaccine, stop smoking. **Secondary**: Screening programme in England for women aged 25–64 years every 3–5 years via liquid-based cytology.

See Section 2C.1 for more detail on screening programmes.

Respiratory diseases

Table 2B.9 Asthma

Clinical characteristics	A chronic, inflammatory condition marked by episodes of shortness of breath, coughing or wheezing, reversible airway obstruction. Triggers vary between individuals.
Public health relevance	Commonest chronic disease in childhood; rising prevalence. Emergency admissions for asthma are included in the *Compendium of Public Health Indicators* as a measure of healthcare performance because admissions can generally be avoided through effective management in primary care or at home (i.e. it is an ambulatory care sensitive [ACS] condition).
Prevalence in the United Kingdom	Lifetime prevalence approximately 1 in 9 [8].
Time	Increasing lifetime prevalence but decreasing incidence.
Place	No clear geographical pattern of asthma occurrence in the United Kingdom but markedly different prevalence across the globe (range, 1%–18%).
Person	**Age**: higher prevalence in children than in adults. **Gender**: commoner in boys than girls. **Family/genetics**: genetic component—higher risk if a family member has atopy (asthma, eczema, or hay fever). **Risk factors** for asthma exacerbations depend on the individual but commonly include the following: • **Lifestyle**: smoking; certain foods (e.g. dairy products, preservatives); exercise; cold air • **Health**: viral infections (e.g. influenza, common cold); stress • **Exposures**: air pollution (e.g. ozone, traffic fumes, tobacco smoke); house dust mite faeces; pollen
Prevention	Secondary avoiding triggers. Annual influenza vaccine. Preventative medications (e.g. inhaled steroids).

Table 2B.10 COPD

Clinical characteristics	COPD is a disease involving chronic bronchitis and emphysema. In contrast to asthma, airflow obstruction is not fully reversible and is usually progressive.
Public health relevance	Potentially avoidable disease since most cases are linked to smoking (80%) or occupational exposure, especially mining and welding. Can remain undiagnosed for years until symptoms are severe. Up to 1 in 8 emergency hospital admissions may be due to COPD. Commonest cause of readmission in many hospitals. High burden of morbidity and mortality (sixth leading cause of death worldwide).
Prevalence in the United Kingdom[a]	Around 1300 per 100,000 people in the United Kingdom have been diagnosed as having COPD (roughly a 1 in 60 lifetime incidence), with many more undiagnosed cases.
Time **Place**	Incidence seems to have peaked recently but prevalence continues to increase (increased survival) [9].
Person	**Gender**: mortality increasing in women, falling in men.[b] **Age**: prevalence increases with increasing age. **Socio-economic circumstances**: more prevalent in lower income groups. **Lifestyle**: smoking. **Other**: occupation, e.g. inhaling airborne particulates.
Prevention	**Primary prevention**: stop-smoking initiatives and avoiding occupational exposure. **Secondary prevention**: medication to control symptoms, home supplemental oxygen, physiotherapy, exercise to reduce disability, influenza and pneumococcal vaccinations.[c]

[a] QOF data.
[b] Mortality of incidence or prevalence?
[c] QOF register?

Other disorders

Table 2B.11 Sickle cell disease

Clinical characteristics	Genetic condition leading to abnormal haemoglobin leads to anaemia, episodic severe pain, immunosuppression, and sometimes chronic kidney disease or bone damage. Carriers (people with sickle cell trait who have only one affected haemoglobin gene) do not have symptoms but may have difficulty with activities requiring exertion or high oxygen demand (e.g. scuba diving, mountain climbing).
Known causes/aetiological mechanisms	Genetic: recessively inherited.
Public health relevance	Health inequalities—in the United Kingdom mainly affects people of African and Caribbean communities. Prenatal testing can be conducted by amniocentesis and chorionic villous sampling (CVS). Antenatal and neonatal screening is recommended for at-risk groups.
Prevalence in the United Kingdom	African and Caribbean descent: 1 in 10–40 has sickle cell trait; 1 in 60–200 has sickle cell disease. UK prevalence around 20 per 100,000 population [9a].
Place	Common in parts of sub-Saharan African and the Caribbean but also the Middle East, parts of the eastern Mediterranean, and Asia.
Person	**Age**: occurs from birth. **Ethnicity**: incidence in people originally from Africa, the Caribbean, the eastern Mediterranean, Middle East, and Asia. **Family**: recessively inherited.
Prevention	Identification of affected fetuses through screening programme.

Table 2B.12 Diabetes

Clinical characteristics	Multisystem disease characterised by hyperglycaemia. Diagnosis according to WHO is fasting plasma glucose >7 mmol/L on two separate occasions or an HbA1c >6.5%.
	Poorly controlled diabetes leads to range of
	• *Acute* complications (e.g. hypoglycaemia, diabetic ketoacidosis)
	• *Chronic* complications, which may be
	  • *Large-vessel* (coronary artery disease, peripheral vascular disease)
	  • *Small-vessel* (retinopathy, nephropathy)
	There are two principal types:
	Type 1—always requires insulin for treatment ('insulin-controlled diabetes')
	Type 2—most common type of diabetes (90% of all cases). May be treated with diet ('diet-controlled diabetes'), oral medication ('tablet-controlled diabetes'), or insulin ('insulin-requiring diabetes')

Known causes/ aetiological mechanisms	Type 1 diabetes is an autoimmune disease in which there is a shortage of insulin-producing islet cells in the pancreas. In type 2 diabetes, the body produces insufficient insulin because of resistance to insulin.
Public health relevance	Incidence increasing, especially type 2 diabetes in children and adolescents. Around 5% of the NHS budget is spent on treating the complications of diabetes.
Prevalence in the United Kingdom	The prevalence of diabetes mellitus in the United Kingdom was approximately 4.45% in 2011 (around 90% type 2 diabetes). Regional prevalence may be estimated using models such as the Association of Public Health Observatories (*APHO*) *Diabetes Prevalence Model*. Diabetes registers in primary care can provide estimates of the diagnosed cases in a GP-registered population; however, people typically have type 2 diabetes for 6–7 years before diagnosis.
Time	Worldwide incidence increasing.
Place	Common in some communities (e.g. Pima Indians, Pacific Islanders, South Asian communities in the United Kingdom).
Person	**Age**: type 1 onset in childhood, declining incidence thereafter; type 2 incidence in adults usually aged 40 or more but increasingly seen in children with obesity. **Ethnicity**: high in populations of South Asian and African–Caribbean origin (e.g. four times more prevalent in people of Bangladeshi descent that in the general population). **Socio-economic circumstances**: more prevalent in people with lower incomes. **Disease/health**: obesity (particularly central obesity) has a strong association with type 2 diabetes; risk of gestational diabetes in pregnancy. **Lifestyle**: inactivity/high-calorific diet. **Family**: particularly for type 1. Also inherited forms of type 2 diabetes.
Prevention	**Primary**: weight management (diet and exercise) can reduce the risk of type 2. **Secondary**: risk of diabetes complications mitigated by exercise, self-management, medication (especially antihypertensives).

2C

Diagnosis and Screening

Diagnosis and screening are linked processes that have implications which span from the individual patient through to entire populations. Screening is an example of a practical public health intervention that has the potential to save thousands of lives. As with any clinical intervention, however, it has the potential to do more harm than good. As we shall see, the question of whether or not to offer a particular screening programme is far more complex than it might at first appear.

2C.1 Screening for diseases

Principles, methods, applications, and organisation of screening for early detection, prevention, treatment, and control of disease.

The aim of screening is to reduce the harm caused by a disease or its complications. Screening is a service in which members of a defined population at risk of the disease are asked a question or offered a test to **identify those individuals who are more likely to be helped than harmed by further tests** or treatment. A screening test does *not* diagnose the disease: this is usually made using a subsequent *diagnostic* test.

Screening programmes vary from country to country in terms of

- Diseases that are screened
- Target age groups
- Frequency of testing
- Tests used

Principles

The UK National Screening Committee (NSC) defines screening as

> *a process of identifying* **apparently healthy people** *who may be at* **increased risk** *of a disease or condition. They can then be offered information, further tests and appropriate treatment* **to reduce their risk** *and/or any complications arising from the disease or condition.*

In order for screening to be successful, certain prerequisites must be met regarding the **disease**, the **test,** the **treatment,** and the **programme.** These are covered in more detail in Section 2C.8 but Table 2C.1

Table 2C.1 Organisation of screening

Consideration	Details	Further reading
Identifying and inviting participants	Agreeing who to target (e.g. what age), identifying individuals (e.g. through practice register, inviting through letter or by sending a test kit).	Section 2C.8
Informing participants	Informing participants of the benefits and risks of participation.	Sections 2C.7 and 2C.8
Selecting the screening test	Based on reliability, acceptability, validity (sensitivity/ specificity), cost-effectiveness, feasibility, availability of resources, etc.	Sections 2C.2 and 2C.8
Setting a threshold	Choosing a threshold for the screening test that best distinguishes 'normal' from 'abnormal'.	Section 2C.2
Diagnostic phase	Although an intervention may directly follow screening, normally a further diagnostic test is done.	Sections 2C.3 and 2C.8
Treatment phase	If a diagnosis is made, treatment is offered.	Section 2C.8
Evaluation	Including both the ongoing quality assurance for continuous improvement of how the programme is running and evaluation of the effectiveness of screening.	See Section 2C.8

provides an overview of the organising principles of a screening programme.

Methods and applications

UK National Screening Programmes

UK In the United Kingdom, the NSC is responsible for decision about whether to introduce, modify, or withdraw a particular screening programme (see Section 2C.10). The committee keeps under review the evidence in favour and against screening for over 100 diseases. The programmes it currently recommends are listed in the tables shown later (Tables 2C.2 through 2C.5).

ENG In England, there are other interventions that are typically referred to as 'screening' but which do not form part of a NSC-approved systematic population screening programme and are not managed by the NSC. Some of these are listed in Table 2C.6.

Programmes in individual countries

AUS Details of the Australian and South African screening programmes are shown in Tables 2C.7 and 2C.8.

Table 2C.2 Antenatal screening programme

Weeks into pregnancy	Screening test	To test for
0–12 (or asap)	Maternal blood test	Infectious diseases (HIV, syphilis, hepatitis B, rubella immunity)
0–12 (or asap)	Maternal blood test for blood group and rhesus D status	Haemolytic diseases, anaemia
0–12 (or asap)	Maternal blood test	Sickle cell and thalassaemia
8–12	Maternal blood test Ultrasound scan (nuchal translucency)	Down's syndrome
18–21	Ultrasound scan	Fetal anomalies (e.g. spina bifida, cleft lip, congenital heart conditions)

Table 2C.3 Newborn screening programme

Time after birth	Screening test	To test for
5 days	Heel-prick (blood spot) test	Phenylketonuria (PKU) Congenital hypothyroidism Sickle cell disease and thalassaemia Cystic fibrosis Medium chain acyl dehydrogenase deficiency (MCADD) (a fatty acid oxidation disorder)
2 weeks	Hearing screening programme	Moderate to profound permanent bilateral deafness
72 h and 8 weeks	Physical examination	Congenital heart disease Congenital cataract Congenital malformation Cryptorchidism Developmental dislocation of the hip

Table 2C.4 Children's screening programmes (performed at school entry)

Programme	To test for
Growth [10] (height, head circumference, weight)	Growth disorders (e.g. Turner's syndrome and growth hormone deficiency)
Hearing [11]	Hearing impairment, deafness not detected by, or developed since, the newborn screen
Vision	Visual impairment

Table 2C.5 Adult screening programmes

Disease	Screening test	Subsequent test	Age group	Frequency
Abdominal aortic aneurysm (AAA) [12]	Abdominal ultrasound	Repeat ultrasound or CT	Men aged 65 years	One-off
Breast cancer	Mammography	Fine-needle aspiration	50–70 (phased extension to age 47–73 by 2016 in England)	3-yearly
Cervical cancer	Liquid-based cytology combined with HPV triage for borderline cytology results	Colposcopy	England and Northern Ireland: 25–49 years 50–64 years Scotland: 20–60 years Wales: 20–64 years	 3-yearly 5-yearly 3-yearly 3-yearly
Bowel cancer	Faecal occult blood	Colonoscopy	60–69	2-yearly
Diabetic retinopathy	Digital photography of the retina plus grading	Fluorescein angiography	12 years and over, with diabetes	yearly

Table 2C.6 Examples of other (non-NSC) screening programmes in England

Disease	Description of screening programme
Cardiovascular disease	The *NHS Health Check* is composed of tests (cholesterol), biometric measurements (blood pressure, BMI), and lifestyle questions (e.g. smoking, alcohol consumption) that are offered in a primary care setting to men and women aged 40–74 years. Together, these assessments are used to gauge a participant's risk of cardiovascular disease and to provide a focus for risk-reduction measures.
Childhood obesity	The National Child Measurement Programme is part of the government's strategy to tackle obesity. All school children aged 4–5 years and 10–11 years are measured for height and weight, and the results are sent to the child's parents. Additional NHS follow-up is provided to children who are identified as being underweight, overweight, or obese.
Chlamydia	As part of the National Chlamydia Screening Programme, all sexually active men and women aged under 25 years are offered chlamydia tests yearly and after partner change.
Prostate cancer	Under the prostate cancer risk management programme, men can request a prostate specific antigen (PSA) test to detect signs of prostate cancer. Note that this is controversial since it is far from clear that the harms of screening are outweighed by the benefits.
TB	Chest radiograph screening is mandatory at the port of entry for individuals arriving from countries with a TB incidence above 40 cases per 100,000 population per year who are planning to stay in the United Kingdom for more than 6 months.

Table 2C.7 AUS Australian screening programmes

Screening programme	Description
Antenatal and newborn screening	Very similar to the United Kingdom.
Breast cancer	Actively offered, by direct invitation, to all women aged 50–69 years at 2-yearly intervals. Breast screening is also freely available to women from age 40 years.
Cervical cancer	Cervical screening is supported by a backup record system that enables reminders, recall, and comparisons with previous histology. There is current debate about changing to 3-yearly and the impact of the new human papillomavirus (HPV) vaccine.
Bowel cancer	Use of an immunochemical faecal occult blood test has been successfully pilot tested. Provided that adequate resources for diagnosis and treatment can be demonstrated, it may be rolled out over the coming years.
Other	Informal screening for melanoma (physical examination) and prostate cancer (PSA testing and digital rectal examination) occurs in the primary care setting—but neither meets the WHO criteria.

Table 2C.8 SA South African screening programmes

Screening programme	Description
Antenatal and newborn screening	Similar to the United Kingdom except no tests for sickle cell disease, thalassaemia, cystic fibrosis, and fatty acid oxidation disorders. Also, because of the high burden of HIV and AIDS, heel-prick (blood spot) tests for HIV PCR are done on all babies born to mothers living with HIV. Although there is an established screening policy in place at antenatal clinics to screen for congenital syphilis, operational difficulties limit the effectiveness of programmes in many settings. Unlike the United Kingdom, the United States, and Canada, South Africa has not developed evidence-based guidelines for detecting retinopathy of prematurity (ROP), which accounts for 11% of blindness in South Africa. There is an initiative to implement screening for ROP. The Health Professionals Council of South Africa (HPCSA) has best practice guidelines for newborn and infant hearing screening in South Africa. The Western Cape Government adopted and implemented a developmental screening programme in collaboration with the developmental disability division of the Child Health Unit at the University of Cape Town. While focused at provincial level, the evaluation has the potential to influence a national developmental screening policy.
Cervical cancer	There is a national programme in place to screen for cervical cancer. The target population is women aged 30 years or older who should have three pap smears in their lifetime. Opportunistic screening is done in the private sector. HPV vaccination of girls has not been implemented due to cost.

2C.2 Statistical aspects of screening

Statistical aspects of screening tests, including knowledge of and ability to calculate, sensitivity, specificity, positive and negative predictive values (PPV and NPV), and the use of receiver operating characteristic (ROC) curves.

The validity or accuracy of a screening test may be expressed in four dimensions, namely, sensitivity, specificity, PPV, and NPV. These metrics are calculated as described in Box 2C.1 and Table 2C.9.

Sensitivity and specificity are test specific (i.e. measures of how well a screening test performs against a gold standard). They are unaffected by the prevalence of the disease in the population. In contrast, PPV and NPV are population specific and do depend on the prevalence of the disease in the population.

There is a trade-off between sensitivity and specificity. A test that is sensitive enough to detect all those with a disease is also likely to incorrectly classify some of those without the disease as having the disease.

An example is shown in Box 2C.2.

Threshold setting

All screening and diagnostic tests require a **threshold** level to be defined, which constitutes the dividing line between a normal and abnormal line. For example, the National Abdominal Aortic Aneurysm Screening Programme in England defines aortic aneurysms ≥3 cm diameter as requiring follow-up and those ≥5.5 cm requiring urgent referral. For many tests, most patients will be clearly normal or abnormal; however, some patients will remain

Box 2C.1 2×2 Table of screening test result versus gold standard

		True disease status (or gold standard) Positive	Negative	Total
Test result	Positive	*a* (true positive)	*b* (false positive)	$a+b$
	Negative	*c* (false negative)	*d* (true negative)	$c+d$
	Total	$a+c$	$b+d$	$a+b+c+d$

Table 2C.9 Screening test dimensions, calculations, and effect of high prevalence

Dimension	Definition	Calculation[a]	Effect of high prevalence
Sensitivity	Proportion of those people who have the disease who are correctly detected by the test (i.e. the ability of a test to detect all those with the disease in the screened population)	$\frac{a}{a+c}$	No effect
Specificity	Proportion of those people who do not have the disease who are correctly left undetected by the test (i.e. the ability of a test to identify correctly all those free of the disease in the screened population)	$\frac{d}{b+d}$	No effect
PPV (*'yield'*)	Proportion of those testing positive who truly have the disease	$\frac{a}{a+b}$	Increases PPV
NPV	Proportion of those testing negative who are truly disease-free	$\frac{d}{c+d}$	Decreases NPV

[a] Note that in the MFPH examination, candidates may need to draw the 2 × 2 matrix provided so that it is laid out in the same format as in Box 2C.1, the letters a–d can be used to generate the correct calculations.

in the grey zone between the two so a line needs to be drawn to determine how the test will perform in practice. The positioning of this line will always constitute a **compromise** between sensitivity (i.e. picking up everyone who has the condition) and specificity (i.e. avoiding healthy people being labelled as positive for the test) (see Table 2C.10). One technique to assist with threshold setting is the use of receiver operating curves (see Box 2C.3).

Parallel and serial testing

Sometimes, two tests are used to screen for the same test in the same individual. These tests may be offered either at the same time (**parallel testing**) or sequentially (**serial testing**). For example, in England, Down's syndrome screening normally consists of a combination of an ultrasound and a blood test conducted between 10 and 14 weeks into pregnancy (**parallel** testing). Where screening indicates a high risk of Down's, a diagnostic test (amniocentesis and chorionic villus sampling [CVS]) is offered. In contrast, in cervical cancer screening with a human papillomavirus (HPV) triage stage, a colposcopy is only offered to patients who have an abnormal smear test *followed* by a positive HPV test (**serial testing**). Parallel testing leads to higher sensitivity but lower specificity, whereas serial testing results in higher specificity [13,14].

Box 2C.2 Example: A cervical cancer screening test

In a population where the prevalence of cervical cancer was 38.6 women per 10,000, 88,084 women were screened for cervical cancer but 73 of the 86,569 women who tested negative turned out to have the disease. What was the sensitivity, specificity, PPV, and NPV of the test?

		Cervical cancer		
		Confirmed	Refuted	Total
Smear test	Positive	267	1,248	**1,515**
	Negative	73	86,496	**86,569**
	Total	**340**	**87,744**	**88084**

Sensitivity = 267 ÷ 340 = 0.785 or **78.5%**

Specificity = 86,496 ÷ 87,744 = 0.986 or **98.6%**

PPV = 267 ÷ 1,515 = 0.176 or **17.6%**

NPV = 86,496 ÷ 86,569 = 0.999 or **99.9%**

Table 2C.10 Trade-off between high sensitivity and high specificity

Reasons for setting the line towards high sensitivity	Reasons for setting the line towards high specificity
Serious disease with definitive treatment	Unpalatable treatment
Risk of infectivity to others	Costly, risky subsequent diagnostic test
Subsequent diagnostic test cheap and low risk	

Box 2C.3 Receiver operated characteristic (ROC) curves

A **ROC** curve is a plot of the trade-off between the sensitivity and specificity of a test across a range of threshold values (e.g. for a range of AAA diameters on ultrasound). The name of the curve derives from its original use in radar technology. The curve displays the proportion of people with the disease who receive a positive test result (sensitivity) plotted against the proportion of people without the disease who receive a positive test result (1−specificity) (see Figure 2C.1). The dotted line shown in the figure represents a useless test that has no discriminatory power.

ROC curves have two main uses:

1. To aid in the setting a threshold value for a test
2. To compare the performance of different screening tests for the same disease

The AUROC, also known as the c-statistic, can be used to compare the performance of different screening tests. The greater AUROC (i.e. the closer the curve follows the left hand border and top border of the plot), the better the test. An AUROC of 1 would indicate a perfectly sensitive and specific test, whereas an AUROC of 0.5 (i.e. following the reference line) indicates that the test is equally likely to produce a true positive as a false positive.

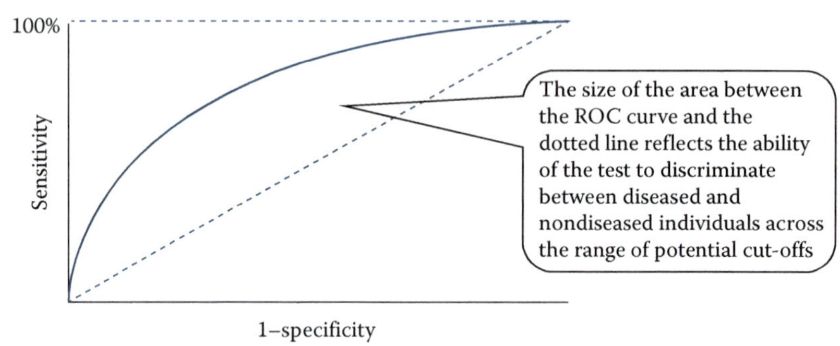

Figure 2C.1 ROC curve.

2C.3 Differences between screening and diagnostic tests and case finding

Screening tests, diagnostic tests, and case finding are related concepts:

- **Screening tests** are used to guide whether or not to offer a diagnostic test. They are offered to asymptomatic people who may or may not have a disease precursor or early disease.
- **Diagnostic tests** are used to determine whether or not a person has a disease. They are offered to people who with an indication that they may have the disease, such as a suggestive history, symptom, sign, or screening test result.

- **Case finding** is the process of identifying individuals or groups of people who are suspected to be at elevated risk of a disease or other adverse outcome, such as unplanned hospital admission.

A comparison between screening and diagnostic tests is given in Table 2C.11.

Case finding

The process of case finding involves searching systematically for high-risk people, rather than waiting passively for them to present themselves to medical attention once symptoms or signs of active disease have occurred.

Examples of case finding include:

- GP practice identification of patients at high risk of CHD (e.g. those over 50 years with body mass index (BMI) >30)
- Genetic testing of relatives who have a family member with a hereditary disease
- Identifying cases in a communicable disease outbreak
- Detecting individuals at high of unplanned hospital admission in the near future (see Box 2C.4)

Note the similarities between case finding and screening: both processes seek to risk stratify the population using a simple and cheap procedure, and both are justified only when better outcomes can be achieved by identifying people with early disease and offering them prompt treatment.

Some advantages and disadvantages of case finding are listed in Table 2C.12.

Table 2C.11 Comparison between screening and diagnostic tests

	Screening test	Diagnostic test
Purpose	To detect early disease or a risk factor for the disease in asymptomatic individuals.	To establish whether symptomatic individuals or asymptomatic individuals with a positive screening test truly have the disease.
Threshold	The cut-off is set towards high sensitivity. As a result, many of the positive results are false. This is acceptable, especially if the screening test is not harmful or expensive.	The cut-off is set towards high specificity. More weight is given to diagnostic precision and accuracy than to the acceptability of the test to patients.
Cost	Since large numbers of people will be screened to identify a very small number of cases, the cost must be considered carefully.	Patients have symptoms that require accurate diagnosis and therefore higher costs are justified.
Result of test	The result of the test is an estimate of the level of risk (e.g. risk of Down's syndrome in antenatal screening is based on a combination of maternal age, AFP, nuchal fold, etc.) and determines whether a diagnostic test (e.g. amniocentesis) is justified.	The test provides a definitive diagnosis (e.g. a definite diagnosis of Down's syndrome through CVS).
Invasiveness	Often non-invasive.	May be invasive.
Population offered the test	Asymptomatic people at risk of the disease where offering the benefits of the test outweigh the risks.	People with an indication that they have the disease.

Box 2C.4 Case finding patients at high risk of hospitalisation

Hospital costs are highly skewed across the population, with a small number of individuals accounting for a high proportion of expenditure. In theory, it is possible to invest considerable resources in these people to improve their health status while making net savings from averted hospital admission. However, there is a rapid turnover of high-risk patients, with current high-risk patients experiencing fewer admissions in future even without intervention (a phenomenon known as regression to the mean).

The evidence suggests that the case finding process might best be performed using a predictive risk model that uses relationships in routinely collected data to forecast which individuals in a population are at high risk of emergency hospital admission in the forthcoming year. Several predictive models are used in the NHS, including the Patients at Risk of Re-hospitalisation (PARR) model and combined predictive model in England, the PRISM tool in Wales, and SPARRA and SPARRA-MH in Scotland. High-risk patients identified by these models may be offered an intervention (e.g. input by a community matron or admission to a 'virtual ward') with the aim of reducing their risk of unplanned hospital admission.

In the United States, efforts are being made to improve the efficiency of the case finding process by identifying the subgroup of high-risk patients who are thought to be most amenable to hospital avoidance care. This second step is known as 'impactibility' modelling:

Types of impactibility model

Type of model	Justification	Effect on efficiency	Effect on inequalities
Identify subgroup of high-risk patients with an ACS condition	The ACS conditions are a group of diagnoses where there is evidence that effective management in the community should avert the need for hospitalisation.	May improve efficiency by concentrating resources on patients with conditions that are known to be amenable to primary and community care	May help reduce healthcare inequalities because ACS conditions tend to have a higher prevalence in more deprived areas
Identify subgroup of high-risk patients with a large number of quality gaps in their care	A quality gap is a recorded difference between best medical practice and the documented care received by the patient. A high gap score may indicate a large number of practical steps that can be taken to reduce risk of hospitalisation.	May improve efficiency by targeting resources on patients in whom there are clear, practical steps for improving the quality of care	May improve efficiency because high-quality primary care is inversely correlated with deprivation (inverse care law)
Exclude patients who are expected to be most difficult to work with	Patients with mental health problems, language difficulties, or dependency on drugs or alcohol may be challenging to work with.	May improve efficiency (e.g. by reducing costs of translation services)	Likely to worsen health inequalities (and may be illegal in the United Kingdom)

Table 2C.12 Advantages and disadvantages of case finding

Advantages	Disadvantages
Cheap. Low personnel demand. Case finding improves the PPV of a diagnostic test by targeting high-risk patients with higher underlying prevalence. By targeting preventative care, case-finding tools can help improve care of individuals and reduce costs for the state. Cost-effective method for identifying cases of familial conditions such as familial hypercholesterolaemia.	Potential to widen health inequalities because some high-risk groups are hard to reach (homeless, refugees, etc.).

2C.4 Likelihood ratios

The likelihood ratio (LR) provides an estimate of how many times more likely individuals with the disease are to have a particular screening test result than individuals without the disease (see Box 2C.5).

The LR for a positive result (LR+) indicates by how much the odds of the disease increase when a test is positive.

The LR for a negative result (LR–) indicates by how much the odds of the disease decrease when a test is negative.

Interpretation of LRs

The further away the LR is from 1, the stronger the evidence for absence or presence of disease, see table 2C.13. For example, an LR of 0.1 would result in a post-test likelihood of disease much smaller than the pre-test, so would provide strong evidence that disease was absent.

The use of LRs to calculate post-test probability is described is Section 2C.5.

Box 2C.5 LR calculation

		True disease status (or gold standard) Positive	Negative	
Test result	**Positive**	*a* (true positive)	*b* (false positive)	*a+b*
	Negative	*c* (false negative)	*d* (true negative)	*c+d*
		a+c	*b+d*	

Positive likelihood ratio (LR+)

$$LR+ = \frac{\text{True positive rate}}{\text{False positive rate}} = \frac{a \div (a+c)}{b \div (b+d)}$$

$$= \frac{\text{Sensitivity}}{1 - \text{Specificity}}$$

Negative likelihood ratio (LR–)

$$LR- = \frac{\text{False negative rate}}{\text{True negative rate}}$$

$$= \frac{c \div (a+c)}{d \div (b+d)} = \frac{1 - \text{Sensitivity}}{\text{Specificity}}$$

Table 2C.13 Interpretation of LRs

Value of LR	Interpretation
<0.1	Large pre- to post-test changes in probability, i.e. provides strong evidence against the diagnosis in most circumstances
0.1–0.2	Moderate pre- to post-test changes in probability
0.2–0.5	Small pre- to post-test changes in probability but may be useful
0.5–2	No useful change in pre- to post-test probability
2–5	Small pre- to post-test changes in probability but may be useful
5–10	Moderate pre- to post-test changes in probability
>10	Large pre- to post-test changes in probability, i.e. provides strong evidence in favour of the diagnosis in most circumstances

2C.5 Pre- and post-test probability

See also Sections 2C.4 and 1B.19.

By comparing the pre- and post-test probabilities, it is possible to determine whether the likelihood of diagnosis has risen (increased post-test probability) or fallen (decreased post-test probability). This comparison helps guide informed choice.

The PPV of a screening test is frequently regarded as a proxy for the post-test probability. However, PPVs are calculated from research studies based on a reference group with a particular prevalence of disease. An individual with a particular risk factor for the disease or from a population with a different disease prevalence may have a different probability of having the disease to the reference population (i.e. a different pre-test probability). If this is the case, then using the PPV may be inappropriate for that individual; instead, the post-test probability should be calculated using LRs.

Pre-test probability

This is the probability—before the diagnostic test is performed—that a patient has the disease. This may be estimated as

- The prevalence of the disease (if no other characteristics are known for the individual)
- The post-test probability (if the individual has had one or more preceding tests)
- An estimation based on the clinical characteristics of the individual

Pre-test probabilities may thus be estimated from routine data, practice data, or clinical judgement.

Post-test probability

The post-test probability may be estimated as the PPV of a screening test, or it may be calculated more accurately for the individual based on their pre-test probability and LRs.

Post-test probability using likelihood ratios

This is an application of Bayesian statistics (see Section 1B.19) since it uses a prior belief (the pre-test probability) to establish the result. In general, this method is preferable to simply using the PPV in case the pre-test probability differs from the prevalence of the disease in the reference group. LRs are calculated from the sensitivity and specificity of a test and therefore do not depend on the prevalence in the reference group (unlike the PPV).

The post-test probability can be estimated from the LR as follows:

$$\text{Pre-test odds} = \frac{\text{Pre-test probability}}{1 - \text{Pre-test probability}}$$

$$\text{Post-test odds} = \text{Pre-test odds} \times \text{Likelihood ratio}$$

$$\text{Post-test probability} = \frac{\text{Post-test odds}}{1 + \text{Post-test odds}}.$$

Note: the positive post-test probability is calculated using LR+ and the negative post-test probability using LR–.

The post-test probability can also be calculated using a Fagan nomogram (see Figure 2C.2). To use the nomogram, plot the pre-test probability and the LR. Join the two points with a straight line and extrapolate to find the post-test probability.

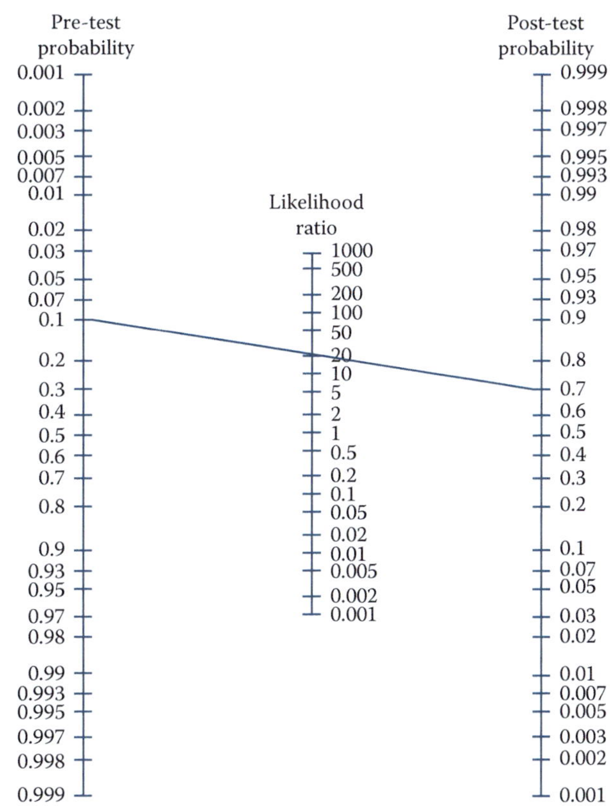

Figure 2C.2 Fagan's nomogram for calculating post-test probabilities. (Reproduced with permission from Fagan, T.J., *New Engl. J. Med.*, 293, 257, 1975.)

2C.6 Ethical, economic, legal, and social aspects of screening

Screening programmes are inherently attractive to the public and to the media because of their potential to *'nip a problem in the bud'* and to downplay the problems associated with false positives and false negatives. This cognitive bias can lead to undue pressure being placed on policymakers to introduce a screening programme without considering the opportunity costs and harms involved. For this reason, public health practitioners must ensure that the ethical, economic, and social consequences have been considered carefully before any new screening programme is introduced.

Ethics

Beauchamp and Childress [16] set out one of the most widely used frameworks in medical ethics, which they first described in 1979. The framework consists of four principles, namely, **beneficence**, **non-malfeasance**, **justice,** and **autonomy** (Table 2C.14). Screening programmes have the potential to violate any or all of these.

Economics

The opportunity costs of a screening programme must always be considered (i.e. the balance of the costs, benefits, and harms of the programme compared to other potential ways in which the funds might have been used to improve population health). The costs of a screening programme may include

- Marketing
- Administration
- Staffing
- Specialist equipment and disposables
- Subsequent diagnostic tests
- Costs of treatment

It is therefore essential to take into account the expected incidence of the disease or its precursor. Against these costs should be balanced the likely reductions in the cost of treatment as people are diagnosed and treated earlier (often considerably less costly than treating advanced disease).

Economic analyses of **adult** screening programmes should specifically address the following points:

- At what age should individuals begin and cease to be offered screening for this disease?
- How often should individuals be offered screening?

Legal aspects

The main legal aspects of screening are described in Table 2C.15.

Social aspects

Social aspects of a screening include those factors that may affect participation, such as those shown in Box 2C.6.

Health beliefs and attitudes are important influences on preventive behaviour, and they tend to vary between different subgroups of the population. These factors should be considered at the planning stage of a new programme in order to avoid exacerbating health inequalities (e.g. between social classes or between different ethnic groups).

Table 2C.14 Beauchamp and Childress's ethical principles applied to screening

Principle	Description
Justice	Screening programmes should be used only when all other primary preventive measures are in place, since primary prevention is likely to be more cost-effective than screening. Another challenge is to ensure that the screening programme does not worsen healthcare inequalities. Steps should be taken to ensure that the uptake of the programme is as good among the deprived populations (who are typically at greatest risk) as it is among more affluent populations. Screening programmes are often examples of the prevention paradox (see Section 2H.4), which states that the majority of the people receiving a preventive intervention will not benefit from that intervention. In fact, Raffle and Gray [17] argue that people often hold the opposite perception, which they call the '**popularity paradox**'. While screening confers a known risk of over-diagnosis and overtreatment, people who receive treatment following screening disproportionately believe it saved their lives. It could be argued that this misperception is unjust.
Autonomy	Individuals should be provided enough information about the potential benefits and harms to make an **informed decision**. However, communicating risk to patients is notoriously difficult (see Section 2F.2), and it is questionable whether the majority of people who partake in a screening programme truly understand the consequences of their participation. This concern is heightened by the fact that the parameters of a screening test are set below 100% accuracy.
Beneficence	All people who are screened are by definition asymptomatic but at risk. Screening programmes offer considerable benefits to those true positive cases that are offered early treatment. However, most participants will not benefit in this way. A particular concern relates to screening for infectious diseases where screening may be introduced primarily for the **benefit of society rather than the individual** screened (e.g. TB screening for residents of sub-Saharan Africa and India who move to the United Kingdom).
Non-malfeasance	Some of the **harms** that may result from a screening programme include • Psychological harm from false positives in the interval before diagnostic testing • Increased anxiety in both true and false positives • Iatrogenic harm from the subsequent diagnostic test (which is often invasive) • Unwarranted reassurance from false negatives (which may cause people to belittle and ignore symptoms that develop later, thinking that they are disease-free) • Unplanned effects of a positive result (e.g. increased insurance premiums) • Over-diagnosis (i.e. detection of disease that would not otherwise have become apparent in a person's lifetime) • Harm of unnecessary treatment in false positives

Table 2C.15 Legal aspects of screening

Access	Many screening tests can only be accessed via an authorised clinician.
Accreditation	In order to assure standards, diagnosticians such as cytopathologists and radiologists must be registered and accredited by a statutory body. To retain their accreditation, diagnosticians must deal with a minimum number of abnormal cases each year.
Vulnerable groups	For certain diagnoses (e.g. genetic screening for Huntington's disease), the right of children *not* to be screened may be protected in law. Likewise, the law offers protection to prisoners and to people with learning difficulties against coercion into screening programmes.
Confidentiality	Data from screening programmes would potentially be valuable to companies offering life insurance. For this reason, the data are carefully protected in accordance with Caldicott guidelines.

Box 2C.6 Factors that affect screening participation

Increase	Decrease
Perception of disease **severity** Perception of **susceptibility** to the disease Perception that screening is beneficial Knowledge of the disease Knowledge of the **availability of treatment**	Disease **phobia** Perception that disease is not serious and/or common High **residential mobility** (postal screening invitation does not reach them) **Unpalatable screening test** (e.g. home faecal occult blood test) Stigma associated with the condition Screening sites inaccessible

2C.7 Informed choice

The principles of informed choice.

An informed choice is a decision based on accurate information regarding rights, risks, and benefits. To constitute an informed choice, this information needs to have been fully understood by the participant.

Requirements for informed choice

UK The General Medical Council advises that patients should be provided with the following information in order to make an informed decision with regard to a screening programme:

Purpose of the screening test

Likelihood of positive and negative findings

Possibility of **false results**

Risks associated with the screening process

Any significant implications of screening for the **particular condition** (medical, social, or financial)

Follow-up plans, including the availability of counselling and support services

It must always be stressed to screened people that a negative test does *not* mean that they are necessarily disease-free and likewise that a positive test does not mean that they necessarily have the disease.

Screening and informed reproductive choice

Screening for genetic carrier status may assist prospective parents in making informed reproductive choices. Likewise, screening for fetal anomalies during pregnancy provides information to forewarn and assist couples in making decisions about further diagnostic tests and whether to continue or terminate a pregnancy.

2C.8 Planning, operation, and evaluation of screening programmes

The introduction of a new screening programme is a major undertaking. The infrastructure, logistics, and workforce issues all need to be planned carefully. An ongoing audit of the screening programme should form an integral part of the plans.

Planning and operation

There are important planning, operation, and evaluation issues to consider for all aspects of a screening programme, including the **disease**, the screening **test,** and the **treatments** to be offered.

Some of the planning and operational considerations include the following:

- **Who is eligible** for screening
- **How often** the screening test should be offered
- How individuals are to be **invited** to take part in screening
- **Quality assurance** mechanisms to ensure the correct results are sent promptly and referrals for further tests made where required

Systematic (register-based) screening requires identifying the eligible population and contacting all of the eligible people on the list. In the United Kingdom, GP registers are most commonly used for this purpose.

The WHO criteria for assessing the viability, effectiveness, and appropriateness of a screening programme were set out by Wilson and Jungner [18] and are summarised in Table 2C.16.

Evaluation

The evaluation of a proposed screening programme involves consideration of (1) the relative burden of the disease, (2) feasibility of screening, (3) effectiveness of the programme, and (4) cost.

1. **Relative Burden of Disease**

   The burden placed on population health and healthcare services will depend both on the severity of the disease and on its prevalence.

2. **Feasibility**

   Feasibility will depend on the following:

   - Relative ease with which the population can be **organised** to attend for screening
   - **Acceptability** of the screening test (see Box 2C.7)
   - Existence of facilities and resources to perform the necessary diagnostic tests and treatments **post-screening**

3. **Effectiveness**

   This is the extent to which implementing a screening programme affects the subsequent outcomes (e.g. morbidity or mortality). This impact is difficult to measure because of three **biases** that must be borne in mind when evaluating a screening programme: selection bias, lead-time bias, and length-time bias (see Table 2C.17).

   Furthermore, there are difficulties in evaluating rates of over-diagnosis as this requires long-term follow-up and in assessing the effect on all cause mortality as this requires very large numbers.

Table 2C.16 Wilson and Jungner's [18] criteria for assessing screening programmes

Disease	**Important** health problem (i.e. common and serious). Well-recognised **preclinical** stage. **Natural history** understood including development from latent to declared disease—detectable risk factor, disease marker. Long **latent period** (i.e. time between first detectable signs and overt disease).
Diagnostic test	**Valid** (sensitive and specific). Simple and **cheap**. Safe and acceptable. Reliable.
Diagnosis and treatment	**Agreed policy** on the further diagnostic investigation of individuals with a positive test result and on the choices available to those individuals. **Facilities** are adequate. Evidence-based **policies** covering which individuals should be offered treatment and the appropriate treatment to be offered. **Treatment available** that is • Effective • Acceptable • Safe • Cost-effective • Sustainable
Overall screening programme	**Evidence** from high-quality RCTs that the screening programme is effective in reducing mortality or morbidity. Evidence that the complete screening programme (test, diagnostic procedures, treatment/intervention) is clinically, socially, and ethically **acceptable** to health professionals and the public. **Opportunity cost** of the screening programme (including testing, diagnosis, and treatment) should be economically balanced in relation to expenditure on medical care as a whole. Adequate **staffing and facilities** for testing, diagnosis, treatment, and programme management should be available prior to the commencement of the screening programme. Clear **management**, monitoring, and quality assurance. Those offered screening must be able to make **informed choices**.

Box 2C.7 Inequalities in uptake of colorectal cancer screening in England

The acceptability and accessibility of a screening programme is often judged on screening uptake (i.e. the proportion of individuals offered a test who accept the offer). A colorectal screening programme was introduced in England in 2006. Faecal occult blood test kits were posted to over 2.6 million men and women aged 60–69 years. Between 2006 and 2009, 54% of people who were eligible returned their kits but there were marked differences by the following:

Socio-economic circumstances: only 35% of those living in the most deprived areas returned a kit compared with 61% in the least deprived areas.

Ethnicity: uptake in the most ethnically diverse areas was just 38% compared with 52%–58% in other areas.

Gender: women were more likely to return a kit than men (56% versus 51%).

If this differential uptake continues, then health inequalities in survival from bowel cancer may widen.

Source: von Wagner, C. et al., *Int. J. Epidemiol.*, 40(3), 712, 2011.

Table 2C.17 Types of biases in screening programmes

Type of bias	Description
Selection bias	Members of the public who participate in screening programmes **differ systematically** from those who do not. This can work both ways: sometimes, people at higher risk may be more likely to attend for screening (e.g. women with a family history of breast cancer may be more likely to attend breast screening); equally, people with lower risk may sometimes be more likely to attend—a phenomenon known as the **healthy screenee effect** (e.g. people from higher socio-economic groups are generally more likely to attend cervical screening despite being at lower risk). Performing an RCT eliminates this form of bias but the findings of a trial may not be generalisable to non-trial conditions.
Lead-time bias	People in the screened group may appear to survive longer after diagnosis than those in the unscreened group when in fact their life expectancy is unchanged. The reason for this phenomenon is that screened patients will be made **aware of their disease earlier** (the lead time) and will thus seem to survive longer. This time factor must be accounted for when making comparisons with the unscreened group (see the following diagram in which the apparent survival time from diagnosis is longer in people whose disease was detected by screening (5 years) than for people where the disease was detected clinically (3 years), whereas in fact the average date of death is the same in both groups. 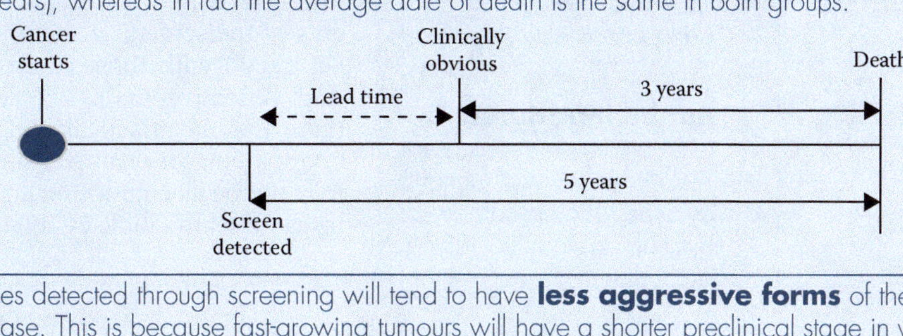
Length-time bias	Cases detected through screening will tend to have **less aggressive forms** of the disease. This is because fast-growing tumours will have a shorter preclinical stage in which to be detected by screening so it is less likely they will be picked up this way. Because such fast-growing tumours also often have a worse prognosis, it means that survival will appear to be better in cases detected by screening than in those detected clinically.

4. **Cost**
   Resources for healthcare will always be scarce relative to competing demands. The cost-effectiveness of a screening programme compared with other forms of healthcare and public health interventions should therefore be considered. The costs to be considered are not only those of the screening programme itself but also the costs relating to the subsequent diagnostic tests and treatment. However, the costs associated with the absence of screening must also be considered (these include the costs that would be incurred in the treatment of patients with more advanced stages of disease).

2C.9 Developing screening policies

Evidence basis needed for developing screening policies and implementing screening programmes, including established programmes such as breast and cervix and those currently in development, being piloted or subject to major research activity.

Evidence for screening programmes determines which of the policy options shown in Table 2C.18 should be taken regarding established and proposed programmes.

Table 2C.18 Policy options for screening programmes

Current programmes	Current programme should: • **continue unchanged** • **continue but be revised** • **be stopped**
Proposed programmes	Proposed programme should • **be introduced**, provided that the resources, both financial and human, are available to ensure adequate quality standards. and • **not be introduced** (e.g. prostate screening not recommended until further evidence shows there to be a reliable test for screening purposes).

Evidence base for screening policies

UK The NSC advises the United Kingdom's four chief medical officers on screening policy. It considers evidence about the benefits, risks, and costs of screening for conditions currently being investigated by research and evaluates this evidence according to their own criteria (based on those set out by Wilson and Jungner [see Section 2C.8]). Final policy decisions on screening are based on rigorous assessment of the health technology—often by means of RCTs. Two examples of diseases for which there has been a lot of debate as to the costs and benefits of screening are described in Boxes 2C.8 and 2C.9.

Before being rolled out nationwide, pilots are first established to compare the theoretical benefits of the screening shown in a research setting ('efficacy') with those in an ordinary service setting ('effectiveness'). This is important because there may be practical issues that were hitherto unapparent, for example, staff in a service setting may not be as committed and skilled as those in a research team (Table 2C.19).

Box 2C.8 Programme subject to major research activity: Breast screening (benefits outweigh the harms?)

Breast cancer screening is one of the United Kingdom's most established screening programmes. However, in recent years, there has been extensive debate about its effectiveness and whether it does more harm than good. In 2012, the DH and Cancer Research UK commissioned an independent review of breast screening to review the evidence.

The review concluded that on balance breast screening has more benefits than harms. They estimated that 'for every 10 000 UK women aged 50 years invited to screening for the next 20 years, 43 deaths from breast cancer would be prevented and 129 cases of breast cancer, invasive and non-invasive, would be over-diagnosed; that is one breast cancer death prevented for about every three over-diagnosed cases identified and treated'. The panel recommended that information to reflect these findings had to be made clear to women attending screening to enable informed decisions to be made.

Source: Independent UK Panel on Breast Cancer Screening, The benefits and harms of breast cancer screening: An independent review. *Lancet*, 380, 1778–1786. http://www.cancerresearchuk.org/cancer-info/publicpolicy/ourpolicypositions/symptom_Awareness/cancer_screening/breast-screening-review/breast-screening-review

Box 2C.9 A decision not to screen: Prostate cancer

There is currently no national screening programme for prostate cancer in the United Kingdom. To date, there have been two trials of prostate cancer screening using PSA testing: the European Randomized Study of Screening for Prostate Cancer (ERSPC) and the Prostate, Lung, Colorectal, and Ovarian Cancer Screening Trial (PLCO). The ERSPC showed a moderate reduction in death from prostate cancer but also a substantial increase in over-diagnosis; the PLCO showed no statistically significant difference in death rates. Mathematical models have also been used to assess the costs and benefits of prostate cancer screening at different ages and frequencies. A policy review in 2010 concluded that based on current evidence, prostate cancer screening was not justifiable for three main reasons: PSA testing has low specificity and sensitivity; it is currently not possible to identify which cancers will progress to severe disease (leading to high rates of over-diagnosis); and, furthermore, it is unclear which treatment is most effective for localised screen detected cancer (radiotherapy, radical surgery, or active surveillance). The current policy is due to be reviewed again in 2013/14.

Source: http://www.screening.nhs.uk/prostatecancer

Table 2C.19 Emerging screening programmes and those under review

Category of screening programme	Examples
Currently in development	Introduction of HPV triage and test of cure as part of cervical screening (England)
Being piloted	Flexible sigmoidoscopy for bowel screening for men and women aged 55–59 (England) [22]
Subject to major research activity	Breast cancer (see Box 2C.8)
Not considered suitable for national screening	Prostate cancer (see Box 2C.9)

2C.10 Ethical, social, and legal implications of genetic screening tests

Genetic testing can influence eligibility for screening. For example, if a woman has a family history of breast cancer, current guidelines suggest she should be referred for genetic testing. If this indicates she has inherited a faulty gene, she should be invited for annual MRI screening.

While all screening programmes have important ethical, social, and legal dimensions (see Section 2C.7), these issues are brought to the fore in the context of genetic testing.

Ethical implications

Autonomy may be compromised if parents test their children for adult-onset diseases. The potential for long-term psychological **harm** from the knowledge of a diagnosis needs to be considered (particularly regarding testing for genes predisposing an increased risk of conditions that are currently incurable, e.g. Huntington's disease or Alzheimer's disease). Furthermore, equitable **access** to genetic tests needs to be ensured.

Reproductive choice

Couples where one partner is affected by, or is a carrier of, a genetic condition should be offered counselling about their reproductive choices. Options may include prenatal genetic screening and possible termination of an affected fetus or in vitro fertilisation (IVF) in combination with pre-implantation genetic diagnosis.

This is an emotive topic and raises arguments that such 'genetic selection' constitutes a form of eugenics. There is often a fear of genetic screening following the legacy of eugenic programmes in early-twentieth-century Europe and America, which aimed to increase the 'genetic fitness' of the population by selective breeding and sometimes even the forced sterilisation or murder of people with genetic diseases. Any population screening programme must have at its heart the aim supporting individual reproductive choices rather than decreasing the prevalence of a genetic condition.

Social implications

Knowing the genetic profile of an individual has the potential to cause psychological harm including through **stigmatisation**. Indeed, public misunderstanding of the risks of developing genetic diseases can increase stigmatisation.

Legal implications

Right not to be screened

For screening of certain genetic diseases such as Huntington's disease, the right of children not to be screened may be protected. For example, children whose parents have Huntington's disease have the legal right not to be screened until they have capacity to decide for themselves whether or not to be tested.

Consent

Certain people are incapable of providing valid consent, for example, people with learning difficulties or prisoners.

Confidentiality

In general, the **confidentiality** of genetic information is assured as part of normal clinical practice. However, there are certain situations where there may be less clarity and here decisions will need to be made about whether the benefits of disclosure outweigh the need for confidentiality. Examples are

- Cases where the results of a relative's test result may have direct implications for an individual (cf. Huntington's disease)
- Pregnant women wanting to know the result of a test taken by the baby's biological father

Use of genetic information

Legislation should ensure **fairness** in the use of genetic information by insurers, employers, courts, schools, adoption agencies, the military, etc., and outlaw the potential for discrimination. **Note:** The UK has moratoria preventing or limiting insurer's access to genetic data for insurance underwriting.

2D

Genetics

Public health genetics is the study—at a population level—of genetics, genomics, and their links to biomedicine. Since almost all diseases have a genetic component, genetics has a profound influence on almost all branches of public health. This influence is set to grow in the coming years as knowledge in this field is expanding rapidly. Links between genetic mutations and disease can be used to identify people at risk of certain conditions and to develop treatments that are tailored to the individual.

The MFPH Part A syllabus requires candidates to understand the basic principles relevant to public health genetics such as **patterns of inheritance** and **gene–environment interactions**. This chapter covers these principles and includes examples of practical relevance to public health.

2D.1 Elementary human genetics

Genetics is the study of how characteristics and diseases are inherited. The related field of genomics is the study of all the genes of an individual at the deoxyribonucleic acid (DNA), protein, cell, or tissue level. Almost every cell type in the human body contains genetic material in the form of DNA. DNA is generally found in **chromosomes** that are located in the cell's nucleus (see Figure 2D.1). In humans, there are 23 pairs of **chromosomes** per cell. Twenty-two of these are **autosomal** (i.e. not sex linked) but there is one pair of **sex chromosomes** for each cell: **XX** in females or **XY** in males. Each chromosome carries a large number of **genes**, which are segments of DNA that encode a particular **protein**. The total number of protein-coding genes in the human **genome** is unknown, but current estimates are roughly 20,000 to 25,000 genes. In addition, a small number of genes are coded by mitochondrial DNA (i.e. DNA found not in the nucleus but in mitochondria). These genes are all inherited from the mother.

DNA consists of four chemical **bases** (also known as '**nucleobases**' or '**nucleotides**'), which are labelled A, G, C, and T, standing for adenine, thymine, cytosine, and guanine. A group of three base pairs (also known as a 'triplet nucleotide sequence' or a '**codon**') represents instructions for a specific **amino acid**, which are the building blocks of **proteins**. For example, CGC codes for the amino acid arginine. Other codons signal the end of the protein. However, only around 2% of human DNA is made up of these protein-coding sections (or **exons**); the remaining 98% was previously referred to as junk DNA. However, in recent years, the importance of regulatory sequences, which control how genes are expressed in different cells, has been discovered. Current estimates suggest that up to 18% of DNA is made up of regulatory sequences [26].

Gene expression

The information stored in a cell's DNA is used to make proteins in a process known as **gene expression**. In this process, DNA acts as a template for ribonucleic acid (**RNA**), which is produced by

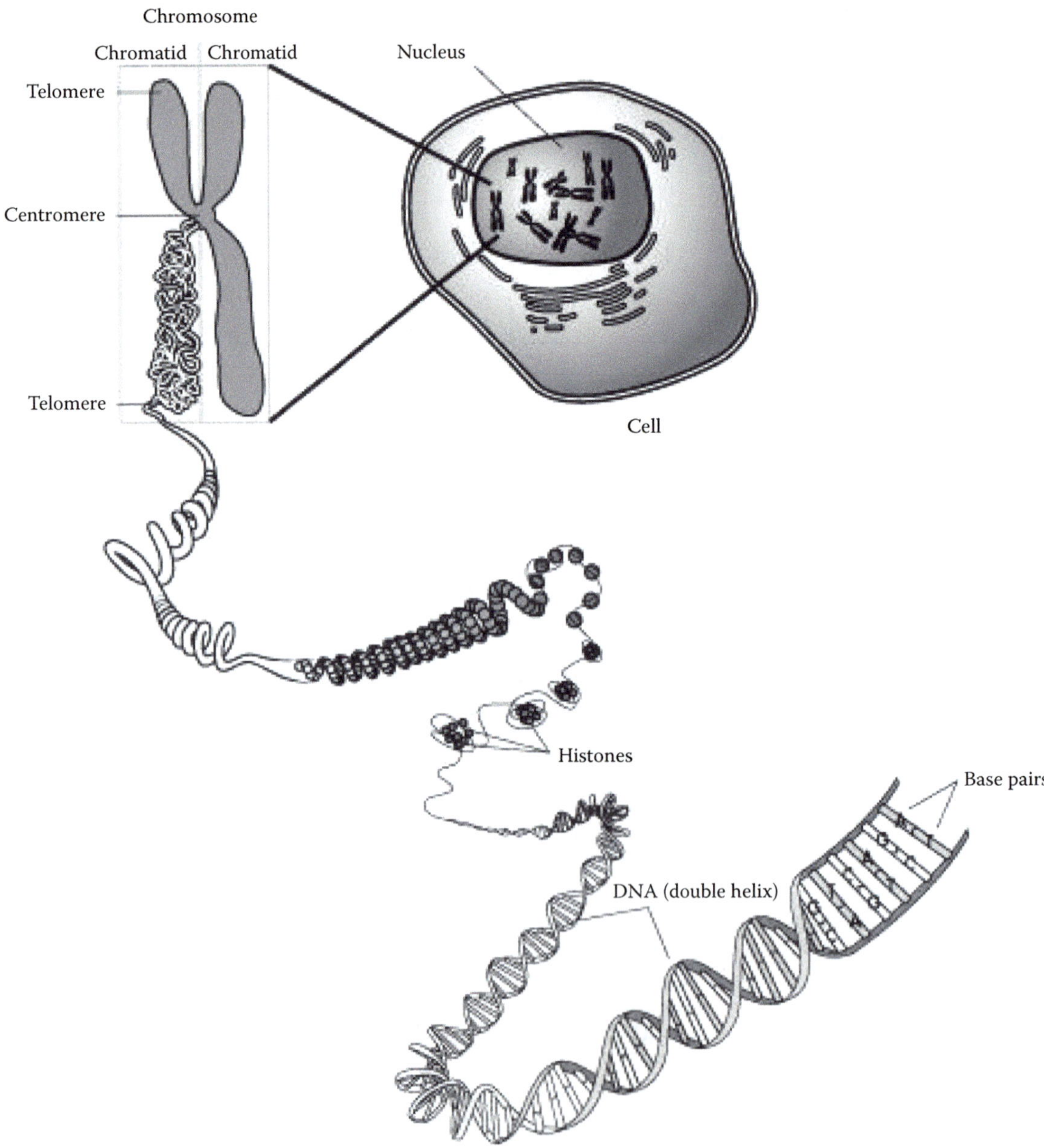

Figure 2D.1 Storage of genetic material in a human cell.

transcription. In turn, RNA is **translated** into **amino acids**. Next, a chain of amino acids is joined together to produce **peptides** or **polypeptides**, which themselves may be joined together to produce **proteins. (Note:** The size boundaries distinguishing peptides, polypeptides, and proteins are arbitrary.) Finally, **protein folding** occurs, during which a polypeptide or protein assumes its 3D, functional form (see Figure 2D.2).

All cells in the body contain the same DNA; however, cells from different tissues clearly have very different functions. These differences occur because different genes are expressed in different types of cell, a process controlled by regulatory DNA sequences.

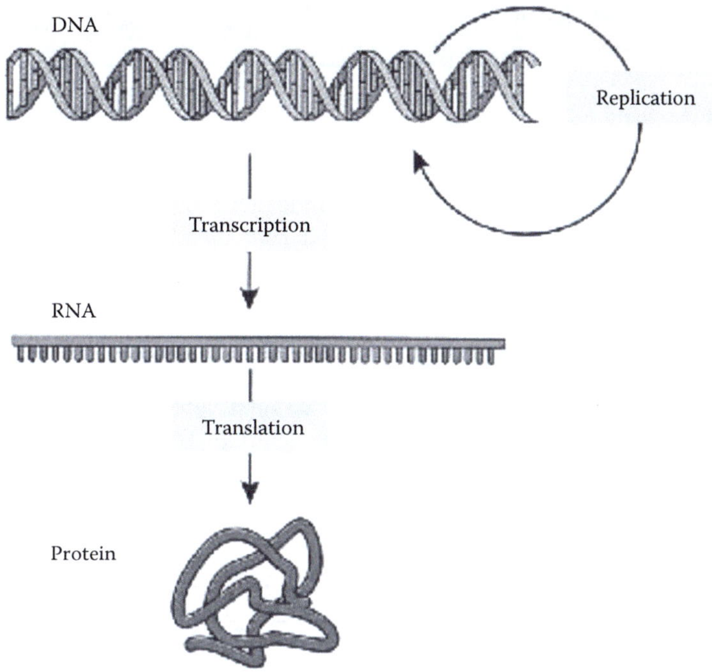

Figure 2D.2 Information stored as DNA is transcribed into RNA, which is then translated into proteins.

Variations in genetic material

The vast bulk (99.9%) of human genetic material is identical across the world's population, with only 0.1% of DNA differing between individuals. However, these differences are responsible for individual characteristics, including the propensity to different diseases.

There are several reasons why genetic material differs between individuals:

1. Half an individual's nuclear genes are **inherited** from their mother and the other half from their father; however, during the process of **meiosis,** the genes are shuffled, thereby producing a different genetic combination in each gamete. Therefore, the specific genes that are inherited from each parent differ from one child to another (except in identical twins).
2. Alterations may occur to the DNA sequence during cell division; normally, these are due to chance but they may also occur due to environmental hazards. Most of these alterations are repaired by cells; however, when they are not, they can lead to changes in a protein encoded by DNA, which can have consequences ranging from no effect to a change in hair colour to a severe genetic disease. Such alterations are known as **mutations** or **polymorphisms**.*
3. There are persistent and heritable alterations in how the genome is expressed that do not involve alterations to the DNA sequence itself. These **epigenetic** changes, such as DNA methylation, can affect the expression of genes and may arise not only during fetal development but may also be influenced by the wider environment (see also gene–environment interactions, 2D.2).

* A genetic polymorphism describes a variation in the genetic sequence that is present in at least 1%–2% of the population. Most polymorphisms do not lead to disease, but some are clear risk factors or protective factors (e.g. genes coding for haemoglobin affect the severity of malaria symptoms). The term gene mutations generally refers to rarer, harmful changes in DNA sequence. If mutations occur in gamete producing cells (those that produce sperm/egg cells), they can be passed on to an individual's offspring.

2D.2 Inherited diseases

Inherited causes of disease in populations.

Most diseases have both genetic and environmental risk factors, but a minority are caused by single-gene mutations or by chromosomal disorders (see Table 2D.1).

Table 2D.1 Inherited causes of disease

Type of inherited disease	Description
Multifactorial diseases	These diseases have multiple genetic and environmental factors. While certain genetic variants may increase the risk of a disease, they do not predict its occurrence absolutely. Diseases of this type include CHD, diabetes, and many cancers. While most genetic variants only lead to a slight increase in risk, others have a more profound effect (e.g. the BRCA 1 mutation is associated with around a 50%–80% lifetime risk of developing breast cancer) (see Section 2D.3).
Single-gene disorders	Also known as **Mendelian** disease, here, one altered gene is responsible for illness. Examples are Huntington's disease and cystic fibrosis. These disease can be further classified (see Table 2D.2) into • Autosomal dominant • Autosomal recessive • X-linked dominant • X-linked recessive • Y-linked
Chromosomal disorders	These disorders affect either whole chromosome or large parts of a chromosome. They include • **Numerical disorders** (e.g. Down's syndrome, where there is an extra chromosome 21) • **Structural abnormalities** (e.g. Charcot–Marie–Tooth disease, which is a neuropathy caused by a duplication of part of chromosome 17) Some, but not all, chromosomal disorders may be inherited.

2D.3 Basic genomic concepts

Basic genomic concepts including patterns of inheritance, penetrance, genotype/phenotype differences, polygenetic disorders, gene–environment interactions, and the role of genes in health and disease.

Genotype and phenotype

An individual carries two copies of each autosomal gene: one on each chromosome. Two different forms of the same gene occurring at the same location (genetic locus) on corresponding chromosomes are known as **alleles**. A person's set of alleles is known as their **genotype**, and the set of characteristics coded by this genotype and expressed in a person (e.g. blue eyes) is called their **phenotype**.

If a person has two identical copies of a particular gene, they are said to be **homozygous** for that gene and will display the phenotype associated with that version of the gene. However, if a person has different copies of the gene (i.e. different alleles), then they are said to be **heterozygous** for that gene. In this case, the characteristic expressed by the gene will depend on which version of the two alleles is **dominant.** For example, the gene for brown eyes is dominant over the gene for blue eyes; therefore, somebody inheriting one of each type of gene will have brown eyes.

Note that the presence of a particular genotype does not necessarily mean that the individual will manifest the associated phenotype. Variable phenotypes arise for many reasons, including the following:

- Incomplete penetrance (see Box 2D.3).
- More than one mutation of the gene associated with a characteristic or disease.
- More than one gene relating to one protein or one characteristic (e.g. cystic fibrosis; see Box 2D.1).

Box 2D.1 Example: Cystic fibrosis—a disease associated with many gene mutations

Cystic fibrosis is an autosomal recessive inherited disorder, which involves a mutation on the gene that codes for a cell membrane channel called the *cystic fibrosis transmembrane conductance regulator* (CFTR) protein. Abnormalities in this protein cause it to malfunction, leading to symptoms that may include

- Respiratory symptoms (due to thickened respiratory secretions)
- Pancreatic insufficiency (caused by an accumulation of thick mucus) causing malabsorption of food
- Elevated levels of chloride in the sweat
- Sterility in men

Hundreds of different mutations have been described on the *CFTR* gene, the most common being DF508, which is a mutation at point 508 on the cystic fibrosis gene. The severity of the disease (i.e. the phenotype) varies considerably between individuals affected by different mutations—particularly with regard to lung function. Some mutations are **non-sense** mutations (i.e. the mutation is so severe that none of the protein is produced) while others are **mis-sense** (i.e. some protein is produced but in small amounts or with altered function). Gene–environment interactions also play a part in cystic fibrosis, with factors such as smoking or malnutrition thought to influence the severity of lung disease. In the future, gene therapy may offer an effective treatment for cystic fibrosis by correcting the *CFTR* gene abnormality.

Source: Reproduced from National Human Genome Research Institute, National Institutes of Health, Learning about cystic fibrosis, www.genome.gov/10001213, 2007.

- Gene–environment interactions mean that the gene is expressed only if certain environmental conditions are satisfied.
- Epigenetic changes in one generation caused by environmental factors (e.g. diet, smoking) may lead to changes in the phenotype of future generations, even though the DNA sequence remains unchanged.

Patterns of inheritance

Inheritance is described as being either **Mendelian** (i.e. following one of the simple patterns of inheritance that were first described by Gregor Mendel) or **non-Mendelian** (i.e. following a more complex pattern of inheritance).

Mendelian inheritance

Mendelian inheritance may be either **autosomal** or **sex linked** and either **dominant** or **recessive** (see Table 2D.2). The application of Mendelian inheritance principles for maximising the effectiveness of a treatment is illustrated in Box 2D.1.

Non-Mendelian inheritance

However, most human diseases do not follow strict Mendelian rules of inheritance and instead described as being **multifactorial** (see *polygenic disorders* and *gene–environment interactions* described later).

Another unusual form of inheritance relates to mitochondrial genes, which are always inherited maternally (see Box 2D.2).

Table 2D.2 Mendelian inheritance

Inheritance pattern	Description	Example
Autosomal dominant	Dominant genetic diseases require only one copy of the gene to be abnormal in order to cause illness. If one parent has the disease, then there is a 50% chance of each child inheriting the disease. Under principles of Mendelian inheritance, there is no 'carrier' state for dominant conditions because the disease affects all individuals who have an abnormal copy of the gene.	Huntington's disease Familial hypercholesterolaemia
Autosomal recessive	Both copies of the gene must be abnormal in order for the individual to be affected by the disorder. A normal gene is able to 'compensate' for the abnormal gene; therefore, individuals with one copy of the abnormal gene are not affected by the gene mutation and are instead described as *asymptomatic carriers*. Where both parents carry one abnormal copy of the gene, there is a 25% chance of each child inheriting the disease. In addition, there is a 50% chance that each child will be a carrier of the disease.	Cystic fibrosis Sickle cell anaemia PKU
X-linked recessive	Here, the mutation is on the X chromosome. Males have only one X chromosome and therefore a mutation in a gene on the X chromosome is more likely to cause disease in men. In contrast, a single recessive mutation on a gene on the X chromosome in women is compensated for by the normal allele on the other X chromosome so that the disease does not occur. Therefore, males are far more likely to be affected with X-linked recessive disorders, and women are more likely to be carriers. Furthermore, in the subsequent generation, all daughters of affected men will be carriers of the condition, while none of their sons will be affected.	Haemophilia Duchenne muscular dystrophy
X-linked dominant	X-linked dominant conditions are all extremely rare but they occur when a single copy of the gene on the X chromosome is mutated.	Coffin–Lowry syndrome
Y-linked	Y-linked disorders are likewise extremely rare.	Male infertility

Box 2D.2 Mitochondrial inheritance

As well as being present in chromosomes within the nucleus, DNA is also found in mitochondria. Mitochondrial DNA encodes enzymes that are responsible for **energy production** in a cell. Accordingly, mitochondrial DNA mutations may lead to a wide range of symptoms associated with energy deficiency in cells, including cardiac disorders and exercise intolerance

Mitochondrial mutations can only be maternally inherited because mitochondria are not passed on in sperm. There is a **threshold effect** with mitochondrial inheritance whereby a child has to inherit a certain proportion of mutated DNA in order to be symptomatic. As a result, there is no predictable inheritance pattern: mothers with mutated mitochondrial DNA can give birth to both affected and non-affected children.

Leigh's disease is an example of a disease caused by mutations in mitochondrial DNA. It affects the central nervous system and causes movement disorders.

Penetrance

Penetrance is defined as the proportion of people with a given genotype that express its phenotype (i.e. the proportion of people with gene for a particular disease who develop that disease). Penetrance varies between different genes (see Box 2D.3).

Polygenic disorders

Family studies have implicated a strong genetic component to many disorders that are not typically thought of as being 'genetic.' As well as **rare single-gene causes** of common diseases (such as diabetes and Alzheimer's disease), far more common are the **polygenic forms** of these diseases (where several gene variants increase susceptibility to the disease).

The patterns of heredity for polygenic disorders are complex and the mechanisms by which the different genes interact tend to be poorly understood. The ways in which the genes interact to cause disease are complicated and involve highly convoluted gene–environment interactions.

Nevertheless, identifying the genes that underlie the polygenic forms of common disorders may be useful for

- Improving the understanding of disease **aetiology**
- **Predicting** who is at risk of illness
- Targeting disease **prevention** or health promotion activities
- Targeting **treatments** to individuals with those genetic variants that most likely to benefit
- Identifying new sites or **biological processes** on which to target therapies

Genetic studies have made some progress in identifying genes implicated in polygenic

Box 2D.3 Examples of variable gene penetrance

Huntington's disease—100% penetrance

Certain Huntington's disease alleles have **full** penetrance. People who carry one *HD* allele with 40 or more CAG triplet repeats will definitely develop the disease.

BRCA-1 or BRCA-2: female breast cancer—50%–80% penetrance

Hereditary breast cancer is linked to several genes. For example, the *BRCA-1* and *BRCA-2* genes have approximately 50%–80% penetrance; therefore, about 5 to 8 out of 10 women carrying one of these genes will develop breast cancer.

Table 2D.3 Challenges to identifying genes in polygenic disorders

Many susceptibility genes	In complex polygenic disorders, there are many susceptibility alleles, each making a small contribution to a person's overall disease susceptibility. In order to detect statistically significant gene effects, very **large sample sizes** are required.
Population heterogeneity	Studies conducted on different populations with the same disorder may not identify the same gene variants. This heterogeneity could be due to variations between **different population gene pools**; equally, it could be because different populations are exposed to **different environmental circumstances** (e.g. diet, pollution).
Incomplete understanding of disease biology	One fruitful approach to finding genes is known as **candidate gene studies**, where particular genes are selected for study because they code for biological functions connected with the disease. However, the selection of candidate genes requires an understanding of disease pathophysiology that is often underdeveloped. So another approach is to conduct a **genome-wide scan**, which does not require the same understanding of disease biology.

disorders (see Section 1A.38). However, few gene variants have been conclusively linked with particular disorders. Scientific progress has been hampered by factors such as those outlined in Table 2D.3.

Gene–environment interactions

Purely genetic diseases, such as Huntington's disease, are relatively rare. In contrast, most common diseases results from a combination of different genetic susceptibility factors interacting with a range of environmental risks. Such diseases are described as **multifactorial**. Environmental factors that may increase the risk of multifactorial diseases include

- Infections (e.g. infection with HIV and Burkitt's lymphoma)
- Chemicals (e.g. carcinogenic chemicals in tobacco smoke and lung cancer)
- Physical hazards (e.g. radiation from radon gas and lung cancer)
- Nutritional exposures (e.g. dietary phenylalanine and phenylketonuria [PKU])
- Behaviours (e.g. physical inactivity and obesity)

This implies that few people inherit these diseases genetically; rather, they inherit susceptibility to a disease, which is modified by their exposure to environmental factors. Understanding the interaction between genes and the environment will help identify high-risk individuals and thereby provide opportunities to target health promotion and disease prevention activities more effectively.

Epigenetics has been proposed as one way of explaining this gene–environment interaction. However, Davey Smith [25] argued that epigenetics offers a 'fashionable contemporary explanation', and as with much epidemiological research, there are challenges to establishing a causal relationship between epigenetic changes and disease occurrence [26].

Genetic disease prevention

Some genetic diseases, such as phenylketonuria (PKU), are only manifested under particular environmental conditions (see Box 2D.4). If these environmental conditions are avoided, then individuals with this genotype will avoid the disease.

Health promotion and genetic disease

Identification of the genetic factors associated with common diseases, and the interplay between

Box 2D.4 Example: Classic phenylketonuria (PKU) presenting a genotype being expressed as a phenotype

PKU is an abnormality in the gene that produces the enzyme phenylalanine hydroxylase which converts the amino acid phenylalanine to tyrosine. Absence of the enzyme leads to accumulation of phenylalanine which is toxic to the brain—leading to mental retardation. The disease is autosomal recessive (i.e. both parents need at least one copy of the faulty gene for a child to have a 25% chance of having the disease and a 50% chance of being a carrier). Babies with PKU are usually detected through the universal screening of newborns but can also be detected antenatally through genetic testing.

If expressed, PKU can cause severe and irreversible learning disability. However, individuals with the *PKU* gene who limit their dietary intake of phenylalanine between birth and adolescence will never develop symptoms.

environmental risks, advances our understanding of the aetiology and epidemiology of common diseases.

By studying gene–environment interactions it may be possible to

- Identify individuals at high genetic risk of disease
- Understand which environmental factors place individuals or groups of individuals at greater risk
- Target health promotion messages and disease prevention interventions to those people who are most likely to benefit

For example, the potential for genetic information to improve the prevention of heart disease is illustrated in Box 2D.5.

Genes in health and disease

In the future, gene characteristics could be used to promote health and to tackle disease. The field of **pharmacogenomics** uses individuals' genetic characteristics as a basis for understanding the relative effectiveness of different pharmaceutical treatments. In particular, people metabolise drugs at different rates, and this heterogeneity

Box 2D.5 Example: Using genetic up-rate to increase the effectiveness of heart disease prevention

Health promotion initiatives to prevent heart disease usually focus on universal messages (e.g. advising the whole population to give up smoking, take regular exercise and eat a healthy diet). However, many people can cite individuals who followed this advice and still suffered from IHD in middle age; equally, they may be able to name individuals who smoked, rarely exercised, ate unhealthy food, and yet lived well into their 80s. Such examples can undermine the public acceptance of health promotion messages.

People who develop IHD often have a family history of the disease, and research has implicated several genes in its aetiology. For example, there are some rare single-gene mutations that increase an individual's risk of dying prematurely from heart disease (e.g. mutated genes that cause familial hypercholesterolaemia). Clearly, it is important to lower cholesterol levels in these individuals through diet and drug treatment, in order to reduce their risk of heart disease.

However, in addition to such known 'high-risk' genotypes, a combination of genetic variations may also increase susceptibility to heart disease and could also be used to identify individuals for more targeted health promotion approaches. For example, one study has suggested that men with a family history of IHD who stop smoking have the potential to decrease their risk of IHD to a greater extent than men without a family history; therefore, it might be worth offering smokers with a family history of IHD even more intensive stop-smoking support than usual.

Sources: Adapted from Hunt, S.C. et al., *Am. J. Prev. Med.*, 24, 136, 2003; McConnachie, A. et al., *BMJ*, 323, 1487, 2001.

Box 2D.6 Gene therapy example: Severe combined immunodeficiency

Severe combined immunodeficiency (SCID) is caused by a single inherited abnormality in the adenosine deaminase (ADA) gene, which leads to the absence of the ADA enzyme. This deficiency leaves children with severely impaired immunity to infections. Gene therapy is now licensed for treating this disorder by inserting modified stem cells into the body using a virus in order to generate the missing enzyme [29].

may explain why a certain dose of a particular drug may be toxic for some people and yet sub-therapeutic for others. A better understanding of these differences might offer opportunities to design treatment regimens based on individual genotypes.

Gene therapy

Gene therapy is an emerging field where vehicles such as viruses or plasmids are used to insert genetic material into the cells of people with a particular disease. One of the few diseases in which this technology has been applied is *severe combined immunodeficiency* (see Box 2D.6).

2D.4 Disease in relatives

Aetiology, distribution, and control of disease in relatives.

The relatives of people who have a disease with a genetic component may wish to know whether or not they are carrying an abnormal gene. Two types of test are particularly relevant in these circumstances (see Box 2D.7). However, genetic testing is fraught with ethical issues (see 2C.10).

Predictive genetic testing or susceptibility testing could be used in future for multifactorial diseases. However, the predictive utility of a genetic test based on a single risk allele is poor. Even using a combination of multiple alleles, the clinical utility of a polygenic test in predicting future disease for the

Box 2D.7 Genetic testing in relatives

Testing method	Description	Example
Predictive genetic testing	This type of test is of value where an individual has a family history of highly penetrative genetic disease that develops in adulthood. The result can help them make informed decisions about having children and, where applicable, to institute measures to reduce their risk from disease.	Huntington's disease BRCA-related breast cancer
Individual carrier testing	This type of test can be offered to asymptomatic individuals who have a relative who is affected by an autosomal or X-linked genetic disorder to help them make informed decisions about having children.	Cystic fibrosis

Box 2D.8 Example: Colorectal cancer using genetic information to target screening

Around 30% of people with colorectal cancer have a family history of the disease. Two syndromes have been identified, which account for 1%–2.5% of inherited colorectal cancer. These syndromes are *familial adenomatous polyposis* (FAP, also known as familial polyposis coli) and *hereditary non-polyposis colorectal cancer* (HNPCC)

Source: Reproduced from Kohlmann, W. and Gruber, S.B. Hereditary non-polyposis colon cancer. www.geneclinics.org, 2004 (updated 2006).

individual may be limited. This is because most individuals are at only slightly increased or decreased risk. Nevertheless, the combination of risk alleles could be used for risk stratification and targeted interventions such as screening [31].

For commoner diseases, population **carrier screening** programmes may be offered.

UK In the UK antenatal screening programme, pregnant women living in high-prevalence areas are offered a blood test to identify whether they are carriers for sickle cell disease or thalassaemia (see Section 2C.11). If the mother is identified as a carrier, then the father is also offered testing.

Control of disease

In healthy relatives, control measures for diseases with a genetic component may include the following:

- **Preimplantation genetic diagnosis**: one to two cells from embryos created by IVF are tested for genetic diseases. Only genetically disease-free embryos are used for implantation.
- **Antenatal testing and screening**: can enable individuals to make informed decisions about whether to continue with a pregnancy if the fetus has a severe genetic disorder (e.g. Edwards syndrome).
- **Earlier screening** or **more frequent screening** or **prophylactic surgery** (e.g. for relatives of people with breast cancer who carry *BCRA-1* or *BCRA-2* mutations or for relatives of people with colorectal cancer) (see Box 2D.8).
- **Treatment to reduce disease risk** (e.g. cholesterol-lowering drugs for people with familial hypercholesterolaemia or tamoxifen for the prevention of breast cancer in people with a strong family history) [32].
- **Genetic counselling** to help people understand the disease and its potential impact and to support people in making decisions about the future.

2D.5 Molecular biology

Elementary molecular biology as related to genetic epidemiology and microbiology.

Molecular biology is the study and manipulation of biological processes and structures at a molecular level. The discipline includes analysing the interrelationships of DNA, RNA, and proteins, and it therefore overlaps with the fields of genetics and biochemistry.

Molecular biological techniques

A range of molecular biological techniques have been developed to enable scientists to identify and study DNA sequences. These techniques include the following:

- The use of **restriction enzymes** to cleave DNA at a particular nucleotide sequence and thus isolate a particular gene or DNA sequence, which can then be replicated and studied
- Amplification of DNA sequences using **polymerase chain reaction** (PCR)

- DNA **sequencing** to identify the order of nucleotides (A, C, G, or T) in a strand of DNA or even whole genome sequencing

Implications of advances in molecular biological techniques for public health [31]

The rapid advances in molecular biological techniques provide a number of potential opportunities for public health. The possibilities of targeting health promotion advice, screening, and medical treatment according to individual genetic profiles are becoming increasingly realistic. Genomic profiling is already being used in areas such as cancer medicine to aid treatment decisions and determination of likely prognosis. There are, however, many challenges including cost, data storage issues, and potential misuse by insurance companies or employers.

Molecular biology applied to microbiology

Molecular biology is important both in the identification of pathogens and for understanding how microbial pathogens function genetically.

Pathogen genetics

There are several notable examples of genes that confer virulence (i.e. provide pathogens with genetic advantages), including the following:

- The use of **reverse transcriptase** by retroviruses such as HIV to incorporate their genetic material into the genome of the host cell, thereby enabling the virus to replicate as part of the host's DNA.
- Extranuclear DNA in the form of **plasmids** may confer a pathogenic advantage such as antibiotic resistance. Plasmids can be exchanged between bacteria, including from one species of bacteria to another.
- Genes that enable **rapid exchange of surface antigens** may prevent recognition of the pathogen by the host's immune system (e.g. influenza virus).

Pathogen identification

The genomes of over 100 pathogens have now been sequenced. This knowledge is invaluable in the study of pathogens, for example, through the following:

- Identification of the **causative organism** in a symptomatic suspected case (e.g. chlamydia and meningococcus)
- Identification of different **genetic strains** of particular pathogens that affect their clinical consequences such as disease severity and susceptibility to medication. For example, the most common genotype of hepatitis C in the United Kingdom—genotype 1—is associated with a lower response to treatment than the other genotypes.
- Improved understanding of disease aetiology through the discovery of **new pathogens**.
- Detection of trends in the occurrence of new strains of disease through the development of **molecular databases** and **surveillance systems** (see Box 2D.9).
- Linkage of infectious disease cases to assist the **investigation of outbreaks**, both suspected and actual.

Box 2D.9 Example: Applying molecular biology to identify TB strains

UK In the United Kingdom, molecular typing is now performed on every positive culture of TB. Positive cultures of TB are sent by local hospitals to a national mycobacterium reference unit, where PCR is used to clone DNA from 15 loci on the TB genome. The analysis of the PCR products is used to

- **Confirm** the bacterium as TB (or another related bacterium)
- Check for antibiotic **resistance**

The technology, which provides results within a few weeks, enables local health protection teams to **link TB patients** who have the same strain of TB. This epidemiological linkage can be used to **trigger an outbreak investigation** if linked patients are found to have strains with the same molecular profile. It can also be useful in **detecting false-positive TB results**, which can occur as a result of laboratory cross-contamination and thereby prevent unnecessary treatment.

A national database, the *UK Mycobacterium tuberculosis Strain Typing Database,* has been created as a national repository for the results. The database is useful for linking strains of TB geographically, as well as for identifying clusters of related strains and for linking molecular characteristics with drug susceptibility.

Source: Reproduced from Health Protection Agency, *Tuberculosis Update, March 2006. The National TB Strain Typing Database – An Update. Information for Action,* Available online at www.hpa.org.uk, 2006.

2E

Health and Social Behaviour

The impact of different lifestyles on health is well recognised, one of the most important lifestyle factors being the diet. The health implications of an unhealthy diet can be severe and are of growing public health importance worldwide. For example, the prevalence of type 2 diabetes in the United Kingdom doubled between 1980 and 2008, with dietary changes being a major contributing factor to this rise.

Influencing behaviour is a complex task that extends well beyond the boundaries of health services into home, work, and leisure activities. Public health specialists have a key role to play in working with other agencies—both national and local—to design, commission, implement, and evaluate interventions that improve health by influencing social behaviour. However, it is not sufficient for public health practitioners simply to know what constitutes a healthy lifestyle. In order to change behaviours, they also need to understand the following:

- The **barriers and motivations** to adopting health lifestyles
- The **evidence** for recommendations and interventions related to diet and lifestyle
- How health and lifestyle are **measured**, including the relative strengths and pitfalls of different evaluation methods

2E.1 Nutrition

Principles of nutrition, nutritional surveillance, and assessment in specific populations including its short- and long-term effects.

Nutrition is the process of securing the dietary requirements of an individual or of a population. The study of nutrition therefore encompasses food production, food choices, appetite and digestion, as well as the metabolism and biochemistry of food for the purposes of growth and tissue replacement.

The components of the diet may be categorised as

- **Macronutrients**, which are required in comparatively large amounts (fat, carbohydrate, protein, and water)
- **Micronutrients**, which are required in far smaller quantities (minerals and vitamins)

Appropriate nutrition is essential for health, and a surplus or deficit of any nutrient can lead to illness. Most of human history was spent as hunter–gatherers and therefore evolution is thought to have rendered the body best suited to this type of diet. Compared with the modern, 'Western' diet, the hunter–gatherer diet contained more carbohydrates, protein, and fibre and considerably less fat.

Nutritional surveillance

Nutritional deficiencies and excesses can lead to long-term ill effects on health; therefore, nutritional surveillance has an important role in monitoring the health of a population. Several techniques are available to assess a population's food intake, as outlined in Box 2E.1. The sources of data are described in greater detail in Table 2E.1.

Short-term nutritional effects

Changes in diet may have short-term effects over the course of several weeks or months. Examples include the following:

- Increase in sugary food intake → dental caries (especially in young children)
- Reduction of salt intake → lower blood pressure
- Lack of protein → kwashiorkor (muscle wasting, protruding belly, fatigue, diarrhoea)
- Lack of protein and calories → marasmus (emaciation)
- Lack of vitamin C → scurvy (listlessness, gum disease, bleeding)
- Lack of B vitamins → beriberi (heart failure with generalised oedema and neuropathy)

Long-term nutritional effects

In the longer term, nutritional influences may manifest themselves only after several decades:

- Central obesity → type 2 diabetes
- Lack of vegetables and fruit → range of diseases including CHD and various cancers
- Lack of dietary calcium → osteoporosis

See also Table 2E.2.

With regard to cancer, dietary factors may have an influence—either beneficial or harmful—at the *promotion* stage of tumour causation (see Figure 2E.1).

Box 2E.1 Study designs to assess population nutrition

Ecological studies

Comparisons may be made between a range of disease outcomes and the diets of different countries or the diet of the same county over time. However, the potential for confounding makes it difficult to draw conclusions. Nevertheless, these types of study are often a fruitful source of hypotheses. For example, the 'French paradox' was an observation that there was a relatively low prevalence of CHD in France, despite a relatively high intake of saturated fats. This observation led to the study of several candidate protective factors, including red wine, fish, and a lack of snacking. However, a subsequent, more careful, study of the prevalence of CHD in France largely dispelled the paradox.

Retrospective case–control studies

Patients with a particular disease are compared with healthy controls regarding a range of dietary influences. As with any retrospective case–control study, these comparisons have the potential for recall bias and for disease onset to influence the diet.

Cohort studies

Data on food intake and other factors are collected from a cohort of people who are initially healthy. Dietary comparisons are then made between individuals who develop a disease and those who do not, with adjustment made for confounding factors.

Randomised trials

A nutrient or another food constituent is given to one group only at random. Disease outcomes in the two groups are compared. As well as being very expensive, the effect sizes seen are usually small—therefore, meta-analyses are often necessary.

Dietary surveys [34]

See Table 2E.1 and Section 2E.3.

Table 2E.1 Sources of nutritional surveillance data

Data source	Description
Food supply data	Data are acquired from multiple sources, including agricultural food production and food imports/exports. This exercise is conducted at a national level for most countries by the Food and Agriculture Organization (FAO) of the United Nations. Ad hoc food mapping exercises may also be conducted. These are a form of needs assessment that involves establishing where people can purchase and eat food. The aim is to identify communities that have the greatest food access needs (so-called food deserts). Often, these are inner-city areas where healthy food is not accessible to residents without cars.
Food expenditure surveys	Most European countries conduct household income and expenditure surveys on a representative sample of households every 1–5 years. These surveys gather detailed data on the food and drinks purchased at shops, restaurants, and other food establishments. The findings can be used to estimate the population's energy and nutrient intake. In the United Kingdom, the ONS *Living Cost and Food Survey* (previously the *Expenditure and Food Survey*) collects food expenditure data on an annual basis using self-reported diaries. This survey covers around 5,000 households across the United Kingdom and forms part of the *Integrated Household Survey* (IHS).
Diet and nutrition surveys	Surveys may involve food diaries, physical measurements (such as BMI and blood pressure), blood analyses, questionnaires, and interviews. Food diaries are often **unreliable** because participants typically underestimate their food consumption; moreover, they are usually **biased** as well because obese people tend to underestimate their intake to a greater degree than non-obese people. As a result, corroborating measurements are usually required to adjust for these inaccuracies [35]. In the United Kingdom, the DH and the Food Standards Agency (FSA) jointly commission the *National Diet and Nutrition Survey*. Data are collected from a representative sample of 1000 adults aged 19–64 years (with ad hoc boosts for people aged <19 years and >64 years). In addition, the *Health Survey for England* collects data every two years on fruit and vegetable intake.
Nutritional surveillance in children	**Breastfeeding surveys**: In the United Kingdom, the *Infant Feeding Survey* is conducted every five years. It collects data from around 15000 mothers on infant nutrition in the first year of life. This includes data on the incidence and duration of breastfeeding. **School meals**: Data are collected on the proportion of children eating school meals. In England, an annual survey by the School Food Trust and the Local Authority Caterers' *Association* includes data on the uptake of school meals. Note that this survey does not include schools which use private (rather than local authority) catering services. **Self-reported surveys**: These collect data directly from children. In the United Kingdom, the *TellUs* Survey was an annual online survey of the views and experiences of children commissioned jointly by the Office for Standards in Education, Children's Services and Skills (OfSted), and the Department for Children, Schools and Families (DCSF). It included questions on the amount of fruit and vegetables that children normally eat, as well as perceptions on the advice that children receive on healthy eating.

Source: National Obesity Observatory, http://www.noo.org.uk/

Table 2E.2 Examples of long term effects of nutritional deficiency

Nutritional deficiency	Clinical effects	Vulnerable groups
Vitamin B_{12} deficiency	Pernicious anaemia, neuropsychiatric symptoms	Alcohol dependency Strict vegetarians/vegans
Vitamin D deficiency	Children: osteomalacia, rickets Adults: osteoporosis	Dark skin colour Religious groups that cover their skin Elderly (lack of sun exposure)
Folate deficiency	Anaemia, depression Birth defects	Alcohol excess Pregnancy and lactation
Iron deficiency	Anaemia	Pregnancy Strict vegetarians/vegans

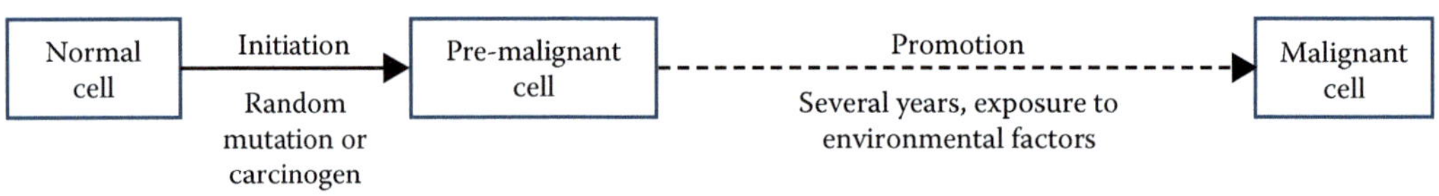

Figure 2E.1 Influence of environmental factors on development of cancer.

2E.2 Malnutrition

The influence of malnutrition in disease aetiology, pregnancy, and in growth and development.

Malnutrition occurs when there is a lack (under-nutrition) or excess (over-nutrition) of any component of the diet. According to WHO, malnutrition is currently the biggest threat to public health worldwide, accounting for some 4 million child deaths each year and 1.5 billion people being overweight.

The mechanisms through which malnutrition causes disease are varied and complex. In the short run, malnutrition can trigger an inflammatory response that involves a release of cytokines. This in turn puts the individual at risk for infections, impaired healing, and organ failure. In the long run, the divergence between modern diets and the hunter–gatherer genome is thought to lead to a vicious cycle of obesity leading to insulin and leptin resistance, which then further exacerbates obesity. This mechanism is thought to underlie the increasing incidence of type 2 diabetes.

It is important to remember, however, that disease can also cause malnutrition. Indeed, the hospital prevalence of malnutrition may be as high as 50% some patient groups. Here, another vicious circle may be established in which disease causes anorexia, leading to decreased oral intake, which exacerbates malnutrition, and thereby increases the risk of illness.

Under-nutrition may occur due to energy deficiency, leading to muscle loss and increasing the risk of infection and disease. **Protein–energy malnutrition** (PEM) accounts for upwards of 5 million deaths per year worldwide. Specific diseases may occur because of micronutrient deficiencies. In particular, deficiencies of iodine, vitamin A, and iron are responsible for a high global burden of disease. While many classic deficiency syndromes such as scurvy and pellagra are uncommon in developed countries, other forms are relatively common among high-risk groups (see Table 2E.2).

Malnutrition in pregnancy

The UK governments recommend that pregnant women eat a balanced diet and avoid certain foods, such as specific cheeses, raw or undercooked eggs and meat, liver, certain types of fish and shellfish, unpasteurised milk, and alcohol.

Women who are considering pregnancy are advised to take a daily supplement of 400 micrograms of folate until the end of the first trimester to reduce the risk of neural tube defects, including spina bifida. They are also advised to take a supplement of 10 micrograms of vitamin D for the duration of pregnancy and when breastfeeding.

Inadequate dietary intake during pregnancy may prevent the fetus from attaining its full potential—a condition known as intrauterine growth restriction (IUGR). IUGR may be defined as an estimated fetal weight below the 10th percentile. It is characterised by a number circulatory changes in the fetus, the effects of which include depriving the brain and heart of oxygen. IUGR is a strong predictor of complications in pregnancy including stillbirth, hypoxic brain injury, and chronic lung disease. It may also lead to long-term effects in adulthood including cardiovascular disease, renal disease, and impaired cognitive development.

Malnutrition in growth and development

There is evidence that nutrition in early childhood has long-term effects on cognitive development, behaviour, physical health, and educational achievement. The WHO has developed child growth standards to assess how well children worldwide are growing, which are widely used in public health and paediatrics. The standards, which require children to be measured regularly for their height and weight, set healthy ranges for children's weight, height/length, BMI, and motor development from birth up to age 5 years.

Childhood malnutrition is associated with a number of adverse outcomes, including obesity, depression, and failure to thrive. It may be classified as

- **Wasting** (acute malnutrition)
- **Stunting** (chronic malnutrition)
- **Underweight** (acute and chronic malnutrition)

The underlying causes of malnutrition include suboptimal breastfeeding, poor household food security, and specific micronutrient deficiencies.

2E.3 Nutritional status

Markers of nutritional status, nutrition, and food; the basis for nutritional interventions and assessment of their impact.

An individual's nutritional status may be measured in a number of ways, including the following:

- **Anthropometry**: (Measuring height and weight to calculate the BMI and plot growth charts, head circumference in infants, and skinfold thickness).
- **Indices of malnutrition**: Such as the Nutritional Risk Index (NRI) or the Malnutrition Universal Screening Tool (MUST).
- **Biochemical tests**: include plasma fatty acid composition, 24-hour urinary sodium, or 24-hour urinary nitrogen as a marker of protein intake. Note that many biochemical tests have limited value in assessing nutritional status as they are compensated for by homeostatic mechanisms; moreover, other diseases can also affect these parameters.
- **Bioelectrical impedance analysis**: can be used for measuring body composition.

- **Imaging**: techniques such as near-infrared interactance and dual-energy x-ray absorptiometry may be used to gauge body fat percentage.
- **Food consumption surveys:** may be prospective or retrospective. Questions may include food frequency and amount questionnaires, food diaries (using household measures or weighed inventory), and the duplicate diet method (i.e. weigh and record two portions of any food that is consumed: one portion is then collected and chemically analysed).

Nutritional interventions

The purpose of nutritional intervention is to reduce morbidity and mortality through dietary change. Many such interventions are relatively cheap in terms of their cost per quality-adjusted life year (QALY). Examples include

- Fluoridation of water
- **Fortification** of foods (e.g. folic acid in flour to reduce the incidence of neural tube defects)
- **Workplace** campaigns (e.g. for more vegetables in canteen meals)
- **Television** series about healthy lifestyles (e.g. Jamie Oliver's school meals campaign)
- Campaigns to promote **home-grown** fruit and vegetables
- Collaboration with supermarkets and with the food industry (see Box 2E.3)
- **Free fruit** in schools

A range of nutritional interventions was deployed in the North Karelia Project (see Box 2E.2) which reduced rates of heart disease in eastern Finland. Specific interventions may be indicated for geographical nutritional deficiencies (e.g. lack of iodine in the Alps; lack of selenium in New Zealand's South Island).

In some countries, there have recently been moves towards collaboration between public health with food and drinks industries; however, there is concern regarding the effectiveness of this approach given the conflicting interests held by these industries (see Box 2E.3).

Box 2E.2 Example: Reducing deaths from heart disease—the North Karelia Project

The North Karelia Project was established in 1972 in response to excessively high rates of heart disease in eastern Finland. The area had a traditional community, with a major dairy farming industry and a range of socio-economic problems.

The project included a wide range of interventions focusing on diet, reducing smoking, and encouraging more exercise. At the individual person level, health practitioners provided disease prevention and health promotion advice, and at the population level, there were TV media campaigns and policy changes. Examples of interventions were

- Cholesterol-lowering **competitions** between villages
- Youth and school projects
- **Collaborations with the food industry** to promote low-fat dairy products and sausages and reducing the salt content of processed foods
- **Encouraging farmers** to grow fruit and vegetables

Surveys conducted every 5 years since 1972 have shown marked changes in the local diet. Health outcomes included

- Reductions in various **risk factors** (cholesterol, **blood pressure levels, and percentage smoking)**
- **Reductions in mortality from heart disease among** adults aged 35–64 years

Source: Adapted from Puska, P. et al., *BMJ*, 287, 1840, 1983; Henkel, G.L., North Karelia project shows the World how to reduce heart disease. www.kantele.com/nwfwebsite/puska_heart.html. New World Finn website, n.d; WHO, *North Karelia Project: From Demonstration Project to National Activity*, Geneva: WHO, Available online at: www.who.int/hpr/successful.prevention.3.html. 2003.

Box 2E.3 Collaboration with industry

In England, the coalition government has encouraged collaboration with industry to improve public health. In 2011, the DH announced the establishment of a number of public health 'responsibility deals' that brought together industry representatives such as food manufacturers and retailers, NGOs, public health bodies, and local government. These partners worked together across five networks to develop a series of 'pledges' for action.

The five networks were

1. Food
2. Alcohol
3. Physical activity
4. Health at work
5. Behavior change

Examples of pledges from the food network included reducing the salt content of foods, providing more information on food and drink content for consumers, and the removal of trans fats from all products.

However, evidence for the effectiveness of voluntary deals to change industry practice and improve population health is weak. As Marteau and colleagues noted, agreements with the food industry in the United Kingdom in the early 2000s (which were reached only with the threat of legislation) led to a 0.9 g reduction in salt intake per person per day—whereas in Japan and Finland, legislated changes led to a 5 g reduction per person per day. Likewise, Cobiac and colleagues reported that mandatory limits on salt content had up to 20 times more impact than voluntary limits.

Notably, several health groups refused to sign up to the responsibility deal on alcohol or left the negotiating table, partly because of a lack of clarity as to what would happen if industry did not adhere to the pledges [40].

Sources: Marteau, T.M. et al., *BMJ*, 342, d288, 2011; Cobiac, L.J. et al., *Heart*, 96, 1920e1925, 2010.

Assessment of impact

The impact of nutritional interventions can be assessed in several ways:

- **Food sales** (e.g. full-fat milk compared with skimmed or semi-skimmed milk)
- **Diet** (using food surveys)
- **Clinical markers** (growth, BMI, blood pressure, dental caries)
- **Biological markers** (serum cholesterol, urinary sodium)
- Morbidity and mortality **endpoints** (MIs, death)
- Psychological indicators (e.g. obesity on self-esteem)

2E.4 Choice of diet

Social, behavioural, and other determinants of the choice of diet.

Individuals' choice of diet is not only influenced by personal preference. Financial and cultural circumstances can play a major role, in particular poverty, ethnicity, and religion.

Social determinants of diet

Poverty

Low-income families often have little disposable income to spend on food. As a result, they tend to have poorer nutrient intake and less food variety and make less healthy food choices. Particular problems include the following:

- Discount stores often have a more limited range of foods available, and less turnover of stock results in older, less nutritious food.
- Tinned and frozen foods are often cheaper than fresh food.
- Lean cuts of meat are usually pricier than fatty ones.
- People with little money for food may not be able afford to experiment with new recipes to vary the diet, since a culinary disaster would result in hunger.

Traditionally, poverty has been more closely associated with poor diet in adults than in their children: parents protected their children, and school meals provided wholesome food. However, concerns remain regarding cooking skills and the nutritional content of school meals leading to childhood malnutrition.

Ethnicity, culture, and religion

While many black and minority ethnic people in the United Kingdom follow Western dietary habits, eating patterns may still be influenced by

- Traditional cuisine
- Festivals and fasts
- Proscription of certain foods
- Demographic and socio-economic factors affecting the population as a whole

As illustrated in Box 2E.4, certain ethnic variations in eating habits were found in the 2004 Health Survey for England.

Education

People with higher levels of education are generally more knowledgeable regarding healthy eating and cooking and are more likely to choose healthier diets.

Behavioural determinants of diet

Attitudes and beliefs

Beliefs regarding the need for a healthy diet vary from one individual to another, with certain groups more likely to consider the need for a healthy diet including females and older adults.

Psychological determinants

Factors such as stress and mood can affect diet, but the mechanisms are complex with some people likely to consume more than average and others likely to consume less.

Box 2E.4 UK Example: Differences in reported eating habits by ethnic group—the 2004 Health Survey for England

The Health Survey for England asks a sample of the population about their eating habits. The 2004 survey found that compared with the general population

- A **higher** proportion of all black and minority ethnic groups (except the Irish) consumed the guideline five portions of **fruit and vegetables**
- All black and minority ethnic groups had a **lower fat intake**
- All black and minority ethnic groups (except the Irish) were more likely to **use salt** in cooking

Source: Reproduced from Sproston, K. and Mindel, J., eds., *Health Survey for England 2004*, Leeds: The Information Centre, Available online at www.ic.nhs.uk/pubs, 2006.

2E.5 Dietary recommendations

Dietary reference values (DRVs), current dietary goals, recommendations, guidelines, and the evidence for them.

The media often provide conflicting, sensationalist messages about healthy diets; therefore, authoritative recommendations are crucial.

Goals

UK In England, the DH issues guidance on healthy eating, including the 'eatwell plate' and eight recommendations for a healthy diet (Box 2E.6), based on advice from the Scientific Advisory Committee on Nutrition.

In Wales, there is more emphasis on policy direction than on goals and targets. For example, a policy entitled 'Food and health guidelines for early years and childcare settings' has recently been produced. Wales also has legislation, such as the 'Healthy Eating in Schools (Wales) Measure 2009', to ensure that healthy eating is promoted and supported in state-funded schools.

Dietary reference values

DRVs issued by the DH are designed for policymakers and professionals, rather than the general public (see Table 2E.3). Their values are set for **healthy people** in various demographic groups, including children at different age bands, adult males and adult females at different age bands, and bands for pregnancy and breastfeeding.

Recommended dietary allowances

IRE The Food Safety Authority of Ireland (FSAI) published recommended dietary allowances (RDAs) in 1999, providing indications of the level of nutrients required to meet the needs of healthy people. The FSAI adopted the EU population reference intake (PRI) values for most nutrients. However, in the case of folate, iron, calcium, and vitamin C, the values for Ireland differ from the EU PRI on the basis of more recent research and a consideration of prevailing Irish conditions (e.g. high incidence of childhood anaemia).

Adequacy of nutrient intake

Surveys of nutrient intake are conducted by weighing and recording all food consumption over a 3-day period and then assessing nutrient intake by using food composition tables. Nutrient intake can then be compared against DRVs.

Good dietary variety

Food usage questionnaires can be used to determine a person's **variety frequency score**. This score is based upon both overall food variety and the variety within each food group.

Table 2E.3 Types of DRVs

Estimated average requirement (EAR)	Average amount needed by a group of people (i.e. 50% of the group's requirements are met)
Reference nutrient intake (RNI)	Amount that is enough to meet the dietary needs of about 97.5% of a group of people (i.e. the majority need less)
Lower reference nutrient intake (LRNI)	Amount that is enough for a small number (2.5%) of people in a group with the smallest needs (most people will need more than this)
Safe intake	Issued when there is insufficient evidence to set an EAR, RNI, or LRNI

Source: Department of Health Committee on Medical Aspects of Food Policy, *Dietary Reference Values for Food Energy and Nutrients for the United Kingdom: Report of the Panel on Dietary Reference Values of the Committee on Medical Aspects of Food Policy.* Stationery Office Books, 1991.

Healthy dietary patterns

Indicators of healthy dietary patterns include:

- Proportions of energy in the diet that are derived from fat and saturated fat
- Healthy diet score (derived from the *frequency of food usage* questionnaire)
- Frequency of eating five or more fruits and vegetables per day

Implementation of the dietary goals

In Scotland, the 2008 policy document *Healthy Eating, Active Living: An action plan to improve diet, increase physical activity and tackle obesity (2008–2011)* was published [45]. This was followed by the publication of *Preventing Overweight and Obesity in Scotland: A Route Map Towards Healthy Weight 2010*, which set out the direction for national and local government decision-making to avoid the predicted increases in obesity and associated health risks. In 2011, the Obesity Route Map Action Plan was published.

WA In Wales [46], the use of the dietary goals to reduce health inequalities is promoted through the implementation of a nutrition strategy for Wales. The *Food and Fitness Plan* seeks to address issues in relation to children and makes seven key recommendations and actions to achieve them, namely,

1. Extend the Welsh Network of Healthy School Schemes (WNHSS)
2. Improve the food and drink consumed throughout the school day
3. Provide high-quality physical education, health-related exercise, and practical cookery skills
4. Provide an environment that will encourage children and young people to take up opportunities for physical activity and healthier foods
5. Develop skills to enable children and young people to take part in physical activity and to prepare healthier foods
6. Develop and deliver training on food and fitness for those working with children and young people
7. Ensure that actions are evidence based, or innovative with evaluation, and that findings are shared

AUS In Australia, as elsewhere, there is an abundance of dietary advice in magazines—mostly not evidence based—against which even the most authoritative recommendations find it hard to compete. In 2005, the *Commonwealth Scientific and Industrial Research Organisation* published *The CSIRO Total Wellbeing Diet*, which has become a best-selling book. This offers scientifically proven, practical advice and contains recipes and 12 weeks of menu plans.

IRE Implementation of Irish national recommendations regarding salt intake is summarised in Box 2E.5.

Box 2E.5 Implementing nutritional recommendations: Salt intake in Ireland

The RDA in Ireland is approximately 4 g salt/day for adults. However, the average daily salt intake is 10 g in adults; it exceeds 5 g in children aged 4–6 years; and it is 6 g in children aged 7–10 years. Clearly, these intakes are all well in excess of physiological requirements. Typical consumption is accounted for as follows:

- 15%–20% of total dietary sodium intake from salt added in cooking or at the table
- 15% from naturally occurring sodium in unprocessed foods
- 65%–70% from manufactured foods

Meat, fish, and bread together account for over 50% of salt intake from foods. The FSAI has worked with bakers to reduce the salt content in bread and the Food Safety Promotions Board has run advertising campaigns to reduce salt consumption.

Source: Reproduced from the Review of the Scientific Evidence and Recommendations for Public Policy in Ireland, available online at: www.fsai.ie, 2005.

Recommendations

ENG Advice to the general public from the NHS is shown in Box 2E.6.

IRE The 'Recommendations for a Food and Nutrition Policy for Ireland' [47] provided guidance on promoting healthy eating that was similar to that issued by the UK advisory agencies. The **food pyramid** has been used for health education, encouraging a balanced consumption of

- Bread, cereal, and potatoes (6+ portions/day)
- Fruit and vegetables (5 portions/day)
- Milk, cheese, and yogurt (3 portions/day)
- Meat, fish, eggs, and alternative (2 portions/day)
- Foods high in fat and/or sugar (choose small amounts)

Box 2E.6 Eight tips for healthy eating

1. Base your meals on starchy foods.
2. Eat lots of fruit and vegetables.
3. Eat more fish—including a portion of oily fish each week.
4. Cut down on saturated fat and sugar.
5. Try to eat less salt—no more than 6 g a day.
6. Get active and try to be a healthy weight.
7. Drink plenty of water.
8. Don't skip breakfast.

Source: NHS, England, December 2012, www.nhs.uk.

AUS In Australia, as elsewhere, there is an abundance of dietary advice in magazines—mostly not evidence based—against which even the most authoritative recommendations find it hard to compete. The Commonwealth Scientific and Industrial Research Organisation (CSIRO) has recently published *The CSIRO Total Wellbeing Diet*, which has become a best-selling book. This offers scientifically proven, practical advice and contains recipes and 12 weeks of menu plans.

Evidence

The evidence for nutritional recommendations comes from a range of sources. However, there are challenges to

Obtaining **undisputed** evidence for nutritional goals for health

Ensuring that the evidence of health risks and benefits is **widely accepted**

Implementing accepted evidence to **change consumption** in the population

Evidence for health-related nutritional goals

Major studies that have generated evidence for the health effects of food substances are listed in Appendix C. Selected studies are also described in more depth as examples in this chapter. Note that there are significant ethical and practical **obstacles** to conducting RCTs involving alterations to the diet of a widespread food substance such as fats. Many of the outcomes of interest, such as cardiovascular events or deaths, occur over the long term, making trials impractical and prohibitively expensive.

International ecological studies, such as **Intersalt** (see Box 2E.7) and **Seven Countries** (see Box 2E.8), have capitalised on the differences in dietary habits that exist between different cultures. They have been useful for indicating which factors affect health (see example boxes). However, as with all ecological studies, they are vulnerable to **ecological fallacies** (see Section 1A.7) and **confounding**. Potentially confounding factors include different genetic susceptibility to disease and unobserved lifestyle variations that could be responsible for the observed observations.

Ensuring that evidence of health risks and benefits is widely accepted

Even where the evidence for a nutritional recommendation is strong, public health practitioners may face **competing commercial interests**. Information about nutrition comes to the public from a range of sources but rarely from peer-reviewed research sources. Common sources include publicity by food manufacturers and retailers, diet books, and magazines. Each of these sources has a vested interest in maintaining or promoting sales in a product. Moreover, advertising for foodstuffs (e.g. showing sports people consuming the product) is often far more powerful an influence on eating habits than the published research.

Implementing accepted evidence to change consumption in the population

People's decisions on what they eat and drink are not always based on long-term health goals. Other priorities often take priority, such as convenience, taste, price, satiating hunger rapidly, or achieving weight loss.

Box 2E.7 Example: Evidence that salt intake is linked to blood pressure

Intersalt is a prime example of a large-scale, cross-sectional study. It investigated the relationship between salt intake (measured by sodium excretion) and blood pressure. The study involved 10 079 men and women in 52 different centres around the world. Each individual's blood pressure and 24 h sodium excretion was measured. Regression analyses suggested that

- Urinary sodium excretion was related to blood pressure at an ecological level
- BMI and alcohol intake were both independently and strongly associated with raised blood pressure

Intersalt's findings were controversial. Several commentaries, including those published by the Salt Institute (an association of salt companies), questioned the study's validity. However, subsequent analyses by the Intersalt group and by other researchers found an even stronger association between blood pressure and sodium levels.

A range of evidence now clearly supports the role of salt in cardiovascular disease [49] (Strazzullo et al. 2009), and a reduction in dietary salt intake is an accepted means of reducing blood pressure. Indeed, a recent Cochrane review found that *'reduction in salt intake lowers blood pressure both in individuals with elevated blood pressure and in those with normal blood pressure'.*

Source: Adapted from Intersalt Cooperative Research Group, *BMJ*, 297, 319, 1988; Hanneman, R.L., *BMJ*, 312, 1283, 1996; He, F.J. and MacGregor, G.A., *Cochrane Database Syst. Rev.* 2004(3), CD004937, 2004.

Box 2E.8 Example: Cholesterol and heart disease—the Seven Countries Study

The Seven Countries Study was inspired by observations that heart disease was a greater problem in the United States than in other countries such as Italy. The chief investigator, Ancel Keys, posed the hypothesis that *'differences among populations in the frequency of heart attacks and stroke would occur in some orderly relation to physical characteristics and lifestyle, particularly composition of the diet, and especially fats in the diet'*.

Settings and methods: The Seven Countries Study involved populations of men aged between 40 and 59. They were surveyed from 1958 to 1970 on their diet and a range of risk factors for heart disease. Men were selected from 18 areas of 7 countries with contrasting dietary habits and different rates of heart disease.

Results: Deaths from heart disease were commoner in countries where animal fat was a major component of the diet, notably Finland, than in countries where olive oil was the main source of fat, e.g. Crete. In addition to academic publications, Ancel Keys also publicised his findings in popular books such as *How to Eat Well and Stay Well: The Mediterranean Way* (1975).

Legacy: The Seven Countries Study was notable for demonstrating links between heart disease and dietary fat at an ecological level and was extremely influential in changing eating patterns across much of the United States and Western Europe. More recently, the focus of concern has shifted towards other types of fat, most notably trans fats. In England, evidence of its harmful effects led to calls from NICE[†] to ban trans fats from the food chain [53].

Adapted from Blackburn (1999) and Keys (1980).

Source: Mozaffarian, D. et al., *N. Engl. J. Med.*, 354, 1601, 2006.

2E.6 Lifestyle

The effects on health of different diets (e.g. 'Western diet'), obesity, physical activity, alcohol, drugs, smoking, sexual behaviour, and sun exposure.

In general, it is difficult to attribute causality between a single aspect of lifestyle and a health effect. This chapter therefore outlines some of the observed relationships. An example is provided in Box 2E.8.

Diet

Table 2E.4 outlines three types of diets and their effects on health

Obesity

Since the 1980s, obesity has risen sharply in the United Kingdom and in many other 'Western' countries among both adults (see Figure 2E.2) and children. For example, in 2010, around 25% of adults and 15% of children were categorised as obese (Health Survey for England) although there is some evidence that the rate of increase in obesity prevalence is now slowing, particularly among children.

Obesity increases the risk of numerous chronic diseases including type 2 diabetes, CHD, hypertension, several cancers, liver disease, and osteoarthritis. In 2007, it was estimated that obesity cost the NHS in England £4.2 billion per year, with the costs to the wider economy as high as £15.8 billion through lost productivity.

Physical activity

Physical activity reduces the risk of obesity and many chronic diseases including CHD, stroke,

Table 2E.4 Factors in different diets and their related health effects

Diet	Composition	Effect on health
Western diet	High total energy High saturated fat (butter, red meat) Low fibre High salt	Energy → obesity Fat → breast cancer, obesity Low fibre → colorectal cancer Salt → stroke
Mediterranean diet	High unsaturated fat (olive oil) High fruit and vegetables Low red meat Moderate red wine	Lower cholesterol/heart disease Lower obesity Lower cancer risk
South Asian diet (in the United Kingdom)	High saturated fat (ghee) High fruit and vegetables	Obesity CHD Stroke Type 2 diabetes

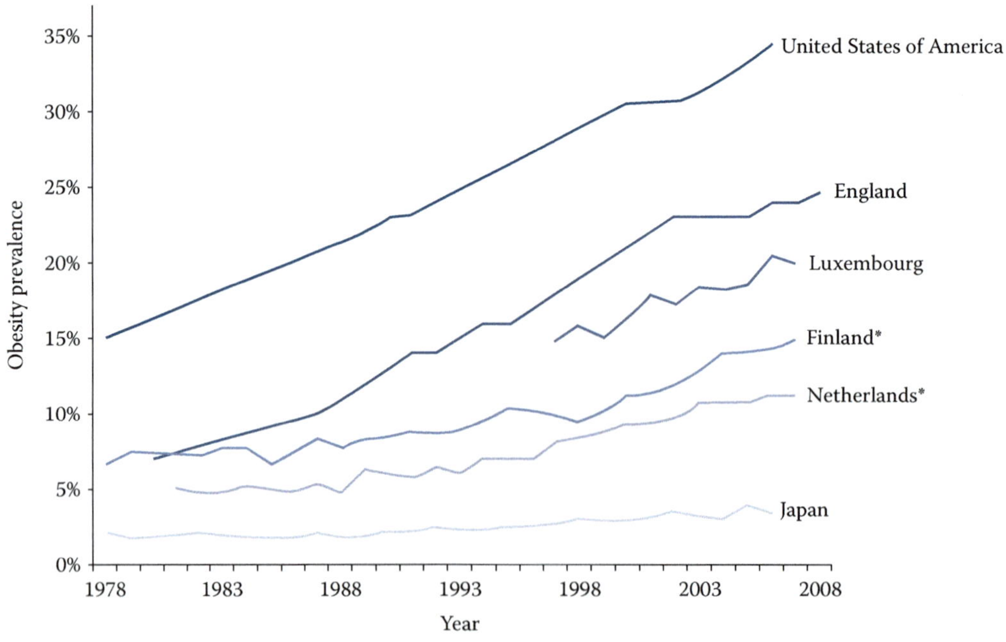

Figure 2E.2 Trends in adult prevalence of obesity (BMI ≥ 30 kg/m²); percentage of the adult population assessed as obese in a selection of countries. *Self-reported data (prevalence for the other countries are based on measured data). (From OECD, http://www.ecosante.org/index2.php?base = OCDE&langs = ENG&langh = ENG; http://www.noo.org.uk/NOO_about_obesity/trends.)

type 2 diabetes, cancer, mental illness, and musculoskeletal disease.

The NHS in England recommends that adults undertake at least 30 minutes of moderate intensity exercise five days a week and that children and young people undertake at least 60 minutes of moderate intensity exercise every day. According to the Health Survey of England (2008), only around 39% of men, 29% of women, 32% of boys, and 24% of girls achieve their physical activity recommendations. The last 20–30 years have been associated with a reduction in physical activity as part of daily routines but an increase in physical activity for leisure.

Alcohol

Some of the effects of alcohol on health are summarised in Table 2E.5.

The NHS in England recommends that men should not regularly drink more than 3–4 units of alcohol a day and that women should not regularly drink more than 2–3 units a day. Pregnant women and those trying to conceive are advised to avoid alcohol; if they do drink, it should be no more than 1–2 units once or twice a week. Data from the General Lifestyle Survey and from alcohol purchasing data suggest that alcohol consumption in the United Kingdom has decreased in the decade up to 2010 following a long-term increase since the 1960s. However, given the lag effect, alcohol-related diseases are continuing to rise.

Table 2E.5 Effects of alcohol on health

Type of alcohol excess	Health effects
Acute excess	Injury Road traffic accidents Violence Social problems Sexually transmitted infections (STIs) Peptic ulcer Liver disease
Chronic excess	Liver disease Pancreatitis Hypertension Stroke CHD Suicide
Excess in pregnancy	Fetal alcohol syndrome

Drugs

Recreational drug use has multiple health effects including

- Psychological effects—addiction, anxiety, depression, psychosis
- Mortality
- Blood-borne viral infections—for example, hepatitis C, HIV
- Poor nutrition
- Social effects—unemployment, homelessness, crime, antisocial behaviour

In England, both illicit drug use and hospital admissions related to drug misuse have declined since the 1990s (Statistics on Drug Misuse: England, 2012—NHS Information Centre). Particularly high-risk groups include young people, prisoners, and homeless people.

Smoking

Smoking is the leading cause of preventable mortality worldwide. It is associated with a wide range of ill health including

- Cardiovascular disease (e.g. CHD, stroke)
- Respiratory disease (e.g. COPD)
- Cancer (including lung, oesophageal, bladder, renal, pancreatic, and cervical cancers)
- Psychological effects (e.g. addiction)
- Pregnancy effects (e.g. IUGR)

Furthermore, tobacco can similar adverse health effects through exposure to second-hand smoke.

Smoking rates are higher in males (except teenagers) and among people in lower socio-economic circumstances. Smoking is also strongly associated with alcohol intake.

Sexual behaviour

Unsafe sex can lead to sexually transmitted infections (STIs) and unintended pregnancies. Both of these phenomena are of high public health importance due to the potential long-term health effects and stigma associated with them. STIs can lead to chronic diseases such as pelvic inflammatory disease, HIV, and cervical cancer due to HPV infection. Certain groups are at increased risk of some STIs, such as men who have sex with men. Such individuals may be offered specific preventative interventions (e.g. hepatitis B vaccination).

Sun exposure

Sun exposure is associated with malignant melanoma and with non-melanomatous skin cancers such as basal cell carcinoma and squamous cell carcinoma. In the United Kingdom, as in many other countries, there has been a large increase in the incidence of malignant melanoma over the last 25 years. In response, Cancer Research UK has run a skin cancer awareness and prevention campaign—*SunSmart*—since 2003 (http://www.sunsmart.org.uk/).

2E.7 Complex interventions

Combating complex problems using a wide range of approaches, including health service interventions and broader cultural interventions.

Several methods have been adopted to tackle complex issues such as poor diet. They include the so-called **medical**, **behavioural,** and **socioenvironmental** approaches:

Medical approach

This approach focuses on disease, with a narrow conception of the causes of disease and the determinants of health. Illness is considered in microbiological or physiological terms. Prevention focuses on known risk factors (e.g. high cholesterol and hypertension as risk factors for cardiovascular disease). Risk reduction focuses on pharmacological interventions (e.g. statins or antihypertensives), and health is equated with the absence of disease and the provision of health services.

Socioenvironmental approach

This approach seeks to improve health by means of strategies that modify the social, political, and economic environment through government and community actions. Health education involves recognition that aspects of home, workplace, and community life may be detrimental to health.

Pros and cons of the socioenvironmental approach are outlined in Table 2E.6.

Behavioural approach

This approach promotes education and free choice, rather than legal or fiscal coercion. Disease prevention can be achieved through the provision of information to populations about lifestyle risk factors (e.g. smoking, drinking, or diet). In particular, many campaigns now make use of **social marketing** to encourage people to adopt healthier eating habits (see Section 2I.3). Social marketing aims to take into account the priorities and perspectives of particular sectors of a target group for health messages. Messages and health promotion campaigns are then targeted accordingly.

A limitation of the behavioural approach is that it tends to disregard sociocultural influences

Table 2E.6 Advantages and disadvantages of the socioenvironmental approach

Advantages	Evidence of **effectiveness** (e.g. legislation to reduce salt in food)
	Potential to reduce **inequalities** (by tackling structural barriers to healthy choices)
Disadvantages	May be perceived as minimising **free will** (the 'nanny state')
	Can lead to **unpopular** policies

on behaviour, such as the way in which dietary choices are influenced by advertising and income. Dietary education may therefore have little impact on poorer families who have no access to affordable fresh fruit and vegetables. This approach has also been criticised for blaming problems on ignorance or on personal choices through the attribution of guilt.

Following the UK General Election in 2010, the new coalition government began promoting a behavioural economics approach to behaviour change. The 2010 public health white paper, 'Healthy Lives, Healthy People', reflects this philosophy by seeking to improve public health while maximising individual autonomy/freedom using the so-called 'nudge' effect (see Box 2E.9).

Box 2E.9 Nudge

Neoclassical microeconomics assumes that individuals always make perfectly rational decisions. In contrast, behavioural economics seeks to recognise the foibles and irrationalities of human nature, including overconfidence, projection bias (blaming others), and the effects of limited attention. These irrationalities can lead to systematically irrational behaviours, such as

Status quo bias (when people prefer to continue a course of action simply because it has been previously pursued)

Social influences (e.g. herd mentality, where people make decisions that following the opinions and choices of others even when demonstrably suboptimal)

Heuristics or 'rules of thumb' (e.g. availability heuristic—perceiving the frequency of an event simply based on the ease with which an example can be brought to mind)

The authors of 'Nudge', Thaler and Sunstein, advocate the doctrine of 'libertarian paternalism'. This is where individuals are given the freedom to make their own choices, but a paternalistic organisation, such as the government, develops a 'choice architecture' that favours the healthiest option. For example, a supermarket might sell a wide range of products and customers are free to purchase any of the foods on offer, including unhealthy foods. However, if healthier options are stocked on the shelves at eye level, then this will have the effect of 'nudging' shoppers into purchasing healthier foods without constraining their liberty. Equally, by making pension schemes opt-out rather than opt-in, the government provides a nudge to higher enrolment, which should help reduce poverty in old age.

The Nudge approach is sometimes criticised as simply devolving responsibility for decision-making to individual citizens. In fact, however, Thaler and Sunstein's vision embraces a responsibility for government to encourage people into making the healthiest selection.

Advantages	Disadvantages
Does not limit individual choice	Relatively ill-defined concept
Low cost	Little evidence at a large scale
Simple and rapid	May be less effective than proscriptive legislation
Some evidence of effectiveness (e.g. placing fruit near checkout increases consumption)	Potential for perverse responses
	Might widen healthcare inequalities

Sources: Thaler, R.H. and Sunstein, C.R., *Nudge: Improving Decisions About Health, Wealth, and Happiness*, Yale University Press, 2008; Marteau, T.M. et al., *BMJ*, 342, d288, 2011.

2F

Environment

There is a growing focus in public health on the impact of human activity on the environment. Climate change, for example, is now widely considered to be the most important threat to the planet. However, the impact of the environment is itself of profound importance to health: where we live, where we work, our air, our water, and our food. Public health specialists therefore need to appreciate the environment from both perspectives:

- **Human impact on the environment** (pollution and climate change)
- **Environmental effects on humans** (the environmental determinants of health)

In particular, they should understand the range of policy levers available to improve the environment and to reduce the impact of environmental hazards on health.

2F.1 Environmental determinants of disease

The field of environmental health traditionally focused on the short-term hazards of different chemical, biological, and physical agents; however, the environment is now generally considered to encompass all external factors including diet, housing, and water quality. Accordingly, in Dahlgren and Whitehead's *rainbow of the wider determinants of health* (see Chapter 2H), the 'environment' can be taken to include all layers of the diagram except the inner layer of 'age, sex, and constitutional factors'. The environmental determinants of health may be subdivided into the categories listed in Table 2F.1.

Environmental burden of disease

As we saw in Sections 2D and 2E, most diseases result from an interaction of hereditary (genetic) and environmental factors. The burden of disease attributable to environmental factors therefore depends on how environmental determinants are defined. In general, however, environmental risk factors are thought to account directly for around 10%–15% of the global burden of disease [61,62].

Table 2F.1 Environmental determinants of health

Global factors	Global warming and climate change (see Section 2F.3) Sustainable development (see Section 2F.4)
Living and working conditions	Housing and the built environment (see Section 2F.5) Transport (see Section 2F.11) Occupational health (see Sections 2F.8 and 2F.9) Water and sanitation (see Section 2F.5) Agriculture and food (see Section 2F.6) Air quality (see Section 2F.6)
Traditional environmental hazards	Physical factors, including temperature, noise, and radiation (see Section 2F.6) Chemical agents (see Section 2F.6) Biological agents (including infectious diseases) (see Chapter 2G)

According to the WHO *2010 Global Burden of Diseases* report, the three environmental determinants that were directly responsible for the greatest loss of DALYs were [63].

- Household air pollution from solid fuels
- Ambient particulate matter air pollution
- Occupational risk factors for injuries

Environmental justice

Exposure to environmental risk factors tends to be greatest among more deprived people—despite the fact that wealthier people tend to be responsible for more pollution and carbon emissions. This is known as **environmental injustice** and it is a cause of health inequalities. Examples of this phenomenon can be seen at a local and a global level. Examples include the following:

- **Local**: Wealthier people cause more pollution from cars; however, the health effects of this air pollution tend to fall disproportionately on deprived groups who live in cheaper housing close to busy roads.
- **Global**: Most carbon dioxide has been released by developed countries; however, it is people living in developing countries that are more likely to suffer the worst effects of climate change (e.g. desertification in parts of Africa and flooding of small island states).

2F.2 Risk and hazard

Environmental **hazards** are factors that have the potential to harm health (e.g. pollution, chemicals, radiation, extreme temperatures), whereas **environmental risk** is the **probability** of an unfavourable event (e.g. radiation exposure, storm, flooding) occurring multiplied by the **consequences** of that event (see Box 2F.1). Note that this definition of risk differs from the epidemiological definition of risk (see Section 1A.10).

Since a hazard only leads to a risk when **exposure** occurs, the field of **risk management** focuses on minimising exposures to hazards (i.e. both the occurrence and impact).

Box 2F.1 Risk vs. hazard

Hazard = Factor that may harm health

Risk = Probability of an unfavourable event × consequence of the event

Risk management

Risk management is important in both community and occupational settings. It involves two key stages: **risk assessment** (or 'risk characterisation') and **risk management** (see Table 2F.2). The risk is first characterised by estimating the occurrence of any adverse health effects in a defined population. This involves three steps: hazard identification, dose–response assessment, and exposure assessment.

Once the risk has been characterised, steps can be taken to limit any effects that a hazard has on health; this risk management includes risk evaluation, risk perception and communication, control of exposure, and risk monitoring.

Risk communication

The manner of risk communication can determine whether an issue is acceptable or not to the public. Successful risk communication relies on a good understanding of the different concepts of risk and the skills and integrity to communicate risk information appropriately and honestly. Poor risk communication not only affects the issue under discussion but may also irreparably damage the trust of the public.

Sandman [64] proposed an alternative concept of risk that takes into account the public's response to a hazard. He defines risk as being what people **feel** is the likelihood of an event rather than the epidemiological likelihood of an

Table 2F.2 Stages of risk management

Stage		Description
Risk assessment	Hazard identification	Identification may be of a • Previously **unknown hazard** through laboratory or epidemiological studies, or through • **Known hazard** in a setting where it had not previously been identified
	Dose–response assessment	Assess the relationship between the **amount of exposure** to a hazard and the **occurrence of adverse health effects** in humans. This estimate may be based on past observational studies or on experimental laboratory studies, e.g. in animals.
	Exposure assessment	Field measurements to estimate • Exposure currently being experienced in a defined population • Exposure that might be expected under different conditions
Risk management	Risk evaluation	Comparison of the risk against known **standards** or guidelines.
	Risk perception and communication	Appreciation of different concepts of risk and communication of this information appropriately and honestly.
	Control of exposure	Control may occur i. At the **source** (e.g. substitution of the hazardous substance with a less hazardous one) ii. Along the **pathway** before the hazard reaches the person (e.g. exhaust abatement) iii. At the **person** level (e.g. personal protective equipment) iv. **Secondary prevention** (i.e. treatment of disease at an early stage before it causes significant morbidity)
	Risk monitoring	A **surveillance** and detection system to ensure that exposure and effects are minimised.

Table 2F.3 Sandman's concept of risk

Concept	Sandman's term	Description	Examples
Technical aspect of risk	Hazard	This epidemiological aspect of risk relates to the **magnitude** and **probability** of the undesirable outcomes. Thus, a hazard can influence how society perceives risks.	An increase in the cancer rate. A catastrophic accident. Number of dead fish in the river. A decline in property values.
Non-technical aspect of risk	Outrage	These are the perceived negative features of the situation itself (as opposed to those of the outcomes).	See Table 2F.4.

event. He divides the 'risk' that people are worried about into two components: **technical** (or 'hazard') and **non-technical** (or 'outrage') (see Table 2F.3). Sandman's concept of risk is therefore the sum of these two aspects (i.e. **Risk = Hazard + Outrage)**.

Sandman suggested that risk communication depends on securing an **appropriate degree of outrage** in the public, so that they are neither unnecessarily frightened nor apathetic about real problems. Sandman listed nine factors that can increase or decrease the level of outrage (see Table 2F.4).

Public health specialists can communicate risk more effectively by **listening** to concerns expressed by the public, including those voiced by of pressure groups, in order to

- Take into account the factors that influence risk perception
- Understand the strength of feeling and the points of view
- Use appropriate media and language to communicate relevant information in a meaningful form

Table 2F.4 Sandman's factors affecting public outrage and hazard perception

Factor	Description
Voluntariness	Since it generates no outrage, a **voluntary** risk is much more acceptable to people than a **coerced** risk. For example, smokers tend to be more accepting of the risks of smoking than exposure to air pollution.
Control	Most people feel safer driving a car than sitting in the passenger seat. When prevention and mitigation are in the individual's hands, the risk (though not the hazard) is seen as being lower than when they are in the hands of others.
Fairness	When people feel that they are subjected to greater risks than their neighbours, they tend to be outraged, especially if the rationale for the extra risk burden is political rather than scientific or random.
Process	Outrage is affected by the public's perception of a public authority (i.e. whether it is perceived as being trustworthy or dishonest, concerned or arrogant). Government agencies can improve public perceptions by proactively informing the public about risks and by responding to the concerns of the community.
Morality	Where a risk has acquired a moral dimension (e.g. childhood cancer), discussion of cost–risk trade-offs is often seen as unacceptably callous. In these circumstances, it would be inappropriate for a public health specialist to argue that an occasional child death was an 'acceptable risk'.
Familiarity	Novel or exotic risks provoke more outrage than familiar risks.
Memorability	Memorable incidents (e.g. Chernobyl, Bhopal, Three Mile Island) make a risk easier to imagine and thus more risky (using Sandman's definition).
Dread	Some illnesses are more dreaded than others. For example, cancer is feared more than heart failure despite a better prognosis in many cases. The long latency of most cancers adds to the dread, as does the inescapability of potential carcinogens.
Diffusion in time and space	If hazard A kills 50 anonymous people a year across the country and hazard B has one chance in 10 of wiping out an entire town of 50,000 people sometime in the next century, then a risk assessment tells us that the two hazards have the same expected annual mortality (50 deaths per year). However, an 'outrage assessment' would show that hazard A is probably acceptable to the public while hazard B is completely unacceptable.

Source: Reproduced from Sandman, P.M., *EPA J.*, 21, 1987.

2F.3 Climate change

The effects of global warming and climate change.

The main causes of anthropogenic (human-induced) climate change are **increased levels of greenhouse gases, especially carbon dioxide** (CO_2) and methane. Most of the heat arriving from the sun is reflected off the earth back into space. But so-called greenhouse gases trap some of this warmth. As the concentration of greenhouse gases increases, so the planet's temperature is predicted to rise. Increased atmospheric levels of CO_2 result from **deforestation** (trees would normally convert CO_2 to oxygen through photosynthesis) and from increased **combustion** of fossil fuels.

Increased energy in the earth's atmosphere is already bringing increased frequency of extreme events, for example, storms, heat waves, periods of cold temperatures (snow and ice), extreme rainfall, as well as rising sea levels and floods. Further climate change [65] in the United Kingdom is expected to bring warmer wetter winters and hotter dryer summers.

Global warming

Average global temperatures have risen over the past century due to both natural and human factors. Climatologists predict that extreme weather such as floods, hurricanes, and droughts will become more frequent because of global warming. Temperatures rose from 1906 to 2005 by 0.74°C on average across the world.

Effects of climate change on health [66]

The health effects of climate change may be direct or indirect (see Box 2F.2).

Responding to climate change

The response to climate change involves both **mitigating** the extent of climate change (by limiting greenhouse gas emissions) and **adapting** to the effects of climate change.

Mitigation

Reducing CO_2 emissions is the most important action to limit anthropogenic climate change. This may be achieved either by

- Using **less energy** from fossil fuels
- **Behaviour change** (e.g. active forms of travel)
- Energy **efficiency measures** (e.g. improving insulation of housing)
- Using **alternative energy** sources (e.g. renewable energy or nuclear power)

Legislation is an important tool for limiting greenhouse gas emissions (e.g. the Kyoto Protocol; see Box 2F.3) and preventing deforestation. Other mechanisms that have been proposed for mitigating climate change include pollution abatement,

Box 2F.2 Direct and indirect effects of climate change

Direct effects	Extreme **heat waves** have led to excess mortality, particularly among old people or those in vulnerable sectors of society Fewer deaths related to **hypothermia** (although paradoxically the temperature in the British Isles may fall due to the effects on the Gulf Stream) **Extreme weather events** (e.g. floods) can lead to injuries, drowning, building collapses.
Indirect effects	Changing epidemiology of **infectious diseases**, e.g. spread of malaria as animals/insects vector borne diseases migrate to different geographical areas (e.g. dengue fever in Madeira in 2012) and more floods, promoting the spread of **water-borne diseases** Changing patterns of **respiratory illness** due to interactions with air pollution and aeroallergens Droughts and changing food availability lead to **starvation, famine and increasing numbers of refugees** Areas submerged under rising sea levels lead to **environmental migrants and increasing numbers of refugees** Reduced agriculture productivity and water resources has **socio-economic impact** on communities Increased pressures on resources, food and water leads to **deaths from conflicts and war** Destruction of earth's protective stratospheric ozone layer leads to increased exposure to ultra-violet radiation and **more skin cancers**

Box 2F.3 The United Nations framework convention on climate change

The United Nations Framework Convention on Climate Change (UN FCCC) was agreed at the United Nations Conference on Environment and Development (the Earth Summit) in Rio de Janeiro in 1992. It had the primary objective of 'stabilis[ing] greenhouse gas concentrations in the atmosphere at a level that would prevent dangerous anthropogenic interference with the climate system'. The UN FCCC is not legally binding; however, it enables legally binding treaties to be negotiated. An annual climate change conference is held during which the 194 signatory countries meet. Some of the key milestones include the following:

Kyoto Protocol 1997 [67]

The protocol is a legally binding agreement for developed countries to cut emissions of the six main greenhouse gases. It came into force in 2005, but while 191 countries have ratified the protocol, one of the biggest producers of greenhouse gases—the United States—rejected the treaty, and Canada renounced the treaty in 2011. The original Kyoto Protocol lasted until 2012.

15th United Nations Climate Change Conference (Copenhagen, 2009)

This conference aimed to establish a new global climate agreement to follow the expiry of the Kyoto Protocol in 2012; however, the agreement was not achieved.

16th United Nations Climate Change Conference (Cancun, 2010)

During this conference, it was agreed that future global warming should be limited to below 2.0°C above preindustrial levels. A $100 billion per year Green Climate Fund was proposed to help poor countries adapt to climate change; however, the funding was not agreed.

17th United Nations Climate Change Conference (Durban, 2011)

This conference resulted in agreement that a new, legally binding deal should be prepared by 2015 to take effect by 2020 to replace the Kyoto Protocol. Many scientists felt that action should begin far sooner than this. There was also some progress made on the Green Climate Fund, including its official launch.

18th United Nations Climate Change Conference (Doha, 2012)

An eight-year extension of the Kyoto Protocol was agreed (until 2020) but only with the scope to influence 15% of global emissions due to the nonparticipation of some key developed countries (Canada, Japan, Russia, Belarus, Ukraine, New Zealand, and the United States) and the fact that developing countries that are major emitters (such as China, India, and Brazil) are not subject to emissions reductions. The concept that developed nations could be financially responsible for other countries for not reducing carbon emissions was strengthened; however, little progress was made on the funding of the Green Climate Fund.

for example, CO_2 scrubbing and **geo-engineering** methods using technologies, such as carbon capture and storage, and releasing reflective particles into the atmosphere.

Adaptation

Various mechanisms may be needed to adapt to the effects of climate change and limit its effects on public health. These include

- Infrastructure developments (e.g. flood barriers, shade, and passive cooling in buildings)
- Information dissemination, for example, warning systems (e.g. heat wave–health warning systems)
- Vaccination against infectious diseases
- Protection from the sun (e.g. 'slip, slap, slop' campaigns using sun creams and clothing)
- Preparing for increased migration

2F.4 Principles of sustainability

Environmental sustainability involves balancing the needs of the present generation with those of future generations. In other words, it involves long-term considerations about how we use resources. Currently, our rate of resource use is unsustainably high, as is our rate of pollution. Examples of unsustainable exploitation of environmental resources include

- The global reduction in productive **soils** for agriculture
- Depletion of ocean **fisheries**
- Use of **fossil fuels** causing global warming

UK The UK Department for Environment, Food and Rural Affairs (DEFRA) adopts a broad view of sustainability, taking into account environmental, social, and economic developments. The department outlines five principles of sustainable development (see Table 2F.5).

Refer to sustainable transport in Section 2F.11.

Table 2F.5 Principles of sustainable development

Principle	Description
Environmental limits	Respecting the limits of the planet's environment, resources, and biodiversity to improve the environment and ensure that all the natural resources needed for life remain for **future generations**
Healthy and just society	Meeting the **diverse needs** of all people in existing and future communities; promoting wellbeing, social cohesion, and inclusion; and creating equal opportunity for all
Good governance	Actively promoting effective, participative systems of **governance** in all levels of society by engaging people's creativity, energy, and diversity
Responsible use of science	Ensuring that policy is developed and implemented on the basis of strong scientific **evidence** while taking into account scientific uncertainty through the **precautionary principle** (see Section 2F.7) as well as public attitudes and values
Sustainable economy	Building a strong, stable, and sustainable economy that provides **prosperity** and opportunities for all, an economy in which environmental and social costs fall on those who impose them (**polluter pays principle**, described in Section 2F.7) and in which incentives are in place to promote efficient resource use

2F.5 Housing and water

Health problems associated with poor housing and home conditions, inadequate water supplies, flooding, poor sanitation, and water pollution.

Housing and health

The relationship between housing and health is complex, with individual exposures not always relating directly to specific morbidities. People living in poor housing conditions typically experience other forms of deprivation as well, such as poor education, unemployment, ill health, and social isolation. This correlation makes it difficult to assess, isolate, or modify the overall health effects of poor housing. In general, housing has implications for both physical and mental health.

Specific hazards of poor housing and their health effects are summarised in Table 2F.6.

ENG The amenities available to a neighbourhood may have a profound impact on health. Amenities such as access to transport, shops, and open spaces affect local levels of safety, isolation, social cohesion, and crime. For example, in England, government policy explicitly recognises the benefits of open spaces in enabling local people to be active and to maintain social links. Local authorities have a duty to consult on any plans affecting open spaces, sports facilities, and related buildings.

Table 2F.6 Housing conditions affecting health

Hazard	Examples and health effects
Temperature	Cold (due to poor insulation and fuel poverty) leading to excess winter deaths, especially in older people. Heat (due to poor ventilation or poorly insulated roofs) again leading to excess mortality, particularly in older people.
Damp and mould	Associated with an increase in aeroallergens (e.g. fungal spores), responsible for respiratory symptoms and general ill health.
Chemicals	Carbon monoxide (due to poorly ventilated or poorly maintained gas boilers and fires) may lead to nausea, fatigue, weakness, and death. Chronic exposure may cause severe harm to the fetus in pregnancy. Lead (e.g. in paint and water pipes) can lead to cognitive impairment and kidney disease, especially in children. Asbestos (e.g. in insulation) is associated with malignancy and respiratory disease.
Radiation	Radon (a naturally occurring radioactive gas) may accumulate in poorly ventilated houses and is associated with lung cancer. High-risk areas include South West England.
Design	Falls are more frequent in poorly designed and poorly maintained homes, especially among older people. Fire may occur more often in poorly maintained homes and may cause more harm because of a lack of fire doors, smoke alarms, fire extinguishers, etc.
Noise	Poor sound insulation may cause noise-related stress, which is associated with poor sleep quality, mental distress, depression, and cardiovascular diseases.
Overcrowding	Psychological distress. Increased spread of communicable diseases such as TB and influenza.

Homelessness

There are strong associations between homelessness and health, especially regarding drug and alcohol abuse, mental health problems, and infectious diseases such as TB and hepatitis. Homelessness includes **sleeping rough** (i.e. sleeping on the street, in doorways, or on night buses) but more commonly involves sleeping on a friend's sofa or spare room, or in a hostel, night shelter, or squat.

Land contamination [68]

Land contamination may occur in **brownfield** sites (i.e. abandoned or underused industrial or commercial land) or in **greenfield** sites (i.e. undeveloped or agricultural land) (see Table 2F.7).

ENG The legal definition of contaminated land is set out in Part 2A of the Environmental Protection Act 1990, which requires that 'significant harm is being caused or there is a significant possibility of such harm being caused' by the contamination. For land identified as being contaminated, the owner or developer is responsible for the costs of **remediation**.

In England, local authorities are responsible for identifying contaminated land in their area. Where an area of land is suspected of being contaminated, the authority will conduct a series of iterative **risk assessments** (see Table 2F.8). The first step of the assessment is to describe a **pathway receptor model** that outlines which people may be at risk of harm, together with the pathways through which they may be exposed to contaminants.

Table 2F.7 Land contamination in brownfield sites and greenfield sites

Site	Cause of land contamination
Brownfield	• Contaminants introduced into the land when it was being used for another purpose in the past
Greenfield	• Spread of chemicals from other areas • Natural contaminants

Water and health

Water is a vital resource for agriculture, industry, drinking, food preparation, and sanitation. Its quantity and quality strongly influence the risk of disease. The availability of water is an issue not just in arid countries but also in developed countries such as the United Kingdom.

Water monitoring and control

UK In the United Kingdom, the Drinking Water Inspectorate (DWI) regulates the quality of water supplied to customers. To ensure that it is safe and acceptable to drink, water undergoes tests for a number of quality characteristics listed in Table 2F.9.

Up to 1 million households in the United Kingdom are not on mains water and have private drinking water supplies (PWS). Regulations came in to force in 2009 controlling PWS. Arsenic concentrations in PWS can be elevated due to underlying geology, causing skin lesions and bladder, skin, and lung cancers.

Water pollution

Water pollution may damage aquatic animal and plant life and makes drinking water more difficult to treat. Common pollutants in water are summarised in Table 2F.10.

Water supply

Water availability is promoted through

- Monitoring **water levels** in ground water, reservoirs, lakes, rivers, and coastal waters
- Requiring water companies to produce a long-term **water resource plan**
- Issuing **abstraction licences** to regulate the amount of water that can be taken from water bodies

At the domestic level, measures to protect water as a resource include

- Hosepipe bans
- Short showers instead of baths
- Short-flush toilets or 'hippo' units in cisterns to reduce the amount of water used during each flush
- Fixing dripping taps and broken pipes
- Reusing water (e.g. from washing vegetables to water plants or flush toilets)

Table 2F.8 Risk assessment for land contamination

<table>
<tr><th colspan="2">Step</th><th>Description</th></tr>
<tr><td rowspan="2">1. Develop pathway receptor model</td><td>a. Identify most vulnerable 'receptor' (person at risk)</td><td>Standard considerations:
• Residential sites: 0–6-year-old female child
• Commercial sites: 16–65-year-old female
(Note: Females are used because their lower body weight means they are at risk of exposure to lower concentrations of chemicals.)
For certain sites, identify specific populations at risk.</td></tr>
<tr><td>b. Identify possible routes of exposure</td><td>Ingestion (metals, e.g. cadmium, arsenic, lead) through
• Hand to mouth route (e.g. by soiled hands, toys)
• Dust
• Attached to vegetables
Public health advice to mitigate/minimise risks. Hygiene practice (e.g. wash hands, better food preparation such as peeling vegetables).
For radiation concerns, also consider the risk of irradiation directly through skin or at a distance.</td></tr>
<tr><td colspan="2">2. Conduct a generic quantitative-risk assessment</td><td>Use of generic risk assessment criteria to screen out sites that do not pose a risk.</td></tr>
<tr><td colspan="2">3. Conduct a detailed quantitative risk assessment</td><td>Use of site-specific assessment criteria to investigate the risk.</td></tr>
</table>

Table 2F.9 Water tests

Water test	Description
Physical characteristics	Taste, colour, smell. The smell of **chlorine** suggests contamination with sewage.
Chemical composition	The concentration of **chlorine** should be kept at around 0.4–0.5 mg/L. The concentration of **nitrogen** is indicative of decomposing organic matter. **Calcium** and **magnesium** are markers of hard water. The absence of **oxygen** signals stagnant water, which can indicate heavy pollution.
Bacteriology	Bacteriological examination is performed to detect faecal organisms such as *E. coli*, cryptosporidia, and other coliforms.

Table 2F.10 Water pollutants

Pollutant	Description
Fertilisers	**Nitrates** and **phosphates**, mostly from agricultural processes, lead to the **eutrophication** of waterways (i.e. the overgrowth of algae and ensuing oxygen depletion).
Metals	**Aluminium** may be naturally occurring, and aluminium sulphate is used in water purification to improve the taste of water. In the Camelford (Cornwall, 1988) incident [69], excessive amounts of aluminium sulphate entered the drinking water causing a range of short-term symptoms (such as diarrhoea, blistering, joint pains, and hair turning blue/green) and long-term neurological effects. **Lead** is usually derived from domestic plumbing systems. Other **heavy metals** may be naturally occurring or may have leached from contaminated soils.
Slurry	Organic waste includes slurries, silage liquor, surplus crops, sewage sludge, and industrial wastes. These may enter the water course if they are poorly stored or are disposed or spread onto land.
Sewage	In the United Kingdom, acceptable sewage regulations are enforced by the Environment Agency (EA) or the Scottish Environment Protection Agency (SEPA).

- Collecting rainwater using water butts
- Fitting water meters

Flooding

Flooding has numerous risks to health including

- Drowning
- Injury
- Mental health effects
- Contamination of drinking water by sewage
- Lack of mains water and electricity (affecting hygiene, heating, and communication)
- Carbon monoxide fumes from indoor use of generators
- Disrupted transport to health services
- Increased infectious disease risk
- Social impacts of relocation, loss of possessions and residence

Water and health in developing countries

Inadequate water supplies remain a major problem for around 15%–20% of the world's population, largely in Asia and sub-Saharan Africa. Poor water security and sanitation problems can result from natural disasters (flood, earthquake, or drought) or from pollution. Moreover, human interventions to reduce water shortages can themselves sometimes exacerbate health problems (e.g. malaria associated with irrigation channels).

Inadequate water supplies can lead to a range of **infectious diseases**, which may be due to

- Ingestion of **faecal contamination**, either due to
  - Lack of water for adequate hygiene (washing hands and food)
  - Ingestion of contaminated water (e.g. diarrhoeal diseases such as cholera)
- **Water-based** microbial agents (e.g. **schistosomiasis**)
- Water-related **vectors** (e.g. malaria)

The United Nations (UN) **Millennium Development Goals** include reducing water shortages and improving sanitation. Reducing the proportion of people without access to safe drinking water and basic sanitation improves health both **directly** and **indirectly** (by reducing the morbidity and mortality of illnesses associated with the water supply, such as diarrhoea).

Sanitation

Sanitation refers to facilities or services for the safe disposal of human urine and faeces and waste water.

Problems with sewage treatment include an odour nuisance to neighbours and annoyance from insects/mosquitoes breeding grounds.

Waste disposal

The **waste hierarchy**, which forms part of the EU's waste management framework, orders the options available for disposing waste from the most desirable to the least desirable. As Figure 2F.1 indicates, the most desirable option is to **reduce** the amount of waste created in the first place. Where reducing use or production of waste is not possible, reusing products should be considered (e.g. domestic reuse of carrier bags). In circumstances where products cannot be reused, they should be recycled. Only where the other options in the hierarchy are unavailable should incineration or landfill be considered.

There are various ways in which the aims of the hierarchy may be achieved. For example, manufacturing industry can adopt low waste processes, and households can use composting to dispose of waste organic material. In the United Kingdom, recycling has increased substantially over the last 10 years, with 43% of domestic waste recycled in 2011/2012 compared to 11% in 2000/2001 [70].

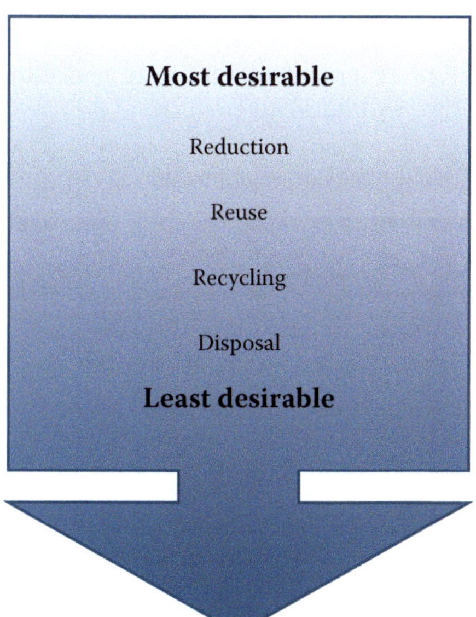

Figure 2F.1 The waste hierarchy.

Incineration

In 2011/2012, approximately 19% of UK waste was incinerated. Incineration may be considered more efficient than landfill because the combustion of waste at high temperatures produces fewer harmful chemicals. However, it is questionable whether incinerators are environmentally sustainable, even those that generate electricity. In comparison, recycling uses considerably less energy because it entails less use of raw materials. Moreover, the ash from incinerators often contains harmful toxins, some of which may be carcinogenic (e.g. dioxins).

Landfill

Around 38% of waste in Britain is disposed of in landfill sites. Landfill presents a number of potentially harmful environmental effects:

- Rotting rubbish emits **explosive gases** such as methane
- **Noxious liquids** from dumps risk polluting local waterways
- Additional **nuisances** including lorry traffic and noise, odours, smoke, dust, airborne litter, and pests (e.g. rats and seagulls)

Hazardous waste

Certain waste items risk causing harm when they are discarded, including batteries, paint tins, fertiliser, and healthcare waste such as body parts, medicines, and sharps. In particular, the inappropriate disposal of radioactive and chemical waste may contaminate the land.

Regulation

UK In the United Kingdom, the Environment Agency (EA) and the Scottish Environment Protection Agency (SEPA) enforce a waste management licensing system to ensure that landfill and incinerator systems do not have an adverse effect on health, the environment, or local amenities.

2F.6 Monitoring and control of environmental hazards

Methods for monitoring and control of environmental hazards including food and water safety, atmospheric pollution and other toxic hazards, noise, and ionising and electromagnetic radiation.

As seen in Section 2F.2, environmental hazards must be monitored in order to reduce the risk of exposures that might lead to adverse health effects. Different monitoring systems are used depending on the hazard, but all systems require surveillance data (see Table 2F.11).

Food safety

See Section 2F.5 for water safety.

Food can affect health not only through its nutritional effects but also through the toxicological safety of any contaminants or additives. Such contaminants may be biological, chemical, or radioactive (see Table 2F.12).

The WHO and the Food and Agriculture Organization (FAO) of the UN set standards for food additives and the use of pesticides in their *Codex Alimentarius*. Within the United Kingdom, the Food Standards Agency (FSA) monitors levels of contamination in food. Food quality may be improved at all stages between food production and consumption (see Table 2F.13).

Atmospheric pollution

Air pollution may be indoor or outdoor (atmospheric or ambient).

Indoor air pollution

Pollution from open solid-fuel stoves is a major public health problem in the developing world. Current efforts to improve insulation are tending to decrease ventilation, thereby exacerbating the problem. Until recently, passive exposure to cigarette smoke was another major problem; however, many countries have now banned such exposure in the workplace and in other enclosed public spaces.

Atmospheric air pollution

Table 2F.14 describes a number of factors responsible for atmospheric air pollution.

Table 2F.11 Environmental surveillance data

Type of surveillance data	Description
Emissions inventories	Records of levels of emissions from specific sources
Environmental data	Measurements of the concentration of pollutants in the air or in water or land (soil)
Biological data	Measurements of toxic substances from environmental hazards in biological samples
Health data	Surveillance data of the health effects of environmental hazards, e.g. infectious disease laboratory reports, hospital episode statistics, or cancer registry data for mesothelioma (associated with asbestos exposure)

Table 2F.12 Food contaminants

Type of contaminant	Examples
Biological	Food-borne infections (e.g. salmonella) (see Section 2G)
Chemical	Pollution (e.g. mercury from industrial waste in fish in Minamata Bay) Food storage/processing (e.g. polychlorinated biphenyls from the inside of silos have been associated with immunosuppression and malignancy)
Radioactive	Contamination of food (e.g. as occurred following the Chernobyl disaster)

Table 2F.13 Opportunities for improving food quality

Stage of food production	Example of a food improvement measure
Production	Reducing pesticide use
Processing	Reducing the risk of biological contamination by drying crops
Preservation and storage	Reducing the risk of biological contamination through irradiation, canning, or freezing
Food preparation	Separating raw and cooked foods and cooking at an appropriate temperature
Food consumption	Consuming within use-by dates

EU Attempts have been made to quantify the mortality and morbidity associated with vehicle pollution in European cities (see COMEAP [71]).

Monitoring and control

UK Air quality is monitored routinely across the United Kingdom. DEFRA's UK-AIR information resource (http://uk-air.defra.gov.uk/) provides information on air pollution nationally and regionally and issues forecasts with health advice, indicating days when levels are above standard levels. The government's Air Quality Strategy for England and Wales sets acceptable levels of the major pollutants. Local authorities are responsible for assessing the air quality in their area and are required to produce an action plan to address any areas where pollution is higher than health-based standards. Currently there are regular exceedances of the NO_2 and PM_{10} standards in the United Kingdom. The European Commission is considering legal action against the UK government (DEFRA) for failure to meet EU air quality regulations.

The UN Economic Commission for Europe supports countries' efforts to reduce pollution levels and manage their natural resources. The UN has also negotiated treaties that require signatory countries to reduce pollution (e.g. the Kyoto Protocol for greenhouse gases and the Montreal Protocol for volatile organic compounds).

Noise

Noise may be defined as **unwanted sound that causes discomfort**. It can lead to health effects such as stress, depression, sleep disturbance, noise-induced deafness, poor school performance, and cardiovascular disease. Noise may originate from a wide range of sources including

- Transport (traffic, railways, airports)
- Industry
- Neighbours (music, car alarms, shouting)
- Workplace (heavy machinery)

In the United Kingdom, the Noise at Work Regulations 2005 ensure that workplaces with high levels of noise monitor noise levels and take action if levels reach 80 decibels (e.g. acoustic treatment of buildings or personal hearing protection for employees). Legislation also exists to restrict noise at night in local communities, including the Anti-Social Behaviour Act 2003.

Radiation

There are two types of radiation (ionising and non-ionising):

- **Ionising radiation** has the ability to ionise atoms (i.e. strip them of electrons) and is characterised by high energy. Ionising radiation is emitted as **alpha particles, beta particles, or gamma rays**.
- **Non-ionising radiation** does not produce sufficient energy to ionise particles. Sources of this type of radiation include sunlight, power lines, and electrical equipment.

Ionising radiation

The most common source of naturally occurring ionising radiation is **radon**, a gas arising from

Table 2F.14 Principal air pollutants

Pollutant	Description and sources	Health effects
Carbon monoxide (CO)	An odourless and invisible gas carbon monoxide (CO) is produced when fossil fuels are burnt with insufficient oxygen. Traffic exhaust fumes and cigarette smoke both contain CO. CO poisoning is usually caused by faulty gas appliances or blocked ventilation. Low-cost carbon monoxide meters are available, but CO poisoning is best avoided by correct installation, maintenance, and proper ventilation of gas appliances.	Highly **poisonous** and causes many deaths each year. Morbidity includes hospital admissions from respiratory disorders; exposure to lower concentrations can cause memory loss, dizziness, and headaches.
Ozone (O_3)	Ozone is found in two regions of the atmosphere: • **Stratospheric** ozone (the *'ozone layer'*) is naturally occurring. • **Ground-level** ozone is produced from reactions between nitrogen oxides, volatile organic chemicals, and sunlight.	• Stratospheric ozone blocks UV radiation and thereby **prevents skin damage** and skin cancers. • Ground-level ozone can cause **respiratory symptoms** and harms plant life.
Nitrogen dioxide (NO_2)	This is a component of vehicle exhaust gases and power station emissions. Environmental levels remain relatively high in many urban areas due to traffic congestion.	Causes **respiratory symptoms**, promotes the formation of ground-level ozone (see earlier), and contributes to acid rain, which damages plant life.
Sulphur dioxide (SO_2)	Sulphur dioxide is mostly produced by coal- and oil-fired power stations. Concentrations have reduced considerably in the United Kingdom since the 1960s.	Causes acid rain, which damages vegetation and can exacerbate **respiratory illness**.
Lead	Lead is produced both through lead extraction and as a by-product of other industrial processes. Lead was formerly added to petrol, but now only unleaded and low-lead fuels are available. Levels in the air have decreased markedly as a result of unleaded petrol.	**Cognitive impairment**, renal disease, and abdominal pains.
Fine particles	Particles 1000th of a millimetre in diameter are generated naturally, by industrial processes, and by traffic emissions—particularly diesel. In the United Kingdom, levels frequently exceed health-based standards.	May exacerbate **respiratory and cardiovascular disease**.
Volatile organic compounds	These include benzene and 1,3-butadiene, which are components of traffic emissions and industrial processes using solvents.	**Carcinogenic** and contribute to ground-level ozone and smog.
Radon	Naturally occurring form of ionising radiation, higher concentrations find in some granites.	Increases the risk of **lung cancer**

Table 2F.15 Measuring radiation [72]

Unit	Symbol	Measure	Illustrative examples
Becquerel	Bq	**Amount** of radioactivity in a material (unit relates to disintegrations per second).	**10 Bq/cm²**: threshold level for contamination of surfaces requiring remediation on health grounds
Gray	Gy	**Absorbed dose**: Energy deposited in each gram of tissue (joules per kg), indicating acute radiation damage to organs.	**10 Gy**: Destroys bone marrow
Sievert	Sv	**Risk of exposure** or **effective dose**: Risk of cancer from chronic or low doses of radiation. Adjusts for the fact that the same absorbed dose from different types of radiation has different capacities to cause cancer. Sieverts take into account the energy transfer according to the type of radiation; thus, 1 Gy of beta or gamma radiation = 1 Sv, but 1 Gy of alpha radiation = 20 Sv.	**0.02 mSv**: 1 chest x-ray [72] **2 mSv**: Average exposure to natural background radiation in 1 year **20 mSv**: Annual dose limit for a radiation worker **1 Sv**: Increases lifetime risk of cancer by approximately 5%

uranium in rocks and soils. Radon accounts for about half of UK residents' radiation dose. Naturally occurring levels of the gas are generally low and are not associated with harm. Higher radon levels are found in the South West England due to the granite geology in the area and have been linked to an increased risk of lung cancer—especially in miners. Householders in areas with high radon levels should monitor and reduce the levels of radon in the home. Radon levels should not exceed 200 Bq/m³. Actions to reduce indoor radon concentrations usually involve improving ventilation to expel radon into the atmosphere.

Naturally occurring ionising radiation accounts for 84% of the radiation exposure in the population. Around 15% comes from healthcare (including radiotherapy and radiology), with the remainder (<1%) coming from industry (e.g. electricity production) and fallout from previous nuclear weapon explosions or nuclear power incidents [72].

Measuring radiation

Radiation is quantified using different methods and different units, based on to the amount of radiation released, the absorbed dose, or the risk to health. The principal methods are shown in Table 2F.15.

Health effects of ionising radiation

The health effects of radiation depend largely on the dose. Health effects are only likely to occur with doses over 1 Gy and are classified as **early** and **late**:

- Early symptoms include **acute radiation sickness** (diarrhoea, vomiting, and skin epilation), sterility, and skin erythema.
- Later effects include cancer, hereditary defects in offspring, and organ damage.
- A single exposure to the whole body of a dose greater than 5 Gy is likely to be fatal.

Table 2F.16 Health impacts of non-ionising radiation

Type of non-ionising radiation	Health impact
UVA	Skin cancer Cataracts Skin ageing
UVB	Skin cancer Cataracts Sunburn

Table 2F.17 Two sources of non-ionising radiation

Source	Description
Mobile telephones	The increasing use of mobile phones has been accompanied by concerns about possible harmful effects on health arising from both exposure to • The radio waves that are produced by **devices** that are held close to the head • From the **base stations** that serve the telephones
Power lines	High-voltage power lines emit extremely low-frequency (ELF) magnetic fields of around 50–60 Hz. Some evidence suggests that ELF radiation may possibly increase the risk of leukaemia in children in homes with high levels of exposure, although other researchers argue that these findings are due to bias or confounding.

UK *Monitoring and control*

Current UK policy in this area is largely set by EU directives. In England, several government bodies are involved in the monitoring and control of radiation:

- The Centre for Radiation, Chemical and Environmental Hazards of Public Health England monitors and researches the effects of radiation in the United Kingdom.
- The EA is a major source of guidance and regulation for a wide range of environmental issues in England and Wales, including radiation.
- DEFRA is responsible for implementing legislation and for regulating of chemicals and environmental threats to health.

Households in high-radon areas are recommended to have radon monitoring for test periods lasting several months. Employees working in settings with high levels of radiation (e.g. medical imaging) should wear personal radiation monitors to monitor their exposure.

Nonionising radiation

Sunlight is the main source of **ultraviolet (UV) radiation** and consists of UV A and B radiation (see Table 2F.16). Exposure to both types of radiation increases the risk of developing cataracts and skin cancer such as melanoma, squamous cell skin cancer, and basal cell cancer.

There have been suggestions that some types of electromagnetic radiation (electromagnetic fields [EMFs]) might be associated with the development of cancer. Two major areas of public concern have been mobile telephones and power lines (see Table 2F.17). However, most research evidence suggests that any risks, if they exist at all, are probably very small.

2F.7 Use of legislation in environmental control

The control of environmental pollution and waste production by businesses requires effective legislation because of potential conflict between economic priorities, protecting the environment and human health effects. This tension is particularly pertinent for small businesses and also in developing countries where the information and expertise to implement environmentally friendly measures may be lacking.

Environmental hazards are seldom limited by geographical boundaries. For example, acid rain caused by UK power plants in the 1970s and 1980s mainly fell in continental Europe. Therefore, legislation and strategies to tackle pollution and waste production should be set at an international level. Within the EU, such legislation may be **primary** (e.g. treaties) or **secondary** (e.g. directives and regulations).

European Union Legislation

EU European environmental legislation is based on two guiding principles: **polluter pays** and the **precautionary principle** (see Table 2F.18).

European legislation aims to restrict levels of pollution and emissions and to ensure the safe disposal of waste through measures outlined in Table 2F.19.

Compliance with the terms of permits and regulations can be enforced through

- **Inspections**, followed by warning letters or formal cautions
- Enforcement or prohibition **notices**
- Suspension, revocation, or modification of **permits**
- **Penalties**, such as fines and imprisonment

Regulatory agencies

UK In the United Kingdom, the EA regulates large and complex industrial processes, while local authorities regulate smaller-scale industries. Other relevant regulatory agencies include the Health and Safety Executive, DWI, Trading Standards, and the FSA. Environmental health officers from the local authority enforce the regulations of the Environmental Protection Act [73] (preventing the sale of contaminated foods, unsafe housing standards, and nuisance), the Clean Air Act, and the Environmental Permitting Regulations.

Table 2F.18 Principles of European environmental legislation

Guiding principle	Description
Polluter pays	This is the principle that the party responsible for creating pollution should pay for the recovery, cleanup, recycling, or disposal of products after use. The payment may also be a tax on business or consumers who use an environmentally unfriendly product, such as certain types of packaging.
Precautionary principle	Credible but unproved health hazards should be treated as real threats until shown otherwise. Decisions affecting the environment should not be delayed while scientific data are collected. Instead, policymakers should err on the side of protecting the environment and health.

Table 2F.19 Measures in European legislation to restrict pollution

Measure	Description
Permits or licences	Issued to companies using natural resources, disposing of waste, or producing pollution (e.g. sewage companies, water companies, and manufacturing industries). Conditions attached to the permit typically set limits on the amount of pollution that may be produced or stipulate the use of specific procedures and **best available techniques** (BAT).
Taxes or levies	By reflecting the environmental costs of production, these penalties aim to discourage the production of emissions. An example is the **climate change levy**.
Trading schemes	Companies participate in a scheme that is committed to reducing emissions. Firms may **buy or sell excess emission allowances** and can thereby compete on the basis of an overall reduction in emissions.
Product labelling schemes	Eco-friendly or **energy efficiency ratings** are displayed on household and office appliances and buildings.

Effectiveness of legislation

Compliance with environmental legislation is variable. There are many reasons for this inconsistency, including

- Business not always being aware of legislative requirements
- Monitoring in some countries being more rigorous than others
- Penalties for non-compliance being comparatively weak (cf. health and safety offences)
- Compliance not always being perceived as central to a firm's survival

2F.8 Health and safety at work

Appreciation of factors affecting health and safety at work (including the control of substances hazardous to health).

Factors affecting health at work include the work **environment**, occupational **equipment,** and other **employees**. Improving occupational health should be in the interest of both employees and employers because, in addition to the health effects, the financial costs of penalties and lost working time may be substantial.

Types of workplace exposures are described in Table 2F.20.

Table 2F.20 Occupational hazards

Type of hazard	Examples
Chemical	Vinyl chloride used in manufacturing industries → liver cancer Exposure to coal dust by coal miners → pneumoconiosis Asbestos exposure in shipyard workers and insulation workers → asbestosis and mesothelioma
Physical	Noise from heavy machinery → hearing impairment Very hot or cold substances → thermal injury/burns Exposure to ionising radiation (see Section 2F.6)
Mechanical	Moving parts of machinery → trauma Lack of barriers on scaffolding → falls Poor work station design → repetitive strain injury or back pain
Biological	Needlestick injury in healthcare workers → exposure to blood-borne viruses (BBVs) Exposure to raw sewage → leptospirosis Exposure to farm animals and waste → brucellosis, anthrax
Psychological	Bullying, harassment, discrimination, lack of control, lack of reward, long working hours → stress, anxiety, or depression

Note: Those at particular risk of exposure to environmental hazards in the workplace or exposure from hazards include temporary workers, women (a higher proportion are in lower status jobs), people working illegally (e.g. asylum seekers), lone workers, staff in small businesses (small businesses can have the most difficulty complying with workplace regulations), and pregnant women.

Prevention

Interventions to minimise exposure to occupational health hazards can be targeted at two key areas (the worker and the work environment):

i. The worker—education and training on health and safety and provision of personal protective equipment (PPE)
ii. The work environment—ensuring that processes are as safe as possible, that harmful substances/machinery are contained, that monitoring systems are in place, and that hazards are minimised

Control of substances hazardous to health

UK The Control of Substances Hazardous to Health (COSHH) regulations [74] limit exposures to the following types of hazardous substances:

- Substances **used** directly in work activities (e.g. adhesives, paints, cleaning agents)
- Substances **generated** during work activities (e.g. fumes from soldering and welding)
- **Naturally occurring** substances (e.g. grain dust)
- **Biological agents** such as bacteria and other microorganisms (e.g. leptospirosis in sewage treatment workers)

These regulations require employers to

- Assess the risk posed by the hazard
- Decide on necessary precautions
- Control or prevent exposure
- Maintain appropriate testing and control measures
- Monitor exposure
- Undertake health surveillance for diseases that may be caused by exposure
- Ensure appropriate education and training of employees
- Prepare for possible incidents

Other occupational health regulations

UK Pertinent regulations include

- Reporting of Injuries, Diseases and Dangerous Occurrences Regulations (RIDDOR) [75], which is required for all serious work-related incidents
- WHO occupational limits for pollutants
- European Working Time Directive regulations (e.g. restricts the working week to 48 hours)

Occupational health agencies

UK Key agencies involved in occupational health in the United Kingdom are listed in Table 2F.21.

Safety at work audits

Procedures to monitor and control health and safety factors at work can be considered in several sequential steps (see Table 2F.22).

Table 2F.21 UK agencies involved with occupational health

Agency	Purpose
Health and safety executive	Sets regulations Monitors workplaces Investigates incidents Enforces workplace regulations
Trade unions	Campaign for workers' rights to healthy working conditions Survey employees' working conditions Provide advice on legal issues concerning health and safety Represent employees with employers on health and safety issues
Local authorities	Local inspection, enforcement of regulations Monitors workplaces Investigates incidents
Employers	Implement regulations Provide safe working conditions
Occupational health departments	Undertake pre employment health checks Advise employers on workplace hazards and their control Advise employees on health and safety issues Monitor sickness absence Offer immunisations if appropriate, e.g. in health and social care settings

Table 2F.22 Steps involved in safety at work audits

Step	Description
1. Assessment	Assessment of hazards in the environment
2. Identification	Identification of those at most risk (e.g. through pre-employment health checks)
3. Surveillance	Surveillance of hazards, incidents, and health-related morbidity (through systems of incident reporting, feedback, and analysis)
4. Mitigation	Action to reduce exposure to hazards (through training, provision of protective equipment to exposure, and emergency planning)
5. Monitoring	Monitoring of the effect of interventions to reduce effects of hazards (e.g. through incidence, sickness, and absence records)

2F.9 Occupation and health

The effects of occupation on health vary according to the

- Type of occupation
- Personal risk factors
- Levels of social support

In general, there are substantial health benefits to being in work, but certain occupations can expose employees to particular risks (see Section 2F.8).

Table 2F.23 Consequences of unemployment

Level of impact	Consequences of unemployment
Individual	• Suicide rates among the unemployed increase within a year of job loss. • Cardiovascular mortality rises over 2 or 3 years and continues for the next 10–15 years.
Family	• Spouses of people out of work can also experience poor health. • Spouses whose partner has been forced to give up work due to illness may additionally be burdened with caring responsibilities. • In families where individuals are seeking work, the effects of poverty appear to be most severe in the short term. In the longer term, families may adapt to unemployment.
Society	• Increased unemployment places a greater burden on society through fewer people making tax contributions and increased social security and health service needs of people without work.

Unemployment

Being out of work is associated with adverse physical, mental, and social effects. These phenomena are related partly to the length of time spent unemployed. Although being out of work may cause morbidity, the causal relationship also works the other way around (i.e. people who are physically or mentally unwell may be more likely to leave jobs or have difficulty working). Studies indicate that ill health and healthcare use are also associated with job insecurity, especially the **anticipation** of job losses.

There are consequences from unemployment on the **individual**, on **families,** and on **society** at large (see Table 2F.23).

2F.10 Health impact assessment for environmental pollution

See Section 1C.17 for details on health impact assessment (HIA) and environmental impact assessment (EIA).

In considering the health impact of pollution, the risk assessment principles introduced in Section 2F.2 should be applied (e.g. hazard identification, assessment of the dose–response effect, and an assessment of the level of exposure).

Although the Environmental Impact Directives [76] do not legally require mandatory HIAs for developments and new polluting industries, the UK Planning Act [77] requires assessments on health for those involving chemicals, poisons, or radiation. For nationally significant infrastructure planning developments, HIAs are increasingly being prepared to consider the impacts on health of developments.

2F.11 Transport policies

Transport policies need to acknowledge the potential **benefits** of increased transport and accessibility, which increase **employment** opportunities, improve the availability of **goods**, and lead to a greater choice of **social activities**. It is also important to recognise the health benefits associated with active transport (walking or cycling), as well as the risks associated with non-active forms of transport (e.g. road, rail, and air) which include

- Air pollution and global warming
- Noise pollution
- Collisions, including road traffic accidents
- Effects on social cohesion (e.g. from a busy dual carriage-way bisecting a community)

Road transport is one of the greatest contributors to air pollution, particularly in towns and cities (see Section 2F.6). However, while emissions from most industrial and transport sources are generally decreasing, the impact of air travel is increasing. According to the European Commission, EU emissions from international aviation now account for 3% of all greenhouse gas emissions in the EU and are projected to increase by around 70% between 2005 and 2020 [78].

Sustainable transport

Sustainable transport policies promote forms of transport that have the potential for maintaining wellbeing in the long term, which has environmental, economic, and social dimensions. Such policies typically focus on environmentally friendly transportation, taxation, reducing car usage, reducing the environmental impact of transport, reducing emissions, and promoting sustainable forms of transport, for example, car sharing and public transport.

Environmental friendly transportation

Alternatives to cars can be encouraged by sustainable transport policies (see Table 2F.24).

Active forms of transport, such as walking and cycling, have health benefits for the **individual**, through increased physical activity, and for the **population** as a whole through reduced air pollution, reduced greenhouse gas emissions, and reduced noise. Cycling also has health risks including exposure to vehicle emissions and risk of road traffic collisions; however, studies in European settings have shown that the health benefits of cycling to the individual outweigh the risks [79].

Table 2F.24 Alternative means of transportation

Transport option	Promotion policies
Walking	Pedestrian zones, walking routes
Cycling	Bicycle lanes, employer cycle loan schemes, city cycle share schemes
Public transport	Subsidised public transport systems, integrated modal transport hubs
Employer commuter clubs	Car sharing schemes, green travel plans

Taxation

Taxation can be used to encourage industry and consumers to adopt more fuel-efficient vehicles and thereby reduce vehicle emissions.

Reducing car usage

This can be achieved through

- Levies or taxes for road use (e.g. London congestion charge)
- Parking restrictions and charges
- Subsidising the cost of public transport
- Encouraging car sharing through introducing share-only lanes and high-volume occupancy lanes
- Reducing the transport of freight via road and increasing rail transport of freight

Reducing the environmental impact of transport

Carbon-offsetting initiatives seek to compensate the environment for emissions of carbon dioxide. Processes that emit carbon dioxide are matched with projects that either reduce the emission of carbon dioxide or remove an equivalent amount of the gas from the air. For example, air passengers can make a donation to a non-governmental organisation (NGO) that will fund projects designed to increase forestation.

Wilkinson [80] described how researchers are exploring the option of **carbon capture** as an alternative approach to reducing the impact of carbon dioxide production. The damage to the environment results from carbon dioxide in the atmosphere. Carbon capture relies on finding locations to store carbon dioxide so that it does not reach the atmosphere. Depleted oil and gas fields could be ideal carbon capture locations since they have increasing storage space, and the insertion of carbon dioxide could make the continued extraction of gas and oil more straightforward. Note that carbon capture would neither result in a reduction in the use of hydrocarbons nor in the production of carbon dioxide. Instead, it may best be regarded as a relatively inexpensive **short-term solution** whose value lies in buying time to develop alternative fuel sources.

Emissions trading schemes

Emissions trading schemes provide economic incentives for industrial polluters to reduce their emissions. One example is the EU Emissions Trading System, which expanded in 2012 to include aviation emissions (see Box 2F.4).

Box 2F.4 EU Example: Air transport—an international perspective to transport policy

Over the last few decades, European air transport policies have focused on expanding the air travel market, rather than on reducing or containing its environmental impact. One such policy is the exemption of aircraft fuel for international flights from all taxes. While individual countries in the EU have the option of charging fuel tax for domestic flights, only the Netherlands currently does so.

Partly as a result of these policies, air transport has expanded rapidly. Although aircraft are becoming more fuel efficient, these gains are more than offset by increased air traffic. However, in 2012 the aviation industry became part of the EU **Emissions Trading Scheme**. Under this scheme, the European Commission places an overall cap on emissions per year. Within these limits, companies are given an emissions allowance. If they are in danger of exceeding their allowance, they have two options: either to reduce their emissions (e.g. by investing in new technology) or to buy part of their competitors' allowances on the open market.

Source: Adapted from http://ec.europa.eu/clima/policies/ets/index_en.htm.

2G

Communicable Diseases

Infectious diseases represent the largest cause of childhood and adolescent deaths worldwide. In 2010, for example, they accounted for over 11 million deaths a year in low- and middle-income countries. In higher-income countries, although infectious diseases have a lower mortality than non-infectious disease, they remain a topic of major public health importance for the following reasons:

- Globalisation (infectious diseases now spread rapidly around the globe)
- Re-emergence of old scourges (e.g. TB)
- Novel infections (e.g. severe acute respiratory syndrome (SARS), novel coronavirus)
- Evolution of existing pathogens leading to new risks (e.g. potential for zoonotic disease threats, pandemic influenzas)
- Resistance to therapeutic agents
- Hospital-acquired infections (e.g. methicillin-resistant *Staphylococcus aureus* [MRSA])
- Burden of long-term conditions (e.g. HIV/AIDS)
- Viral cause of certain cancers (e.g. cervical cancer)

2G.1 States in the development of infectious diseases

Definitions including incubation, communicability, and latent period; susceptibility, immunity, and herd immunity.

Figure 2G.1 [79] sets out some of the key stages in the time course of an infectious disease. See Table 2G.1 for further details.

An individual may progress through several states in terms of their vulnerability and experience of the disease (see Table 2G.2).

In addition, there are population-level measures to consider (see Table 2G.3).

See also Section 1A.30 for further details of epidemiological investigation of infectious diseases.

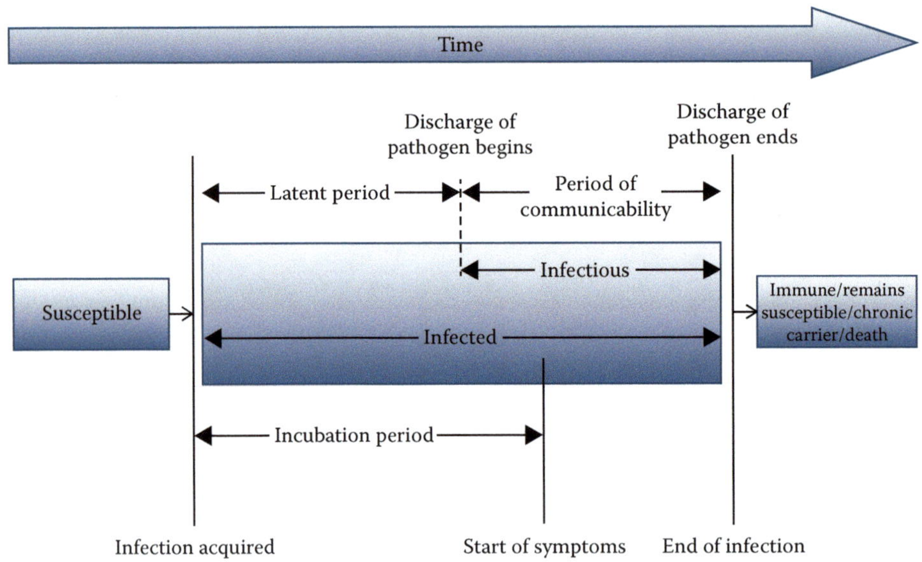

Figure 2G.1 Temporal phases in an infectious disease.

Table 2G.1 Description of key temporal phases in a single infection

Temporal phase	Description
Incubation period	Also known as the 'subclinical period', this is the time between infection and the onset of clinical symptoms. Its duration may be affected by the infecting dose. Establishing the incubation period helps epidemiologists to determine when infection occurred and thus who might be a contact.
Latent period	This is the time between initial infection and the start of infectiousness. Typically, this period is slightly shorter than the incubation period.
Period of communicability	Also known as the 'infectious period', this is the time during which the infected person is capable of transmitting the infective agent. The infectious period often begins before the onset of symptoms.

Table 2G.2 States of host individuals

Host state	Description
Susceptible	Able to become infected by the pathogen if exposed (i.e. lacking immune resistance against the pathogen).
Immune	The state of having sufficient biological defences to avoid infection. Immunity can be considered as passive or active: • **Passive immunity**: short-term immunity acquired either by transplacental transfer of IgG antibodies from the mother or by inoculation with antibodies as a therapy or prophylaxis against infection • **Active immunity**: longer-term immunity due to a prior encounter with an antigen, either from previous infection or vaccination
Infected	Presence of the pathogen within the host. An infected person may be • **Incubating** • **Diseased** • **Carrier**
Case	Somebody who could be infected. A case may be • Possible • Probable • Confirmed Each case must be defined in terms of time, place, and person, based on their symptoms and/or laboratory findings.
Contact	A person who has the potential to become infected due to exposure to a case or other source of infection.

Table 2G.3 Characteristics of the host population

Population measure	Description
Epidemic threshold	The number of susceptible people that is needed in a population in order for an **epidemic** to occur.
Herd immunity	A phenomenon of reduced spread of an infection in a population due to a relatively high proportion of immune individuals and thus low numbers of potentially infectious cases. The **herd immunity threshold** is the proportion of immune people in a population above which the incidence of infection will decrease. For many childhood infections, such as measles, roughly 95% of children must be vaccinated in order to achieve herd immunity.

2G.2 Surveillance

Use and evaluation of national and international surveillance.

Surveillance is the ongoing systematic **collection, collation, analysis,** and **interpretation** of data and the **dissemination** of the information generated to facilitate disease prevention. In summary, surveillance provides information for action. See Table 2G.4 for the different stages in surveillance and Table 2G.5 for the different types of surveillance.

National surveillance

UK Public Health England is responsible for coordinating communicable disease surveillance across England, taking over the functions previously performed by the HPA. In Wales, this function is undertaken by Public Health Wales, and in Scotland, by Health Protection Scotland (HPS). Certain key infectious diseases are kept under constant surveillance in order to

- Detect **trends**
- **Evaluate** prevention and control measures
- **Alert** appropriate professionals and organisations to infectious disease threats

See Table 2G.6.

IRE In Ireland, the Health Protection Surveillance Centre (HPSC) is a unit within the Population Health Directorate of the Health Service Executive (HSE). The HPSC operates the *Computerised Infectious Disease Re*porting (CIDR) system to manage the surveillance and control of infectious diseases in Ireland and to monitor antimicrobial resistance. Health personnel return notification, outbreak, and enhanced surveillance

Table 2G.4 Principles of surveillance

Surveillance stage	Description
Case definition	Definition based on clinical or microbiological criteria
Cases identified through variety of sources	Clinicians or laboratories in primary, secondary, or tertiary care
Data collection tools	Electronic databases Special forms (e.g. Legionella questionnaire)
Systematic collection of data for cases that satisfy the case definition	Passive or active (see Table 2G.5)
Analysis of data and summary statistics	See Section 1B.9
Feedback to data providers and distribution to officials who require it for action	Disseminate—through existing mechanisms (e.g. newsletters, bulletins) or specific articles and reports
Use of surveillance data	Monitoring secular trends Detection of emerging outbreaks Evaluating interventions Monitoring changes in infectious agents Evidence base for policies and guidance Research and modelling

Table 2G.5 Types of surveillance

Method	Description
Passive surveillance	This is the most common form of surveillance and involves the automatic collection of data from **routine sources** (e.g. laboratory reports or hospital episodes). It is simple but is often incomplete.
Active surveillance	This involves making a concerted effort to increase the completeness and accuracy of data (e.g. through **follow-up** phone calls). Such actions may be justified for rare but serious diseases or for disease targeted for elimination. Often, negative reporting is required, whereby laboratories or clinicians must actively report that they have had no cases.
Enhanced surveillance	This involves collecting **additional data** about cases. This may be done for a short period for a specific task (e.g. a research study or the evaluation of new guidelines).
Sentinel surveillance	Surveillance of a sample as a **subset of the population** as a whole. This may be a geographical sample (e.g. sentinel GP practices for influenza surveillance) or a particular risk group (e.g. hepatitis B surveillance among men who have sex with men).
Syndromic surveillance	Surveillance of **symptoms** rather than confirmed cases (e.g. watery diarrhoea or jaundice). This type of surveillance may be useful in emergencies or to investigate an outbreak.

forms electronically. The data are used to generate weekly infectious diseases and outbreak reports, which are published by the HPSC.

International surveillance

The value of global surveillance and of information sharing lies in

- Detecting the emergence of **resistance** in key pathogens
- Guiding **infection control** policies
- Engaging and prompting dialogue with policymakers
- Developing advocacy and **educational programmes**
- Stimulating **research**

Global surveillance serves as an **early warning system** for epidemics and provides a rationale for coordinated public health intervention. When followed by swift public health intervention, the early detection of communicable diseases can reduce morbidity and mortality and mitigate the overall negative effects on international travel and trade.

Global **surveillance** depends on strong **national surveillance systems**. For example, Public Health England houses the WHO reference laboratories for various infections (e.g. influenza; see Box 2G.1, TB, SARS), and it is the European Co-ordinating Centre for the Global Programme on Drug Resistant Tuberculosis.

Examples of other international surveillance systems include the following:

- European Centre of Disease Control (ECDC) infectious disease surveillance.
- European Antimicrobial Resistance Surveillance Network (EARSNet).
- Global Public Health Intelligence Network (GPHIN)—developed by Health Canada, this system trawls the Internet for communicable disease reports in various forums and news wires.
- Global Outbreak Alert and Response Network (GOARN)—a network of networks organised by the WHO—collects information from other sources, for example, GPHIN, WHO collaborating centres, and Pro-Med.

Two examples of global programmes are shown in Boxes 2G.1 and 2G.2.

Table 2G.6 Principal sources of information for national surveillance

Source	Description
Notifiable diseases	By law, certain diseases are deemed '*notifiable*', meaning that doctors have a statutory duty to report them. These reports should be made on the basis of clinical suspicion, rather than waiting for laboratory confirmation. See Section 2G.9 for a list of notifiable diseases in the United Kingdom.
Reports/ special forms/ returns	Laboratory results • **Case reports** (rare diseases, e.g. CJD) • Incident reports (outbreaks) • **Syndromic surveillance systems** (e.g. Royal College of General Practitioners weekly returns for a range of conditions including respiratory and gastrointestinal diseases) • **Sexual health clinic statistics** collected through an electronic surveillance system called the *Genitourinary Medicine Clinic Activity Database* (GUMCAD), which replaced the KC60 system. Chlamydia testing and diagnoses are also collected from STI clinics and community settings through the National Chlamydia Screening Programme • **Vaccine coverage**: collected through the *Cover Of Vaccination Evaluated Rapidly* (COVER) system and in Scotland by *Information Services Data* (ISD) statistics • Death registrations • **HES** (information about inpatient admissions, diagnoses and procedures; A&E and outpatient data are more limited) • **Sentinel surveillance** (e.g. the Nottingham University Primary Care Surveillance Schemes such as *Q Flu* and *Q Research*) • **Enhanced surveillance** including enhanced TB surveillance (e.g. London TB register), enhanced meningococcal surveillance
Surveys	• HIV/AIDS Reporting System (HARS) in England and the Survey of Prevalent HIV Infections Diagnosed (SOPHID) in Wales and Northern Ireland • Seroprevalence surveys • Unlinked anonymous surveys (e.g. blood borne viruses [BBVs] in injecting drug users and BBV in antenatal women)

Box 2G.1 Example: Enhanced surveillance for pandemic influenza

The WHO [82] Global Influenza Surveillance and Response System (GISRS) is a network of over 100 national influenza centres that monitor influenza. It was renamed in 2011 as part of an initiative to strengthen the global response to future potential influenza pandemics. The *Flunet* system interprets the epidemiological information derived from GISRS to generate and distribute real-time maps and graphs of virological activity in all WHO regions [83].

Source: Adapted from World Health Organization, Global Influenza Surveillance and Response System (GISRS), webpages. Accessed July 21, 2014 at: http://www.who.int/influenza/gisrs_laboratory/en/.

Box 2G.2 Example: The WHO information for action—global programme for vaccines and immunisation

The programme monitors and assesses the impact of initiatives for reducing the morbidity and mortality of vaccine-preventable diseases. Its global goals by 2010 included achieving 90% coverage of diphtheria–tetanus–pertussis (DTP) vaccine in all children—a goal that was achieved in over two-thirds of WHO member states. However, there are still significant numbers of unvaccinated children in countries such as the Democratic Republic of the Congo, India, and Nigeria.

Source: Reproduced from WHO, Immunization surveillance, assessment and monitoring, available online at www.who.int/immunization_monitoring/en.

Evaluating a surveillance system

An evaluation of a surveillance system should consider

- The public health **importance** of the disease under surveillance
- The **case definition** (e.g. is it clear and consistent?)
- Details of the **surveillance system** (e.g. its objectives and components)
- Details of the **analysis** and reporting system
- **Usefulness** of surveillance (e.g. the actions that have been taken as a result of its findings)
- Conclusions and **recommendations** to improve the system

In particular, the evaluation should consider each of the attributes shown in Box 2G.3.

Box 2G.3 Attributes of a surveillance system

Qualitative	Simplicity Flexibility Acceptability Representativeness Completeness
Quantitative	Accuracy (e.g. sensitivity, PPV, C-statistic) Timeliness Resource use (direct costs)

2G.3 Methods of control

Communicable disease control aims to prevent the spread of infection in the population. In a healthcare setting, it is termed **infection control** and it aims to prevent **cross-contamination**, which may be

- Between patients
- From healthcare workers to patients
- From patients to healthcare workers

Prevention measures may be targeted at the case, the contacts, or at other potential sources of infection (see Table 2G.7).

Table 2G.7 Methods of communicable disease control

Method	Description
Universal precautions	• Hand washing (e.g. hand hygiene campaigns) • Avoidance of contact with patients' bodily fluids, using PPE including items such as medical gloves, goggles, and face shields
Isolation	• Single room isolation (e.g. MRSA) • Negative pressure room for source isolation (e.g. TB) • Positive pressure room for protective isolation (e.g. for severely immunocompromised patients)
Decontamination	• Decontamination of persons and fomites • Disinfection of equipment and the environment
Quarantine	• Quarantine of contacts (e.g. plague)
Immunisation	• Vaccine prophylaxis of exposed individuals (e.g. hepatitis B)
Chemoprophylaxis	• Antibiotics offered to people who have come into contact with an infectious disease (e.g. meningococcal meningitis or anthrax)
Source removal	• Biociding the water in a cooling tower to control an outbreak of Legionnaires' disease • Product recall • Closure of a restaurant

2G.4 Design, evaluation, and management of immunisation programmes

Note that the terms **vaccination** and **immunisation**, while used interchangeably in common parlance, are in fact slightly different (see Table 2G.8).

Development of a vaccination programme

In developing a new vaccination programme, the following areas of work must be considered:

- Scientific evidence
- Programme strategy
- Administration
- Finance
- Vaccine purchase and distribution
- Communication
- Informatics

Table 2G.8 Vaccination and immunisation definitions

Vaccination	Administration of a vaccine
Immunisation	Administration of a vaccine plus the development of an immune response by the body

UK In England, the DH has overall responsibility for immunisation policy. It is supported by Public Health England, which undertakes vaccine research, epidemiological research, and surveillance and NHS England, which is responsible for planning immunisation. The Joint Committee on Vaccination and Immunisation (JCVI) is an independent expert advisory committee that advises the government on matters relating to communicable diseases. This committee receives papers and hears presentations and must make its recommendations in light of a cost–benefit analysis.

IRE **In Ireland,** the HSE National Immunisation Office website has up-to-date information for parents and professionals on the childhood immunisation schedule and on related topics, such as immunisation for travel (www.immunisation.ie/en).

The Irish DH and the HSE take guidance from the Immunisation Advisory Committee of the Royal College of Physicians of Ireland, which in turn has representatives from DH, the HSE, the RCPI, the Northern Ireland DH and Social Services, and other relevant organisations. The committee's guidance on immunisation is available on the HPSC website (www.ndsc.ie/hpsc).

Vaccination strategies

The WHO's vaccine recommendations are summarised in Table 2G.9.

Immunisation schedules vary by country and vary according to local epidemiology, funding, a consideration of the risk, and efficacy of each vaccine for different age groups. An annual report published jointly by WHO and UNICEF lists the vaccination schedules of every country (WHO 2014).

Table 2G.9 WHO recommendations for immunisations as part of national strategies

Target group	Vaccination
Entire population	TB (BCG) Diphtheria, tetanus, pertussis (DTP) Rotavirus Hepatitis B Measles Rubella Polio Haemophilus influenzae type B (Hib) Pneumococcal conjugate HPV
Selected subpopulations	High-risk **regions** • Yellow fever • Japanese encephalitis • Tick-borne encephalitis High-risk **individuals** • Typhoid • Cholera • Meningococcus (A, C, conjugate) • Hepatitis A • Rabies In certain programmes • Influenza • Mumps

Source: http://www.who.int/immunization/givs/en/index.html; http://www.who.int/immunization/documents/positionpapers/.

Table 2G.10 Targeted immunisation

Circumstances		Example
Travel		Hepatitis A
Occupational		Hepatitis B
Outbreak/incident		Meningitis C
Mass infection	**Eradicate**	Smallpox
	Eliminate	Polio
	Contain	Deliberate release of smallpox

In addition to national strategies, targeted vaccination strategies may be implemented in certain circumstances. Some examples are shown in Table 2G.10.

Implementation of a vaccination policy

In general, vaccine programmes are implemented at a local level using funds allocated by central government.

Changes to the vaccination schedule

After resources have been secured, vaccine manufacturers are invited to submit bids through a competitive procedure. Criteria for successful bidding are safety, efficacy, availability, price, and record of the company against previous contracts. Wherever possible, more than one supplier is chosen to minimise the likelihood of vaccine shortages.

The communication of any changes to the vaccination policy in England is achieved through

- Letters from the chief medical officer, chief nursing officer, and chief pharmacist to all registered doctors, nurses, and pharmacists, respectively
- Website publicity
- Updates to the DH's 'Immunisation Against Infectious Disease' book (known as *'The Green Book'*)
- Outreach activities by a network of *immunisation coordinators*
- Public promotion and marketing

A new promotion programme is then developed for the public, which may include leaflets; fact sheets; press, television, and radio advertisements; videos; and Internet materials such as 'question and answer' formats, frequently asked questions (FAQs), and feedback facilities for questions.

All new materials are pretested with the appropriate target audience, then amended accordingly, and their impact monitored. New data collection arrangements are set up in advance so that the vaccine coverage of a new initiative can be monitored.

Evaluation activities may include

- New **disease surveillance arrangements** to measure the impact of a new policy through laboratory-based data and/or disease notification data
- Seroepidemiological surveillance for gauging population impacts
- **Market testing** to evaluate the impact of any advertising that accompanied the introduction of new vaccines
- **Adverse events** are monitored by
    - **Expert groups** that investigate any reported serious adverse events
    - Records linkage (adverse clinical events recorded in hospital and/or primary care records are linked with immunisation data so that risks of adverse outcomes can be assessed)

Local implementation activities may include

- A **local implementation group**, usually led by an immunisation coordinator, which may include a consultant in communicable disease control (CCDC) or consultant in health protection (CHP), a pharmacist, health visitor, community paediatrician, and a representative from primary care
- A **local training programme** for health professionals

2G.5 Choices in developing an immunisation strategy

Issues for policymakers to consider when developing immunisation policy are listed in Box 2G.4 and are described in Tables 2G.11 and 2G.12.

For example, oral polio vaccine (which is a live attenuated vaccine) leads to greater control of polio because it is more effective but can result in vaccine-related paralysis. Inactivated injected polio vaccine is safer and is therefore used by many countries in which polio has been eradicated (although there is the facility in an outbreak situation for reversion to the live vaccine).

Box 2G.4 Immunisation strategy: Issues of policy makers

- Mass versus selective immunisation
- Live versus inactivated vaccine
- Age at vaccination
- Dose interval and the need for booster doses
- Outbreak response (including whether to create a vaccine stockpile)
- Surveillance
- Containment
- Investment in future research

Table 2G.11 Mass versus selective immunisation

	Mass immunisation	Selective immunisation
Description	Aims to vaccinate all members of the population.	Vaccination of the most at-risk groups, on the basis of factors such as sex, age, occupation, travel, or lifestyle.
Rationale	Leads to herd immunity.	Less costly and reduces the number of adverse events as there are fewer people being vaccinated.
Example	Rubella only causes severe illness to a fetus (congenital rubella syndrome); however, a decision was made to vaccinate both sexes in order to benefit from herd immunity.	HPV vaccination on the other hand is only given to girls in order to reduce their risk of cervical cancer despite arguments that it should also be given to boys to increase herd immunity as well as reduce the risk of genital warts.

Table 2G.12 Different types of vaccine

	Live attenuated	Inactivated (killed)	Conjugate	Subunit	Toxoid	Polysaccharide
Description	Contain live microorganisms whose virulent properties have been disabled.	Contain micro-organisms that were previously virulent but have been killed.	The surfaces of some bacteria are poorly immunogenic, but by linking them to proteins, the body's immune system can develop an immune response to the bacterial outer coat.	Contains only a fragment of the microorganism (e.g. the surface antigens of a virus).	Contain inactivated toxic compounds rather than the micro-organism	Contain polysaccharides from the surface capsule of bacteria.
Example	BCG, MMR, typhoid, yellow fever, oral polio (Sabin), rotavirus, influenza (Fluenz)	Inactivated polio (Salk), hepatitis A, influenza, cholera, rabies, plague	Hib, Men C, Men ACWY, PCV	Hepatitis B, HPV, acellular pertussis	Tetanus, diphtheria	PPV, typhoid

Outbreak response

Vaccines are sometimes introduced in an attempt to control an epidemic. For example, in 2012, the DH in England decided that women should be offered pertussis vaccination after surveillance data showed a considerably higher incidence in both infants and the general population compared with the previous year. The pertussis was, therefore, offered late in pregnancy to protect neonates both through transferred maternal antibodies and by limiting their potential exposure to infected individuals [87].

2G.6 Outbreak investigations

The steps in outbreak investigation, including the use of relevant epidemiological methods.

An outbreak may be defined as

- Two or more related cases of the same disease
- The occurrence of **more cases of disease than expected** in a given area, or among a specific group of people, over a particular period of time
- A single case of a disease of **high public health importance**, for example, anthrax, plague, SARS, diphtheria

The objectives of controlling an outbreak are to

- Minimise the number of **primary cases** of illness through prompt recognition of the outbreak and through the identification and control of the source of the infection or contamination
- Minimise the number of **secondary cases** of infection by identifying cases and taking appropriate action to prevent any spread
- Prevent further episodes of illness by identifying **continuing hazards** and eliminating them or minimising the risk that they pose
- Introduce measures to **prevent future outbreaks**

Outbreak control plans

Outbreak control plans should include

- A description of the **roles** and **responsibilities** of each of the participating organisations and individuals
- Arrangements for **informing** and **consulting** the key personnel (e.g. directors of public health, the regional epidemiologist, relevant reference laboratories, senior managers from the health service and PHE, and the DH)
- Arrangements for **liaison** with local government, hospitals, and health authorities
- **Facilities** required to manage an incident (e.g. an incident room equipped with telephones, fax machines, and other efficient electronic communication systems—including arrangements for outside normal working hours)

Outbreak control group

An outbreak control group should generally be convened when an outbreak occurs and any of the following features apply:

- The disease poses an **immediate health hazard** to the local population
- There are a **large number** of cases
- Unexpected cases appear in **several districts**
- The disease is **unusual** and **severe**

Investigation of an outbreak

The management of an outbreak consists of four tasks that should be conducted **concurrently**—one of which is an epidemiological sequence that should be conducted **serially** (see Figure 2G.2).

Four concurrent tasks

1. Epidemiological sequence
2. Control measures
3. Convene outbreak control group
4. Communication

Follow epidemiological sequence

1. Establish **case definition**
2. Confirm cases are real
3. Determine **background rate** of disease
4. Assess whether this is an outbreak
5. **Find cases**
6. Describe **epidemiological characteristics** of cases—time, place, person, clinical characteristics, laboratory information
7. Plot the **epidemic curve**
8. Generate a **hypothesis**
9. **Test the hypothesis** by means of an analytical study
10. Consider further studies
11. Generate conclusions

Instigate control measures

- Control the source (animal, human, or environmental)
- Control the mode of **spread**
- **Protect** persons at risk
- Continue **surveillance** of control measures
- Declare the **outbreak over** once the number of new cases has returned to background levels
- Introduce measures to prevent future outbreaks (e.g. prosecute, legislate)

Convene outbreak control group

The membership will vary but may include

1. Consultant in communicable disease control/health protection
2. Environmental health officer
3. Consultant microbiologist or virologist
4. Administrative and secretarial support
5. Food chemist
6. Member of state veterinary service
7. Toxicologist
8. Food microbiologist
9. Regional epidemiologist
10. Director of public health
11. Press officer
12. Representative from the HPA, PHE, CFI, e.g. national expert in the specific infection
13. Manager of the institution
14. Food standards authority
15. Water company
16. Occupational health physician
17. GP

Communication

- Consider the best **media** of communication with colleagues, patients, and the public
- Ensure **accuracy** and timeliness
- Include all those who need to know
- Use the media **constructively**

Figure 2G.2 Investigation of an outbreak.

2G.7 Emergency preparedness and response to natural and man-made disasters

Natural and man-made disasters have the potential to cause widespread loss of life and long-lasting damage to health. Multi-agency response systems are required in order to plan and prepare for such disasters. Organisations that may be involved include

- Emergency services (police, fire, and ambulance)
- Health services
- Public health services
- Local government
- National government
- Meteorological organisations or other organisations with specialist knowledge, for example, Environmental Agency and the British Geological Survey
- International partners

Natural disasters

These include extreme weather events and other natural disasters such as

- Temperature extremes
- Flooding
- Drought
- Storms
- Tsunamis
- Wildfires
- Earthquakes
- Volcanoes

As well as their effects on **physical** and/or **mental health,** such events often interrupt utilities such as electricity and water and may hamper access to health services.

Man-made disasters

These include bombings, shootings, and the deliberate or accidental release of chemical, biological, and radiological hazards. Actual and potential examples of such agents include

- Chemical: hydrogen cyanide, chlorine gas, nerve agents (such as sarin)
- Biological: anthrax, plague, smallpox
- Radioactive material

The heightened threat of global terrorism requires thorough preparation to deal with deliberate releases of such substances.

Preparation and response to disasters

The acute response to any disaster should be coordinated by a multidisciplinary incident control team. The WHO's *disaster management cycle* may be used as a framework to help plan for and manage such incidents (see Box 2G.5). This cycle (which starts with prevention and ends with recovery) can be used alongside the risk management strategies outlined in Section 2F.2.

Box 2G.5 WHO disaster management cycle [88]

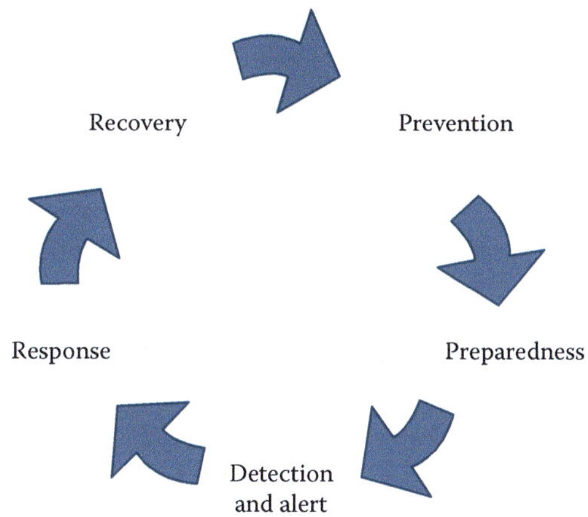

1. Prevention

Prevention entails taking steps to minimise the likelihood of an incident occurring; this may include the replacement of potentially hazardous substances, the installation of defences (e.g. flood barriers), legislation and regulation to minimise risks, and education and publicity to raise awareness.

2. Preparedness

Preparedness involves gathering information on potential hazards, such as at-risk sites, developing an incident response plan, and training response teams including scenario exercises.

3. Detection and alert

This phase uses detection, surveillance, and alert channels to identify any incidents as early as possible. Examples of such systems include earthquake detection systems, health surveillance systems, and environmental monitoring.

4. Response

There are multiple potential interventions that may need to be implemented in response to a disaster, including the mobilisation of emergency services, terminating the release of any hazardous substance, and communication to the press and members of the public (see Figure 2G.2).

5. Recovery

After the immediate effects of the disaster are over, further actions will be needed in order to return to normality and to learn from any mistakes. Actions may include providing support to victims, conducting risk assessments and health outcome assessments, and investigating of the cause of the incident.

2G.8 Important infectious diseases

Knowledge of natural history, clinical presentation, methods of diagnosis, and control of infections of local and international public health importance: including emerging diseases and those with consequences for effective control.

The infectious diseases of public health importance may be grouped into the following categories (although many diseases will fall into two or more categories):

Vaccine-preventable diseases
Nosocomial infections
Gastrointestinal infections
Viral hepatitides
Respiratory infections
STIs
Vector-borne diseases
Other communicable diseases

UK Note in the following tables that references to notifiable disease status pertain to England and Wales (see Section 2G.9).

Vaccine-preventable diseases

See Table 2G.13.

Nosocomial infections

Nosocomial (Healthcare-Acquired) Infections
Healthcare-associated infections (HCAIs) are infections acquired as a result of healthcare. Examples are MRSA, *Clostridium difficile*, glycopeptide-resistant enterococci (GRE), and *Acinetobacter* species.

HCAI risk factors include

- Higher numbers of **susceptible patients** being treated (elderly patients or patients with severe or chronic diseases)
- **Invasive procedures** (e.g. indwelling lines, artificial ventilation)
- **Immunosuppression** (e.g. chemotherapy, post-transplant regimens)
- Increased patient movement between wards or between hospitals (often due to pressures on hospital beds)
- Wider use of **antibiotics** and the emergence of antibiotic-resistant microorganisms

Higher rates of HCAIs are often found in specialist hospitals such as orthopaedic centres. However, with the move towards performing invasive procedures such as minor surgery in the community, primary care HCAIs may become more common.

Some of the impacts of HACAIs are described in Table 2G.14.

Measures to control of HCAIs include the following:

- **Hand washing** is generally the most important prevention activity. For example, in the United Kingdom, the *'clean your hands'* campaign raised awareness among staff, patients, and the public.
- Universal precautions.
- Prudent antibiotic **prescribing.**
- **Surveillance** (e.g. the UK surveillance systems for MRSA, surgical site infection).
- **Isolation** and cohort nursing (Table 2G.15).

Gastrointestinal infections

Four groups of people are identified as posing an increased risk of spreading gastrointestinal infection compared to the general population. See Tables 2G.16 and 2G.17.

Viral hepatitides (Table 2G.18)

Hepatitis B serology

Laboratory reports for hepatitis B contain details of a number of markers; their interpretation is outlined in Table 2G.19.

Respiratory infections

See Table 2G.20.

Table 2G.13 Vaccine preventable diseases

Disease (organism)	Epidemiology	Diagnosis	Reservoir	Transmission	Surveillance	Control
Diphtheria (diphtheria toxin produced by toxigenic *Corynebacterium diphtheriae* or by *C. ulcerans*) **Clinical features** Acute upper respiratory tract infection, enlarged lymph nodes, and 'bull-neck' appearance. May cause respiratory obstruction, paralysis and cardiac failure—fatal if untreated. Many cases vaccinated, so rarely recognised on clinical grounds. There is also a milder cutaneous form.	Rare in countries with routine immunisation. Outbreaks in the former USSR countries in the 1990s. Mortality is greatest in children and those aged >40 years.	Nasal, throat, skin ulcer swabs—identify *C. diphtheriae* (toxigenic). Occasionally toxigenic *C. ulcerans*. Confirmation of toxigenicity from reference laboratory—can be obtained within few hours by PCR.	C. diphtheriae—human reservoir. Reservoir of *C. ulcerans* is cattle.	Direct contact or airborne droplets. Animal contact or consumption of unpasteurised dairy products for *C. ulcerans*.	Statutory notifications, vaccine coverage.	Primary vaccine coverage (three doses) for children aged 2 has been 94% since 2001, just below the WHO target of 95%. Cases barrier nursed, antibiotic treatment, antitoxin, booster or primary vaccination. Contact in the previous 7 days with a case of infection caused by toxigenic *C. diphtheriae* or *C. ulcerans* should be considered at risk. Contacts—swabbed, food handlers/unvaccinated children excluded, antibiotic, booster/primary vaccination. No public health action required if non-toxigenic *C. diphtheriae*.

(continued)

Table 2G.13 *(Continued)* Vaccine preventable diseases

Disease (organism)	Epidemiology	Diagnosis	Reservoir	Transmission	Surveillance	Control
Pertussis (whooping cough) ***(Bordetella pertussis)*** **Clinical features** Cough, cold, fever progressing to paroxysmal cough and bouts of coughing ending with a whoop or vomiting. Last 2–3 months. Can be fatal in infants <6 months. Adults—milder symptoms—recognised as a cause for chronic cough.	Epidemics occur at 3–4 yearly intervals. Large epidemic in England in 2012 prompting introduction of vaccination of pregnant women.	Culture nasal swab—but low sensitivity and high specificity. PCR EIA	Human	Droplet spread	Statutory notifications, vaccine coverage.	**Prevention:** Acellular pertussis vaccine is given in the primary course with diphtheria, tetanus, polio, and Hib, as DTaP/IPV/Hib, at 2, 3, and 4 months of age. A further booster dose with acellular pertussis, as dTaP/IPV, is given with the preschool boosters between the ages of 3 and 5. Vaccination of pregnant women from 28 weeks gestation was introduced in England in 2012 to transfer immunity to the newborn and minimise potentially infectious contacts. **Control:** Cases treated with antibiotic, isolated, vaccinated (if not vaccinated). If a vulnerable contact is present in a household, all offered antibiotic prophylaxis and vaccinate those under 10 and unimmunised. If no vulnerable contacts, no prophylaxis required. Outbreaks—community-wide vaccination if coverage low/case finding/antibiotic treatment.

Tetanus *(Clostridium tetani)* **Clinical features** Painful muscular contractions—especially of neck and jaw. Often history of tetanus-prone wound.	Decreasing in the United Kingdom since immunisation introduced in the 1960s. Occasional infections in IV drug users from contaminated needles. Neonatal tetanus from infection of the umbilical stump remains a major cause of morbidity in Africa and Asia.	Toxin in serum sample—but rarely obtained.	Animal and human intestines Spores in soil contaminated with animal faeces	Dirty wounds Contaminated needles Abdominal surgery	Statutory notifications, vaccine coverage.	**Prevention:** Vaccine—in UK schedule = three doses at 2, 3, and 4 months, boosters at 3–5 years and 13–18 years. Case—vaccinated primary or booster—if 10 years or more since last vaccine or if acquired tetanus-prone wound. **Control of outbreak:** Look for source, e.g. surgery, intravenous drug users.
Poliomyelitis (**poliovirus** 3 serogroups, type 2 most virulent) **Clinical features** Normally asymptomatic or mild pyrexia, headache, or gastrointestinal symptoms. Rarely causes paralysis.	The last UK case was in 2000 (vaccine associated). Worldwide, it has been decreasing since the eradication campaign and is now only present in Nigeria, India, Pakistan, and Afghanistan. The majority of cases are in children under 5 years.	Viral culture/ antibodies	Human	Mainly faecal–oral	Statutory notifications, vaccine coverage.	Oral polio vaccine in endemic countries. Countries where polio has been eradicated for several years may use the inactivated vaccine.

(*continued*)

Table 2G.13 *(Continued)* Vaccine preventable diseases

Disease (organism)	Epidemiology	Diagnosis	Reservoir	Transmission	Surveillance	Control
H. influenzae type b (Hib) **Clinical features** Invasive disease. Commonest presentation is meningitis; others—pneumonia, epiglottitis, bone and joint infection, facial cellulitis.	Prior to the introduction of vaccination, Hib was a major cause of meningitis in infants and young children in the United Kingdom. It is now rare.	Blood/CSF culture PCR Reference laboratory for confirmation and typing	Humans	Droplet spread/direct contact Unvaccinated—higher carriage rate—common in young children	Enhanced surveillance questionnaire in England. Lab reports. Acute meningitis is notifiable. Vaccine coverage data.	**Prevention:** Vaccine in the United Kingdom given at 2, 3, and 4 months with diphtheria/tetanus/pertussis and polio vaccines. Vaccination prevents carriage. **Control:** Notifiable. Unvaccinated household children contacts vaccinated and adults given chemoprophylaxis, including case. Vaccination programme in cluster if coverage low.
Pneumococcus *(Streptococcus pneumoniae)* **Clinical features** Can cause pneumonia, meningitis, or septicaemia.	Mainly affects infants and the elderly. Winter peaks. Reductions in serotypes in vaccine since its introduction in 2006 (England).	Culture (blood/CSF) Urinary antigen Reference lab for serotyping	Human	Direct contact with respiratory secretions	Enhanced surveillance in England (all isolates sent to reference lab). Vaccine coverage data.	Routine vaccination with PCV (7 commonest serotypes) for children, PPV (23 serotypes) recommended for all age >65 years. Chemoprophylaxis and vaccination of close contacts of a case if a cluster/outbreak in an institution.

Meningococcal disease *(Neisseria meningitidis)* —*6 serogroups cause serious disease: A, B, C, W-135, X, and Y* **Clinical features** Non-specific early phase. Babies—floppy, fever, vomiting. Photophobia, neck stiffness. Petechial rash, septicaemia, death. Complications—deafness/convulsions/limb amputation/mental impairment.	Endemic worldwide—highly seasonal. Europe —winter epidemics. Africa—dry season. Associated with mass gatherings, e.g. Hajj pilgrimage. Type C decreased in the United Kingdom since introduction of vaccine. 85% cases now type B.	Blood/CSF culture PCR Reference laboratory for confirmation and typing	Humans	Direct or indirect person to person spread	Acute meningitis and meningococcal septicaemia notifiable. Vaccine coverage.	**Prevention:** Vaccines against serogroups A, C, W135, and Y—short-lived vaccine. Men C vaccine given in the United Kingdom at 2, 3, and 4 months (children >1 year single dose). As of 2014, JCVI recommended the introduction of Men B vaccine from 2 months. **Control:** Chemoprophylaxis—close contacts. Vaccinate if vaccine-preventable strain.

(continued)

Table 2G.13 *(Continued)* Vaccine preventable diseases

Disease (organism)	Epidemiology	Diagnosis	Reservoir	Transmission	Surveillance	Control
Mycobacterium tuberculosis (MTB) (occasionally *M. bovis* and *M. africanum*) **Clinical features** Long incubation period produces chronic disease with risk of reactivation (particularly with age) and fatal without treatment. Most commonly affects lungs; symptoms can include: • Cough • Blood in sputum • Weight loss • Night sweats • Mortality Improves rapidly after introduction of effective chemotherapy.	In the United Kingdom: more common in immigrant ethnic groups with the highest rates found in London. Worldwide, there have been increases since the 1980s associated with the HIV epidemic.	Chest radiograph Sputum smear Sputum culture Microscopy—sputum Sensitivity testing for multidrug-resistant TB (MDR-TB) Molecular typing for identifying clusters	Animals, humans	Direct spread from infected case Bovine TB from ingesting raw milk from infected cows	Notifiable, enhanced surveillance, vaccine coverage.	**Prevention:** BCG vaccine: UK government recommends that the following risk groups be offered BCG vaccination: All infants living in areas where the incidence of TB is 40 per 100,000 or greater Infants whose parents or grandparents were born in a country with a TB incidence of 40 per 100,000 or higher Previously unvaccinated new immigrants from high-prevalence countries for TB. **Control:** Cases with pulmonary TB are followed up by chest clinics to ensure that adequate treatment is given and that contacts are identified, screened, and given prophylaxis where necessary Measures to maximise compliance such as directly observed treatment (DOT). Port health.

Mumps (paramyxovirus) **Clinical features** Tenderness and parotid swelling Meningitis (commonest cause of viral meningitis pre-vaccine era) Orchitis Pancreatitis	Decreases in the United Kingdom since MMR vaccination introduced. Increases in 2003–2006 and 2009–2010—possibly due to reduced vaccination after the Wakefield publications and to waning immunity. Mainly affects children.	Saliva, CSF, urine culture Serology	Humans	Direct contact with saliva or droplets of saliva of an infected person	Notifiable, vaccine coverage data.	**Prevention:** Vaccine in the United Kingdom given at 12–15 months and 3–5 years (in combination with measles and rubella). **Control:** Notifiable. As vaccination rates drop, resurgence and possible outbreaks of these diseases are increasingly likely. Exclusion. Check vaccination status for case. Consider community-wide programme if coverage low in outbreaks.

(continued)

Table 2G.13 *(Continued)* Vaccine preventable diseases

Disease (organism)	Epidemiology	Diagnosis	Reservoir	Transmission	Surveillance	Control
Measles (a paramyxovirus) **Clinical features** Prodromal flu-like symptoms. Koplik's spots inside the mouth. Rash starts on days 3–4, over face, trunk, and limbs. Not itchy. Complications include: Pneumonitis Acute otitis media Pneumonia Encephalitis In pregnancy associated with miscarriage and LBW	Endemic in developing countries, particularly among children under 5 years. Still around 5000 notifications per year in the United Kingdom; this is a large decrease since MMR introduced.	Salivary test kit for measles IgM Serology	Human	Direct contact with saliva or droplets of saliva of an infected person Person to person Measles is highly infectious; therefore, contact is defined as 10–15 minutes in the same room.	Notifiable, vaccine coverage data.	See mumps. Human normal immunoglobulins (HNIG) for the following: Pregnant contacts who are measles IgG negative Babies less than 6 months old—maternal IgG negative Exclusion
Rubella (rubella virus—a member of Togaviridae) **Clinical features** Moderately infectious.	Reduced since MMR introduced, but increase in 2012. Prior to this, only women of childbearing age were vaccinated.	Serum or saliva detection of IgM Viral culture from urine or serum	Human	Direct person to person	Notifiable, vaccine coverage data.	See mumps. Pregnant women in contact with case—tested; if susceptible, offer vaccination postpartum.

Pre-vaccination era. Affecting primary school-aged children, susceptible pregnant women—congenital rubella syndrome Pharyngitis Conjunctivitis Fever Rash	Congenital rubella syndrome now very rare.					
HPV (>100 types—13 types associated with cervical cancer) **Clinical features** Associated with **Cervical cancer** (>70% cases associated with types 16 or 18) **Genital warts** (mainly types 6 and 11) Also associated with penile, vulval, vaginal, anal, and oropharyngeal cancers.	Around 50% of sexually active women are infected with HPV. Cervical cancer has been decreasing in the United Kingdom since 1990 but the prevalence of genital warts has been increasing.	HPV tested using PCR in women with borderline abnormal smears during cervical screening to triage further investigations.	Human	Depends on type (e.g. hand warts by close contact), types associated with genital warts or cervical cancer—sexually transmitted	Cancer registries, GUMCAD returns, vaccine coverage.	Routine vaccination of teenage girls for types 16, 18, 6, and 11 introduced in the United Kingdom in 2012 (prior to this, bivalent vaccine against types 16 and 18). Cervical cancer screening.

Table 2G.14 The impact of HCAIs

Effects on patients	Effects on the health service
Severe or chronic illness Pain, anxiety, depression, Longer stay in hospital Reduced quality of life Loss of earnings Death	Extended lengths of stay. Costs of diagnosis and treatment of the infections and their complications. Costs of specific infection control measures—cleaning, disinfection, cohort nursing, etc. Bed and ward closures and postponed admissions. Provision of isolation facility/rooms. Antibiotic costs may be further increased if the infection is also due to a resistant microorganism.

Sexually transmitted infections

The prevention of Sexually transmitted infections (STIs) involves

- Health and sex education
- Availability of low-cost condoms
- Early detection and prompt effective treatment
- Contact tracing and treating contacts
- Opportunistic or routine screening
- Surveillance: England through returns from genitourinary medicine (GUM) clinics and non-GUM commissioned enhanced sexual health services (see Table 2G.21).

Vector-borne diseases

See Table 2G.22.

Other communicable diseases

See Table 2G.23.

New and emerging infections

Emerging infectious diseases are commonly defined as those that have either newly appeared in a population or have existed but in either case are **rapidly increasing in incidence or geographical range**.

The pattern of communicable disease occurrence is in constant flux. Current influences leading to emerging infections include

- Global travel
- Climate change
- Global trade and importation
- Urbanisation
- Population displacement
- Animal movements
- Changes in agriculture
- Emerging zoonoses
- Deforestation
- Bird migration
- Human conflict
- Antimicrobial resistance
- Genetic mutation/recombination
- Deliberate release

Current concerns

Diseases attracting particular research attention and interest in health protection control policy include

- Smallpox
- Anthrax
- SARS
- Avian influenza and pandemic influenza
- West Nile virus
- Changes in vector distribution
- Pet travel scheme
- Leishmaniasis
- Hantavirus
- MRSA
- Vancomycin-resistant enterococci (VRE)
- Novel coronavirus

Table 2G.15 Nosocomial infections

Disease (organism)	Epidemiology	Diagnosis	Reservoir	Transmission	Surveillance	Control
Methicillin-resistant *Staphylococcus aureus* (MRSA) **Clinical features** Range from skin infection and conjunctivitis, to pneumonia and life-threatening septicaemia.	Proportion of *S. aureus* that is MRSA is increasing. 30% of the general population are colonised by *S. aureus*. In hospitals, the percentage is higher because of more likely contact with infected cases.	Gram stain, culture and sensitivity testing on appropriate specimen 16 strains EMRSA-15 and EMRSA-16 are the dominant UK stains.	Humans, rarely animals	Direct contact	Mandatory surveillance scheme for hospital trusts in England	**Prevention:** Good personal hygiene—hand washing Compliance with infection control measures Hand washing/aseptic techniques/handling waste/waste disposal/ward or equipment cleaning **Control:** Mandatory surveillance schemes in the United Kingdom: • Mandatory *S. aureus* bacteraemia surveillance • Mandatory MRSA bacteraemia-enhanced surveillance scheme Infection control policies—central and local Central government initiatives (DH)—Towards Cleaner Hospitals and Lower Rates of Infection, Saving Lives Delivery Programme to reduce HCAIs, including MRSA antibiotic prescribing policy

(continued)

Table 2G.15 (*Continued*) Nosocomial infections

Disease (organism)	Epidemiology	Diagnosis	Reservoir	Transmission	Surveillance	Control
Clostridium difficile **Clinical features** Diarrhoea post antibiotics, pseudomembranous colitis, fever	Increasing (could be increased investigation/reporting) Hospital outbreaks Elderly at greater risk	Cl. difficile toxin in stool Culture and sensitivity	Human (only causes disease when competing normal gut flora killed by antibiotics)	Direct contact Fomites (e.g. commodes)	Surveillance by NHS trusts is mandatory.	Infection control procedures (hand washing, disposable gloves, and apron for staff and visitors) Early diagnosis and isolation of patients Control of antibiotic use

Table 2G.16 Gastrointestinal risk groups

Group A	People of **doubtful personal hygiene** or whose toilet, hand-washing, or hand-drying **facilities are inadequate** either at home, work, or school
Group B	**Children** who attend preschool groups or nurseries
Group C	People whose work involves **preparing or serving unwrapped foods** that are not subjected to further heating
Group D	**Clinical and social care staff** who have direct contact with highly susceptible patients or persons in whom a gastrointestinal infection would have particularly **serious consequences**

Australia and New Zealand: Important infections

NZ In addition to the lists earlier, certain infectious diseases are of particular importance in Australia and New Zealand, including those described in Table 2G.24.

South Africa: Important infections

Current communicable disease concerns in South Africa are discussed in Table 2G.25.

Table 2G.17 Food-borne gastrointestinal diseases

Disease (organism)	Epidemiology	Diagnosis	Reservoir	Transmission	Surveillance	Control
Campylobacter (mainly *C. jejuni*, also *C. coli*, *C. fetus*) **Clinical features** Ranges from asymptomatic to severe diarrhoea (~50% cases bloody stools)	Increasing in the United Kingdom, the most common bacterial GI infection	Stool culture (high sensitivity with same-day sample) Microscopy (sensitivity lower than culture)	Gastrointestinal tract of birds (particularly poultry) and animals, cattle, and domestic pets	Animal to person (water or food contaminated with faeces) Person to person (direct contact with feces of index case, e.g. person changing soiled nappies) Raw or undercooked meat (especially poultry), non-pasteurised milk	Notifiable, lab reports	**Preventive measures:** Chlorination of drinking water supplies Milk pasteurisation Adequate hygiene, domestic and commercial Kitchens Adequate cooking of poultry Hand hygiene Advice to travellers abroad Control of patient, contacts, and immediate environment Exclusion of symptomatic cases Food hygiene and hand hygiene Avoid non-pasteurised milk and untreated water
Cholera **(toxin-producing *Vibrio cholerae* 01)** **Clinical features** Watery diarrhoea Vomiting 50% case fatality—severe untreated cases	Endemic in many developing countries. Rare in the United Kingdom—all travel associated	Determine if toxin producing Stool culture Direct microscopy of stools PCR	Untreated/ polluted water	Consumption of untreated water, contaminated shellfish and foods eaten raw or washed in contaminated water. Person-to-person spread (by faecal–oral route) is likely to be a threat only when hygiene is very poor and sanitary facilities are inadequate.		

				Cholera rarely occurs in the United Kingdom—most cases are imported; therefore, ask about travel history in week before onset.	Notifiable disease	Secondary spread is rare if hygiene is good. Cases should be excluded until 48 h after first normal stool. Fatalities rare in the United Kingdom: ensure oral rehydration and appropriate antibiotics. Food advice to travellers. **Prevention:** Predominantly education, and adequate hygiene and sanitation, especially for travellers. Advice for travellers to countries with epidemic cholera: a simple rule of thumb is *'Boil it, cook it, peel it or forget it.'* Vaccination: killed whole-cell vaccine leads to poor short-lasting cover and is of little value. Not available in the United Kingdom and is no longer a requirement for travel to any country. **Control:** Safe drinking water supplies

(continued)

Table 2G.17 *(Continued)* Food-borne gastrointestinal diseases

Disease (organism)	Epidemiology	Diagnosis	Reservoir	Transmission	Surveillance	Control
Cryptosporidiosis (*Cryptosporidium parvum*) **Clinical features** Healthy individuals—self-limiting. Immunocompromised—severe illness may lead to death. Diarrhoea—may be bloody.	Seasonal (autumn peak in the United Kingdom). Most common in children	Stool microscopy Intestinal biopsy Serology Genotyping techniques	Gastrointestinal tract of humans and animals (particularly farm and domesticated); water contaminated with faeces Humans	Person to person Animal to person Swimming pool outbreaks	Lab reports	**Prevention:** Hand hygiene Adequate water treatment Monitoring water quality Immunocompromised—avoid contact with farm animals, drink boiled water, avoid contact with infected cases Disinfectants, e.g. hydrogen peroxide **Control:** Exclusion of cases until 48 h after first normal stool Cases should avoid swimming for 2 weeks Contact tracing History of raw water consumption Good practice guideline—nursery/farm/swimming pool/hospitals
Shigellae **(*Shigella sonnei*—common in the United Kingdom and mild)** **(S. *dysenteriae*, S. *flexneri*, S. *boydii*—imported and more severe)**	Stool culture. Reference lab for typing	Isolation of organism from stools Serotyping Phage typing		Person to person Contaminated food/water Faecal–oral route	Food poisoning and HUS notifiable. Enhanced surveillance of non-sonnei Shigella in the United Kingdom	**Prevention:** Hand hygiene Adequate cleaning of toilet area Treatment of drinking and swimming water Advice to travellers

Clinical features *S. sonnei*—mild diarrhoea Others: Watery diarrhoea, vomiting 50% bloody stools *S. dysenteriae* 1—toxic megacolon/ haemolytic—uraemic disease and death					(particularly given increased rates of *S. flexneri* in MSM population in 2012)	**Control:** *S. sonnei:* exclusion of case for 48 h after first normal stool
(*S. dysenteriae* type 1—produce exotoxin—severe illness)						Other *Shigella* species: exclusion of case for 48 h after first normal stool (unless the case is in a risk group—when clearance is needed, i.e. two negative stools taken at least 48 h apart; contacts in risk groups also need microbiological clearance) Contact tracing Reinforce hygiene measures
***E. coli* (verocytotoxin producing).** Most common serotype in the United Kingdom is *E. coli* O157.H7. **Clinical features** *E. coli* O157—asymptomatic/diarrhoeal illness/haemolytic–uraemic syndrome (HUS—particularly in children)/death	Food-borne outbreaks. Greatest in spring/summer. Highest rates in children	Food, environmental, animal samples Stool culture Biochemical and serological testing—isolates Reference labs for VTEC	Gastrointestinal tract of cattle (and possibly other domesticated animals) particularly goats	Contaminated food/ water Animal to person Person to person	Food poisoning and HUS notifiable. Lab reports	**Prevention:** Hand hygiene. Adequate cleaning (kitchen, toilet). Precautions during farm visits. Well-cooked beef, lamb, venison products. Good practice—food processing and food service industries.

(*continued*)

Table 2G.17 *(Continued)* Food-borne gastrointestinal diseases

Disease (organism)	Epidemiology	Diagnosis	Reservoir	Transmission	Surveillance	Control
						Control: Hygiene advice cases/contacts/food service industry. Cases not in risk groups are excluded for 48 h after first normal stool. Cases in risk groups are excluded until microbiological clearance—two consecutive stool samples 2 days apart. Household contacts in risk groups are screened microbiologically.
Salmonellae (*S. enteritidis* PT4—associated with eggs and poultry) **(*S. typhimurium* DT104—increased antibiotic resistance)** **Clinical features** Diarrhoea. Rare complication is abscess formation and septicaemia.	Large outbreaks may occur. Endemic worldwide	Stool culture or rectal swab Blood culture Reference laboratory Serotyping Phage typing	Gastrointestinal tracts of wild and domestic animals, birds (especially poultry), 'exotic' pets (terrapins and iguana), and occasionally humans	Animal to person—contaminated food Person to person—faecal–oral	Food poisoning notifiable, lab reports	**Prevention:** Vaccination of poultry flock Food processing industry systems to identify, control, and monitor potential hazards Personal/food hygiene measures (home, institutions) **Control:** Hand/food hygiene advice Exclude cases for 48 h after first normal stool

Enteric fever (typhoid and paratyphoid) **(*Salmonella typhi and paratyphi* A (80% in the United Kingdom), B (20% in the United Kingdom), and C)** **Clinical features** Gastroenteritis Fever Early disease may involve constipation—later—diarrhoea, vomiting Spots 5% relapse	Endemic in many developing countries. Mainly travel associated in the United Kingdom (South Asia and Africa)	Blood, urine, faeces, bone marrow aspirate culture	Humans	Food borne Person to person in poor hygiene conditions	Enteric fever notifiable, lab reports, enhanced surveillance	**Prevention:** Sanitation. Clean water. Personal hygiene. No effective vaccine. **Control:** Notifiable. Isolation in hospital is advisable. Screen all household contacts. Hygiene advice. Exclude food handlers and other risk groups (1 week after antibiotic therapy, require three clear consecutive samples—48 hours apart). Exclude cases not in risk groups until 48 hours after normal stools.
Norovirus **Clinical features** Diarrhoea and vomiting, normally only lasting a few days. Self-limiting in healthy individuals.	Seasonal with winter epidemics. Frequent institutional outbreaks.	Stool PCR	Humans	Faecal–oral, fomites, and contaminated food (especially molluscs) Transmission risk high because virus survives in the environment for many days; immunity short lived	Lab reports	Infection control precautions including hand washing Food hygiene Cleaning and disinfection Exclusion for 48 hours after symptoms resolved

Table 2G.18 Viral hepatitides

Disease (organism)	Epidemiology	Diagnosis	Reservoir	Transmission	Surveillance	Control
Hepatitis A (HAV) **Clinical features** Ranges from asymptomatic to fulminant hepatitis. Young children are commonly asymptomatic. Adults are more likely to have symptoms—75% of adults develop jaundice. Infectious from 2 weeks before jaundice develops	Endemic in developing countries	Salivary IgM and IgG—useful in outbreak investigations. Detection of IgM (serum/saliva) = acute infection. IgG persists for life. Persistent IgG—past infection/immunisation.	Human gastrointestinal tract	Person to person spread—via faecal–oral route and contaminated food Consumption of food grown or washed in contaminated water (e.g. shellfish, fruit, and vegetables)	Notifiable as acute infectious hepatitis	Use of immunoglobulin (Ig) or vaccination for close, household, and sexual contacts should be offered via GP. Risk groups and all cases should be excluded for 7 days after onset of jaundice and/or symptoms. Travel advice for those to areas of endemicity.
Hepatitis B (HBV) **Clinical features** Non-specific prodromal illness Jaundice (often after fever) Can lead to long-term carriage (carriage rate in UK population ~0.5%) Cirrhosis Hepatocellular carcinoma Co-infection with hepatitis subviral satellite D	Endemic in parts of Asia and sub-Saharan Africa. More common among IV drug users and men who have sex with men	See Table 2G.19 (HBV marker interpretation).	Humans	Person to person by blood-borne routes. Intravenous drug users, sex, bites, scratches Perinatal most common in high-prevalence countries	Notifiable as acute infectious hepatitis	Vaccination of high-risk group—all healthcare workers should be immunised against hepatitis B infection and should be shown to have made a serological response to the vaccine. UK schedule 0, 1, and 6 months. Accelerated schedule 0, 1, 2, and 12 months. If susceptible, vaccinate household and sexual contacts.

						Screening of blood supply in the United Kingdom. Antenatal screening and immunisation of babies at risk.
Hepatitis C (HCV) **Clinical features** Asymptomatic Mild infection Jaundice—unusual 80% carriers 80% chronic hepatitis 10%–20% cirrhosis 1% liver cancer		Enzyme immunoassay—detect HCAb Recombinant immunoblot assay (RIBA) confirms HCAb HCAb +—previous exposure PCR—detect infection (HCV RNA)	Humans	Historical: blood products until screened since 1991. Now intravenous drug users: 80%. Sharing razors or toothbrushes. Body piercing (like tattooing or acupuncture). Vertical transmission rare. Risk is highest in HIV mothers and those who have high viral load. Insufficient evidence to assess the risk of transmission via breast milk.	Notifiable as acute infectious hepatitis. Hepatitis C National Register was established in 1998. Aim of the register is to inform the natural history of HCV infection in the United Kingdom. Majority of these cases are transfusion recipients who were traced during the national HCV look-back programme.	No vaccine Interferon and ribavirin treatment for chronic infection with HCV Needle exchange, safe blood transfusion (e.g. screening blood donors)

(*continued*)

Table 2G.18 *(Continued)* Viral hepatitides

Disease (organism)	Epidemiology	Diagnosis	Reservoir	Transmission	Surveillance	Control
Hepatitis D (HDV) **Clinical features** Exists only in conjunction with HBV. Known also as the 'delta agent' Increases risk of cirrhosis		Serology	Humans	As for HBV		As for HBV
Hepatitis E (HEV) **Clinical features** Illness similar to HAV without chronic sequelae or carriage Most cases—young-/middle-aged adults High case fatality in third trimester of pregnancy		Serology Specific IgM testing		Faecal–oral Person to person—low spread		Provision of safe water supplies. Pregnant and older people, those with weakened immune systems, and people with chronic liver disease might need closer observation for deterioration in liver function. No vaccination.

Table 2G.19 Interpretation of hepatitis B markers

Laboratory abbreviation	Serological marker	Description	Implication
HBsAg	Hepatitis B surface antigen	Serological marker on surface of HBV that is present in serum during acute or chronic infection	Person is infectious. Presence for >6 months implies chronic carrier status.
Anti-HBs	Hepatitis B surface antibody	Antibody to surface antigen that is usually produced as part of the normal immune response	Person is immune (either due to recovery from prior infection or due to vaccination).
Total anti-HBc	Total hepatitis B core antibody	Antibodies (of all classes) to a component of HBV	Previous or ongoing infection.
IgM anti-HBc	IgM hepatitis B core antibody	IgM class of antibody that persists for 6 months following exposure	Acute or recent infection.
HBeAg	Hepatitis B e-antigen	Marker present soon after exposure, then absent within 3 months	High infectivity.
Anti-HBeAb	Hepatitis B e-antibody	Develops after HBeAg (except in chronic carriers who may not raise antibody)	Low infectivity.

Disease (organism)	Clinical features	Epidemiology	Diagnosis	Reservoir	Transmission	Surveillance	Control
Influenza virus 3 types: A, B, C A and B cause most clinical disease in humans Type A is more severe and causes most outbreaks/ epidemics	Normally causes a mild upper respiratory tract infection, sometimes with diarrhoea and vomiting. Can lead to severe disease (particularly in the elderly) complicated by bacterial pneumonia which may be fatal	3 distinct types: **1. Seasonal influenza** Winter peaks, elderly/chronically unwell most at risk **2. Pandemic influenza** 4 major pandemics in the last 100 years: 1918 A/ H_1N_1 (killed around 45 million people worldwide), 1957 A/H_2N_2, 1968 A/H_3N_2, 2009 A/H_1N_1. Some pandemics (e.g. 1918) mainly affected young adults **3. Avian influenza** H_5N_1, associated with close contact with birds. Mainly seen in SE Asia. There have been >300 human cases, around 200 of which were fatal. Concerns that this could lead to a pandemic if develops human-human transmission	PCR Antibody testing	Human for most human infections New subtypes from birds/ mammals (e.g. swine)	Airborne (droplet)	Sentinel GP practice surveillance Flu Survey (conducted by London School of Hygiene and Tropical Medicine) NHS Direct syndromic surveillance Laboratory reports COVER vaccine coverage data	Annual vaccine with 3 subtypes changes each-year based on WHO recommendations (due to antigenic drift) Vaccination recommended for all age>65 years, pregnant women and other risk groups International surveillance

Legionella pneumophilia	Atypical pneumonia resistant to usual antibiotics 10-15% mortality Also causes a milder febrile illness (pontiac fever)	Sporadic cases or clusters ~300 cases per year in the UK ~50% acquired abroad At risk groups: Males>females, elderly, chronic illness	Urinary antigen Sputum culture	Environmental water	Airborne droplets/ aerosols (e.g. cooling towes, air-con units, jacuzzis)	Notifiable in the UK National surveillance scheme	Regular maintenance and inspection of water systems backed up by legal enforcement Investigation of clusters

Table 2G.21 Sexually transmitted diseases

Disease (organism)	Epidemiology	Diagnosis	Reservoir	Transmission	Surveillance	Control
Chlamydia trachomatis **Clinical features** Commonest bacterial STI in the United Kingdom Highest rates in young people (especially under 24 years) Majority asymptomatic Untreated may lead to pelvic inflammatory disease (PID), ectopic pregnancy, and ophthalmia neonatorum	Most commonly diagnosed STI in GUM clinics in the United Kingdom. Highest among those aged 16–24 years	PCR or culture of urethral, vulvovaginal, cervical, or urine samples	Human	Sexually Mother to baby	GUMCAD returns Chlamydia Testing Activity Dataset (disaggregated data on all NHS and NHS-commissioned Chlamydia testing carried out in England)	**Prevention:** National Chlamydia Screening Programme commenced in 2002 in England Antibiotic treatment Contact tracing and treating partners Education and awareness raising Condom distribution
Gonorrhoea (*N. gonorrhoeae*) **Clinical features** Second most common bacterial STI in the United Kingdom Men more likely to have symptoms than women Complications: • PID, ectopic pregnancies • Septic arthritis • Ophthalmia neonatorum	Second commonest bacterial STI diagnosed in GUM clinics in the United Kingdom. Highest among those aged 16–24 years. Highest rates in urban areas (especially London)	Microscopy or culture of urethral, cervical swabs, in higher prevalence settings, may be tested using PCR of urine samples, or vulvovaginal swabs	Human	Sexually	GUMCAD returns GRASP (gonococcal resistance to antimicrobial surveillance programme)	**Prevention** Antibiotic treatment—but many strains resistant to commonly used antibiotics Contact tracing and treating partners Outbreak control Education and awareness raising Condom distribution

Syphilis **(*Treponema pallidum*)** **Clinical features** Primary ulcer: third of cases develop secondary eruption. Late lesions of skin, bone, central nervous system, heart	More common in large cities and sea ports. Risk groups include men who have sex with men and young adults.	Microscopy in early syphilis Serological tests[a]—treponemal (e.g. TPHA) and non-treponemal (e.g. VDRL) test	Human	Sexually Mother to baby Blood transfusion	GUMCAD returns Enhanced Surveillance—mainly due to outbreaks seen in Manchester, London, Bristol, and Brighton among gay men and heterosexual men and women	**Prevention**: Routine antenatal screening Antibiotic treatment Contact tracing Outbreak control Late syphilis—test for HIV also Education and awareness raising among high-risk groups (e.g. gay men in urban areas) Condom distribution
Human immunodeficiency virus (HIV) **Clinical features** Leads to immunosuppression (loss of CD4 cells). Early symptoms: flu-like symptoms though some people are asymptomatic. Reduced CD4 count associated with higher risk of and from a range of serious morbidities (e.g. TB) that have high costs of treatment and care, significant mortality, and a high number of potential years of life lost (YLL).	Emerged as new epidemic in the 1980s. Big decrease following public education campaigns in the 1980s and 1990s. Around 24% is thought to be undiagnosed. Highest rates among men who have sex with men and black Africans.	HIV antibody test P24 antigen—for early tests and screening blood Viral load/ CD4 count	Human	Person to person Sexually Blood transfusion Sharing needles Mother to baby Risk of transmission higher in people infected with other STIs, HCV, TB	HIV and AIDS Reporting System (HARS) returns, lab reports	**Prevention:** Surveillance Routine antenatal screening Education, condom distribution particularly among high-risk groups Contact tracing Antiretroviral treatment (reduces viral load and therefore risk of transmission) (no vaccine yet)

(continued)

Table 2G.21 *(Continued)* Sexually transmitted diseases

Disease (organism)	Epidemiology	Diagnosis	Reservoir	Transmission	Surveillance	Control
Human immunodeficiency virus (HIV) **Clinical features** With regular check-ups, treatment (when required), and healthy lifestyle, HIV is no longer fatal but a manageable long-term condition.	Prevalence increasing partly due to people with HIV living longer. Rate of new diagnoses decreasing due in part to reduced incidence in heterosexual people from high-prevalence countries, but rates rising in men who have sex with men.					Post-exposure prophylaxis Secondary prevention: CD4 count monitoring, lifestyle/ nutrition advice and support

[a] TPHA, Treponema pallidum haemagglutination assay; VDRL, Venereal Disease Reference Laboratory.

Table 2G.22 Vector borne diseases

Disease (organism)	Epidemiology	Diagnosis	Reservoir	Transmission	Surveillance	Control
Malaria Caused by the protozoa ***Plasmodium falciparum, P. vivax, P. ovale, P. malariae, P. knowlesi*** **Clinical features** Variable severity (*P. falciparum* causes the most fatalities) Non-specific flu-like symptoms Can cause weight loss, renal failure, and respiratory distress	Only travel associated in the United Kingdom (~1500–2000 cases per year). Highest burden in Africa (major cause of childhood mortality). High-risk groups include children and pregnant women. Sickle cell trait is protective.	Microscopy (blood smear) Rapid diagnostic test (antigen) PCR	Humans (*P. knowlesi*—macaques)	Vector—anopheles mosquito	Notifiable in the United Kingdom Lab reports	Travel advice, e.g. ABCD: **A**wareness of risk, **B**ite prevention (DEET, bed nets), **C**hemoprophylaxis, early **D**iagnosis (awareness of flu-like symptoms after travel)
Dengue fever Caused by a flavivirus (DEN-1, DEN-2, DEN-3, DEN-4) **Clinical features** Fever, headache, myalgia, vomiting, rash Usually non-severe Can cause haemorrhagic fever in children	Global prevalence increasing Endemic in tropics Only travel associated in the United Kingdom Outbreak in Madeira in 2012 and transmissions seen in other parts of Europe (e.g. Greece) More severe in children	PCR	Humans	Vector—Aedes mosquito	Viral haemorrhagic fever (VHF) is notifiable Lab reports	Travel advice as per malaria. Aedes aegypti is a day biting mosquito; therefore, additional precaution is also needed during the day.

(*continued*)

Table 2G.22 *(Continued)* Vector bone diseases

Disease (organism)	Epidemiology	Diagnosis	Reservoir	Transmission	Surveillance	Control
Lyme disease Caused by the spirochaete bacterium ***Borrelia burgdorferi*** **Clinical features** Early symptoms: fever, headache, erythema migrans rash Late symptoms if untreated: arthritis, neurological symptoms, cardiovascular symptoms	Increasing in the United Kingdom (possibly partly because of increased diagnosis and reporting) ~900 cases in 2010 In the United Kingdom, some of the areas with highest rates include Exmoor, New Forest, Lake District, and Scottish Highlands. At-risk groups include walkers and forestry workers.	Serology	Mice and other rodents, deer	Vector—Ixodes tick	Lab reports Enhanced surveillance	Tick awareness + early removal DEET Keeping to footpaths

Table 2G.23 Other communicable diseases

Disease (Organism)	Epidemiology	Diagnosis	Reservoir	Transmission	Surveillance	Control
Chickenpox/ shingles **Clinical features** Chickenpox: normally a mild fever followed by a vesicular rash	Endemic worldwide.	Clinical	Human	Direct contact/ airborne droplet	GP sentinel surveillance	Vaccine is available: used for healthcare professionals and contacts of immunocompromised patients if no previous exposure.
Caused by ***Varicella zoster virus*** (a herpesvirus) **Clinical features** Shingles: painful rash with a dermatomal rash. Can cause severe diseases in neonates and pregnant women (including pneumonia and congenital varicella syndrome)	Chickenpox mainly affects young children. Shingles mainly affects elderly.			Very infectious until all lesions crusted		Routine vaccination being considered in the United Kingdom. Exclude affected children from school until 5 days from rash onset or until all vesicles dried (this is sometimes longer than 5 days). Exposed pregnant women are offered immunoglobulin.

(continued)

Table 2G.23 *(Continued)* Other communicable diseases

Disease (Organism)	Epidemiology	Diagnosis	Reservoir	Transmission	Surveillance	Control
Creutzfeldt–Jakob disease (CJD) Caused by a prion protein **Clinical features** Neurological symptoms, dementia Fatal within 1–2 years of onset	Classical CJD is most common (though still rare)—cases may be sporadic (~85%) or due to inherited mutations (~15%). New variant CJD (vCJD) caused an outbreak in the United Kingdom and some parts of Europe following consumption of bovine spongiform encephalopathy (BSE)-infected cattle.	Clinical Post-mortem brain examination	vCJD—BSE-infected cattle	Consumption of infected cattle Contaminated surgical instruments (but CJD mainly sporadic)	CJD research and surveillance unit	CJD: Disposal of surgical instruments (difficult to destroy the prion with normal decontamination processes) vCJD: Slaughtering cattle, ending the use of meat and bone meal feed
Scabies Infestation caused by the mite ***Sarcoptes scabiei*** **Clinical features** Itchy rash, especially between fingers and toes Itching most intense at night	Pandemics (1918, 1945, 1990s) Winter outbreaks (e.g. nursing homes) Children and young adults most at risk	Hand lens/ microscopy of skin scrapings	Humans	Close contact		Treatment of cases and household contacts with permethrin/malathion. Washing clothes and sheets. Cases are infectious until treated.

Note: See *Communicable Disease Control and Health Protection Handbook* by Hawker et al. for other diseases.

Table 2G.24 Important infections in Australia and New Zealand

Infection	Description
Leptospirosis	Also known as **Weil's disease**, this zoonotic infection follows exposure to urine from infected animals and urine-contaminated surface water. It is an important occupational zoonotic disease for farmers and abattoir workers in New Zealand. Individual cases and outbreaks are common in developing countries, particularly following flooding.
Rheumatic fever	Acute rheumatic fever may occur following streptococcal throat infection and may result in serious damage to heart valves, leading to chronic rheumatic heart disease (CRHD). Acute rheumatic fever and CRHD remain important causes of morbidity and mortality for indigenous people in New Zealand (Maori), Australia (Aborigines), and the Pacific Islands.
Q Fever	Caused by Coxiella burnetii, this infection may present acutely as a severe flu-like illness that is sometimes associated with hepatitis and pneumonia, or it may progress to a chronic form with endocarditis. Infection usually occurs through aerosol or dust inhalation when working with infected animals, animal tissues, or animal products. The main carriers of the disease are farm animals such as cattle, sheep, and goats, but other animals such as kangaroos, bandicoots, and domestic pets (such as dogs and cats) can also be infected.
Murray Valley encephalitis	The majority of infections are subclinical. Symptoms may include fever, rash, confusion, paralysis, and seizures. Permanent neurological disease or death may also occur. Mosquitoes infected with the virus transmit the disease to humans, with birds providing the natural reservoir. Intermittent outbreaks occur and environmental activity is monitored in sentinel chicken flocks.

Table 2G.25 Important infections in South Africa

Infection	Description
HIV and TB	The duel epidemics of HIV and HIV-associated TB continue to place a huge burden on South Africa's healthcare resources. This is also now complicated by the additional burden of MDR-TB and extreme drug-resistant tuberculosis (XDR-TB) epidemics. The National DH in conjunction with the National Institute for Communicable Diseases is undertaking a nationally representative survey in 2013 to determine the prevalence and trends of MDR-TB in all 9 of South Africa's province.
Tick-bite fever	The incidence rates of tick-bite fever infection have been estimated to be in the region of 4%–5% in visitors from Europe, which are higher than those for other febrile illnesses such as malaria and typhoid fever. There is a large population at risk, e.g. game reserve visitors, hunters, soldiers, and farmers.
Rabies	Although there is a safe and effective vaccine against rabies, there are still cases reported in the rural areas of Africa where access to animal health facilities are limited, stray dogs are common, and fewer pets are regularly vaccinated against rabies.

2G.9 Organisation of infection control

Organisation is required at several levels, including national and local government, and health services including hospitals and community services.

National government

National Centres, such as Public Health England's *Centre for Infections* (CFI), are responsible for

- Infectious disease surveillance
- Providing specialist and reference microbiology and microbial epidemiology
- Coordinating investigation and cause of national and uncommon outbreaks
- Helping advise government on the risks posed by various infections
- Responding to international health alerts

Department of Health

ENG The devolved governments have overall responsibility for all health policy matters, including those relating to infection control. In England, the chief medical officer and chief nursing officer develop policies, guidance, and tools for the NHS. They seek advice from experts within and outside the DH to advise them on infection control matters, including

- Aseptic technique
- Cleaning
- Decontamination
- Hand washing
- Invasive devices (installing catheters)
- Isolation
- Laboratory specimen guidance
- Laundry and linen handling/management
- Handling of sharps
- Waste disposal/management

Examples of recent initiatives are given in Box 2G.6.

Local government

A local authority's environmental health service has a duty to register, inspect, and investigate food premises. Environmental health officers have legal powers of enforcement and prosecution.

In England, local authorities have the power to take action to control notifiable diseases within their boundaries. Councils are required to appoint a 'proper officer' who is usually a CCDC/CHP.

In Scotland, the Public Health etc. (Scotland) Act 2008 came into effect in 2010 and requires health boards and local authorities to designate sufficient competent persons to exercise health protection functions on behalf of the board.

Health services

As part of their remit to promote health and prevent disease, health authorities/boards are responsible for the surveillance of disease and for identifying problems and establishing planning measures.

Box 2G.6 Examples: Recent Department of Health initiatives on infection control

- Code of Practice for the Prevention and Control of Infections (2010) sets out 10 criteria against which the Care Quality Commission (CQC) will assess both NHS and independent providers of health and social care on infection control.
- Health Bill (2006)—Includes Hygiene Code of Practice for the Prevention and Control of HCAIs.
- Saving Lives—A delivery programme to reduce HCAIs, including MRSA (2005).
- A Matron's Charter—An action plan to cleaner hospitals (2004).
- Getting Ahead of the Curve—A strategy for combating infectious diseases (including other aspects of health protection) (2002).

Table 2G.26 Activities of the infection control team (ICT)

Planning	Developing policies and procedures Accommodation Purchasing equipment Clinical waste
Education	Education of staff Audit Hand washing
Surveillance	Antibiotic use
Outbreak	Advise on outbreaks Use of isolation facilities

Hospitals

In England, NHS hospitals are required to have in place an infection control team (ICT) consisting of an infection control physician or microbiologist and an infection control nurse (ICN), one of whom will act as the Director of Infection Prevention and Control (DIPC). In Scotland, every health board has an executive lead for HCAIs and an infection control manager (ICM) who is responsible for managing the ICT and for coordinating all aspects of infection control, including HCAIs. The activities of the ICT are listed in Table 2G.26.

The ICT reports to the hospital infection control committee, the members of which may include the chief executive (or a director-level deputy) and a CCDC/CHP. The committee meets regularly to review infection control matters.

Community services

Community ICNs encourage collaboration among community staff, ICTs, and CCDC/CHPs, as well as with care homes, prisons, nurseries, and schools.

Notifiable diseases

WA + ENG The diseases in Table 2G.27 are statutorily notifiable in England and Wales: all doctors working in these countries are required

Table 2G.27 Notifiable diseases in England and Wales

Acute encephalitis	HUS	Rubella
Acute infectious hepatitis	Infectious bloody diarrhoea	SARS
Acute meningitis	Invasive group A streptococcal disease	Scarlet fever
Acute poliomyelitis	Legionnaires' disease	Smallpox
Anthrax	Leprosy	Tetanus
Botulism	Malaria	TB
Brucellosis	Measles	Typhus
Cholera	Meningococcal septicaemia	VHF
Diphtheria	Mumps	Whooping cough
Enteric fever (typhoid or paratyphoid fever)	Plague	Yellow fever
Food poisoning	Rabies	

Source: http://www.hpa.org.uk/Topics/InfectiousDiseases/InfectionsAZ/NotificationsOfInfectiousDiseases/ListOfNotifiableDiseases/.

Note: Since Health Protection Regulations on notifiable diseases were updated in 2010 (following the changes in the Health and Social Care Act [2008]), there is now a duty for doctors also to notify where they suspect a patient has been contaminated in a manner that presents (or could present) a significant harm to human health. A list of causative agents (infectious, chemical, and radiological) is also included in the regulations (e.g. *Campylobacter* spp., *Giardia lamblia*, hepatitis A virus [HAV]).

to report any suspected cases to the proper officer of the local authority. The proper officer is required to provide anonymous details to Public Health England or Public Health Wales, respectively, every two weeks.

SCOT In Scotland, notifiable diseases are reported to HPS based on a clinical diagnosis by the medical practitioner, while notifiable organisms are reported based on the laboratory identification of the pathogen from an appropriate clinical sample. A list of notifiable diseases and organisms is available at http://www.legislation.gov.uk/asp/2008/5/schedule/1.

NI In Northern Ireland, a similar system operates to the rest of the United Kingdom (i.e. when a GP or other doctor in attendance suspects that a patient has a notifiable disease, he or she is legally required to inform the director of public health at the public health agency). **Note:** In Northern Ireland, **chickenpox** and **gastroenteritis (in persons aged <2 years)** are notifiable diseases in addition to those listed earlier [90].

2G.10 Microbiological techniques

Basic understanding of the biological basis, strengths, and weaknesses of routine and reference microbiological techniques.

There are two main methods of microbiological analysis—the traditional method involves growing a culture of the specimen in order to isolate and identify the microorganism (bacteria, fungi, viruses, and parasites). The alternative is a range of modern molecular methods that involve the identification of specific DNA or RNA (e.g. RNA transcriptase) within the specimen. Tuberculosis (TB), for example, once took 12 weeks to diagnose; now using molecular methods, it takes 24 h.

Main categories of methods used in microbiology laboratories

- Microscopy (including immunofluorescence)
- Culture
- Identification (e.g. typing of bacterial strain)
- Isolation of virus
- Drug sensitivity
- Serology (including immunoassay for antigen and antibody)

Routine microbiological techniques

Local hospital laboratories have tended to use traditional techniques, the strengths and weaknesses of which are listed in Table 2G.28.

Reference microbiological techniques

Molecular biological techniques form the basis of detecting and characterising an ever-increasing range of viruses, bacteria, fungi, and protozoa.

Nucleic acid probes are commercially available for CMV, HPV, hepatitis B virus (HBV), hepatitis C virus (HCV), *Chlamydia trachomatis, Neisseria gonorrhoeae, Streptococcus pyogenes,* and mycobacteria, among others.

Nucleic acid amplification systems are available for the direct detection in clinical specimens of HCV, HIV, *Mycobacterium tuberculosis (MTB), C. trachomatis,* and *N. gonorrhoeae.*

Strengths and weaknesses of these techniques are listed in Table 2G.29.

Immunoassays

These are used in the detection of microbial antigens and offer the potential for rapid diagnosis. Examples include **enzyme-linked immunoassays** and **direct immunofluorescence antibody assays**. Table 2G.30 lists strengths and weaknesses of immunoassays.

Table 2G.28 Strengths and weaknesses of routine microbiological techniques

Strengths	Weaknesses
Relatively low cost Can provide definitive diagnosis	Limited ability of laboratories to provide doctors with timely and clinically relevant information. Low sensitivity, e.g. samples taken after antibiotic has been given may test negative. Samples taken after onset of illness may result in difficulty isolating pathogen, e.g. viruses. Limited range of tests available—may not be able to provide full identification, e.g. toxin-producing strains.

Table 2G.29 Strengths and weaknesses of reference microbiological techniques

Strengths	Weaknesses
Increased speed Increased sensitivity and specificity Identify organisms that do not grow (or grow only slowly) in culture Identify genes that result in resistance to antibiotics 'Fingerprint' individual isolates for epidemiological tracking Recognition of newly emerging infectious diseases Control of antibiotic resistance in *S. pneumoniae*, *H. influenzae*, *S. aureus*, and common Gram-negative bacilli	Need for specialised equipment. Segregated rooms in laboratories. Currently detect only microorganisms. Turnaround times for existing tests are much longer than can potentially be achieved using molecular methods.

Table 2G.30 Strengths and weaknesses of immunoassays

Strengths	Weaknesses
Technical simplicity Rapidity Specificity Cost-effectiveness	Poor sensitivity Low NPV Low PPV

Automated and semi-automated systems

These fall into two main groups:

- Identification and susceptibility testing (some can provide results within a single working day)
- Blood culture systems (most true positive results are detected within 24–36 h)

Some blood culture systems have been adapted for automated or semi-automated culture (e.g. for *M. tuberculosis* and other mycobacteria). These enable the identification and susceptibility results to be processed from large numbers of blood culture samples.

Table 2G.31 lists the strengths and weaknesses of automated and semi-automated systems.

Molecular methods undoubtedly have enormous potential in diagnosing infectious diseases. New molecular methods will be widely accepted and implemented routinely within the next decade.

Table 2G.31 Strengths and weaknesses of automated and semi-automated systems

Strengths	Weaknesses
Reduce the traditional dependence on biochemical reactions to identify organisms	Organisms may be incorrectly identified, e.g. database does not include the correct identification.
Avoid the many labour-intensive steps between isolating and reporting clinically significant bacteria	Bacteria with heteroresistance to b-lactam drugs, inducible resistance mechanisms, or susceptibility gene mutation may be misclassified.
Provide rapid results Perform tests more reproducibly	May miss resistance of an organism to antibiotic, e.g. enterococci to glycopeptides; use supplemental testing with manual methods for problematic combinations of organisms and drugs.

2G.11 International aspects of communicable disease control

International aspects of communicable disease control, including port health.

Globalisation has increased the risk of international spread of infectious diseases. Historically, the most important measures to stop the importation of infectious diseases were **quarantine** and **trade embargoes**. Increasingly, however, public health specialists are expected to balance the protection of public health with the avoidance of unnecessary disruption to trade and travel. Therefore, **multilateral obligations** and more nuanced **port health** measures are becoming increasingly important.

International obligations

International Health Regulations

This is a multilateral initiative by countries to develop a global tool for the surveillance of cross-border transmission of diseases.

Core obligations for WHO member states

Countries are obliged to notify the WHO of public health emergencies of international concern, such as all cases of smallpox, SARS, wild-type polio, or a new subtype of human influenza. They must also

- Respond to requests for **verification** of information regarding urgent national risks
- **Control** urgent national public health risks that threaten to transmit disease to other member states
- Provide routine **port** inspection and control activities to prevent international disease transmission
- Apply the **measures** recommended by the WHO during public health emergencies

Core obligations of the WHO

In return, the WHO has a duty to respond to the needs of member states regarding the interpretation and implementation of its regulations. It must update these regulations (and their supporting guides) so that they remain scientifically valid. In addition, the WHO must publish recommendations for use by member states during public health emergencies of international concern.

Port health

In the United Kingdom, the regulations for ships, aircraft, and international trains give local authorities and port health authorities the power to appoint medical and non-medical port health officers who can prevent the entry of communicable diseases into the country.

Circumstances requiring the intervention of port health staff include

- **Outbreak** of food- or water-borne disease on board a vessel
- **Contamination** of aircraft by faeces or vomitus

- Pests (rodents or insects) on board a vessel
- Passengers or crew who are suspected of being infected with viral haemorrhagic fever (VHF), yellow fever, plague, cholera, diphtheria, or TB

The port medical inspector advises immigration officers on matters of health protection. Immigration officers may refer passengers who are immigrating to the United Kingdom, long-stay visitors and people visiting the country for health reasons. Some of these passengers may be required to have a chest x-ray, with the findings being passed to the CCDC/CHP.

2H

Principles and Practice of Health Promotion

Health promotion is the science and art of encouraging people to adopt actions to reduce their risk of developing disease. It is increasingly being recognised that health promotion is most effective when it focuses on enabling people to increase **control** over their own health. For this reason, it is often helpful to regard the discipline as a **sociopolitical process**.

2H.1 Responsibility for health

Collective and individual responsibilities for health, both physical and mental.

There are different views about the extent to which health is a collective or an individual responsibility. These perspectives determine how societies organise themselves to improve health:

- **Social responsibility** (or 'collectivism') is a **doctrine** that holds that an entity (be it state, government, corporation, organisation, or individual) has a responsibility to society as a whole. This responsibility can be **positive** (i.e. a responsibility to act) or **negative** (i.e. a responsibility to refrain from acting).
- In contrast, **individualism** (or 'libertarianism') is a moral, political, and social **philosophy**, which emphasises the importance of the individual. Its central tenets are individual liberty, personal independence, and the *'virtues of self-reliance'*.

Proponents of social responsibility and public initiatives argue that their policies are beneficial to the individual and that excessive individualism may actually be detrimental to the individuals themselves. In contrast, individualists hold that public initiatives may have unintended consequences beyond the issues that they are intended to address. Many commentators find the *'beneficial to the individual'* argument condescending and argue that individualism is not about individual benefit so much as individual choice.

It generally falls to politicians to decide which paradigm dominates health policy in any one country at a given time. For example, the absence of a universal health service in the United States has its roots in the political belief that individuals, rather than society, should be responsible for healthcare.

Collective responsibilities

UK Approaches that emphasise collective responsibilities for health encompass population-wide measures such as legislation and regulation (see Table 2H.1, which uses examples from the United Kingdom).

Individual responsibilities

Approaches based on **individual responsibility** focus on initiatives to enable individuals to make an **informed choice** (see Table 2H.2).

A further example of an approach that seeks to maximise individual choice is the **nudge** approach, or *'paternalistic libertarianism'* (see Box 2E.9).

Table 2H.1 Healthcare policies that emphasise collective responsibility

Policy	Example
Legislation	Drink-driving laws exist not just to protect the individual but also to ensure that the individual does not put others at risk.
Regulation	Health and safety legislation and regulations enable external bodies such as the Health and Safety Executive to inspect businesses and ensure that they are protecting their employees.
Population-wide measures	Fluoridation of the water supply.
Progressive health service funding systems	Universal taxation, where high earners provide a larger contribution for NHS costs, despite the fact that people earning least often use the service more intensively.

Table 2H.2 Healthcare policies that emphasise individual responsibility

Policy	Example
Information provision	Advertising safe drinking limits, which allows individuals to choose how much to drink given their knowledge of the health consequences.
Deregulation	Relaxation of licensing laws to allow pubs and shops to sell alcohol 24 h a day, which relies on individual choice regarding when and how much to drink.
Choice in healthcare	Private healthcare insurance enables individuals to choose whether or not to insure their health and where and when they receive healthcare.

2H.2 Determinants of health

Interaction between genetics and the environment (including social, political, economic, physical, and personal factors) as determinants of health, including mental health.

See also Section 2I.2.

The factors with the greatest influence on health are termed the **determinants of health**. While healthcare and social care services focus largely on dealing with the consequences of poor health, most of the positive determinants of health lie **outside the direct influence** of these services. One of the first proponents of this concept was Thomas McKeown, who studied trends in population growth and mortality. He found that large declines in mortality from major infections **predated** the development of effective treatment for these diseases. He concluded that the following factors had a greater influence on reductions in mortality than specific preventative and therapeutic measures, namely, limitation of **family size**, an improvement in **food supplies,** and a healthier **physical environment**. More recently, genetic and epidemiological studies have improved our understanding of the relative contributions of factors such as education, employment, housing, and environmental policy to health and illness. This insight is useful when developing health promotion interventions, in particular

- Whether to use **targeted** or **universal** programmes
- How to allocate resources
- Predicting susceptibility
- Predicting **uptake** of health promotion in the population

Several theories exist for considering the range of influences on health. This multiplicity is potentially confusing, but it reflects the rapid advances that have been made in this important field over the last half century, as well as the changing political and cultural perspectives from which the theories arise. Four of the key frameworks are summarised in Table 2H.3 and will then be discussed in turn.

Lalonde health field concept (1974)

Marc Lalonde, who was the Health Minister of Canada between 1972 and 1977, proposed the health field concept in 1974 in a seminal report titled *A New Perspective on the Health of Canadians.* Building on the ideas of McKeown, it used evidence of mortality and morbidity in Canadians to argue that healthcare services were not the most important determinant of health. Lalonde identified four fields—**biology**, **lifestyle**, **environment,** and **healthcare**—as the determinants of health

Table 2H.3 Frameworks for the determinants of health

Framework	Author(s)	Year	Summary
Health field concept	Lalonde	1974	Healthcare is not the sole determinant of health. The four health fields are biology, lifestyle, environment, and healthcare.
Policy rainbow	Dahlgren and Whitehead	1991	Determinants of health exist as **interrelated layers** of influence.
Health field model	Evans and Stoddart	1990	Health is not only the absence of disease but also takes into account **functional status** and wellbeing.
Social determinants model	Diderichsen and Hallqvist	1998	Social conditions affect individuals' **social situations**, which in turn determine their health risks.

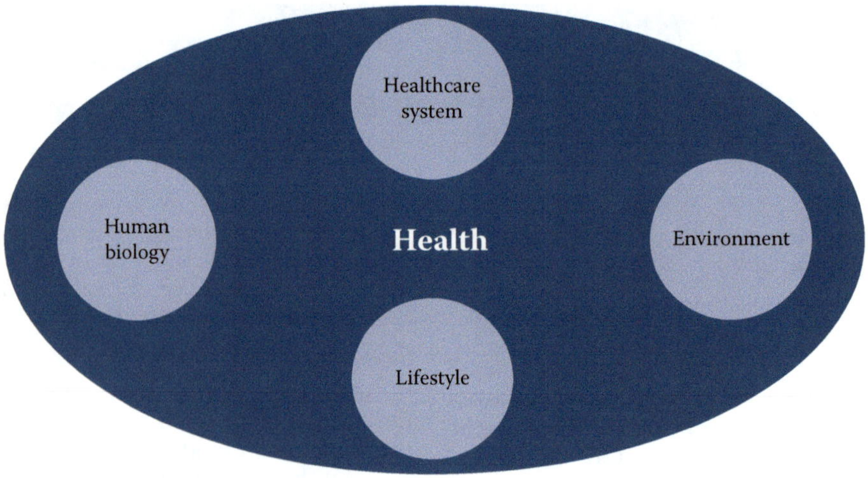

Figure 2H.1 Lalonde health field concept. (Reproduced from Lalonde, M., A new perspective on the health of Canadians: A working document, www.phacaspc.gc.ca/ph-sp/phdd/pdf/perspective.pdf, 1974.)

(see Figure 2H.1). The report set a new direction for Canadian health policy, in which

> *The Government of Canada now intends to give to human biology, the environment and lifestyle as much attention as it has to the financing of the healthcare organisation so that all four avenues to improved health are pursued with equal vigour.*
>
> Reproduced from Lalonde [91]

The model was modified in response to criticism that it was too focused on lifestyle and gave insufficient attention to the environment. However, the Lalonde model has been hugely influential throughout the world and was pivotal in the growth of health promotion as a discipline.

Dahlgren and Whitehead [92]

Dahlgren and Whitehead's health policy 'rainbow' identifies a range of determinants of health (see Figure 2H.2). It recognises that some determinants are not modifiable (e.g. age and sex) but that many others can potentially be altered. Dahlgren and Whitehead built on previous models by giving an indication of the **different levels** at which health is affected (see Box 2H.1). The model makes no attempt to explain the relationships between elements in the different tiers nor between factors in the same tier. Instead, it aims to stimulate discussion about the interrelationship of different layers and the relative importance of each layer and each element to health. In addition, the model aims to promote debate regarding potential opportunities for intervention in each layer for improving health and reducing inequalities. Table 2H.4 illustrates how the rainbow has been used to develop policy.

The relative importance of the factors in each layer varies according to the health issue or population under consideration.

Evans and Stoddart [94]: The health field model

In the health field model, health is explicitly conceptualised as being not only the presence or absence of disease but also includes **functional status** and **wellbeing**. By setting out a relationship between the determinants of health, the health field model helps practitioners understand how the determinants are themselves influenced and therefore how they might be modified (see Figure 2H.3).

Evans and Stoddart's framework of health fields encompasses a range of factors, including those shown in Table 2H.5.

Social determinants frameworks

The associations between social conditions and health have been thoroughly explored. Research

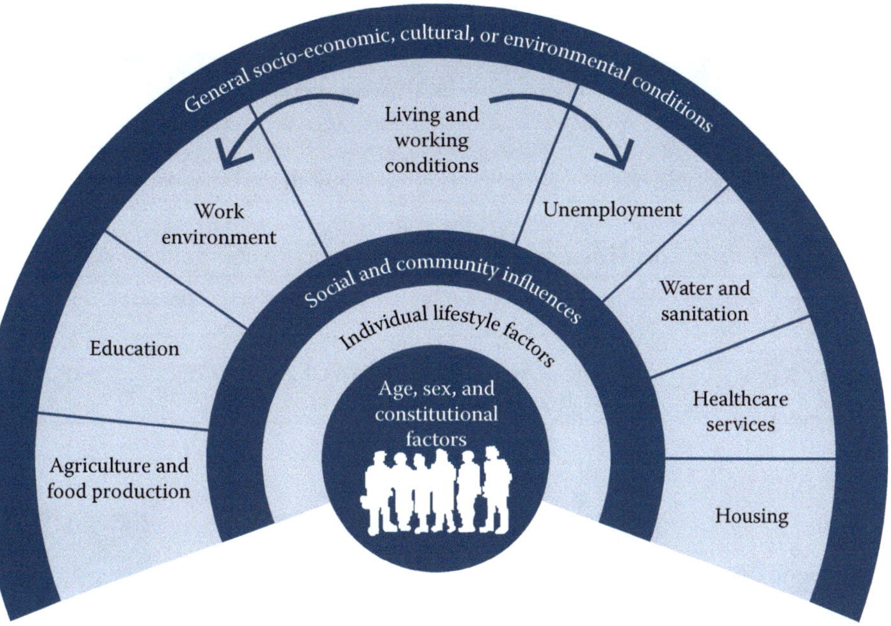

Figure 2H.2 Dahlgren and Whitehead's health rainbow. (Reproduced from Dahlgren, G. and Whitehead, M., *Policies and Strategies to Promote Social Equity in Health*, Stockholm, Sweden: Institute for Futures Studies, 1991.)

Box 2H.1 ENG Example: London Health Commission reports

The work of the London Health Commission was informed by Dahlgren and Whitehead's policy rainbow. The commission produced an annual report on the health of Londoners, focusing on variations on ten indicators including

- **Health outcomes** (e.g. life expectancy, infant mortality, and self-reported health status)
- Determinants of health
- Social and community influences (e.g. levels of crime)
- Living and working conditions (e.g. employment, education and housing)
- Environmental factors (e.g. road safety and air pollution)

The commission's analysis linked individual constitutional factors with the determinants in higher levels. For example, there are clear physical and biological reasons why very young and very old people are more susceptible to disease and injury than adults of working age. The report also considered the changes in people's living conditions as they age, particularly the following:

- **Housing**: Young households (where the oldest member is 16–24) were most likely to live in poor housing and households with residents aged over 75 were also likely to live in poor housing.
- **Employment**: 16–19-year-olds had the highest unemployment rates.
- **Crime**: Young households were most likely to be burgled.

Poor socio-economic conditions often affect old and young people in different ways. For example, while young people may be physically robust enough to withstand the health risks of poor living conditions, older people tend to be more susceptible.

Source: Reproduced from London Health Commission, *Health in London: 2002 Review of the London Health Strategy High-Level Indicators*. London, UK: London Health Commission, Available online at: www.londonshealth.gov.uk/pdf/hinl2002.pdf, 2002.

Table 2H.4 Dahlgren and Whitehead's health policy rainbow applied to health promotion

Layer	Example of a health promotion intervention
Individuals	Although some individual factors are fixed (e.g. age), others can be influenced (e.g. lifestyle and behaviour). Influences at this layer include **information** and **education** and also influences from the **distal** determinants in the other layers.
Communities	Strengthening communities through action to improve the local **environment** and **living conditions** or through *'bottom-up'* action led by local community groups.
Access	Improving access to services such as **healthcare**, **leisure**, and **transport** in terms of location, cost, and appropriateness.
Macroeconomics	Instituting **macroeconomic** or **cultural** change at national or global levels, possibly through legislation.

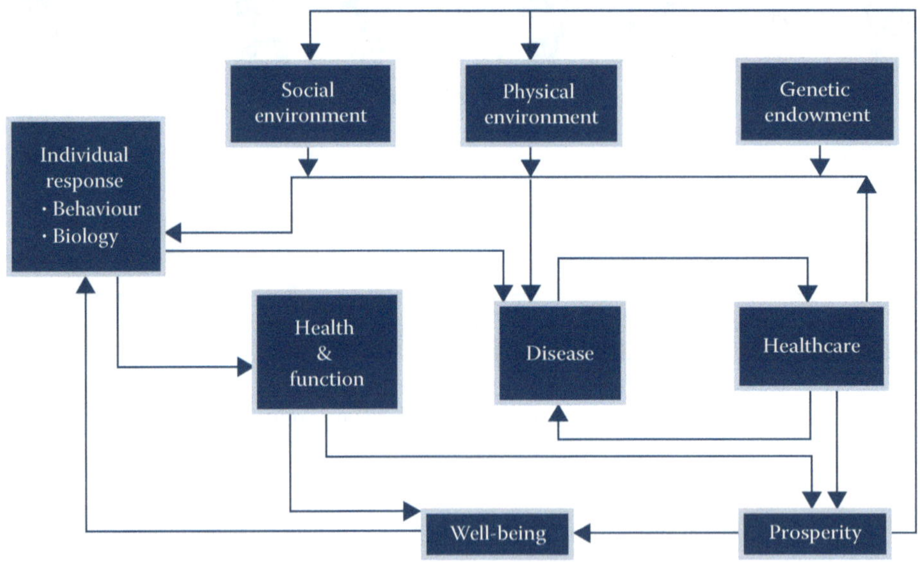

Figure 2H.3 The health field model. (Reproduced with permission from Evans, R. and Stoddart, G., *Soc. Sci. Med.*, 31, 1347, 1990.)

has strongly linked adverse health outcomes (e.g. premature mortality, vulnerability to illness and injury, self-reported health, and wellbeing) to **education** and **employment**. For example, the **Whitehall study** found that people employed in the lower grades of the British civil service were more likely to die prematurely than their colleagues employed in higher grades. Indeed, there are several models that place social conditions as the predominant determinant of health and health inequalities.

Diderichsen and Hallqvist [95] devised one of the most commonly cited *'social determinants'* frameworks. Their model identifies four broad conceptual mechanisms:

1. **Social stratification** (social conditions, such as education and employment, will determine people's social situation) leading to
2. Differential exposure and
3. **Differential vulnerability** which together result in
4. Differential consequences

These mechanisms work synergistically to generate health inequities. For each mechanism, the possible entry points for policy interventions can be identified in the model (see Figure 2H.4).

Table 2H.5 Evans and Stoddart health field model

Health field	Examples
Social environment	Education, employment, family, poverty.
Physical environment	Poor housing, proximity to hazards, waste, and conflict.
Genetics	Genetic factors that interact with environmental conditions.
Behaviour	Viewed as an '*intermediate*' determinant (i.e. not simply a voluntary act), behaviour is shaped by a range of determinants, including education, access to facilities, and financial considerations.
Healthcare	Another '*intermediate*' determinant, this encompasses access and quality of healthcare.

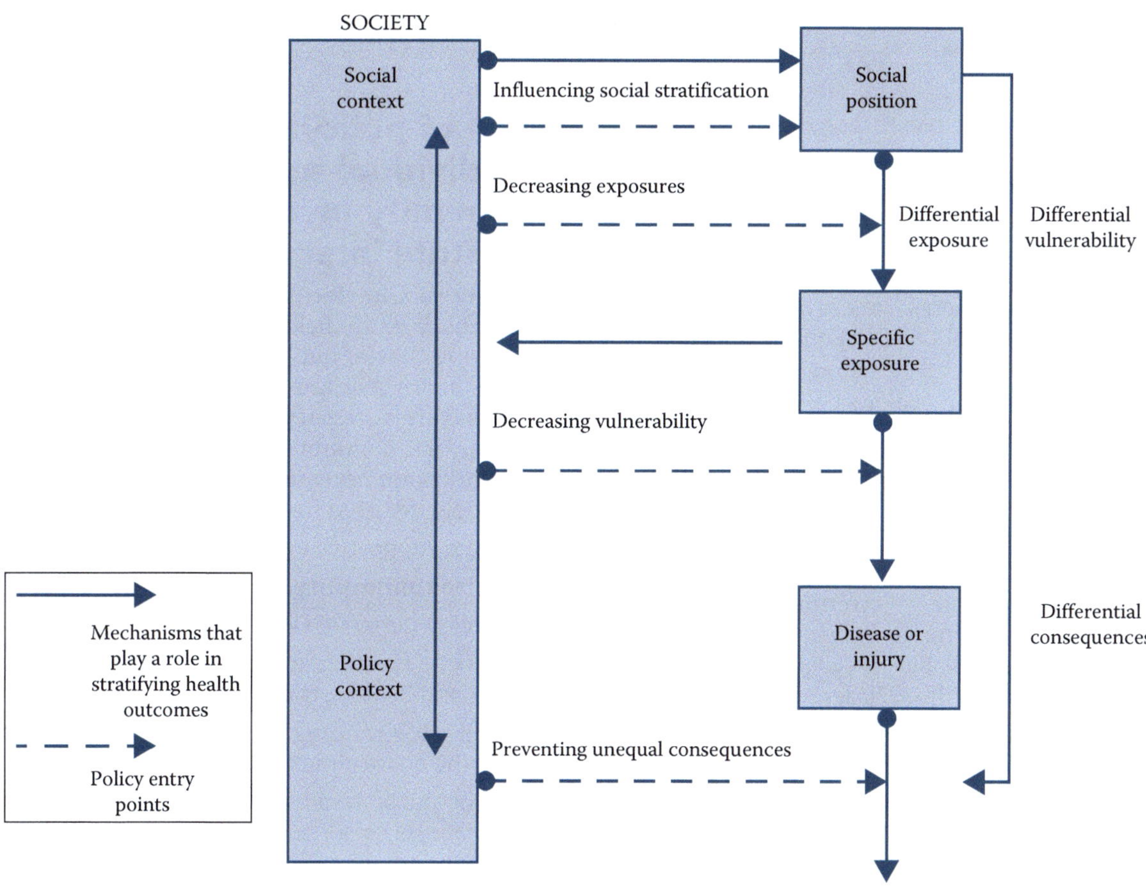

Figure 2H.4 The social determinants frameworks. (Adapted from Diderichsen, F. and Hallqvist, J., Social inequalities in health: Some methodological considerations for the study of social position and social context, in Arve-Parès, B., ed., *Inequality in Health: A Swedish Perspective*, Stockholm, Sweden: Swedish Council for Social Research, pp. 25–39, 1998.)

Other models focusing on social determinants of health include explicit recognition that

- Health influences a person's social position, as well as vice versa
- There are interacting effects between social and biological pathways
- Access to—and the quality of—healthcare are related to the social determinants

More recently, the focus for action has been on the **social inequalities** of health, which Dahlgren [96] defined as

> *Systematic differences in health between socio-economic groups [which] are socially produced, modifiable and unfair.*

This reflects the growing disparity in life expectancy and health status between different socioeconomic groups, at a time when, overall, the average health status and life expectancy continue to improve.

2H.3 Policy dilemmas

Ideological dilemmas and policy assumptions underlying different approaches to health promotion.

While the aims of healthcare treatment are usually relatively clear, the aims of health promotion may be contentious. Health promotion can reach beyond the traditional boundaries of healthcare into policymaking, personal choice, and community development. The incursion of health promotion into these spheres is more acceptable in some contexts than others and depends on factors such as the following:

- **Prevailing policy**: Two contrasting health policy statements (e.g. *Health for All* [1986] and *Choosing Health* [2004]) exemplified how approaches to health promotion could be shaped by views regarding personal autonomy and the role of communities
- **Socio-economic circumstances** affect both the community's health needs and the resources available to promote health (e.g. Naidoo and Wills [97] described the dilemma of health promotion for people whose primary problem was economic poverty).
- The characteristics of the particular **health issue** (e.g. the epidemiology and perceptions of HIV and AIDS have dictated the focus of health promotion activities in this area)

Effect of policy: Balance of individual autonomy, community involvement, and state intervention

The **Ottawa Charter [98]** applied WHO's *Health for All* policy to the field of health promotion. The aims of the charter implicitly assumes that certain circumstances that are beyond the control of the individual are necessary to support health promotion (i.e. that community involvement and state intervention are necessary). The charter advocates that people involved in health promotion should

- Create supportive **environments**
- Enable **community** participation
- Develop personal **skills** for health
- Reorient healthcare services towards **prevention** and health promotion
- Build wide-ranging **public policies** that protect the environment and promote health

ENG The public health white paper Healthy Lives, Healthy People (2010) aimed to maximise individual choice through the 'nudge' effect (see Section 2E).

Table 2H.6 Needs and entitlements by role

Role	Needs and entitlements
Patient	Receives intervention only; does not need to provide further input into the way that programmes and services are delivered
Consumer	Needs sufficient information to make an informed choice about whether to accept or reject a health-promoting behaviour or intervention
Empowered participant	Needs adequate skills and resources to enable participation and has responsibilities in shaping and delivering health promotion

Individual roles

A person can assume different roles (e.g. patient, consumer, participant). Each role has different expectations and requirements in terms of information, skills, and involvement (see Table 2H.6).

Tackle poverty or address narrower determinants of health?

An ideological dilemma of health promotion is whether its aim is to

- Reduce inequalities in **access to health services**
- Reduce inequalities in **health** (which would require wider actions outside the health remit)

The **Black Report** [99] argued that poverty was one of four possible explanations for the widening health inequalities observed in Britain over the course of the twentieth century.

See Sections 4A.8 and 4C.10.

Poverty

Poverty (both relative and absolute) is a major determinant of ill health. Low pay, inadequate benefits, or unemployment lead to various types of poverty, such as food and fuel poverty, poor housing and transport, and social isolation. These in turn lead to

- **Physical** problems (e.g. low birthweight (LBW) babies, respiratory disease)
- **Psychological** problems (e.g. stress, depression, anxiety)
- **Behavioural** changes (e.g. smoking, insufficient exercise, poor diet)

Barriers

Some of the barriers to effective health promotion in the context of poverty include the following:

- Intrinsic **victim blaming** culture.
- Focusing on knowledge, attitudes, and behaviour ignores the **constraints on choice** associated with poverty, which make healthy choices more difficult.
- Focusing on **one-to-one interventions** can ignore wider social influences and may underestimate the effect of poverty.
- The lack of a **common approach** to poverty in health promotion.
- Initiatives that may alleviate poverty (e.g. increasing access to employment) are **outside the remit of healthcare**.

Policies

Policies to reduce poverty and reduce morbidity include

- **Macro**-level changes (e.g. minimum wage)
- Collection of **data** on the wider social and economic determinants of health
- **Multi-sector action** (e.g. basing benefits advisors in health clinics)
- **Community development** in addition to health advice (e.g. food cooperatives to support healthy eating messages)

Targeted or universal health promotion?

Targeting offers an opportunity to **prioritise resources** and to **tailor messages** and activities to the particular characteristics of the people who need them the most. However, there are disadvantages associated with targeting health promotion, outlined in Table 2H.7. The problems associated with both targeting and universal health promotion approaches are illustrated with respect to HIV/AIDS in Box 2H.2.

An alternative strategy to targeting is to attempt to reduce risk across the whole population (see Section 1C.16). Where a risk factor is widespread in society, universal approaches can have a larger effect than targeted interventions. For example, universal approaches to reducing dietary salt (e.g. lobbying manufacturers to reduce levels of salt in their products) can reduce the population's average blood pressure and thereby reduce the burden of CHD. In this case, however, while the population's risk of disease may be substantially reduced, the average individual risk of disease is barely affected. This is known as the **prevention paradox** and its recognition can cause the public to lose credibility in universal approaches (see Section 2H.4).

Table 2H.7 Disadvantages of targeting health promotion

Targeted focus	Examples	Disadvantages
Behaviour	Smoking, eating, car driving	This risks **widening health inequalities** by appealing to people with the resources and circumstances available to change their behaviour. For example, advice to eat more fruit is easier to follow by people who can afford fruit and who live in an area where fruit can readily be purchased.
Group	Children, older people, gay men	Assumes that groups are **homogeneous** (e.g. that all gay men indulge in promiscuous, unprotected sex and that men who self-identify as straight do not have sex with men). Can lead to **culture blaming** (i.e. ascribing the risk to an inherent aspect of culture rather than a problem to be tackled jointly by the community and public health specialists). For example, the Asian rickets campaign focused on health education messages about increasing vitamin D in the diet, thereby placing the blame for vitamin D deficiency on Asian families. In contrast, when vitamin D deficiencies were first recognised in the 1950s as a general health problem, the response was to fortify core foods. Groups that are deemed to be at risk of a certain condition (e.g. sickle cell disease in people of African descent) may be **neglected** with regard to broader health problems (e.g. CHD).
Condition	Hypertension, diabetes	As part of the **prevention paradox**, many healthy people will be '**pathologised**' unnecessarily (e.g. hypertension will be diagnosed and treated in many people who will never become ill as a result of elevated blood pressure but will be caused unnecessary worry and suffer the side effects of antihypertensive treatment). In contrast, focusing only on people at high risk can **miss** many people who are actually at risk. For example, more people who are normotensive die from CHD than people with hypertension. Moreover, concentrating on high-risk attributes while ignoring broader social influences may be less successful than whole-population initiatives.

Box 2H.2 USA + UK Example: Changing approaches with the changing perceptions and epidemiology of HIV/AIDS

When the HIV/AIDS epidemic began in the 1980s in the United Kingdom and the United States, health promotion messages were initially targeted at gay men. This led to

- An illusion that heterosexual people were immune to HIV/AIDS
- Increased homophobia
- Difficulties in attracting funding and resources for what became seen as a 'marginal' illness

By the mid-1980s, the epidemic had changed and HIV was recognised as an infection that could potentially affect anyone. As a result, a whole-population approach for HIV/AIDS health promotion was adopted. However, this caused

- A shift in resources from gay projects to professionally led, mainstream interventions
- Explicit, detailed guidance on safer sexual behaviour that would previously have been unacceptable to the general public
- A change in messages from minimal behaviour change (sex, but safe sex) towards more conservative messages (monogamy)
- Ignored the fact that gay men were still at disproportionately high risk
- Downgraded the strong activist/support networks that had been built up

The debate still continues with HIV about whether to focus resources on the whole population or on the groups that are most at risk (i.e. people from sub-Saharan Africa and men who have sex with men).

Source: Reproduced from Naidoo, J. and Wills, J., *Practising Health Promotion: Dilemmas and Challenges*, London, UK, Baillière Tindall, 1998.

2H.4 Prevention paradox

As described in Section 2H.3, public health practitioners often face a dilemma over whether to target people at greatest risk of a disease or attempt to lower the risk across the whole population. The **Rose hypothesis** and the **prevention paradox** consider the arguments for and against a population-based approach.

Rose hypothesis

In the 1980s, Geoffrey Rose argued that because risk factors for diseases are often normally distributed (i.e. more disease will occur among the large number of people at low or medium risk than the few at high risk), universal programmes will have a greater overall effect on health at the population level than targeted approaches (see Section 1C.16).

Prevention paradox

The prevention paradox describes the phenomenon whereby actions to reduce the risk of a disease across the population may successfully reduce the population's overall risk while providing only a minimal benefit to each individual. For example, the mandatory wearing of seat belts is a policy that affects all car users but prevents death only in the small minority involved in a road traffic collision. As Rose [100] put it, 'A preventive measure that brings large benefits to the community offers few benefits to each participating individual'.

Implications for health promotion

Because an individual only tends to receive a minimal benefit from a universal intervention, the alternative, targeted approach may seem more attractive because the prevention paradox can cause a loss of credibility in health promotion materials (see Section 2H.3). For example, health promotion advice recommends reducing fat in the diet in order to minimise the risk of CHD. If it is evident that some people who eat a high-fat diet do not develop heart disease, there may be less incentive for other people in the community to reduce their dietary fat intake. Hunt and Emslie [101] describe what happens when health promotion materials do not take into account the prevention paradox:

> *The failure to acknowledge the prevention paradox more directly in health education material... can lead, at best, to greater mistrust among the general public of the messages contained, and at worst to their outright rejection.*

2H.5 Health education

Health education and other methods of influencing personal lifestyles which affect health.

Health education is sometimes erroneously taken to be synonymous with health promotion—the flawed assumption being that if people were sufficiently well informed about health, then they would make healthy choices. Frameworks of the determinants of health illustrate that health is actually affected by more than simply an individual's personal choices (see Section 2H.2). This reality is echoed in models such as Ewles and Simnett's [102] five approaches to health promotion, which explicitly include other activities, such as social change, within the remit of health promotion (see Section 2H.7).

Nevertheless, education is a major component of health promotion. Formal health education programmes usually aim to influence people's beliefs, attitudes, and behaviours and enable them to make an informed decision about the aspects of their lifestyle that affect their health.

However, people do not receive their health education only from planned, conventional, health promotion practitioners, and materials. Rather, there is a range of other routes, including friends, family, television, and magazines, as illustrated by the example of children's knowledge of drugs and alcohol (see Box 2H.3).

Box 2H.3 ENG Example: Schoolchildren's knowledge and use of drugs and alcohol

Regular surveys are conducted in England to explore secondary schoolchildren's smoking habits and their knowledge and use of drugs and alcohol. The 2011 survey included 6,500 pupils aged 11–15.

Sources of information

The 2011 survey suggested that informal sources play as great, or a greater, role in where pupils receive their information about drugs and alcohol compared with formal education. It concluded that

'Pupils were more likely to cite their parents as a useful source of information for smoking and drinking than for drug taking: parents were cited as providing useful information on smoking and drinking alcohol by 77% and 79% of pupils respectively, but 66% said their parents gave them useful information on drug taking. A similar pattern was seen for the TV, with 73% saying the TV provided useful information on smoking and 70% saying the TV provided useful information on drinking alcohol, compared with 64% for drug use'.

Sex and ethnicity

Girls were more likely than boys to smoke regularly but boys were more likely to take drugs. While white pupils were more likely to smoke and drink alcohol, black pupils were more likely to report taking drugs.

Source: Reproduced from the Health and Social Care Information Centre, Lifestyle Statistics, Smoking, drinking and drug use among young people in England in 2011, http://www.ic.nhs.uk, 2012.

2H.6 Settings for health promotion

Appropriate settings for health promotion (e.g. schools, the workplace).

Some key locations for conducting health promotion include

- Workplaces
- Schools
- Primary care
- Prisons
- Universities

These settings offer the **structure** (e.g. physical building), **resources** (e.g. staff), and **access** to people (who spend considerable time in these settings) for health promotion to improve health and productivity. The provision of health promotion in these settings may improve the performance of the organisation as a whole, as well as improving the health of individuals.

See Table 2H.8 for further details.

Table 2H.8 Settings for health promotion

	Schools	Workplaces	Primary care
Target	Children and adolescents	Employees	Patients
Others	Parents	Employees' relatives and friends	Customers (e.g. in pharmacies), patients' relatives and friends, staff
Potential hazards at the setting	**Physical** Exposure to unhealthy food **Psychological** Peer pressure Stress from assessments and examinations Bullying	**Biological** Exposure to toxic chemicals and fumes **Physical** Musculoskeletal symptoms lifting and handling Sedentary lifestyle, e.g. office work **Psychological** Stress, bullying and harassment	Workplace hazards (apply to staff)
Potential benefits to the organisation and individual	**Performance** Better educational results **Wellbeing** Stronger links between school and home Prevention or delay in risk-taking behaviours (e.g. drugs)	**Performance** Recruitment, morale, retention Reduced absenteeism **Wellbeing** Exposure to healthy social norms (e.g. no-smoking workplaces) Reduce hazards	**Performance** Overall cost savings Reduced consultation rate Reduced referral rates Reduced emergency care
Resources available to support health promotion	**Staff** Teachers School nurses **Facilities** Playing fields (if any) Classrooms	**Employees** Occupational health Health and safety officers Managers Workers **Partners** Unions **Facilities** Office space, financial	**Staff** GP Practice nurses Receptionists Community nurses Pharmacist Dentist Optometrist **Facilities** Practice/shop space

Table 2H.8 *(Continued)* Settings for health promotion

	Schools	Workplaces	Primary care
Examples of major policies or activities	Local areas can implement or adapt **'Healthy Schools'**, which encompasses Personal, social, and health education Healthy eating Physical activity Emotional health and wellbeing **Ofsted** National inspections cover preparing children and young people for the next stage in their lives and spiritual, moral, social, and cultural provision.	**Health and Safety Executive** **COSHH** (see Chapter 2F) **Policies** Harassment Smoking **Training** Health and safety Manual handling **Subsidised or free:** Counselling Bike loans Canteens with healthy menus Gym membership Vaccinations for at-risk workers (e.g. hepatitis B and influenza offered to healthcare workers)	**General practice** Vaccinations Lifestyle advice Screening Disease prevention treatment **Pharmacies** Display leaflets Provide smoking cessation Monitor blood pressure, cholesterol **Dentists and optometrists** Smoking advice
Advantages	Most children in school. 'Captive audience'. Children are in school for several years so changes can be tracked over time. Opportunities for progressive programme.	Protect health Access to health workers (who would not attend health settings and therefore may not otherwise have access to health messages)	Patients seeking primary care may be more **receptive** to health messages. Most people have **contact** with primary care at some point. People are more receptive to health messages from senior health professionals.
Limitations	**Work pressures** may affect implementation. What about children **excluded** or away from school for other reasons? Staff (particularly non-health professionals) need to **develop skills** and confidence to deliver health messages.	**Work pressures** may affect implementation. **Priorities for employees** may differ from health at work (e.g. earning money). **Priorities for employers** may conflict with health priorities, particularly in **low-paid** or **illegal** work. **Unemployed** people are not covered.	**Short consultations** mean insufficient time to discuss health promotion. If the intervention is not in the contract/not prioritised, then it may not take place. Some staff not convinced of benefits or trained to deliver health promotion. **Work pressures** may affect implementation.

2H.7 Models of health promotion

The value of models in explaining and predicting health-related behaviour.

Models of health promotion have been developed to

- Define the **scope and aims** of the discipline
- Enable health promotion practitioners to **understand what motivates** individuals and/or communities to adopt health-seeking/harming behaviours
- Inform the **development** of health promotion programmes to influence health behaviours

The principal health promotion models are summarised in Table 2H.9.

Health belief model [104]

The health belief model (HBM), shown in Box 2H.4, was first developed by American social psychologists Hochbaum, Rosenstock, and Kegels in response to the failure of a free TB health-screening programme and has evolved over time. The HBM is based on the understanding that a person will take a health-related action if that person believes all of the statements shown in Box 2H.5. Interventions may act as a 'cue to action' to influence any or all of these perceptions.

Some strengths and weaknesses of the HBM are listed in Table 2H.10.

Social cognitive theory

Developed by Bandura in the 1970s and 1980s, and also known as the **social learning theory,** this model focuses on three influences on behaviour [105] (see Table 2H.11).

Observational learning is the concept that humans learn not just by **doing** (participation) but also by **watching** other people's behaviour and the rewards that they receive from their behaviours.

Table 2H.9 Health promotion models

Name	Author	Year	Brief description
Health belief model (HBM)	Hochbaum et al.	1958	Individuals will adopt health-related actions if they believe that they are faced with risk and have the potential to reduce the risk.
Social learning theory	Bandura	1977	Behaviour is influenced by social norms, expectations, observations, and perceived ability to control behaviour.
Theory of planned behaviour	Azjen and Fishbein	1980	The belief of what others expect (subjective norm) also affects attitudes that change behaviour.
Stages of change	Prochaska and DiClemente	1984	Individuals go through several stages to change behaviour.
Spheres of health promotion	Tannahill	1985	Overlapping spheres of protection, prevention, and education.
Beattie model	Beattie	1991	Four approaches covering a range of levels of authority and individuality.
Ewles and Simnett model	Ewles and Simnett	2003	Multidisciplinary perspective, from biomedicine to sociopolitical change.

Box 2H.4 Health belief model

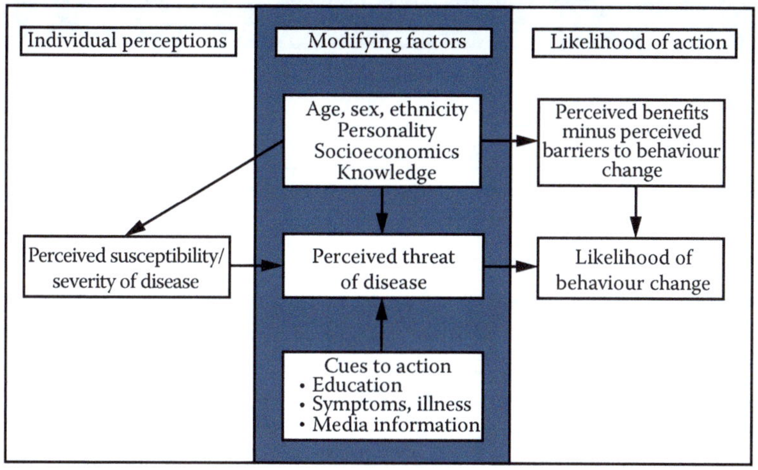

Source: Reproduced from Strecher, V.J., and Rosenstock, I.M., The health belief model. In *1997 Cambridge Handbook of Psychology, Health and Medicine*, Baum A. et al. (eds), Cambridge University Press, Cambridge, pp. 113–117, 1997.

Box 2H.5 Criteria of behaviour change according to the health belief model

Belief	Description
1. Susceptibility	They are susceptible to the condition or problem.
2. Severity	It could have potentially serious consequences.
3. Course of action	A course of action is available to reduce the risks.
4. Benefits outweigh costs	The benefits of the action outweigh the costs or barriers.
5. Ability[a]	The individual perceives that they have the ability to carry out the action (i.e. 'self-efficacy').

[a] Note that the final parameter, self-efficacy, was added later by Rosenstock et al. [106]. This addition is thought to improve the way that the HBM meets the challenges of changing *habitual* unhealthy behaviours such as being sedentary, smoking, or overeating.

Table 2H.10 Strengths and weaknesses of the HBM

Strengths	Weaknesses
Most useful for less entrenched, simpler **preventive** behaviour changes (e.g. uptake of immunisations, screening)	Less useful for **complex**, long-term behaviours (e.g. alcohol dependence).
Evidence supports the usefulness of the model in predicting behaviour or improving the effectiveness of some interventions.	It does not account for other forces circumstances that influence behaviour aside from individuals' beliefs (e.g. societal norms, provision of health care).

Table 2H.11 Social cognitive theory

Influence on health behaviour	Description
Reciprocal determinism	The continuous, subtle, and complex interactions between people's behaviour and their environment.
Social norms	The effect of social and cultural conventions on behaviour.
Cognitive factors	These encompass observational learning, expectations, and self-efficacy.

Table 2H.12 Strengths and weaknesses of social cognitive theory

Strengths	Weaknesses
• Realistically **complex** solutions to health problems (i.e. not too simplistic). • Unlike the *stages of change* model and the *HBM*, it explicitly recognises the impact of **environmental, social and behavioural factors**. • Widens the role of health promotion beyond individual persuasion about a discrete behaviour to cover the entire social environment and **wider personal beliefs**.	• Can be difficult to implement because of its broad scope and complexity

The term '**expectations**' is used to describe the capacity of a person to anticipate and value the outcomes of a particular behaviour. This capacity varies between individuals, which underlines the importance of exploring personal attitudes and beliefs when seeking to change behaviour. For example, young women who believe that smoking helps with weight loss are more likely to be persuaded to give up if they are given information about other ways to control weight, rather than by warning them about the risks of smoking and lung disease.

Self-efficacy is a person's perceived ability to control their own behaviour. This phenomenon is both person specific and environment specific. For example, a person may be very confident of their ability to avoid alcohol at home but less so in a social situation.

Some of the strengths and weaknesses of social learning theory are listed in Table 2H.12.

Theory of planned behaviour

This model was first developed by Azjen and Fishbein in 1980 (see Figure 2H.5). In this model, the person's belief of **what others expect** (i.e. the 'subjective norm') leads to attitudes that change behaviour. It is therefore important to challenge these beliefs, for

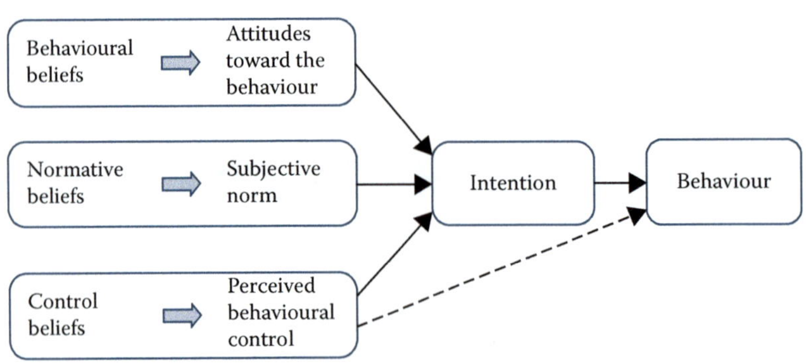

Figure 2H.5 Theory of planned behaviour.

Box 2H.6 Stages of change

- Pre-contemplation
- Contemplation
- Determination
- Action
- Maintenance
- (Termination)

example, by countering the belief among teenagers that all of their peers are taking drugs. As with social cognitive theory, the theory of planned behaviour highlights the importance of self-efficacy (i.e. perceived behavioural control) on behaviour change. Some school programmes use this model to emphasise how children can control their own actions (e.g. how to say no to drugs and deal with peer pressure).

Stages of change model

Developed by Prochaska and DiClemente [107], this model is also known as the **trans-theoretical model**. It describes behaviour change as a process (i.e. not a one-off event) and it predicts that people who change their behaviour will progress through the stages shown in Box 2H.6.

People can enter or exit at any point—and they can **stall** at any stage. The model can be applied to people who initiate change themselves, as well to people in organised programmes. Programmes based on this model require an initial understanding of the stage or stages at which participants may enter the programme.

Strengths and weaknesses of this model are listed in Table 2H.13.

Spheres of health promotion

Tannahill [108] considered health promotion to be defined by *'three overlapping spheres of activity'* (see Figure 2H.6):

- Health education
- **Protection** against harm and enhancing wellbeing
- **Prevention** of disease, disability, and injury

Examples of the contents of areas of the overlapping spheres are shown in Table 2H.14.

The strengths and weaknesses of Tannahill's model are summarised in Table 2H.15.

Table 2H.13 Strengths and weaknesses of the stages of change model

Strengths	Weaknesses
• Useful for long-term, **complex** behaviour changes (e.g. giving up smoking, weight management) • Useful for practitioners who wish to **tailor their counselling** (and their expectations for change) according to the stage of the model in which the individual is currently located • Useful for **programme planning**, to organise interventions sequentially and to match interventions to stages of the population	• Less useful for programmes aimed at **whole communities**

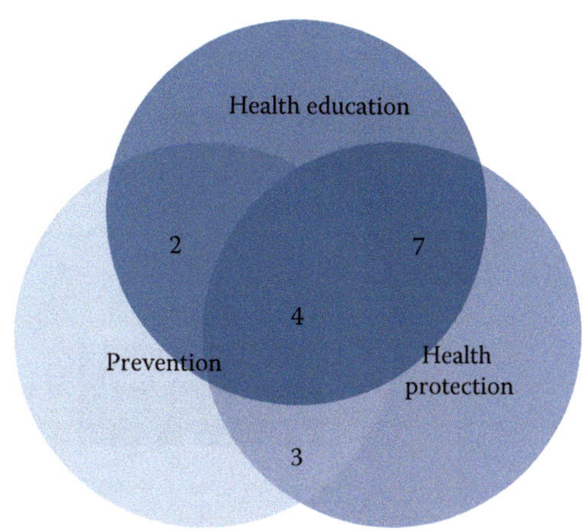

Figure 2H.6 Spheres of health promotion. (From Tannahill, A. What is health promotion? *Health Education Journal*, 44; 167–168, 1985.)

Table 2H.14 Spheres of health promotion

Sphere	Contents
Prevention	Organised, preventive healthcare programmes (e.g. immunisation)
Health education	Health education to prevent disease onset (e.g. smoking cessation advice and information)
Health protection	Health protection legislation to prevent illness or injury (e.g. fluoridation of water)

Table 2H.15 Strengths and weaknesses of Tannahill's health promotion model

Strengths	Weaknesses
• **Simple** to understand • **Widely adopted** for defining what constitutes health promotion and for informing health promotion practitioners how to plan and conduct their work • **Encompasses wellbeing** not simply the absence of disease	• Distinction between protection and prevention is **arbitrary** at times.

Beattie model

Beattie's model of health promotion (summarised in Naidoo and Wills [109]) considers not just the activities involved in health promotion but also how they are delivered (i.e. from the top down or from the bottom up). It is a useful tool for critically evaluating health promotion programmes, particularly regarding the balance of authoritative and negotiated approaches.

Beattie outlined four approaches to health promotion:

1. Health **persuasion**
2. Personal **counselling** for health

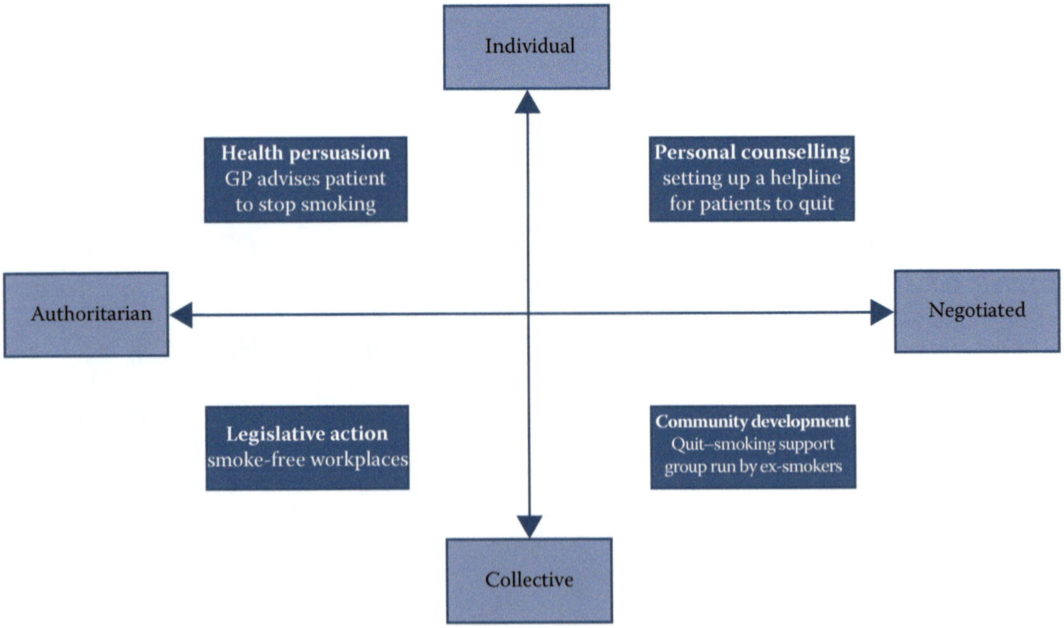

Figure 2H.7 Beattie's model of health promotion.

Table 2H.16 Ewles and Simnett's health promotion approaches

Approach	Description	Example
Medical	Focused on disease and biomedical explanations of health Narrow concept of disease (ignores social and environmental dimensions)	Immunisation Screening
Behavioural	Encourages individuals to adopt healthy behaviours	Healthy cooking classes
Educational	Provision of knowledge and information and assists development of skills for individuals to make informed decisions	Schools
Empowerment	Helps individuals to identify their own concerns and needs Health educator as facilitator	Community development work
Social change	Focus on socio-economic environment in determining health Involves lobbying, policy planning, negotiating	Lobbying Policy planning Negotiating

3. **Legislative** action
4. Community development

Which approach should be used in a particular circumstance depends on

- The **mode** of the programme (ranging from authoritative [top down] to negotiated [bottom up])
- The **focus** of the programme (individual or collective)

See Figure 2H.7.

Ewles and Simnett

The model proposed by Ewles and Simnett [102] considers health promotion from a multidisciplinary perspective. It explicitly incorporates biomedical approaches and activities in order to achieve policy and social change within the broader scope of the discipline. This model considers five approaches, and the most appropriate combination of these approaches depends on the **starting point** of the health promotion initiative (see Table 2H.16).

2H.8 Risk behaviour

Risk behaviour in health and the effect of interventions in influencing health-related behaviour in professionals, patients, and the public.

A person's aversion or predilection to risky behaviour is influenced by several factors, including the following:

- **Familiarity** with the **outcome** of the risky behaviour.
- Degree of **personal control** over the risk factor—in contrast to environmental risks, individuals tend to downplay personal risks. This tendency is due to beliefs of personal invulnerability and that other people are at greater risk *('It won't happen to me')*.
- **Demographics** (age, gender, and ethnicity)—young people are more likely to take risks (partly due to greater peer pressure) and women are more likely to be risk averse.

Health risk factors

Factors known to be risks to health include those shown in Box 2H.7.

Box 2H.7 Types of health risk

Type of risk	Examples
Harm	Smoking
Harm and benefits	Alcohol or food
Harm to others	Unprotected sexual intercourse, driving while intoxicated

Risk interventions

Interventions can be implemented at different levels:

- **Professionals**—to reorient services
- **Patients**—to receive preventive treatment, make lifestyle changes
- The **public**—to make healthy choices and protect or promote the health of society

For risk communication, see also Section 2F.2.

2H.9 Communication in health education

Theory and practice of communication with regard to health education.

For health education to be effective, it needs to

- Be received
- Be understood
- Stimulate a change in **attitude**
- **Provoke** a change in behaviour

The success of a health education message depends not simply on **what** is said but on **how** it is said and which **media** are used to communicate it.

Health messages

McGuire [110] proposed five communication inputs for health messages aimed at changing behaviour, namely, the **source**, **message**, **channel**, **receiver,** and **destination** (see Figure 2H.8).

Source

This is the person or organisation that generates the message. The credibility of a source depends on several factors, including

- Source's position in society
- Training and **qualifications** of the source
- **Shared characteristics** with the recipient (e.g. age, culture)
- Perceived conflict of interests

For example, a health advice message from a health minister may not be as credible as one from a doctor.

Message

What is said and how it is said. A message may be **verbal** or **non-verbal,** and it may be **horizontal** or **vertical** (see Box 2H.8). Finally, health promotion messages can be designed to **persuade** or to **empower** the recipient.

Channel

This is the medium or **media** through which a message is conveyed. Channels include

- One to one (e.g. midwife–patient consultation)
- Small groups (e.g. antenatal classes)

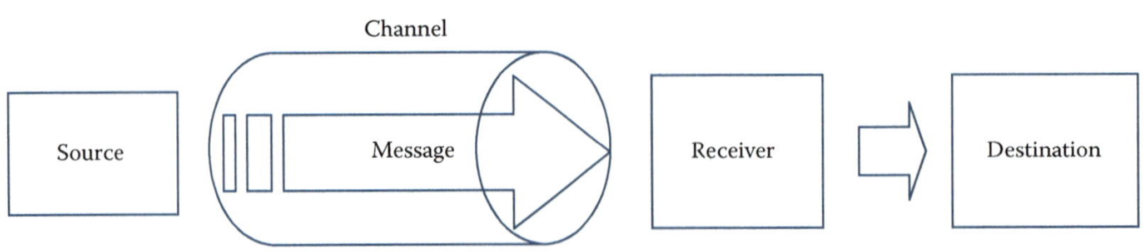

Figure 2H.8 Components of health messages.

Box 2H.8 Types of message

Type of message	Description
Verbal	Written or spoken words
Non-verbal	Images or sounds
Horizontal	General lifestyle improvement messages (e.g. eating a healthy diet)
Vertical	Specific issue messages (e.g. advice not to binge-drink)

- Drama, storytelling, or songs
- Mass media (broadcast, Internet, newspapers, leaflets)

The most appropriate **setting** for the communication to take place will depend on the message. Examples include

- Home
- Schools
- Community centres
- Workplaces

Integrated marketing communication (IMC) may achieve greater efficacy through

- Using a mixture of channels
- Use of public relations, advertising, and promotion

Receiver

The target audience should be the prime consideration of any communication. Messages may be targeted, for example, at

- Individuals, families, or communities
- Adults, adolescents, or children
- Men or women

Destination

- This is the desired outcome of the communication, be it a change in attitudes, a change in beliefs, or a change in behaviour.

Successful communication outputs

In order for a communication to improve health, it has to fulfil several requirements—the requirements listed in Table 2H.17.

Media

Different channels of communication may be better suited to different aims and different settings. Often, however, they will be most effective when used in **combination**. Table 2H.18 compares some features of mass communication methods with small group methods.

Table 2H.17 Requirements for successful communication

Requirement	Description	Example
Be seen or heard	Will the target audience see/hear the message?	A poster for young people is displayed in places where young people go such as schools and colleges.
Attract attention	Will the target audience notice the message?	A newspaper insert is sufficiently enticing for readers to notice it rather than throw it away unread.
Be understood	Is the language intelligible to the target audience?	The wording and images on a leaflet are pretested on a sample of the intended audience to ensure that it is readable and unambiguous.
Be accepted	Does the message reinforce current attitudes and beliefs?	Stop-smoking advertising is often effective in influencing smokers who have already decided that they wish to quit. It is less effective on those who do not want to give up.
Change behaviour	Are all the factors that could prevent behaviour change being addressed?	In order to change their diet, people on low incomes may require messages about healthy nutrition to be supported by food subsidies.

Table 2H.18 Features of mass versus small group communication

Feature	Mass media	Individual or small group
Methods	Broadcast: TV, radio, cinema. Print: Newspapers, magazines, posters, and leaflets. Electronic: Websites, e-mail lists, social media, e.g. Twitter.	Face to face: Motivational interviewing, CBT, consultations, classes, groups. At a distance: Telephone, e-mail, text, direct messaging.
Scope	Many recipients.	Few recipients.
Flexibility	Low: One style produced for all recipients (electronic media excepted).	High (message can be tailored to the individual or group).
Feedback	Low.	High—Integral part of the process.
Strengths	Useful for reinforcing attitudes and behaviours. Simple, unambiguous messages (e.g. stop smoking). Ensures that same message reaches all recipients.	Can be used to challenge current attitudes and behaviours. Useful for conveying complex messages (e.g. benefits and risks of alcohol). May use techniques to support self-efficacy.
Weaknesses	Weak link between mass media production and the receipt of information (e.g. the information broadcast on TV may not be watched, and even if watched, it may not be listened to or understood). Limited scope to tailor information so that it is more suitable for particular individuals or groups. Expensive: Mass media may be unaffordable for local campaigns.	Can reach only small numbers, so it is less well suited to messages that need to reach whole populations. Low profile without the mass media. Hard to control how information is disseminated by individual practitioners.

2H.10 Legislation and health promotion

Role of legislative, fiscal, and other social policy measures in the promotion of health.

Health promotion can make use of a range of levers at the national and community levels to create a supportive environment that encourages health-seeking behaviour (see Table 2H.19).

Social policy

Social policy measures encompass a wide range of arrangements and structures designed to **increase harmonisation** in society—be it at an international, national, or local level [111]. While some policies will specifically be targeted at promoting health, other policies, on a wide range of other issues, will also influence health.

A society's dominant **ideology** will influence its policy development and the degree to which state intervention will be acceptable in that society. For example, cultures that prize the individual freedoms may be less inclined to promote policies of collective actions, such as banning the possession of handguns.

Table 2H.19 Levers for encouraging health-seeking behaviour

Measures	Description	Example
Legislative	These include bans and restrictions to discourage behaviours known to have a damaging effect on health. Other legislative measures include injury control measures, pollution control, health and safety at work regulations, food additive requirements, and communicable disease laws.	Ban on children purchasing cigarettes Seat belt requirements Speed limits Clean air acts
Fiscal	Systems of taxation to discourage certain behaviours and subsidies to encourage others.	Alcohol duty
Other social policies	Other local, national, or international health cultures and policies.	Healthy workplaces HIAs of policies Research support and funding

Bans and restrictions

Restrictions or bans on activities or goods may target the availability, use, sale, and advertising of the harmful commodity.

Availability

ENG + WA + SCOT Cigarettes to young people: In the United Kingdom, the Children and Young Persons Act 1993 (http://www.legislation.gov.uk/ukpga/Geo5/23-24/12) made it illegal to sell cigarettes to those under 16 years. The Children and Young Persons (Protection from Tobacco) Act 1991 (http://www.legislation.gov.uk/ukpga/1991/23/section/1) strengthened the existing legislation by increasing penalties and made provisions for enforcement by local authorities. The Children and Young Persons (Sale of Tobacco etc.) Order 2007 (http://www.legislation.gov.uk/uksi/2007/767/made) increased the age limit from 16 to 18 years.

ENG + WA Alcohol at particular times of day: In England and Wales, the Licensing Act 2003 liberalised the times at which alcohol may be sold. Many establishments now potentially sell alcohol 24 hours a day.

UK Drugs/medicines: The Medicines Act 1968 controls the availability of medicines, ranging from drugs that are on general sale to medications that are available only on prescription.

Usage

UK Smoke-free public places: In Ireland, this became law in 2004. Similar legislation was enacted in Scotland in 2006 and in Wales, Northern Ireland, and England in 2007 (www.ash.org.uk).

Sales

UK Illicit drugs: The Misuse of Drugs Act 1971 designates controlled drugs (both 'medicinal' drugs and drugs with no known therapeutic benefit) into three classes—A, B, or C—with corresponding restrictions on their availability and penalties for selling or being in possession of the drug. The most severe sentences are for class A drugs and the least severe for class C.

Advertising and information

ENG + WA + NI Tobacco warnings: Compulsory labelling of cigarette packets with health warnings is stipulated in the Tobacco Advertising and Promotion (Point of Sale) Regulations 2004, which also banned tobacco advertising except at the point of sale (www.opsi.gov.uk/si/si2004/20040765.htm). Following the Health Act 2009, a tobacco point-of-sale display ban came into force in large stores in 2012 and will include small stores from 2015.

These measures often require legislation, although voluntary industry codes of practice also exist (e.g. major soft drink retailers have voluntarily pledged not to target adverts at children). Restrictions and bans are only successful if they are supported by favourable public opinion or by enforcement.

Fiscal measures

Fiscal measures generally take place at a state level and can involve either **taxes** or **subsidies**. Such measures alter the price of goods to reflect the **externalities** associated with the particular action or goods. An externality is a cost or benefit from consumption that falls on someone other than the consumer. For example, herd immunity is a positive externality of immunisation (a positive externality is beneficial).

Taxation

Taxation can serve two purposes:

1. To raise revenue
2. To **decrease demand** by increasing the price of the good to the consumer (or sometimes to the producer, e.g. the *polluter pays* principle)

In the United Kingdom, taxation to influence health is largely limited to alcohol and tobacco. Its success depends on the **price elasticity** of the goods (i.e. by how much the demand for a product is affected by its price). The price elasticity of goods will be different for different groups within society. So, for example, tax rises on tobacco products have had the greatest effects on young people and people on lower incomes.

Section 4D.1 covers in more depth concepts of economics including elasticity and externality.

Specific fees for particular activities can also be used to increase the price of producing or consuming goods (e.g. the **congestion charge** levied for driving into central London during busy times of day). The arguments for and against taxation as a health promotion measure are illustrated with respect to fatty foods in Boxes 2H.9 and 2H.10.

Subsidies

Subsidies decrease the price of consumption of goods to the consumer in order to adjust for the **positive externalities** associated with consuming them. An example in health policy in England is the *Healthy Start Scheme*, where families with young children receive vouchers for liquid milk, infant formula milk, or fresh fruit and vegetables to encourage the consumption of these foods by children.

Note that there may be **unintentional health effects** associated with subsidies. For example, the Common Agricultural Policy has subsidised tobacco farmers across Europe in a way that has encouraged tobacco production. This subsidy is gradually being phased out, and in the short term, it is being revised so that subsidies are no longer linked to the amount of tobacco produced.

Box 2H.9 UK Example: Should fatty foods be taxed?

In 2011, the UK Prime Minister stated that a fat tax should be considered to tackle growing levels of obesity. This followed the introduction of a policy in Denmark placing a surcharge on food with more than 2.3% saturated fats. Marshall and colleagues [112] explored the benefits of taxing foods high in saturated fats and found that

- There are **precedents** for taxation to influence health (e.g. increasing tobacco duties)
- Diet is partly responsible for ischaemic heart disease (**IHD**)
- The costs of consumption are therefore partly borne by **health services**
- Increasing the price of fat could decrease the consumption of high-fat foods (assuming that these goods are indeed **price elastic**)
- The effects may be greatest on people with low incomes, who would be most sensitive to price changes and who are at higher risk of heart disease

In contrast to the taxation of tobacco, however, the argument for foods may be less persuasive because the relationship between fats and heart disease is complex. Some fats are necessary and beneficial, and people are affected by fat to a greater or lesser extent according to their genetic make-up.

Other elements of the diet that could be targeted include salts and refined sugars.

Box 2H.10 Example: Australia's approach to tobacco control

Australia's Tobacco Control Programme: Timeline

1960s	Commencement: **Publicity** about effects of smoking following the first consolidated evidence about the harms caused by smoking
1970s	**Labelling**: Health warnings placed at the bottom of cigarette packs (1973) and **Advertising restrictions**: Tobacco advertising banned on television and radio (1976).
1980s	**Resourcing**: Government sponsored quit campaigns progressively introduced throughout Australia. All state cancer societies supported an anti-tobacco lobbying agency, ASH (Australia). **Legislation**: States and territories commenced bans on smoking in enclosed public places.
1990s and 2000s	**Taxation and fiscal measures**: Federal Government changed tobacco excise tax to remove tobacco companies' freedom to offer smokers 'bonus' cigarettes at discounted prices in Australia (1999). Fiscal measures developed to reduce affordability of smoking.
2012	**Legislation**: First country to introduce plain packaging laws which prohibit use of logos, brand imagery, and promotional text on tobacco products and packaging and include restrictions on colour, size, format, and materials of packaging, as well as the appearance of brand names.

Source: Scollo, M.M. and Winstanley, M.H. (eds.), *Tobacco in Australia: Facts and Issues*, 3rd edn, Melbourne: Cancer Council Victoria, 2008, Available from http://www.tobaccoinaustralia.org.au.

2H.11 Programmes of health promotion

Methods of development and implementation of health promotion programmes.

Health promotion programmes can be developed at local, national, and international levels and therefore vary greatly in their scope and aims. Many tools exist to assist in planning and developing health promotion programmes, such as the **PRECEDE–PROCEED** model and the **European Quality Instrument for Health Promotion.** The broad stages in developing a health promotion programme may be summarised using the mnemonic 'AS ROME' (see Table 2H.20).

Approaches to health promotion

Programmes often include a combination of the following approaches:

- Changes in **policy** to shift culture and/or behaviour (see Section 2H.10)
- Distribution or redistribution of **resources** to provide incentives or remove barriers to change
- Community development (see Section 2H.12)

Table 2H.20 Steps in the development of a health promotion programme

Step	Description
Assess need	This may involve the use of epidemiological, demographic, and socio-demographic data, assessing the **felt need** of the target audience and the **perceived need** of professionals. (See Section 1C.1)
Stakeholders	Stakeholder analysis and engagement, including both **primary stakeholders** (potential beneficiaries) and **secondary stakeholders** (who may be involved in project delivery). (See also Section 5B.3)
Resources	Identifying the **human** and **financial** resources needed for the programme and setting a budget. This process may involve prioritising some areas above others.
Objectives/Aims	Considering what the programme hopes to achieve (e.g. a health improvement or a behaviour change), with **numerical targets** if appropriate.
Methodology	Actions that will be taken to achieve the aims and the techniques that will be used. This may be based on health promotion theories (see Section 2H.7) and evidence from epidemiological studies.
Evaluation	Assessing how well the desired outcomes were achieved (see Section 2H.14).

- **Information**, communication, and education to inform people of the risks and benefits associated with behaviours and to influence attitudes towards change (see Section 2H.9)

Implementation

Frontline clinical staff and members of the community conduct far more health promotion than do health promotion or public health staff. Implementation therefore requires working with diverse practitioners to ensure that they are equipped to carry out health promotion programmes. Some considerations are set out in Table 2H.21 and the issues in practice are described with reference to smoking cessation in Box 2H.11.

In order to ensure that a programme has been implemented effectively, it should be **evaluated** during or after the programme's completion (see Section 2H.14).

Table 2H.21 Issues affecting implementation of health promotion

Values	Do participants have the **cultural** and **professional values** to support the programme's aims? For example, if members of the community are opposed to sex outside of marriage, then they will be unlikely to publicise or support community-based testing for STIs in young people.
Motivation	What is the **motivation** for staff not connected with health improvement to change their practice to improve health? This could involve providing incentives (e.g. financial bonuses related to programme implementation).
Guidance	Is it clear from the **policies** and **guidance** what exactly is required of staff and community members? People may support a programme in principle but, if their role is unclear, then the programme may not be implemented successfully.
Skills	Do participants have the relevant **skills** and **competencies** to carry out their roles? If staff are required to perform tasks that they have not conducted before, then they may need additional training.
Time	Is there **enough time** to put changes in place? While consultations in general practice could be an ideal opportunity to discuss behaviour changes with patients, it may not be feasible to do this in a 10 min consultation (or shorter).

Box 2H.11 UK Example: Reducing smoking among NHS staff

In an NHS trust, a programme to reduce smoking among staff involved

- Responding to **national policy** and targets regarding smoking
- Staff **surveys** to find out the smoking prevalence and the attitudes of smokers towards giving up
- **Research** into guidelines, evidence of effectiveness, and case studies of other organisations' experience
- Application of relevant health promotion **theory** (e.g. *stages of change* model)
- Consideration of the **resources** available to support the programme

The implementation comprised the following steps:

- Creation of a **policy** regarding smoking at work, with staff involvement to ensure that the policy was workable and that staff felt some ownership of it.
- **Dissemination** of the smoking policy to ensure that staff were aware of whether they could smoke at work and the support available to help them stop.
- This was followed by **monitoring** and **enforcement** of the policy (e.g. recording occasions where the policy was not adhered to and disciplinary action for staff smoking in no-smoking areas).
- Ensuring a strong **partnership** with the local NHS stop-smoking service, with time being made available to enable smokers to attend support groups.
- Sufficient **incentives** for staff to give up (e.g. free or subsidised nicotine replacement therapy, stop-smoking support groups, and one-to-one help).
- Recruitment and training of sufficient smoking cessation **advisers** at the trust to support staff giving up.

2H.12 Community development methods

Building stronger communities is a key strategy for **health improvement** and for **reducing health inequalities**. Community development

- Is fundamental to **building healthy environments** and providing individuals with the social support to adopt and maintain health-seeking behaviours
- Encompasses a **range of activities** to generate social networks and to empower people to shape their local services and have an input into their community
- Can stimulate innovative and **creative solutions** to problems that are not amenable to conventional health promotion programmes
- Must ensure that people in greatest need of stronger communities do actually benefit

Defining the community

A community is not a static entity. Rather, it consists of groups of people with a common characteristic at a particular time, most commonly

- **Geographical** (e.g. housing estates, villages)
- **Social** (e.g. workers' groups, student unions, lesbian/gay communities)
- **Cultural** (e.g. religious, ethnic)

Terms such as **community development**, **community participation,** and **community renewal** are often used interchangeably. In contrast to social planning and other initiatives aimed at changing communities, community development is a 'bottom-up' approach, whereas social planning would be described as 'top down'.

Methods

Community development uses a combination of activities. Smithies and Adams [114] suggest that there are five core activities of community development (see Table 2H.22).

A key priority in community development is the **empowerment** of community members to take **ownership** of projects. This process may involve a facilitator initiating projects, but ideas and decisions should gradually be transferred to the community.

Projects may progress from one type of activity to another as they mature, as illustrated in Box 2H.12.

Advantages and challenges of community development

The advantages and disadvantages of community development are outlined in Table 2H.23.

Table 2H.22 Activities of community development

Activity	Description	Examples
Formal participation	Formal participation in decision-making.	Focus groups Consultation days
Community action	Priorities are developed by community groups.	Lobbying Self-help activities
Facilitation	Health service employees promote community activities.	Provision of meeting rooms and refreshments
Interface	Statutory services working closely with communities and community leaders.	Consultation with local imams
Strategy	Strategic support from national initiatives.	Neighbourhood renewal funds Local strategic partnerships (LSPs)

Box 2H.12 Example of community empowerment: Cooking skills in the community

	Top-down target	Tackling obesity.
	Formal participation	A decision by the local authority or council to fund training in cooking skills for local people following consultation with mothers who attend the local children's centre in a deprived area.
	Facilitation	Local mothers attend cooking skills course funded by the NHS and local authority.
⇒ More user-led	Community action	Trained mothers organise and provide training for other local mothers.

Table 2H.23 Advantages and disadvantages of community development

Component	Advantages	Disadvantages
Initiating projects	User-led—Can achieve better community support if based on community priorities.	Resource intensive. Time-consuming. Can be difficult to secure funding (especially given the unknown outputs).
Goals	Can focus on root causes of ill health rather than simply lifestyle choice (e.g. organising a food cooperative rather than just providing dietary advice).	Long timescales: It may take years for health outcomes to appear and for communities to change.
Evaluation/ outputs	The process of enabling communities to participate is an end in itself. Enhances self-esteem, confidence, and control.	Results are often intangible and unquantifiable.
Communities involved	Can reach disadvantaged or excluded groups that conventional interventions would miss (see Section 2H.6).	There may be a conflict of accountability for community development workers: do they work for the community or for the statutory service?

2H.13 Partnerships

Working with people outside the field of public health is essential for delivering effective health promotion.

Partnerships in public health

As illustrated in Dahlgren and Whitehead's health policy rainbow and Lalonde's health field concept (Section 2H.2), the determinants of health include factors such as the wider environment, lifestyle, housing, and transport as well as healthcare. Public health specialists must therefore work with people or organisations from many different fields including clinicians, other local authority departments, and local businesses.

Other reasons why partnership work is important include

- Avoiding duplication
- **Pooling resources**—Funding, experience, contacts, information, skills
- **Political imperatives**—Duty to work together (e.g. health and social care provided to patients discharged from hospital)

Partners

Public health practitioners need to work with partners from a range of disciplines and organisations (see Table 2H.24).

Types of partnership working

Public health practitioners work in partnership in a number of ways (see Table 2H.25).

Barriers and challenges to successful partnership working

Partnership working can be challenging and it can be easy to blame problems on the other members of the partnership. However, many of the difficulties involved in partnership working are due to a mismatch in the ways that the organisations or individuals within them work. Table 2H.26 outlines some of these factors as well as some questions that might help identify why partnerships may not be working effectively.

Table 2H.24 Different types of partners in public health

Type of partner	Examples
Within organisation	Other local authority departments (children and young people, social care, trading standards, environmental health, communications, finance, HR) ENG Other teams in Public Health England (health protection, health intelligence, screening)
ENG Health organisations	Acute hospitals, mental health hospitals, clinical commissioning groups (CCGs), academic departments, NHS England Community health services (e.g. health visiting, weight management services, stop-smoking services)
Within the community	Police, fire service, voluntary sector, local businesses

Table 2H.25 Different methods of working in partnership

Type of partnership	Example
Statutory committees	ENG Health and wellbeing boards.
Shared targets and monitoring	Local area agreements. Community strategies. WA Health, social care, and wellbeing strategies. Wales has had joint NHS, local authority, and third sector strategies, underpinned by joint needs assessments since 2003.
Joint projects	Production of joint reports (e.g. *Health in London* was jointly produced by the London Health Observatory, the Health Development Agency, and the Greater London Authority).
Specifically resourced initiatives	Sure Start. Healthy Schools. Teenage Pregnancy Partnerships.
Shared posts	ENG Director of Public Health employed jointly by a local authority and Public Health England. Joint service and academic posts.
Shared budgets	ENG A cluster of CCGs may choose to commission programmes across all partners' areas, with pooled budgets and pooled resources.

Measuring success

Partnerships, like other aspects of health promotion, should be evaluated to ensure that they are meeting their aims. There are a number of tools that could be used to do this but Donabedian's evaluation model (see Section 1C.9) is a useful approach for considering what a partnership has achieved (see Table 2H.27).

Table 2H.26 Challenges to partnership working

Challenge	Pertinent questions to consider
Aspirations	Do all partners want the same outcomes from a partnership? Are partners working to different, or even conflicting, performance drivers? (e.g. the NHS is driven by health outcomes, whereas private industry is driven by profit) Are all partners clear about what the objectives of the partnership are?
Processes	Organisational cultures: Do different organisations function in the same ways? Consider Handy's work (see Sections 5B.1 and 5B.3). Are there compatible systems for making decisions? Do some members need to take decisions back to in-house committees or boards? Can representatives authorise spending or actions at the meeting on behalf of their organisation? Team working: How do different members of the partnership work in a team? Consider Belbin's team roles (see Sections 5A.1).
Commitment	The opportunity to build up a relationship can be lost if there is no continuity of people attending meetings. Who attends the meetings? Are they the right people? Do they attend regularly? Do the same people attend each meeting?
Influence	Are people from equal levels of seniority attending the meeting? As there may be no direct leverage over members of the partnership through line management, how can it be ensured that group members deliver on what they promise?
Power	Big fish/little fish situations (e.g. statutory agencies versus user groups in the community). How is the agenda developed? Are all parties given plenty of time to contribute? Where are meetings held: always in NHS premises? Or out in the community?

Table 2H.27 Evaluation of partnerships

Type of evaluation	Examples
Structure	Joint funding. Joint posts.
Process	Internal and partnership plans are aligned. Meetings well attended.
Outcome	Objectives and milestones are achieved. Outputs (e.g. reports) are used and valued by the partners and by the local community.

2H.14 Evaluation

Evaluation of health promotion, public health, or public policy interventions.

The principles of evaluation outlined in Section 1C.10 can also be applied to health promotion, public health, and health policy interventions.

2H.15 International initiatives

International initiatives in health promotion.

The principal actors in international health promotion have changed since the middle of the twentieth century, when there were relatively few agencies working across countries. At the time, the WHO (a subsidiary of the UN) had the greatest role and was largely uncontested in its activities. Now, as Walt [115] and Lincoln and Nutbeam [116] describe, international health promotion is characterised by

- A smaller, more contested role for the WHO
- A range of other UN organisations with a remit for health (e.g. UNICEF, the UN Population Fund, and the World Bank—which is currently the largest donor for health projects)
- Increasing activity from NGOs, particularly from the private sector
- Bilateral activity between two countries' governments (e.g. host country and the UK Department for International Development [DFID])
- Resurgent interest in 'vertical' programmes that focus on discrete diseases (e.g. the Gates Foundation's activity focuses on particular diseases)

Timeline

Some key health promotion landmarks are summarised in Table 2H.28. Box 2H.13 provides examples of the application of other major global health policy developments.

Table 2H.28 Key health promotion landmarks

Landmark	Setting	Year	Description
Lalonde Report	Canada	1974	Commissioned by the then Canadian Health Minister, Marc Lalonde, and generally regarded as a key turning point in health promotion. Established the **health field** concept of health (see Section 2H.2).
Health for All: Declaration of Alma-Ata	WHO	1978	WHO stated the aim of providing universally accessible primary care, which included health education.
Health for All 2000: Ottawa Charter	WHO	1986	WHO established the core **principles of health promotion** internationally.
Millennium Development Goals	UN	2000	**Eight targets** aimed at improving the lives of the world's poorest peoples.
Global Fund	International	**2000**	Global partnership among governments, civil society, the private sector, and affected communities to combat AIDS, TB, and malaria.
Global Strategy	WHO	2004	Global strategy on **diet, physical activity, and health** provides member states with a range of global policy options to address the growing problems of unhealthy diet and physical inactivity.
Bangkok Charter	WHO	2005	WHO recognised the growing burden of communicable and non-communicable diseases and called for greater coherence across governments, international organisations, and civil society.
High-level meeting on non-communicable disease prevention and control	UN	2011	Only the second UN high-level meeting on health. Aimed to elevate the attention and resources targeted at non-communicable diseases including cardiovascular disease, diabetes, cancer, and chronic respiratory disease.

Box 2H.13 Examples: Application of global health policies

Healthy Cities [116]

This initiative was launched by WHO Europe to support cities in prioritising health improvement and to provide resources and guidance for cities to improve health. Over 1000 European cities now participate, linked through national and international networks. The programme sets priorities for 5-year periods. A recent phase had three core themes: **healthy ageing**, healthy **urban planning**, and **HIA**. In addition, all participating cities focus on the topic of physical activity.

Framework Convention on Tobacco Control [118]

This framework was WHO's first treaty. It is a binding international legal instrument with broad commitments and governance for national governments regarding tobacco control. It sets international standards on a range of tobacco-related issues, including tobacco price and tax, tobacco advertising and sponsorship, labelling, illicit trade, and second-hand tobacco smoke.

UNICEF Baby-Friendly Initiative [119]

The WHO and UNICEF set up the Baby-Friendly Initiative programme in 1992 to encourage maternity hospitals to help mothers breastfeed. It sets 'ten steps to successful breastfeeding', from setting an organisation-wide policy, ensuring staff have the knowledge, skills, and facilities to implement it and providing support to women.

Sources: WHO, *Healthy Cities and Urban Governance*. Geneva, Switzerland: WHO, Available online at www.euro.who.int/healthy-cities, 2006; WHO, *Framework Convention on Tobacco Control*. Geneva, Switzerland: WHO, Available online at www.who.int/tobacco/framework/en/, 2005b; http://www.unicef.org.uk/BabyFriendly/.

2H.16 International health promotion initiatives

Opportunities for learning from international experience.

International agencies such as the WHO are central for disseminating and publicizing key health promotion issues and may use any or all of the methods shown in Table 2H.29.

Note that an approach that was successful in one country may be unsuccessful in another country for reasons such as different

- Cultures
- Health systems
- Funding of healthcare
- Demographic structures
- Disease epidemiology and health needs

The example described in Box 2H.14 describes some of the problems in transferring lessons learnt about HIV health promotion from Western Europe to Central and Eastern Europe.

Table 2H.29 Methods of disseminating health promotion initiatives

Method	Applciation
Guidance and toolkits	Where practice and evidence exists.
Consensus statements	Where evidence is not conclusive but advice is helpful.
Expert networks	Where opinion at an international level is required (see Section 1C.13).
Other	Other systems for sharing experience include international scholarships, study visits, conferences, and the Internet.

Box 2H.14 Example: Transferring lessons learnt regarding HIV/AIDS prevention from Western Europe to Central and Eastern Europe

The HIV epidemic has been relatively minor so far in Central and Eastern European countries, providing an opportunity for instituting preventive measures and for learning lessons from HIV prevention in Western Europe. Wright [120], however, highlights the fact that there are diversities within Europe that may affect the extent to which Western European approaches can be used. One key issue is the cultural difference between some groups of men who have sex with men and the gay identity.

In Western Europe, the central role of the gay community in leading health promotion to prevent the spread of HIV/AIDS was one of the 'success stories'. In Eastern European countries, however, it cannot be assumed that there is an established gay culture among men who have sex with men. For example, legal restrictions on homosexuality are severe in parts of Central and Eastern Europe.

Wright argues that the focus should therefore be on

'Assisting each country to adapt basic principles of HIV prevention to their current political and social situation'.

Source: Reproduced from Wright, M., *Health Promot. Int.*, 20, 91, 2005.

21

Disease Prevention and Models of Behaviour Change

Following on closely from the theories explored in Section 2H, this chapter tackles the challenges, approaches, and priorities involved in improving health in practice. We will explore the principal tools used to improve health and prevent disease, which range from **social marketing** (a relatively new technique that is becoming increasingly widespread) to **target setting** (which has become integral to the delivery of many modern health services). **Preventive actions** are arguably most important in children and families, whose health can be particularly vulnerable to the effects of living in **deprivation**. However, as we shall see, robust evaluation of such strategies is often lacking.

21.1 Prevention in the early years

Evaluation of preventive actions, including the evidence base for early interventions on children and families and support for social and emotional development.

The goal of most public health interventions is to prevent disease and maximise health. Interventions aimed at pregnant women, babies, and young children have the potential to influence health and wellbeing throughout life. However, working with these groups presents some particular challenges, not least because the outcomes are often realised only decades later.

Evaluation of preventive actions

The principles of evaluation are covered in Section 1C.9, and Section 1A.17 provides an overview of the study designs used for evaluating preventive interventions.

The evaluation of any public health intervention may be complicated by various factors (see Table 21.1, which includes examples relating to early years interventions).

Table 21.1 Complicating issues regarding the evaluation of public health interventions

Issue	Description	Example relating to early years
Study design	Some authors have argued that RCTs may be difficult to justify ethically for preventive studies. Moreover, RCTs may not be possible in certain circumstances (e.g. interventions delivered as a result of a policy change such as the introduction of the smoking ban in public places).[a]	The Scottish FSA recommends mandatory fortification of flour[b] to improve pregnancy outcomes. While the effect of eating fortified bread could be evaluated using an experimental design, it would be extremely difficult to evaluate the introduction of mandatory regulation using an experimental design.
Lack of control group	Poorly designed studies are prone to biases and confounders, making it difficult to determine whether the intervention was truly associated with the observed impact on health.	There is some RCT evidence from the United States that compared with controls, recipients of an intervention such as the Nurse Family Partnership or Head Start as young children committed fewer crimes as young adults (see Box 21.4).
Measuring an absence	It is not always possible to predict or model the course of events if a preventive action was not put into practice. For example, it is impossible to tell what the disease occurrence would have been had a vaccine programme not been delivered.	Without a trial design, it would be very difficult to attribute the observed effect to the early years interventions, since it is impossible to project with any accuracy what the load on the criminal justice system would be 20 years and therefore whether any criminal behaviour had been prevented.
Lead times	Long time delays between an intervention and the manifestation of its effects can require lengthy (and therefore costly and complex) studies (e.g. effect of early years' education on achievement at 18 years of age or effect of smoking cessation on lifetime risk of cancer). Where effects are not observed in the short term, it can be difficult to ensure continued support for preventive actions.	In addition, these benefits have taken decades to become apparent.

[a] Tones [121].
[b] http://www.food.gov.uk/scotland/scotnut/folicfortification/#.uo6Qlg_ZYsi.

Evidence base

Studies that investigate the impact of early interventions on children and families may be considered under five principal headings, namely,

1. Education
2. Health and nutrition
3. Socio-economic benefits
4. Emotional and social support
5. Combined programmes

Education of the child and parents

Preschool education can improve children's social and intellectual development, as well as their long-term outcomes (see Box 21.1).

Education for parents can include **parenting skills** and ensuring that young parents have access to **adult education** programmes.

Box 21.1 EU The Effective Provision of Pre-School Education (EPPE) project

A cohort study of 3000 children across Europe considered the effects at age 6–7 of preschool education and the home learning environment on children's

- Literacy
- Numeracy
- Social development (e.g. anxiety, antisocial behaviour and positive social behaviours)
- Social inequalities

The key findings included

1. Children who attended preschool showed **higher educational and social attainment**, even after adjusting for home and social circumstances.
2. The **quality** of preschool education influenced the educational levels achieved.
3. Although the home environment was important, parents' **socio-economic status did not affect children's benefit** from preschool education.
4. The report concluded that 'what parents do is more important than who they are …. Children whose parents read to them, taught them letters and numbers, songs and nursery rhymes, and took them to the library had better outcomes at 6 and 7 years'.

Source: Reproduced from Sylva, K., et al., *The Effective Provision of Pre-School Education (EPPE) Project. EPPE findings from the Early Primary Years.* London, UK: DFES. Available online at www.surestart.gov.uk/research/keyresearch/eppe, 2004.

Health and nutrition

Low birthweight

Health promotion in the early years starts before birth with interventions designed to reduce the risk of **LBW** babies. LBW is associated with higher infant mortality and long-term effects, such as a higher risk of chronic conditions in adult life (e.g. diabetes, heart disease). LBW is more common in lower socio-economic groups. An evidence review [124] identified two major modifiable factors that influence LBW, which are as follows:

1. Poor **maternal nutrition** at conception and during pregnancy can lead to LBW babies. While there is evidence that **calcium** supplements and **folate** can be effective in mitigating risk, there is little evidence about the effectiveness of any other supplements.
2. **Smoking during pregnancy** doubles the risk of having a LBW baby. Formal smoking cessation programmes with nicotine replacement therapy help some pregnant women to give up smoking. However, other factors (e.g. partner's smoking status and the mother's socio-economic group) affect the success of such programmes.

Breastfeeding

Research suggests that **breastfeeding** can improve the health and wellbeing of infants and mothers as follows [125]:

- Reduced risk of infections through **passive immunity** (antibodies in the colostrum) and other mechanisms
- Lower rates of SIDS
- Reduced rates of **obesity** in the child and possible reductions in the rates of **diabetes**
- Lower rates of **atopy**
- Greater mother–baby **bonding** (mediated through hormone release)
- Reduced rates of **breast and ovarian cancer** in the mother

Breastfeeding is less common in lower socio-economic groups and rates are falling in certain minority ethnic groups that traditionally breastfed their babies. Prenatal support and education for mothers have been shown to improve breastfeeding rates. In the early years, interventions to promote maternal and child nutrition include:

- **Education** (e.g. improved diet, cooking skills)
- **Subsidies** (e.g. free school meals, free fruit in schools)

Box 21.2 UK The Healthy Start scheme

The *Healthy Start* programme is a government scheme to provide food and vitamin vouchers for disadvantaged pregnant women and young children. The vouchers can be spent at local retailers on certain food items, including milk, formula milk, fruit, and vegetables. Coupons are also provided to women for 'healthy start vitamins' in pregnancy (folic acid, vitamin C, and vitamin D) and early childhood (vitamin A, vitamin C, and vitamin D).

An evaluation commissioned by the DH found that the scheme was working well—misuse is rare, retailers accept the vouchers, and beneficiaries use vouchers for the correct products.

Source: Healthy Start scheme research published, July 2012. http://www.dh.gov.uk/health/category/policy-areas/public-health/maternity-public-health/healthystart

- **Supplements** (e.g. fluoridation of water supplies, nutritional supplements in staple foods, such as bread)

An example of an early years nutritional intervention is shown in Box 21.2.

Childhood immunisations

See 2G.4–5.

Interventions to prevent childhood injuries

Numerous interventions exist to reduce the risk of injury in childhood; these include:

- Education campaigns (e.g. focusing on burns, poisonings, and falls)
- Playground renovation
- Increased supervision
- Seat belts
- Cycle helmets

While there is strong evidence for specific interventions such as seat belts or cycle helmets, other multi-agency mixed programmes are often difficult to evaluate for the reasons outlined in Table 21.1 [127].

Socio-economic benefits

In the United Kingdom, the **Acheson Report** [128] concluded that families with young children were at increased risk of poverty. Many of these families found themselves in a 'benefit-dependent poverty trap' where they were unable to seek work because affordable childcare was unavailable. The report recommended reducing poverty in young families by

- Providing accessible and affordable **childcare**
- Increasing **benefits** and the **uptake of benefits** offered to pregnant women and to families with young children

Emotional/social support

Family support programmes can be based at the **community level** (e.g. addressing poverty, social isolation, and lack of community resources) or at the small group or individual level (e.g. home visiting during pregnancy and after birth).

The aims of such support are to

- Improve **parental** wellbeing (e.g. provide parents with respite, problem-solving skills, and decrease incidence of postnatal depression)
- Improve **children's** physical, emotional, and cognitive development
- Prevent child abuse

Few studies have evaluated the long-term outcomes of family support. However, in 2005, the European Early Promotion Project (a cohort study of approximately 1000 families across Europe) identified that **training healthcare workers** to support early parent–infant relationships led to fewer psychosocial problems in young children.

Combined programmes

Combined programmes include elements from more than one of the four types of intervention described earlier. They are often run by multi-agency teams. An example in England from the

1990s was the *Sure Start* programme, which has now developed into children's centres. This programme provides childcare, early education, health, and family support in disadvantaged areas. An ongoing evaluation (the National Evaluation of Sure Start) has produced regular reports on the success of Sure Start (see Box 21.3).

A similar programme—Head Start—has been running over a longer period in the United States (see Boxes 21.4 and 21.5).

Box 21.3 Evaluation of Sure Start

An initial evaluation of Sure Start in 2005 found little benefit for children living in Sure Start Local Programme (SSLP) areas and in some cases found that educational achievements in SSLP areas were worse than in control areas.

However, a later evaluation in 2008 found a number of benefits associated with living in a SSLP area by the time children reached 3 years of age. These improvements included better social development, improved parenting, more positive social behaviour, greater rates of immunisation, and lower rates of accidental injuries.

More recently, a 2012 report found that by the age of 7, children in Sure Start areas had greater improvements in home learning environments, greater decreases in harsh punishment by parents, and greater improvements in life satisfaction of parents.

Box 21.4 USA Head Start: Long-term effects of comprehensive child development in the early years

The Head Start programme is a preschool education scheme run for disadvantaged families and children in the United States to reduce social, educational, and health inequalities between children from disadvantaged backgrounds and their more affluent peers. As well as preschool education, Head Start provides a range of other services, including

- Facilitating use of medical care for children (e.g. immunisations and dental health)
- Provision of healthy food and snacks
- Encouragement of parents' involvement in their children's education

Because Head Start was established in the 1960s, it has been now possible to evaluate its long-term outcomes. A large-scale survey of social, health, and economic behaviours (the Panel Survey of Income Dynamics) has been conducted in a cohort of 8000 families since 1968. In 1995, adults aged 18–30 were asked as part of the survey whether they participated in Head Start or another preschool as a child. The survey found that adults who had attended Head Start were more likely to **complete high school** and **attend college** than their siblings who attended other preschools.

The effects of the Head Start programme are not restricted to educational achievement but also encompass **crime** and **economic benefits**. For example, Head Start graduates of African-American origin were less likely to have been charged or convicted of a crime than their siblings who attended other preschool programmes. Also, white graduates in their 20s who had attended Head Start earned higher incomes than comparator groups.

Sources: Reproduced from Administration for Children and Families, Head Start General Information, available online at www.acf.hhs.gov/programs/hsb/2006; Garces, G.T. et al., *Am. Econ. Rev.*, 92, 999, 2002; Fight Crime: Invest in Kids, *Head Start Reduces Crime and Improves Achievement*, New York: Fight Crime: Invest in Kids, Available online at www.fightcrime.org/reports/headstartbrief.pdf, 2006.

Box 21.5 Family nurse partnership RCT evidence for a preventive intervention in the early years

The Family Nurse Partnership (FNP) is a preventive programme for vulnerable young first-time mothers. It offers intensive and structured home visiting, delivered by specially trained nurses, from early pregnancy until age two.

The programme uses in-depth methods to work with young parents on attachment, relationships, and psychological preparation for parenthood. Family nurses build supportive relationships with families and guide first-time teenage parents so that they adopt healthier lifestyles (for themselves and their babies), provide good care for their babies, and plan their futures.

The FNP is based on the Nurse Family Partnership, a similar programme that has been delivered and tested extensively in the United States over the last 30 years. Evidence from three RCTs of the FNP showed significant benefits for vulnerable young families in the short, medium and long term across a wide range of health and social outcomes, including

Improvements in antenatal health

Reductions in children's injuries, neglect, and abuse

- Improved parenting practices and behaviour
- Improved early language development, school readiness, and academic achievement
- Fewer subsequent pregnancies and greater intervals between births
- Increased maternal employment and reduced welfare use

Overall, the cost savings in the United States ranged from $17,000 to $34,000 per child by the time they reached 15 years, with a $3–5 return for every $1 invested.

In England, FNP was tested in a 3-year formative evaluation beginning in 2007. Subsequently, a large-scale RCT was established, whose preliminary findings are due in 2014.

Source: UK Department of Health, www.dh.gov.uk.

21.2 Pre-determinants of health

Pre-determinants of health, including the effect of social cohesion on health outcomes.

The pre-determinants of health are **factors that portend the determinants of health**. However, the distinction between pre-determinants and determinants is variable (e.g. income can be seen both as a determinant of health or as a pre-determinant of a determinant such as housing) (see Section 2H.2).

Pre-determinants can be considered at the individual and community levels and may be grouped as material goods, policies, and societal factors (see Table 21.2).

Impact of pre-determinants of health

Kahan [132] described how the pre-determinants of health are mediated through various routes. An example is shown in Figure 21.1.

Social cohesion and health outcomes

A society with strong **social cohesion** has strong interactions, is mutually supportive, and has few inequalities. In contrast, a lack of social cohesion

Table 21.2 Pre determinants of health

Material	Policies	Society
Sufficient and healthy food	Minimum wage	Social cohesion (i.e. the extent to which a society is mutually supportive and minimises inequalities)
Pure water	Health at work	
Clean air	Maternal services	Values and attitudes (e.g. the balance between competitive and cooperative approaches)
Income	Childcare	
Housing	Benefits	Ethnic diversity and the tolerance of different cultures
Green spaces	General education	Language ability

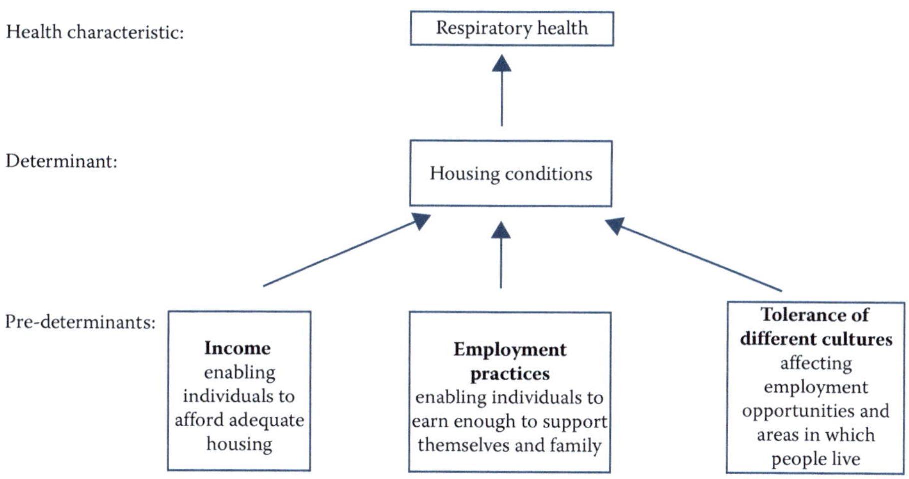

Figure 21.1 Example of pre-determinants impacting on respiratory health.

Box 21.6 EU Social cohesion as a pre-determinant of health

The Council of Europe directs member states to consider social cohesion as *'an essential condition for democratic security and sustainable development'*. As such, its policies are designed to reduce inequalities and to increase active participation in the community.

The Council recognises not only that social cohesion influences the incidence of disease and death but also that it **can be influenced by health policy**. For example, the funding of healthcare through private insurance systems may cause more inequalities than social insurance or tax-based systems. Hence, private insurance may adversely affect social cohesion.

Source: Reproduced from Council of Europe, Social cohesion strategy. Available at www.coe.int/T/E/social_cohesion, 2006.

can lead to social isolation and insecurity, which in turn can affect both physical and psychological health. Wilkinson [133] suggested that reduced income differentials, a greater sense of solidarity, and greater social cohesion all lead to improvements in life expectancy [133]. An illustration of social cohesion in improving health in Europe is described in Box 21.6.

2I.3 Individual behaviour change

Approaches to individual behaviour change including economic and other incentives.

Interventions to influence health behaviour may be implemented at multiple levels, ranging from the whole population down to the individual level. Individual, or small-scale, interventions include face-to-face health promotion techniques and incentives to encourage healthy behaviour.

Face-to-face methods: Motivational interviewing [135,136]

Motivational interviewing, developed by Rollnick and Miller in the 1990s, is a style of counselling based on the stages of change model (see 2H.7). It is a patient-centred method that aims to develop an individual's motivation to change by exploring the **reasons why they may be ambivalent** about behaviour change. Motivational interviewing has a growing evidence base of effectiveness in a number of therapeutic areas including drug misuse, eating disorders, and smoking cessation. Its characteristics are to

- Use **empathy** with reflective listening
- **Highlight discrepancies** between patient's most deeply held values (e.g. desire to be 'good') and current ('unhealthy') behaviours
- **'Roll with resistance'** (i.e. respond with understanding rather than confrontation)
- **Build the patient's self-efficacy** and confidence that they can effect change themselves

Cognitive behavioural therapy

Cognitive behavioural therapy (CBT) aims to interrupt habitual cycles of unhealthy behaviour by replacing them with healthy ones. CBT involves similar techniques to motivational interviewing but also incorporates **cognitive exercises** such as imagining the scenario of being offered a cigarette and how to behave in this scenario.

Use of incentives to encourage healthy behaviour

Fiscal measures to encourage healthy behaviour at a population level are described in Section 2H.10; however, personal financial incentives may also be used to encourage behaviour change. Marteau and colleagues [137] describe some examples of incentive schemes, such as

- Vouchers to encourage smoking cessation (United Kingdom)
- Money towards healthcare costs for adherence to diabetes treatment (United States)
- Financial rewards for avoiding STIs (Tanzania)
- Financial rewards for achieving weight loss targets (Italy)
- A points scheme for healthy school meals (United Kingdom)

Research suggests that financial incentives do tend to be effective in the short term and they may also be effective in the long term if accompanied with other health promotion advice. However, such initiatives are associated with a number of moral concerns, including whether they are a form of bribery, are overly paternalistic, and are a poor use of public funds.

2I.4 Role of social marketing

The term **social marketing** describes the use of techniques of commercial marketing to **sell a health message** in order to benefit individuals and society [138]. Social marketing approaches involve the seven steps described in Table 2I.3 (see also www.nsms.org.uk).

As with the sale of any commodity, selling a health promotion message involves a consideration of the four Ps of marketing, namely, the **product**, its **price**, **placement,** and **promotion** (see Table 2I.4).

Social marketing has a number of strengths and weaknesses, as shown in Table 2I.5.

Table 21.3 The social marketing process

Step	Description
1. Identify the target group	In contrast to traditional health approaches, segmented groups by risk, or disease categories (e.g. diabetic patients, HIV+, or socio-demographic characteristics such as age group or income bracket), marketing approaches use **segmentation tactics** such as psychographic classification, lifestyle characteristics, and consumption patterns.
2. Research target group	**Surveys and focus groups** are used to assess ● Attitudes and beliefs ● Habits and lifestyles ● Needs
3. Competitive analysis	The **competition** in this context may include the tendency to continue current behaviours and the influence of unhealthy industries (e.g. the tactics of the tobacco industry).
4. Set objectives	Clear **objectives** are needed for the campaign (e.g. raise awareness or change behaviour).
5. Develop the message	The **message** needs to be thoroughly pretested with target group to ensure that it is credible.
6. Sell the message	**Sell** the message through a mixture of considerations (e.g. the 4 Ps; see Table 21.4).
7. Evaluate	The campaign should be **evaluated** so as to monitor success and to guide refinements during the campaign.

Table 21.4 The 4 Ps of marketing

4 × Ps	Description
Product	It must be clear what exactly is being 'sold'. For example, in a campaign to boost the proportion of children receiving MMR, the product could be the **procedure** (delivery of vaccine), the **service** (visit to nurse), or the **outcome** (immunity from measles). Each of these items will have different appeals for different groups.
Price	This is the relationship between the costs and benefits of the programme to the behaviour change. For example, in the case of vaccination, some parents do not see measles as a serious disease and therefore may not value the benefits of immunity. The price should be considered in economic terms (i.e. not simply the financial cost but also the **opportunity cost**).
Place	The **channel** used will affect who has exposure to the message and therefore the levels of awareness of the message among the audience. The type of message will also affect which channels should be used.
Promotion	Promotion can be achieved through various **media** and **advertising**. Marketing campaigns can include e-mails, mail-outs, text messages, events, merchandising (e.g. red ribbons for AIDS), and partnerships with commercial companies and third sector organisations.

Table 21.5 Strengths and weaknesses of social marketing

Strengths	Weaknesses
• Based on an objective understanding of the **target group**, not on the health promoter's perceptions of the group. • **Clear objectives** are integral to the approach. • Makes use of techniques that have been successfully applied **commercially**.	• Assumes that the individual is fully able to choose to change behaviour (i.e. that health is an **individual choice** and that socio-economic barriers are not a factor in health choices). • As in commercial marketing, there is a danger of portraying only **partial information** in an effort to change behaviour (e.g. 'Just Say No' is catchier message than a rounded picture of the positives and harms of drug taking). • Danger of reinforcing the same **stereotypes** and attributes used by commercial marketing to sell products, such as equating health with physical characteristics (e.g. youth, attractiveness, health, being thin) or with moral attributes (e.g. being in control).

21.5 Involving the public

Involvement of the general public in health programmes and their effect on healthcare.

Reasons for including the public in health programmes are shown in Table 21.6.

Levels of involvement

Brager and Specht [139] described a **health ladder** that specifies different levels of community involvement (see Table 21.7).

One criticism of the health ladder approach is that it implies that organisations should be striving to reach the top of the ladder in every community. However, full involvement of the community may not always be feasible or desirable, and often the appropriate level of involvement will be lower down the ladder.

Many partnership structures (e.g. prescribing committees, mental health forums, CHD networks, cancer networks) contain individuals who will represent themselves and their experiences to the professionals running the groups. Such people may not be typical of people with the same conditions. Members will often need support from the chair of such groups to participate fully, but the perspective that service users offer can be invaluable. Examples of patient involvement are described in Box 21.7.

Table 21.6 Reasons to involve the public

Reason	Details
Improved treatment outcomes	Patients who are not informed or involved in treatment decisions are less likely to be **concordant** with treatment.
Empowerment	The process of participation can empower individuals and communities to understand their own situations and to assume increased **control** over the factors affecting their lives. This process can, in turn, enhance people's sense of wellbeing and quality of life.
Democracy	Community participation in decision-making, planning, and action is a **human right**.
Integrated approaches	Communities that are not restricted in their thinking by organisational boundaries can help to develop integrated, holistic, and cross-cutting approaches to address complex issues.
Better decisions	Involving people can result in more responsive, effective, and appropriate services.
Acceptability	People are likely to be more accepting of programmes that they have been involved in and are thus more likely to adopt any health messages.
Ownership and sustainability	Community participation is essential if interventions and programmes aimed at promoting health, wellbeing, quality of life, and environmental protection are to be widely owned and sustainable.

Table 21.7 Brager and Specht health ladder of involvement

Control	Participants' actions	Examples
High	Has control	Organisation asks a community to identify the problems and make all key decisions on goals and means; it is willing to help the community at each step to accomplish goals.
	Has delegated authority	Organisation identifies and presents a problem to the community; it defines limits and asks community to make a series of decisions that can be embodied in a plan which it will accept.
	Plans jointly	Organisation presents tentative plans that are open to change by those that are affected; it expects to change its plans at least slightly and perhaps more subsequently.
	Advises	Organisation presents a plan and invites questions; it is willing to change plans only if absolutely necessary.
	Is consulted	Organisation tries to promote a plan; it seeks to develop support to facilitate acceptance.
	Receives information	Organisation makes a plan and announces it; the community is informed and compliance is expected.
Low	None	Community told nothing.

Box 21.7 ENG Hospital design

Example: Evelina Children's Hospital

A children's board composed of children treated at the previous hospital and local children helped to design the new Evelina Hospital building. There is clear evidence of how children's views influenced the building design. For example, children said that they did not want long straight corridors, so instead the building has a curvy 'snake' floor plan.

Source: Reproduced from the Evelina Children's Hospital Appeal, available online at www.evelinaappeal.org/hospital/index.html.

21.6 Deprivation and its effect on health

Concept of deprivation and its effect on health of children and adults.

Deprivation can be **material** or **social** in nature and can encompass all aspects of life. It is associated with

- Lower life expectancy
- Higher risk of tobacco, alcohol, and drug dependence
- Higher chance of developing a long-term illness

See Section 1C.8 for measures of deprivation.

Table 21.8 Manifestations of deprivation

Domain	Issues
Housing	Temporary accommodation; damp, overcrowded, or poorly maintained housing
Environment	High levels of crime; poor access to facilities and transport
Income	Low income
Employment	Low status posts, hazardous work, and job insecurity
Education	Lack of high-quality education during childhood and adolescence
Social exclusion	Isolation, poor social support, or abusive relationships

Concepts of deprivation

Deprivation manifests itself in a number of ways (Table 21.8), and the longer that people are exposed to deprivation, the greater its effects.

Poverty can be **absolute** or **relative** (see Table 21.9).

Table 21.9 Types of poverty

Type of poverty	Definition
Absolute poverty	Lacks the basic material necessities for life
Relative poverty	Lives on under 60% of the median national income

Factors that reinforce deprivation

A number of phenomena are known to result from and exacerbate the effects of deprivation (see Table 21.10).

Table 21.10 Factors that reinforce the effects of deprivation

Reinforcing factor	Description
Social exclusion	Relative poverty leads to exclusion from society (e.g. exclusion from decent housing).
Discrimination	Racism, homophobia, ageism, and discrimination against people who have received psychiatric treatment or who have been in prison or care all serve to exclude people from accessing services. These prejudices act as barriers to the opportunities open to other people, such as access to jobs, housing, and social networks.
Employment	**Unemployment** and job insecurity lead to stress and health effects. The **degree of control** and level of demand in a job both influence health. There is a **gradient** across high-, middle-, and low-ranking staff even when employed by the same employer (e.g. as shown by the Whitehall study).
Stress	The effects of continuing anxiety, insecurity, low self-esteem, social isolation, and lack of control have both **psychological** and **physiological** effects, such as increased risk of heart disease.
Antenatal effects	Stress and lifestyle factors during pregnancy (e.g. smoking or ill health) have an effect on the fetus, which may manifest as fetal abnormalities and LBW. LBW is associated with increased risk in adult life of diseases such as diabetes and CHD (see also Sections 2A.1, 2B.1.5 and 2B.1.11).

21.7 Community development

Benefits and means of community development, including the roles and cultures of partner organisations.

See Section 2H.12.

21.8 Health impact assessment

HIA of social and other policies.

See 1C.17 for principles and practices of HIA. Box 21.8 provides an example of the use of HIA on policies in London.

Box 21.8 HIA of policies in London

The London Health Commission conducted rapid HIAs of the mayor of London's draft strategies aimed at improving the lives of Londoners. These strategies included policies on social issues such as culture, children and young people.

The HIAs took a largely pragmatic approach to meet time and resource constraints. They involved workshops with key stakeholders, written submissions, and the synthesis and review of available evidence.

An evaluation noted that the HIAs succeeded in

- Influencing strategy: officials drafting the strategy considered health because they knew that it would be subject to an HIA and they later made revisions as a result of HIA recommendations
- Involving a wider group of stakeholders than would otherwise have been involved in the policies
- Providing the evidence base for decision-makers to make choices
- Raising the profile of HIAs

Challenges included:

- Short timescales
- No established quality standards for HIAs
- Gaps in research evidence
- Involving the right stakeholders
- Relative priority of different types of research

Sources: Reproduced from HIA Gateway, available online at: www.nice.org.uk; London Health Commission, available online at: www.londonshealth.gov.uk/hia.htm#Top.

21.9 Strategic partnerships

Role of strategic partnerships and the added value of organisations working together.

2H.13 describes examples where it may be particularly beneficial for organisations to work together, as well as examples of levers to create partnerships, different partnership types, and the barriers and facilitators of partnership working.

ENG Local strategic partnerships

Local strategic partnerships (LSPs) were statutory multi-agency bodies that functioned over an area of local government or social care. They were established to encourage collaborative working and community involvement when addressing complex problems that could not be tackled by one organisation working alone (e.g. neighbourhood renewal strategies to improve jobs, education, health, housing, and tackling crime). The membership of LSPs included representatives from the statutory, voluntary, community, and private sectors. They provided a forum where local chief executives could meet to discuss inter-agency working and to hold partnership structures in an area to account.

21.10 Setting targets

The role of target setting, targets, and goals.

See also Section 4D.4 and Section 1C.6.

Reasons for setting targets in healthcare include:

- Adoption of management practices and culture in health services
- Improvement of performance and accountability
- Ensuring consistency across services

Targets can relate to each component of Donabedian's framework (i.e. **structure**, **process**, **output**, or **outcome**) (see Table 21.11).

Targets can be set at the **micro**, **meso**, or **macro** level (see Table 21.12).

Characteristics of 'good' targets

'SMART' targets comply with the points in the mnemonic of Table 21.13.

Table 21.11 Donabedian's framework applied to target setting

Indicator	Example
Structure	Director of public health in post at 85% of local authorities.
Process	80% of GP practices maintain a register of their patients with diabetes.
Output	98% of patients seen within four hours of arrival in A&E.
Outcome	Cancer deaths reduced by 20% by 2010 relative to 1990 baseline.

Table 21.12 Levels of target setting

Level	Example
Individual	Personal development plan (PDP) agreed with line manager.
Organisational	Local authority targets for the provision of affordable housing.
National	Public Service Agreement (PSA). In return for investment, the government sets minimum standards to be delivered across a range of public services, including health, education, and crime prevention [142].
International	WHO's *Health For All* targets.

Table 21.13 Characteristics of a good target

Characteristic		Description
S	**Specific**	Target relates to what the target setter wants to achieve.
M	**Measurable**	Indicator is defined precisely (quantitatively if possible).
A	**Achievable**	Target is achievable but challenging.
R	**Relevant**	Target is relevant to current performance (e.g. lung cancer deaths are mainly due to smoking practices 30 years ago rather than current health service interventions).
T	**Timescales**	Timescales must be defined in advance for each target.

Table 21.14 Strengths and weaknesses of using targets

Strengths	Weaknesses
• Provide a focus to performance improvement. • Priorities are set explicitly. • Create a level playing field for the organisations under comparison (e.g. hospitals, local authorities). • Number and domains of targets can be set to reflect organisational priorities and goals. • Opportunity for sharing good practice and learning. • Can lead to greater managerial interest in target areas.	• Information is often unavailable for measuring meaningful health outcomes. • Distortions of practice or gaming. For example, some hospitals attempted to reclassify their A&E trolleys as beds in order to meet the waiting time target. Elsewhere, ambulance services were de-prioritising people in rural areas because they knew that they had no chance of meeting transport time target. • Distort priorities—those areas of healthcare that are not amenable to targets are paid insufficient attention. • Disengagement of clinicians if targets are set externally or set from the top down.

Rewards for meeting, and punishments for not meeting, targets mean that these areas of healthcare tend to receive increased managerial interest. However, the high stakes involved (e.g. risk of job losses or attainment of foundation trust status) can lead to gaming and distortion of priorities.

Advantages and disadvantages of targets

The principal strengths and weaknesses of using targets are described in Table 21.14.

References

1. Global Burden of Disease study 2010.
2. http://www.healthmetricsandevaluation.org/gbd/visualizations/gbd-2010-patterns-broad-cause-group?unit=pc&sex=B&metric=daly&stackBy=region&year=5.
3. Ohberg, A. and Lonnqvist, J. (1998) Suicides hidden among undetermined deaths. *Acta Psychiatrica Scandinavica* 98, 214–218.
4. Barr, B. et al. (2012) Suicides associated with the 2008–10 economic recession in England: Time trend analysis. *BMJ* 2012, 345.
5. http://www.bhf.org.uk/plugins/PublicationsSearchResults/DownloadFile.aspx?docid=e3b705eb-ceb3-42e2-937d-45ec48f6a797&version=-1&title=England+CHD+Statistics+Factsheet+2012&resource=FactsheetEngland.
6. NHS Choices. Stroke webpages. Accessed July 21, 2014. http://www.nhs.uk/actfast/Pages/know-the-signs.aspx.
7. Cancer Research UK. (2014) Cancer incidence for common cancers. Accessed July 21, 2014 http://www.cancerresearchuk.org/cancer-info/cancerstats/incidence/commoncancers/.
8. Simpson, C.R. and Sheikh, A. (2010) Trends in the epidemiology of asthma in England: A national study of 333,294 patients. *Journal of the Royal Society of Medicine* 103(3), 98–106.
9. Simpson, C.R., Hippisley-Cox, J., and Sheikh, A. (2010) Trends in the epidemiology of chronic obstructive pulmonary disease in England: A national study of 51 804 patients. *Brit J Gen Pract* 60(576), e277–e284.

9a. Lucas, S.B., Mason, D.G., Mason, M., and Weyman, D. (2008) *A Sickle Crisis? A report of the National Confidential Enquiry into Patient Outcome and Death.* http://www.ncepod.org.uk/2008report1/Downloads/Sickle_report.pdf.

10. http://www.screening.nhs.uk/growth.
11. http://www.screening.nhs.uk/hearing-child.

12. Healthy Weight Healthy Lives: National Child Measurement Programme guidance for primary care trusts 2010/2011. http://www.dh.gov.uk/prod_consum_dh/groups/dh_digitalassets/documents/digitalasset/dh_115112.pdf.
13. NHS Choices. (2012) Down's syndrome screening. Accessed July 21, 2014 http://healthguides.mapofmedicine.com/choices/map/down_s_syndrome_screening1.html
14. Public Health England. NHS cervical screening programme webpages. Accessed July 21, 2014 http://www.cancerscreening.nhs.uk/cervical/
15. Fagan, T.J. (1975) Nomogram from Bayes's theorem (letter). *New Engl J Med* 293, 257.
16. Beauchamp, T.L. and Childress, J.F. (2001) *Principles of Biomedical Ethics*, 5th edn. Oxford: Oxford University Press.
17. Raffle, A. and Gray, M. (2007) *What Screening Does in: Screening: Evidence and Practice*, Chapter 3. Oxford: Oxford University Press, p. 68.
18. Wilson, J.M. and Jungner, G. (1968) *Principles and Practice of Screening for Diseases*. Geneva, Switzerland: WHO.
19. von Wagner, C., Baio, G., Raine, R. et al. (2011) Inequalities in participation in an organized national colorectal cancer screening programme: Results from the first 2.6 million invitations in England. *Int J Epidemiol* 40, 1–7. Accessed 21 July 2014 at http://ije.oxfordjournals.org/content/early/2011/02/16/ije.dyr008.
20. Independent UK Panel on Breast Cancer Screening. (2012) The benefits and harms of breast cancer screening: An independent review. *Lancet* 380, 1778–1786. http://www.cancerresearchuk.org/cancer-info/publicpolicy/ourpolicypositions/symptom_Awareness/cancer_screening/breast-screening-review/breast-screening-review.
21. http://www.screening.nhs.uk/prostatecancer.
22. Public Health England. UK flexible sigmoidoscopy screening trial. Accessed July 21, 2014 http://www.cancerscreening.nhs.uk/bowel/flexible-sigmoidoscopy-screening-trial.html.
23. National Human Genome Research Institute, National Institutes of Health. (2007) Learning about cystic fibrosis. www.genome.gov/10001213.
24. The ENCODE Project. Encyclopedia of DNA elements. http://www.genome.gov/10005107.
25. Davey Smith, G. (2011) Epidemiology, epigenetics and the 'Gloomy Prospect': Embracing randomness in population health research and practice. *Int J Epidemiol* 40, 537–562. http://ije.oxfordjournals.org/content/40/3/537.full.
26. Relton, C.L. and Davey Smith, G. (2010) Epigenetic epidemiology of common complex disease: Prospects for prediction, prevention, and treatment. *PLoS Med* 7(10), e1000356. doi:10.1371/journal.pmed.1000356. http: //www.plosmedicine.org/article/info%3Adoi%2F10.1371%2Fjournal.pmed.1000356.
27. Hunt, S.C., Gwinn, M., and Adams, T.D. (2003) Family history assessment: Strategies for prevention of cardiovascular disease. *Am J Prev Med* 24, 136–142.
28. McConnachie, A., Hunt, K., Emslie, C. et al. (2001) Unwarranted survivals' and 'anomalous deaths' from coronary heart disease: Prospective survey of general population. *BMJ* 323, 1487–1491.
29. http://www.nature.com/news/gene-therapies-need-new-development-models-1.11521.
30. Kohlmann, W. and Gruber, S.B. (2004, updated 2006) Hereditary non-polyposis colon cancer. www.geneclinics.org.
31. Zimmern, R.L. (2011) Genomics and individuals in public health practice: are we luddites or can we meet the challenge? *J Public Health* 33(4), 477–482.
32. http://www.cancer researchuk.org/cancer-help/trials/ibis-international-breast-cancer-intervention-study.
33. Health Protection Agency (2006) *Tuberculosis Update, March 2006. The National TB Strain Typing Database—An Update. Information for Action*. Available online at: www.hpa.org.uk.
34. Public Health England. (undated) Nutrition data sources. Accessed July 21, 2014 http://www.noo.org.uk/data_sources/Nutrition.
35. Livingstone, M., Barbara, E., and Black, A.E. (2003) Markers of the validity of reported energy intake. *J Nutr*, 133 (3), 895S–920.
36. National Obesity Observatory, http://www.noo.org.uk/.
37. Puska, P., Salonen, J.T., Nissinen, A. et al. (1983) Change in risk factors for coronary heart disease during 10 years of a community intervention programme (North Karelia project). *BMJ* 287 1840–1844.

38. Henkel, G.L. (undated) North Karelia project shows the World how to reduce heart disease. www.kantele.com/nwfwebsite/puska_heart.html. New World Finn website.

39. WHO. (2003) *North Karelia Project: From Demonstration Project to National Activity*. Geneva: WHO. Available online at www.who.int/hpr/successful.prevention.3.html.

40. Triggle, N. (2011) Health groups reject 'responsibility deal' on alcohol. BBC website. Accessed July 21, 2014 http://www.bbc.co.uk/news/health-12728629.

41. Marteau, T.M., Ogilvie, D., Roland, M., Cuhrcke, M., and Kelly, M.P. (2011) Judging nudging: Can nudging improve population health? *BMJ* 342, d288.

42. Cobiac, L.J., Vos, T., and Veerman, J.L. (2010) Cost-effectiveness of interventions to reduce dietary salt intake. *Heart* 96, 1920e1925. doi:10.1136/hrt.2010.199240.

43. Sproston, K. and Mindel, J. (eds). (2006) Health Survey for England 2004. Leeds: The Information Centre. Available online at: www.ic.nhs.uk/pubs.

44. Department of Health Committee on Medical Aspects of Food Policy. (1991) *Dietary Reference Values for Food Energy and Nutrients for the United Kingdom: Report of the Panel on Dietary Reference Values of the Committee on Medical Aspects of Food Policy*. Stationery Office Books. ISBN-10 0113213972.

45. The Scottish Government, Healthy eating, active living: An action plan to improve diet, increase physical activity and tackle obesity (2008–2011). The Scottish Government Publications, 2008. Available from http://www.scotland.gov.uk/publications/2008/06/20155902/0; The Scottish Government. overweight and obesity in Scotland: A route map towards healthy weight 2010. The Scottish Government Publications, 2010. Available from http://www.scotland.gov.uk/Publications/2010/02/17140721/19; The Scottish Government. Obesity route map—Action plan version 1. The Scottish Government Publications, 2011. Available fromhttp://www.scotland.gov.uk/Resource/Doc/346007/0115166.pdf.

46. http://www.wales.gov.uk/topics/educationandskills/schoolshome/curriculuminwales/guidanceresources/foodandfitness/?lang=en.

47. Nutrional Advisory Group. (1995) *Recommendations for a Food and Nutrition Policy for Ireland*. Dublin, Ireland: Stationery Office.

48. Review of the Scientific Evidence and Recommendations for Public Policy in Ireland. (2005), available online at: www.fsai.ie.

49. Strazullo, P. et al. (2009) Salt intake, stroke, and cardiovascular disease: Meta-analysis of prospective studies. *BMJ* 339, b4567, doi: 10.1136/bmj.b4567.

50. Intersalt Cooperative Research Group. (1988) Intersalt: An international study of electrolyte excretion and blood pressure. Results for 24 hour urinary sodium and potassium excretion. *BMJ* 297, 319–328.

51. Hanneman, R.L. (1996) Intersalt: Hypertension rise with age revisited. *BMJ* 312, 1283–1284

52. He, F.J. and MacGregor, G.A. (2004) Effect of longer-term modest salt reduction on blood pressure. *Cochrane Database Syst Rev* 2004(3), CD004937.

53. NICE. Taking further steps to tackle the risk from heart attacks and strokes webpages. Accessed 21 July 2014 http://www.nice.org.uk/nicemedia/live/13024/49273/49273.pdf.

54. Blackburn, H. (1999) On the Trail of Heart Attacks in Seven Countries. www.epi.umn.edu/research/7countries/index.shtm.

55. Keys, A. (1980) *Seven Countries: A Multivariance Analysis of Death and Coronary Heart Disease*. Cambridge, MA: Harvard University Press.

56. Mozaffarian, D., Katan, M.B., Ascherio, A., Stampfer, M.J., and Willett, W.C. (2006) Trans fatty acids and cardiovascular disease. *N Engl J Med*, 354, 1601–1613.

57. OECD, http://www.ecosante.org/index2.php?base=OCDE&langs=ENG&langh=ENG.

58. http://www.noo.org.uk/NOO_about_obesity/trends.

59. Thaler, R.H. and Sunstein, C.R. (2008) *Nudge: Improving Decisions About Health, Wealth, and Happiness*. New Heaven, CT: Yale University Press.

60. Donaldson, L.J. and Gabriel Scally. (2009) *Donaldsons' Essential Public Health*. : New York: Radcliffe Publishing.

61. Health Protection Agency (2005). *Hepatitis C in England: The First Health Protection Agency Annual Report 2005*. London: Health Protection Agency. Available online at: www.hpa.org.uk.

62. Lim, S. S. et al. (2013) A comparative risk assessment of burden of disease and injury attributable to 67 risk factors and risk factor clusters in

21 regions, 1990–2010: A systematic analysis for the Global Burden of Disease Study 2010. *The Lancet* 380(9859): 2224–2260.

63. The Lancet. Global Burden of Diseases, Injuries, and Risk Factors Study 2013 webpages. Accessed 21 July 2014 http://www.thelancet.com/themed/global-burden-of-disease.
64. Sandman, P.M. (November 1987) Risk communication: Facing public outrage. *EPA J* 21–22. Available online at: www.psandman.com/articles/facing.htm.
65. UKCIP Climate impacts webpages. Accessed July 21, 2014 http://www.ukcip.org.uk/essentials/climate-impact/.
66. Reference key HPA report 'Health effects of climate change in the UK 2012'.
67. United Nations. (1997) Kyoto Protocol to the United Nations Framework Convention on Climate Change. UN Doc FCCC/CP/1997/7/Add.1, Dec. 10, 1997; 37 ILM 22 (1998).
68. http://www.hpa.org.uk/webc/HPAweb File/HPAweb_C/1242198452810;An introduction to land contamination for public health, Professionals www.hpa.org.uk.
69. http://en.wikipedia.org/wiki/Camelford_water_pollution_incident.
70. Department for Environment, Food & Rural Affairs (2013). Local authority collected waste management—Annual results. Accessed July 21, 2014 http://www.defra.gov.uk/statistics/environment/waste/wrfg23-wrmsannual/.
71. COMEAP (Committee on the Medical Effects of Air Pollution), http://www.hpa.org.uk/webc/HPAwebFile/HPAweb_C/1317137023144 HPAweb&Page&HPAwebAutoListName/Page/1158934607609?p=1158934607609.
72. Watson, S.J., Jones, A.L., Oatway, W.B., and Hughes, J.S. (2005) *Ionising Radiation Exposure of the UK Population: 2005 Review.* HPA-RPD-001, Chilton.
73. Environmental Protection Act. (1990) http://www.legislation.gov.uk/ukpga/1990/43/contents.
74. The Control of Substances Hazardous to Health Regulations 2002. (2002) http://www.legislation.gov.uk/uksi/2002/2677/contents/made.
75. Reporting of Injuries, Diseases and Dangerous Occurrences Regulations 2013. (2013) http://www.legislation.gov.uk/uksi/2013/1471/contents/made.
76. The Planning Inspectorate website. Accessed July 21, 2014. http://infrastructure.planningportal.gov.uk/
77. UK Planning Act (2008) http://www.legislation.gov.uk/ukpga/2008/29/contents.
78. European Commission. (2014) Climate action: Reducing emissions from aviation. Accessed July 21, 2014 at:http://ec.europa.eu/clima/policies/transport/aviation/index_en.htm.
79. de Hartog et al. (2010) Do the health benefits of cycling outweigh the risks? *Environ. Health Persp* 118(8), 1109.
80. Wilkinson, M. (2006) Carbon capture and storage. www.co2storage.org.uk.
81. European Commission. The EU Emissions Trading System (EUETS) webpages. Accessed July 21, 2014 http://ec.europa.eu/clima/policies/ets/index_en.htm.
82. World Health organization. Global Influenza Surveillance and Response System (GISRS) webpages. Accessed July 21, 2014 at: http://www.who.int/influenza/gisrs_laboratory/en/.
83. World Health organization. Global Immunization Vision and Strategy webpages. Accessed July 21, 2014 at: http://www.who.int/immunization/givs/en/index.html;
84. WHO, Immunization surveillance, assessment and monitoring, available online at: www.who.int/immunization_monitoring/en.
85. http://www.who.int/immunization/givs/en/index.html.
86. http://www.who.int/immunization/documents/positionpapers/.
87. http://www.dh.gov.uk/health/2012/09/whooping-cough/.
88. http://www.who.int/environmental_health_emergencies/publications/FINAL-PHM-Chemical-Incidents_web.pdf.
89. http://www.hpa.org.uk/Topics/InfectiousDiseases/InfectionsAZ/NotificationsOfInfectiousDiseases/ListOfNotifiableDiseases/.
90. http://www.infectioncontrolmanual.co.ni/.
91. Lalonde, M. (1974) A new perspective on the health of Canadians: A working document. www.phac-aspc.gc.ca/ph-sp/phdd/pdf/perspective.pdf.
92. Dahlgren, G. and Whitehead, M. (1991) *Policies and Strategies to Promote Social Equity in Health.* Stockholm, Sweden: Institute for Futures Studies.

93. London Health Commission. (2002) *Health in London: 2002 Review of the London Health Strategy High-Level Indicators*. London, UK: London Health Commission Available online at: www.londonshealth.gov.uk/pdf/hinl2002.pdf.

94. Evans, R. and Stoddart, G. (1990) Producing health, consuming resources. *Social Science and Medicine* 31, 1347–1363.

95. Diderichsen, F. and Hallqvist, J. (1998) Social inequalities in health: Some methodological considerations for the study of social position and social context. In: Arve-Parès, B. (ed.) *Inequality in Health: A Swedish Perspective*. Stockholm, Sweden: Swedish Council for Social Research, pp. 25–39.

96. Koller, T. (2006) *WHO Interview with Prof Goran Dahlgren* – www.euro.who.int/socialdeterminants/socmarketing/20060221_6.

97. Naidoo, J. and Wills, J. (1998) *Practising Health Promotion: Dilemmas and Challenges*. London, UK: Baillière Tindall.

98. WHO. (November 21, 1986) Ottawa Charter for Health Promotion. *First International Conference on Health Promotion*, Ottawa, Ontario, Canada, WHO/HPR/HEP/95.1. Geneva, Switzerland: WHO. Available online at: www.who.int/hpr/NPH/docs/ottawa_charter_hp.pdf.

99. Black, D., Morris, J.N., Smith, C. et al. (1980) *Inequalities in Health: Report of a Research Working Group* (Black Report). London: Department of Health and Social Security. Available online at: www.sochealth.co.uk/history/black.htm.

100. Rose, G. (1981) Strategy of prevention: Lessons from cardiovascular disease. *BMJ* 282, 1847–1851.

101. Hunt, K. and Emslie, C. (2001) Commentary: The prevention paradox in lay epidemiology—Rose revisited. *Int J Epidemiol* 30, 442–446.

102. Ewles, L. and Simnet, I. (2003) *Promoting Health: A Practical Guide* (5th edn.). London, UK: Ballière Tindall.

103. Health and Social Care Information Centre, Lifestyle Statistics. (2012) Smoking, drinking and drug use among young people in England in 2011. http://www.ic.nhs.uk/searchcatalogue?productid=7911&q=title%3a%22smoking+drinking+and+drug+use%22&sort=Relevance&size=10&page=1#top.

104. Hochbaum, G.M. (1958) *Public Participation in Medical Screening Programs: A Socio-Psychological Study*. PHS publication No. 572. Washington, DC: US Government Printing Office.

105. Bandura, A. (1977) *Social Learning Theory*. New York: General Learning Press.

106. Rosenstock, I.M., Strecher, V.J., and Becker, M.H. (1998) Social learning theory and the Health Belief Model. *Health Education Quarterly* 15, 175–183.

107. Prochaska, J.O. and DiClemente, C.C. (1984) Self-change processes, self-efficacy and decisional balance across five stages of smoking cessation. In: *Advances in Cancer Control: 1983*. New York: Alan R. Liss, Inc.

108. Tannahill, A. (1985) What is health promotion? *Health Educ J* 44, 167–168.

109. Naidoo, J. and Wills, J. (2000) *Health Promotion: Foundations for Practice* (2nd edn.). London, UK: Baillière Tindall.

110. Mcguire, W.J. (1989) Theoretical foundations of campaigns. In: Rice, E.R. and y Atkin, C.K. (eds.) *Public Communications Campaigns* (2nd edn.). Newbury Park, CA: Sage, pp. 43–65.

111. Bunton, R. (2002) Health promotion as social policy. In: Bunton, R. and Macdonald, G. (eds.) *Health Promotion: Disciplines and Diversity* (2nd edn.). London, UK: Routledge.

112. Marshall, T., Kennedy, E., and Offutt, S. (2000) Exploring a fiscal food policy: The case of diet and ischaemic heart disease. Commentary: Alternative nutrition and outcomes using a fiscal food policy. *BMJ* 320, 304–305.

113. Scollo, M.M. and Winstanley, M.H. (eds.). (2008) *Tobacco in Australia: Facts and Issues*, 3rd edn, Melbourne: Cancer Council Victoria. Available from http://www.tobaccoinaustralia.org.au.

114. Smithies, J. and Adams, L. (1990) *Community Participation in Health Promotion*. London, UK: Health Education Authority.

115. Walt, G. (2001) Global cooperation in international health. In: Merson, M., Black, R.E., and Mills, A.J. (eds.) *International Public Health: Diseases, Programs, Systems, and Policies*. New York: Aspen Publishers.

116. Lincoln, P. and Nutbeam, D. (2005) WHO and international initiatives. In: Davies, M. and Macdowell, W. (eds.) *Health Promotion Theory*. London, UK: McGraw-Hill.

117. WHO. (2006) *Healthy Cities and Urban Governance*. Geneva, Switzerland: WHO. Available online at: www.euro.who.int/healthy-cities.

118. WHO. (2005b) *Framework Convention on Tobacco Control*. Geneva, Switzerland: WHO. Available online at: www.who.int/tobacco/framework/en/.

119. Unicef Baby Friendly Initiative webpages. Accessed July 21, 2014 http://www.unicef.org.uk/BabyFriendly/http://www.unicef.org.uk/BabyFriendly/.
120. Wright, M. (2005) Homosexuality and HIV/AIDS prevention: The challenge of transferring lessons learned from Western Europe to Central and Eastern European Countries. *Health Promotion International* 20, 91–98.
121. Tones, K. (2000) Evaluating health promotion – beyond the RCT. In: Norheim, L., Waller, M., (eds.) *Best Practices, Quality and Effectiveness of Health Promotion*. Helsinki, Finland: Finnish Centre for Health Promotion, pp. 86–101.
122. Food Stanards Agency (Undated). Folic acid fortification. Accessed July 21, 2014 http://www.food.gov.uk/scotland/scotnut/folicfortification/#.UO6QLG_ZYsI.
123. Sylva, K., Melhuish, E., Sammons, P. et al. (2004) *The Effective Provision of Pre-School Education (EPPE) Project. EPPE findings from the Early Primary Years*. London, UK: DFES. Available online at: www.surestart.gov.uk/research/keyresearch/eppe.
124. Bull, J., Mulvihill, C., and Quigley, R. (2003) *Prevention of Low Birth Weight: A Review of Reviews for the Effectiveness of Smoking Cessation and Nutritional Interventions*. London, UK: Health Development Agency.
125. Chung, M., Raman, G., Chew, P., Magula, N., Trikalinos, T., and Lau, J. (2007) Breastfeeding and maternal and infant health outcomes in developed countries. *Evid Technol Asses (Full Rep)* 153, 1–186.
126. Department of Health. (2012) Healthy start: Retailer research summary. https://www.gov.uk/government/publications/healthy-start-scheme-research.
127. Elizabeth, T. and Therese, D. (2002) Community-based childhood injury prevention interventions: What works? *Health Promot Int* 17(3), 273–284.
128. Acheson, D. (1998) *Independent Inquiry into Inequalities in Health Report*. London: TSO. Available online at www. archive.official-documents.co.uk/document/doh/ih/ih.htm.
129. Administration for Children and Families. (2006) Head start general information website. www.acf.hhs.gov/programs/hsb/.
130. Garces, G.T., Thomas, D., Currie, J. (2002) Longer-term effects of HeadStart. *Am Econ Rev* 92, 999–1012.
131. Fight Crime: Invest in Kids. (2006) *Head Start Reduces Crime and Improves Achievement*. New York: Fight Crime: Invest in Kids. Available online at: www.fightcrime.org/reports/headstartbrief.pdf.
132. Kahan, B. (2005/2006) Interactive domain model best practices: The pre-determinants of the social determinants of health. www.idmbestpractices.ca/idm.php?content=archjottings#brkOctober05.
133. Wilkinson, R.G. (1996) *Unhealthy Societies: The Afflictions of Inequality*. London: Routledge.
134. Council of Europe. (2006) Social cohesion strategy. Available at: www.coe.int/T/E/social_cohesion.
135. Treasure, J. (2004) Motivational interviewing. *Adv Psychiatr Treat* 10, 331–337.
136. Lai, D.T. et al. (2010) Motivational interviewing for smoking cessation. *Cochrane Database Syst Rev* 1, CD006936.
137. Marteau, T.M., Ashcroft, R.E., and Oliver, A. (2009) Using financial incentives to achieve healthy behaviour. *BMJ* 338, 1415.
138. Kotler, P. and Zaltman, G. (1971) Social marketing: An approach to planned social change. *J Mark* 35, 3–12.
139. Brager, G. and Specht, H. (1973) quoted in World Health Organization (2002) *Community Participation in Local Health and Sustainable Development: Approaches and Techniques*. Available online at: www.euro.who.int/document/e78652.pdf.
140. Evelina Children's Hospital Appeal, available online at www.evelinaappeal.org/hospital/index.html.
141. HIA Gateway, available online at: www.nice.org.uk, London Health Commission, available online at: www.londonshealth.gov.uk/hia.htm#Top.
142. HM Treasury. (2007) Public service agreements. London, UK: HSMO. Available online at: www.hm-treasury.gov.uk/pbr_csr/psa/pbr_csr07_psaopportunity.cfm.

Section 3

HEALTH INFORMATION

Health information is essential for planning, operating, and evaluating health services. Without reliable and meaningful data, services would be unaware of and unresponsive to changes in circumstances. Managers would find it challenging to make predictions and introduce changes aimed at improving efficiency.

In many developed countries, there is a vast array of information available on populations, sickness, and health. However, the quality and appropriateness of this information often varies widely.

Section 3 provides public health practitioners with an appreciation of what types of information are available, how data are collected, and some of the advantages and disadvantages of the use of different types of data in public health.

Throughout Section 3, we largely focus on applications in the English or UK context. However, the general principles apply more widely, and where there are pertinent differences, other international examples are also given.

3A

Populations

Public health practitioners require an understanding of the population, for example, calculating rates and risk ratios requires a viable denominator as well as a count of disease occurrences. The population size, **demography**, and social characteristics in most developed countries are now enumerated by regular censuses. This chapter discusses the methods by which **census** information is obtained and, where this information is not available or sufficient, the methods by which **populations are estimated**. It also summarises **trends** in population structures across time, comparisons between different regions, and approaches to address the health consequences of **population changes**.

3A.1 Conduct of censuses

A census is a snapshot **enumeration survey** of an entire defined population. The term most commonly refers to a national census, which is used to determine the population of a country on a defined date. Although imperfect, it provides the most complete set of population data available, and its findings find widespread use within the health, housing, education transport, and other sectors for

- Making **comparisons** between regions
- Resource allocation
- Analysing **trends** over time
- Being **denominator** data for health and other population statistics

Many developed countries hold a census every 5–10 years, often enshrined in the constitution. Censuses can be conducted either by **interviewing** members of the population or by **self-enumeration** plus a post-enumeration survey (to assess under-enumeration).

Questionnaires can be delivered and collected by the following means:

Traditional 'drop-off' and 'pick-up'
Post-out and post-back
The Internet

UK censuses UK

The first UK census was held in 1801, and they have been held decennially since then, except during wartime. The Census Act makes completion of the census form compulsory, with non-responders facing a large fine. The organisations responsible for conducting the UK census, as well as analysing

Table 3A.1 Summary of the conduct of the 2011 census

Preparation	Planning began with a **consultation exercise** and the publication of a White Paper in 2008 There was then a parliamentary **debate** on the choice of questions, followed by a **publicity** exercise Census forms were designed for **self-completion** by the so-called householder and included both household and individual questions **Household questions** • Type, owner occupied or rented, number of rooms, type of heating, etc. • Number of cars or vans • Household members and their relationships **Individual questions** • Demographics: age, sex, marital/civil partnership status, country of birth, ethnicity • Migration (length of time in the United Kingdom) • Health: self-reported general health status, activity limitation due to ill health or disability, provision of unpaid care • Qualifications, employment, journey to work • In Wales, there was also a question about the Welsh language
Delivery	Census forms were posted to all households using a newly developed national address register The forms requested information about 'every person who usually lives in the household'. There were also visitor questions for 'all other people staying overnight' on the night of the census Census questionnaires could be completed online or returned by post. A questionnaire tracking system was used to enable targeted follow-up of households that had not returned the questionnaire. The estimated person response rate was 94%
Analysis	Completed forms were first **scanned** Scanned forms were then **coded** using automated and manual systems Paper forms were destroyed (with the scanned images being stored to be **made public** 100 years later) Coverage was assessed using a census follow-up survey, and adjustments were made to account for under-enumeration Data were **quality assured** Results were then tabulated into **databases** according to output areas (OAs) and SOAs (see Section 1A.18 for details), ready for analysis A **Census Output Prospectus** was published setting out the release plans for the census statistics

census data and disseminating its findings, are as follows:

- The ONS (England and Wales)
- General Register Office for Scotland (Scotland)
- Northern Ireland Statistics and Research Agency (Northern Ireland)

2011 Census

UK Table 3A.1 provides an overview of the 2011 UK census, including the preparatory, delivery, and analysis phases.

At the time of writing, the UK government is deliberating whether the 2011 census may be the last of its type. Future options being considered include a rolling census, an aggregation of routine data, sampling of a proportion of the population or some combination of these.

Census small areas

UK Historically, census information was collected by **enumeration district**, and local data were generally analysed at the level of the **electoral ward**. However, enumeration districts and electoral wards varied greatly in size (the latter ranging from 100 residents to over 30,000) and were subject to frequent boundary changes, which caused problems for longitudinal comparisons.

For the 2001 census, OAs were designed (using a geographic information system [GIS]) that were as follows:

Coterminous with postcodes
Uniform in population size
Compact in shape
Socially homogeneous

A new hierarchy of SOA groups is now used, which groups OAs into units that are similar in population size and are highly stable over time. There are three levels of SOA, the lower SOA representing four to six OAs: see Box 3A.1.

Collection in other countries

HK In Hong Kong, censuses are conducted every 10 years, with bi-censuses in the middle of the intercensal periods. For example, the 2006 bi-census involved interviews at 1 in 10 households.

Box 3A.1 Super output areas

Unit	Approximate population size
Upper SOA	25,000
Middle SOA	7,000
Lower SOA	1,500
OA	300

The 2001 population census used two types of questionnaires:

1. A short form (six in seven households) on basic characteristics. Self-enumeration forms were mailed to the householders and collected by enumerators.
2. A long form (one in seven households) collecting data on a broad range of socio-economic characteristics through face-to-face interviews.

A further data collection tool, the THS, is used in Hong Kong. This instrument gathers information on health status, patterns of health service utilisation, and healthcare service expenditure profiles. The tool was used in 1999, 2001, 2002, and 2005.

NZ + AUS In New Zealand and Australia, censuses are administered using a similar approach to the United Kingdom.

Every 5 years, the Australian Bureau of Statistics and Statistics NZ conduct a nationwide census, which is available online and in paper form.

Limitations of national censuses

The major limitations relate to cost, under-enumeration, timeliness, and misreporting.

1. **Cost**
   The 2011 UK census costs almost £500m and is one of the major reasons why the UK government is considering the alternatives.
2. **Under-enumeration**
   Certain groups tend to be particularly difficult to enumerate, including the following:
   - Young, inner-city men
   - Multiple-occupancy buildings and student houses

Box 3A.2 Population registers

Advantages	Disadvantages
More up-to-date results Linked statistical database allows multivariate analysis Improved planning, provision, and monitoring of surveys More consistent statistics Supports evidence-based policy Improved efficiency and quality from permanent systems	Not a snapshot, so complicated to compare regions Loss of 'brand' • lower response rates • results have less impact Depends on quality and availability of administrative data Actual risk of confidentiality breaches Perceived risk of confidentiality breaches

   - People who do not speak the official language(s) of the country
   - Babies
   - Very elderly people
   - Military personnel
   - Homeless people
   - Traveller communities
3. **Timeliness**
   Since they are typically conducted every 10 years, census data are often out of date. Furthermore, the data from a census can take a long time to be released.
4. **Misreporting**
   Being self-reported, the accuracy of a census can be difficult to assess. Examples of misreporting include the following:
   - Elderly people often round age to the nearest 5 years.
   - Divorced men tend to report that they are single rather than divorced.
   - Women tend to misreport their age.

Alternatives to traditional censuses

Between census years, planners must compromise using either out-of-date results from the most recent census (with or without projections) or more up-to-date results from less robust sources. The subsequent census often leads to dramatic revisions in statistics. For these reasons, some European countries are switching to **rolling censuses, population projections, and/or population registers** (see Box 3A.2).

3A.2 Collection of routine and ad hoc data

Raw population data used by researchers and public health practitioners either can come from routine sources (see Section 1A.1) or may be specifically commissioned and collected.

Routine data

Databases containing routinely collected data are a plentiful source of health information—often covering entire populations and spanning many years. The advantages and disadvantages of routine data are listed in Box 3A.3.

Ad hoc data

Ad hoc data are obtained either by commissioning a specific data collection exercise (e.g. a patient survey) or by requesting ad hoc extracts from a routine data source (e.g. from a cancer registry). Advantages and disadvantages of such data are listed in Box 3A.4.

Box 3A.3 Routine data

Advantages	Disadvantages
Readily available Cheap Can be complete (e.g. register of births) Large numbers of subjects Particularly useful when different data sources are linked Can provide baseline data on expected levels of health or disease	Limited to what is actually collected and when (therefore the data may not align with the purpose you are intending) Difficult to assess quality Access sometimes restricted Potential delays in publication Data linkage is often complex May be incomplete Often poorly presented and analysed

Box 3A.4 Ad-hoc data

Advantages	Disadvantages
Can specify exactly what data are to be collected Can target data collection to the subgroup of interest Can collect qualitative data Can be responsive to emerging needs Quality can be assessed Flexible mode of administration (e.g. face-to-face, telephone, postal, the Internet) Enables greater depth of statistical analysis	Sampling frame may be unknown Potentially costly May be difficult to link to routine data sources Typically the number of subjects is small Data linkage is complex Greater potential for selection bias Validity and/or reliability may be poor

3A.3 Demography

Demography is the study of the characteristics and dynamics of human populations. Population change may arise because of any of the following four factors:

1. Births
2. Deaths
3. Migration
4. Ageing

Table 3A.2 provides a summary of the key demographic concepts.

The calculation of these parameters is a prerequisite to making population projections (see Section 3A.7).

Table 3A.2 Important demographic concepts

Concept	Description
Total population size	Population size is measured definitively at each census. Differences from one census to the next reflect the historical trend in population growth or shrinkage
Age structure	Ages are divided into a series of bands (e.g. 0–4 years, 5–9 years), and the population is described according to the number of people in each band
Fertility	This is the number of offspring per female by age band Overall fertility rate = Number of live offspring per 1000 per year in women aged 15–49 (**Note: Fecundity** = Number of offspring biologically possible per female)
Mortality	This is the count of the number of deaths per year by age bands. It is the calculated probability that a person in a particular age band will die each year: $= \frac{(\text{Number that died per year}) \times (\text{Length of age band})}{(\text{Total number of individuals in each age band})}$
Survival	Probability of survival = (1 – Probability of dying)

3A.4 Major demographic differences

Important regional and international differences in populations, in respect of age, sex, occupation, social class, ethnicity, and other characteristics.

UK Some of the principal demographic differences between the home nations of the United Kingdom are shown in Table 3A.3.

Age

Age distributions can be represented graphically as **population pyramids**: see Figures 3A.1 through 3A.3.

Different age groups are unevenly distributed across the United Kingdom, with the youngest median ages in London (34.7 years) and Northern Ireland (36.3 years) and the oldest in the South West of England (41.7 years) and in Wales (40.8 years).

Gender

UK In the United Kingdom, slightly more boys are born each year than girls (in 2011, there were 2 million boys aged 0–4 years, while just over 1.9 million girls of the same age), but overall there are fewer males than females in the UK population (31 million males in the United Kingdom in 2011, compared with 32 million females). This is because from age 22 upwards, there are more women in each age group due to higher female immigration and lower female deaths from accidents and suicide. The gap narrows for people in their 40s (more immigration of men in this age group) and then widens again for older age groups (due to longer female life expectancy and the impact of World War II).

There are also differences in the male-to-female ratio across ethnic groups: see Box 3A.5.

Occupation

In terms of employment, developed countries tend to rely less on the **primary** sector jobs (agriculture, raw materials, etc.) and the **secondary** sector (manufacturing, construction, etc.) and

Table 3A.3 Differences in demographics between different parts of the United Kingdom

Constituent country	Number of people at 2011 census	Percentage of UK population (63 181 775)	Percentage population growth 2001–2011	Population density (number/km²)
England	53,012,456	83.9	+7.8	407
Northern Ireland	1,810,863	2.9	+7.5	133
Scotland	5,295,000	8.4	+4.6	67
Wales	3,063,456	4.8	+5.5	148

Source: Reproduced from ONS, 2011 Census for England and Wales, http://www.ons.gov.uk/ons/guide-method/census/2011/index.html, 2011.

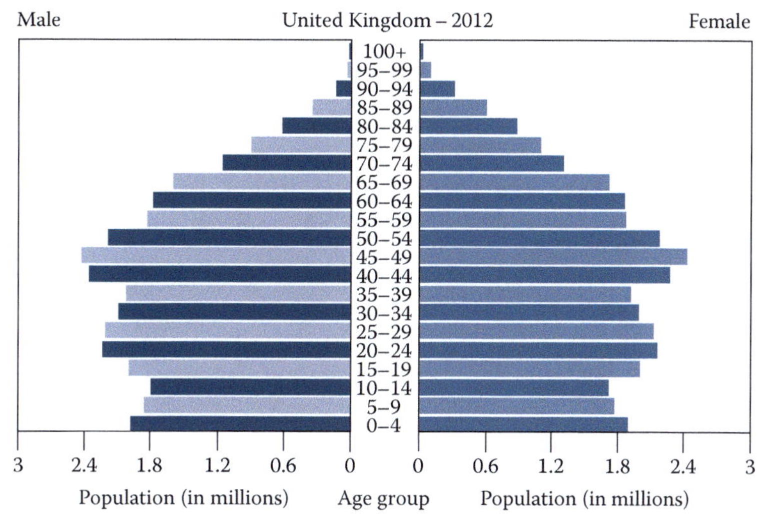

Figure 3A.1 UK population structure 2012. (From US Census Bureau, International Data Base.)

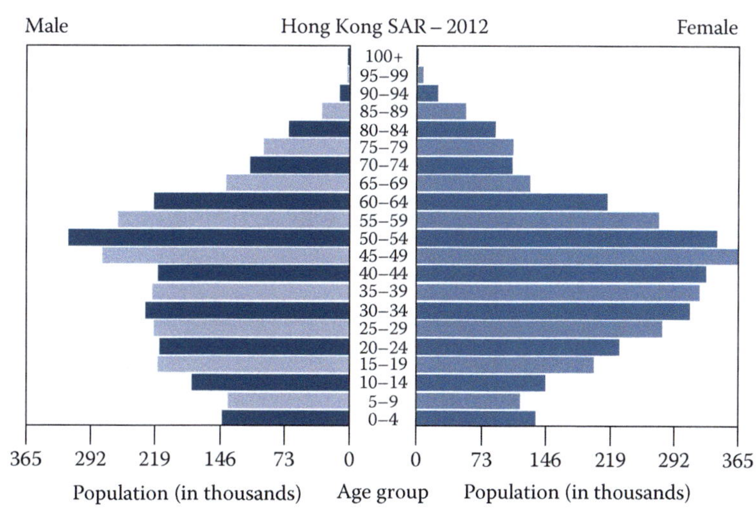

Figure 3A.2 Hong Kong population structure 2012. (From US Census Bureau, International Data Base.)

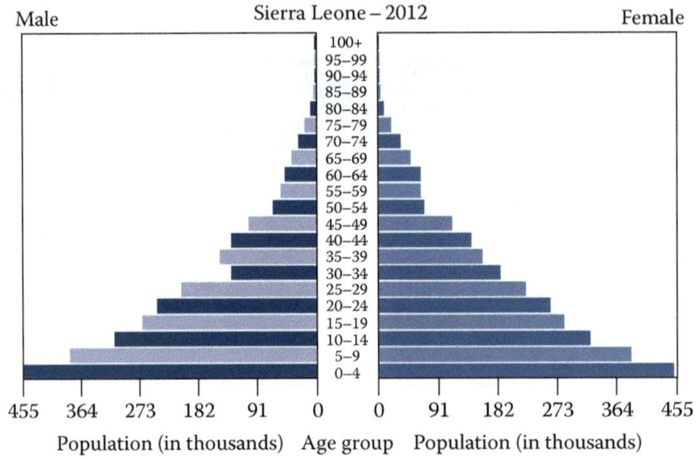

Figure 3A.3 Population structure Sierra Leone 2012. (From US Census Bureau, International Data Base.)

Box 3A.5 Gender differences

More men	More women
Pakistani	White
Bangladeshi	Black
Chinese	Indian

more on the **tertiary** (services) and **quaternary** (research and development) sectors. There tend to be regional hubs for service sectors, for example, London (United Kingdom), Zurich (Switzerland), and the Northern Cape (South Africa), and research and development sectors (e.g. so-called *Silicon Fen* around Cambridge).

Ethnicity

ENG + WA Ethnic diversity increased substantially between 2001 and 2011, particularly in London where white ethnic groups now make up 59.8% of the population (down from 71.2% in 2001) (see Table 3A.4). Non-white groups tend to have younger age structures than the white population, resulting from past immigration and fertility patterns.

Measuring ethnicity

UK The 2011 census question on ethnicity asked, ***'What is your ethnic group?'***, and allowed respondents to choose from one of the 16 options shown in Table 3A.5.

Table 3A.4 2011 Ethnic groups in England and Wales

	England	London	Wales
White (%)	85.5	59.8	95.6
Mixed/multiple ethnic group (%)	2.2	5.0	1.0
Asian/Asian British (%)	7.7	18.4	2.2
Black/African/Caribbean/Black British (%)	3.4	13.3	0.6
Others (%)	1.0	3.4	0.5

Source: Reproduced from ONS, 2011 Census for England and Wales, http://www.ons.gov.uk/ons/guide-method/census/2011/index.html, 2011.

Table 3A.5 Classification of ethnicity according to the 2011 UK census

		England and Wales	Scotland	Northern Ireland
A	White	English/Welsh/Scottish/Northern Irish/British Irish Gypsy or Irish Traveller Any other white (write in)	Scottish Other British Irish Gypsy Traveller Polish Any other white (write in)	White Irish Traveller
B	Mixed	White and black Caribbean White and black African White and Asian Any other mixed (write in)	Any mixed or multiple ethnic groups (write in)	White and black Caribbean White and black African White and Asian Any other (write in)
C	Asian or Asian British	Indian Pakistani Bangladeshi Chinese Any other Asian (write in)	Pakistani, Pakistani Scottish or Pakistani British Indian, Indian Scottish, or Indian British Bangladeshi, Bangladeshi Scottish, or Bangladeshi British Chinese, Chinese Scottish, or Chinese British Any other Asian (write in)	Indian Pakistani Bangladeshi Chinese Any other Asian (write in)
D	Black or black British	Caribbean African Any other black (write in)	African, African Scottish, or African British Any other African (write in) Caribbean, Caribbean Scottish, or Caribbean British Black, black Scottish, or black British	African Caribbean Any other black/African/Caribbean (write in)
E	Other ethnic groups	Arab Any other (write in)	Arab, Arab Scottish, or Arab British Any other (write in)	Arab Any other (write in)

As different ethnic populations mix and intermarry, the fastest-growing ethnic group is now people of mixed ethnicity. The 2001 UK census was the first census to ask about the backgrounds of this ethnic group, but the groupings then changed slightly in 2011, making comparisons between censuses difficult.

Other related questions were, *'What is your country of birth?'* and *'What is your religion?'* The latter was a voluntary question.

3A.5 Methods of population estimation and projection

UK Because the national census is only conducted every 10 years, other methods are required for estimating the population size in the intercensal years. The ONS produces mid-year population estimates on June 30 each year. These are approximations of the resident population and are calculated using the cohort component method.

Cohort component method

See Table 3A.6.

Mid-year population estimates are essential for local planning needs (e.g. planning for employment, housing, education, healthcare, and access to services). However, the estimates may be inaccurate because of difficulty in accessing reliable data on both local and international migration, especially regarding short-term migrants. This issue is particularly pertinent given that migration is now the major driver of population change in the United Kingdom.

Special groups

Certain mobile subpopulations are not included in the general population calculation, but are instead estimated separately and then taken into account when the total is calculated. These groups include prisoners, members of the armed forces, and boarding school pupils.

Estimates

UK Population estimates are generated for the populations listed in Box 3A.6, stratified according to age, sex, and marital status.

Projections

UK In the United Kingdom, population projections are produced by the ONS and are used for planning across government sectors. The core function of the ONS is to produce 25-year projections of the UK population and its constituent nations every 2 years, stratified according to age, sex, and marital status. These figures are also used to produce sub-national projections. Less accurate, 70-year projections are also made.

Box 3A.6 Geographies for population estimates

- UK as whole
- Constituent countries
- Government office regions
- Local authorities
- Health authority areas
- Primary care areas

Table 3A.6 Cohort component method for mid-year population estimates

Steps	Data sources
1. Take the previous mid-year estimate	Previous mid-year estimate (or the census findings in census years[a])
2. Increase the population's age by 1 year	
3. Add births	ONS
4. Subtract deaths	ONS
5. Adjust for external migration	International Passenger Survey Irish National Household Survey (for migration between the United Kingdom and the Republic of Ireland)
6. Adjust for internal migration	GP registration data (linked by NHS number)
7. Conduct quality control checks	For internal consistency and against previous estimates

[a] Population estimates are more reliable in census years: in these years, the cohort component method is still used, but the census population needs to be adjusted only by the number of weeks between the census and June 30.

Box 3A.7 Factors used in population projections

Factor	Basis of forecast
Birth sex ratio	Stable at 1.05 males per female
Mortality	Extrapolate historical trends
Fertility	Judgement
Migration	Judgement

Population projections are usually based on the estimates and trends shown in Box 3A.7.

The uncertainty is greatest regarding fertility and migration. Traditionally, all factors have been forecast along smooth paths, but there is now a move towards **stochastic predictions**, where the probabilities of random fluctuations are incorporated. Likewise, the uncertainty regarding population forecasts has traditionally been expressed as a range (lower to upper), but **probabilistic population forecasting** (with 95% confidence intervals) is now superseding this.

3A.6 Life tables

Life tables and their demographic applications.

Life tables, also known as **mortality tables**, list the probabilities that a person will die before their next birthday based on their age and sex. In the United Kingdom, these tables are generated by the ONS for the country as a whole and for its constituent nations.

Construction of life tables

Age-specific mortality rates are applied to a hypothetical population (e.g. of 100,000). The probability of dying in each period is applied to the number of people surviving to the beginning of that period, so that the number remaining in the population gradually decreases towards 0. This enables the number of people in the cohort who would survive each year to be calculated, as well as the number who would die and the average number of years that somebody would live at each age (i.e. their life expectancy). A worked example is shown in Table 3A.7.

Period and cohort life tables

Life tables are of two principal types: **period** and **cohort**.

Period life tables

These tables are calculated using the age-specific mortality rates for a given historical period (either a single year or a run of years), with no allowance made for any later actual or projected changes in mortality. A period life table displays the life expectancy of people of a given age in a given year if they experienced **that year's age-specific mortality rates** for the rest of their lives (e.g. mortality rate for 70-year-olds in 2012, for 71-year-olds in 2012, and for 72-year-olds in 2012). **Note:** Official life tables that relate to past years are generally period life tables.

Cohort life tables

In contrast, cohort life tables are calculated using age-specific mortality rates which do allow for known or projected changes in mortality in later years. A cohort life table displays the average life expectancy of a group of people of a given age in a given year if they experienced the projected future age-specific mortality rates from the series of future years in which they would actually live at each succeeding age if they survived (e.g. mortality rate for 70-year-olds in 2012, for 71-year-olds in 2013, and for 72-year-olds in 2014). Therefore, if mortality rates were projected to fall in the future, then the cohort life expectancy at a given age would be longer than the period life expectancy for that age. **Note:** Cohort life tables are also used (in a slightly different way) in survival analysis (see Section 1B.18).

Table 3A.7 Excerpt from an example of a life table of people aged 70+

Age	Central rate of mortality	Probability that someone will die before their next birthday	Number of people who survive to age x	Number of people who die at age x	Number of person years lived between age x to x + 1	Total number of person years lived above age x	Average life-expectancy at age x
x	m_x	q_x	l_x	d_x	L_x	T_x	e_x
70	0.027274	0.026907	100,000	2,690.7	98,654.7	12,86,000	12.86
71	0.030869	0.0304	97,309.3	2,958.2	95,830.2	11,87,173	12.20
72	0.034271	0.033694	94,351.1	3,179.1	92,761.6	10,90,699	11.56

Formulae, definitions and notes

m_x = Number of deaths in people aged x over the past 3 years divided by the average population at that age in the same period.

$q_x = 1 - e^{(-m_x)}$ Note that q_x is not the same as m_x; q_x is the age-specific risk of death.

$l_x = l_{x-1} - d_{x-1}$

$d_x = l_x \times q_x$

$L_x = l_x - (d_x/2)$ Assumes that people who die that year on average die halfway through the year, hence dx/2 (i.e. there is an equal chance of dying at any time of year, which is not typically the case).

$T_x = L_x + L_{x+1} + \cdots + L_{x+n}$

$e_x = T_x/l_x$ To calculate T_x (and thus life expectancy) the table would need to be continued until l_x reaches 0.

Applications of life tables

Several metrics can be derived from life tables, including the following:

- Proportion of people born in different years who are still alive.
- Remaining life expectancy of people at a particular age.
- Probability of surviving to a particular age.
- Life expectancy can in turn be used to derive other measures such as the HALE, DALYs, and PYLL.

Life tables are used for planning in all sectors of government, but particularly with regard to pensions and social insurance. As well as separate life tables for men and women, it is also possible to distinguish other factors that affect mortality, including ethnicity, social class, and smoking status. Life tables are also used for making international comparisons.

3A.7 Population projections

UK See Section 3A.5 for methods of population projections.

Note that when making official predictions, the ONS assumes that there will be improvements in mortality and increases in net immigration. A summary of the main estimates used in the 2010 UK population projections is shown in Box 3A.8.

Box 3A.8 Estimates used in 2010 UK population projections

1. The UK population was projected to increase by 4.9 million over 10 years from 62.3 million (2010) to 67.2 million (2020) with an annual average growth rate of 0.8%.
2. Over 25 years, the population was projected to increase by 10.9 million to 73.2 million (2035):
   a. Forty-seven percent of this projected increase was directly attributable to migration.
   b. Fifty-three percent was due to natural change (births > deaths), of which 32% would have occurred without migration and the remaining 21% was due to the effect of net migration on natural change.
   c. Therefore, 68% of population growth was projected to be attributable either directly or indirectly to migration.
3. The population was projected to continue ageing, with the median age set to increase from 39.7 years (2010) to 42.2 years (2035).
4. Projected increases for different age groups:
   a. Children <16 years: Increase by 12% from 11.6 million (2010) to 13.0 million (2035)
   b. Working-age people: Increase by 16% from 38.5 million (2010) to 44.7 million (2035)
   c. Pensionable age people: Increase by 28% from 12.2 million (2010) to 15.6 million (2035)
   d. Age >80 years: Increase by 100% from 2.9 million (2010) to 5.9 million (2035)

3A.8 Effects on population structure of fertility, mortality, and migration

Fertility

The main fertility measures are summarised in Table 3A.8

In the absence of migration, the growth or decline of a population depends on sustained patterns in replacement fertility. Changes in replacement fertility are slow to take effect because of population momentum (i.e. large cohorts of the population in childbearing years will continue to have high numbers of births even if fertility falls).

Replacement fertility values vary between countries (see Box 3A.9), and the commonly quoted

Table 3A.8 Fertility measures

Fertility measure	Description
TPFR	Also known as the *total fertility rate*, this is the average number of children that would be born to a woman during her lifetime, assuming that she were to experience current age-specific fertility rates and that she were to survive to the end of her reproductive life TPFR = The sum of age-specific fertility rates at a given time
General fertility rate	This is the annual number of live births per 1000 women of childbearing age: General fertility rate = (Number of live births/Number of women aged 15–44) × 1000[a]
Replacement fertility	This is the total fertility rate at which newborn girls would have on average exactly one daughter over their lifetimes (i.e. where women have just enough female babies to replace themselves). This needs to be higher than two children per female in order to compensate for • **Mortality** before the end of reproductive age • **Unbalanced sex ratio** at birth (in the United Kingdom, the ratio of male births to female births is approximately 1.05:1)

[a] Sometimes taken as aged 15–49.

Box 3A.9 Replacement fertility

Place	Replacement fertility
Island of Reunion	2.05
Western Europe	2.10
Africa	2.70
Sierra Leone	3.43

figure of 2.1 children applies only to the developed world. International variation is mostly due to mortality differences, particularly with respect to HIV/AIDS.

UK In the United Kingdom, replacement fertility has fallen because of the decreasing mortality of young people. Again ignoring immigration, if the TPFR drops below replacement fertility, then the size of the population will eventually fall. However, population decline may not be observed immediately because of the buffering effects of other factors, including the following:

- Age structure of the population
- Changes in age-specific mortality rates
- Childbearing postponement

The last of these phenomena has occurred in several developed countries in recent decades. It has the effect of stretching out the population into the future. TPFR in the United Kingdom is currently around 1.7.

Mortality

Clearly, increased mortality leads to a reduction in the size of the population in the age band in which the mortality occurs. The ages with greatest mortality have historically been in infancy and old age, although certain events have led to declines in other age groups (e.g. 'Spanish flu' disproportionately affected young adults, and war affects young men).

Population time bomb

The process of **demographic transition** (see Figure 3A.4) can result a **population time bomb**: As the number of people who are economically active falls relative to people requiring health and social care, the resulting effects may have profound implications for society.

In economic terms, a country achieves its optimum population when productivity per capita is highest. By definition, **underpopulated countries** can increase their productivity by increasing their population, whereas **overpopulated countries** can increase productivity by reducing their population size.

Migration

See Section 4C.10.

Net migration is the difference between the number of people out-migrating (emigrating) and in-migrating (immigrating). Both immigration and emigration occur most commonly among young adults, with slightly more males than females migrating each year overall.

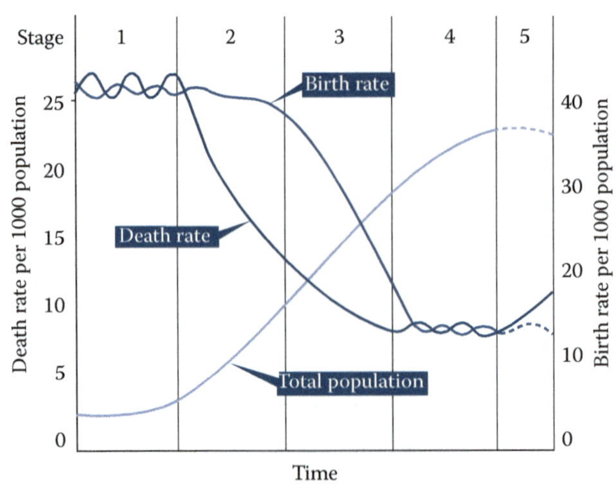

Figure 3A.4 Demographic transition.

UK In the United Kingdom, both immigration and emigration have increased in recent years. The countries from which the highest proportion of UK immigrants came in 2010 were India (11.9%), Pakistan (5.8%), Poland (5.4%), Australia (5.2%), and China (5.2%). Emigration from the United Kingdom has been mostly in people from the 25–44 age group and has mainly been to other EU countries, Australia, and New Zealand.

3A.9 Historical changes in population size and structure and factors underlying them

Over the course of several centuries, large populations have changed with regard to their age structure and geographical distribution. The populations of many countries have followed three distinct phases, namely, pre-industrial, industrial, and post-industrial. See Table 3A.9.

This is underpinned by the '**demographic transition model**' which is made up of five phases:

1. Pre-industrial
2. Developing
3. Urbanisation
4. Developed
5. Deindustrialised (i.e. switch from manufacturing to service-based economy)

The American demographer Warren Thompson (1887–1973) developed this model in 1929 (see Figure 3A.4).

United Kingdom

UK The UK population of around 63 million (2011 census) increased in size by 25% since 1951 due to births exceeding deaths. There were more births than deaths in the United Kingdom in every year since 1901 (with the exception of 1976, see the following discussion). Net immigration has also been a factor since the mid-1990s.

Underlying factors affecting population size include changes in **fertility**, **migration,** and increasing **urbanisation**: see Box 3A.10.

Table 3A.9 Phases of population transition

	Population growth	Fertility and mortality	Age
Pre-industrial	Slow	High	Young
Industrial	Fast	Intermediate	Intermediate
Post-industrial	Slow	Low	Old

Box 3A.10 UK demographic trends

Fertility	There are fewer people aged under 16s and more over 65s **Birth rates** rose after both world wars, with a 'baby boom' in the1960s. Rates then steadily fell until reaching a nadir in the 1970s, with some increases in the 1980s and 1990s before falling again in the early 2000s The average age at which women give birth to their first child has been increasing. More women remain childless (1 in 5 now compared with 1 in 10 for women born in the mid-1940s). See also Section 3B.4
Migration	**Net immigration** into the United Kingdom is an increasingly important factor in population size. Immigration has been relatively high since the 1950s, particularly in urban areas such as London and Birmingham
Urbanisation	England is one of the most crowded countries in the world. Over **90% of inhabitants live in urban areas** that cover just 8% of the land area

World

The UN Population Division previously expected the absolute number of the world's infants to begin falling in 2015 and the number of children under 15 to begin falling by 2025. Other forecasters had calculated that the world's population would peak at **9 billion** in **2070**, with the average age of the population steadily rising. The UN (2011) projects that the population global population will reach 10.1 billion by 2100 and continue growing; this change is mostly due to lower than expected declines in fertility in Africa.

3A.10 Effects of demographic change on healthcare

The significance of demographic changes for the health of the population and on the need for health and related services.

See Table 3A.10.

Table 3A.10 Changes in population size and structure and effects on the need for healthcare

Demographic changes		Effect on health and need for health and related services
Population structure	Age	An ageing population will generate greater demand for geriatric, intermediate, and social/personal care
	Ethnicity	Greater ethnic diversity will lead to different risk factors for diseases, different patterns of disease, and demand for different models of care provision (e.g. bilingual healthcare workers, culturally specific services such as women-only group sessions) Access to healthcare should be monitored to ensure that there is no discrimination due to language, cultural, or knowledge barriers
Population mobility	Short term (travel)	Increased global spread of infectious disease and pandemics (e.g. SARS in the early 2000s)
	Longer term (migration) (see Section 4C.11)	International spread of emerging diseases (e.g. TB). Healthy migrant effect Migration of healthcare workers
Urbanisation		Increased spread of infectious diseases
Housing	People living longer More people living alone Lower building rates	Demand for new homes has increased over the past 30 years Housing shortages in southeast England are acute, leading to a shortage of workers. The situation is due to worsen if current trends continue Risk of health problems associated with overcrowding/poor housing (e.g. respiratory illnesses)

3A.11 Policies to address population growth nationally and internationally

Policies in a particular country are shaped by the nature of the demographic challenges faced by that country. In many developed countries, relatively low birth rates require policymakers to address issues associated with an ageing population; worldwide, however, there is a need for policies to restrict or limit population growth while recognising that there will be an increasingly ageing population.

United Kingdom

UK The ageing population of the United Kingdom means that there will be a relative shortage of working-age adults compared with the demand from the total population. This is particularly the case regarding people with professional qualifications such as clinical staff.

Policymakers can increase the number of working-age adults by the following:

- Incentivising people to have larger families by means of **family-friendly policies** (e.g. subsidised paternity and maternity leave, tax allowances for parents)
- Encouraging people of working age to move to the United Kingdom through **managed migration** strategies
- Increasing the state pension age (e.g. in 2011, the UK government announced an increase in the state pension age to 67 years by 2028)

Demand for affordable housing is increasing and could be met by the following:

- Increasing the supply and affordability of housing in areas of high demand (e.g. Thames Gateway)
- Key worker policies (providing subsidised housing for staff, e.g. science teachers)
- Neighbourhood renewal to tackle problems in declining areas
- Sustainable development

International

According to circumstances, strategies may be aimed at the following:

- Restricting population growth (e.g. China's one-child policy)
- Encouraging a lower rate of growth (e.g. developing countries promoting birth control by improving family planning services and providing subsidised contraception or sterilisation)
- Focusing on gender equality and increasing educational and employment opportunities for women (independent women are more likely to have smaller families, thereby promoting gender equality and empowering women, which is one of the UN's millennium development goals)
- Targeting resources into the research of diseases associated with ageing (e.g. Alzheimer's disease)
- Tackling environmental problems and the demand for natural resources (e.g. through international treaties)

3B

Sickness and Health

Information regarding sickness and health can be derived from a variety of sources, not only from health service data. To use this information effectively, public health specialists require a familiarity with the major data resources, an understanding of the limitations to data validity, and an appreciation of the methods available for linking one set of data to another.

3B.1 Routine mortality and morbidity data

Sources of routine mortality and morbidity data, including primary care data, and how they are collected and published at international, national, regional, and local levels.

Routine information is **collected regularly** and made partially or fully available. In most countries, it provides information about health service use, mortality, and morbidity in a standardised format (see Section 3A.2). The sources described below relate mainly to national systems used in England and Wales, although similar systems exist in Scotland and other countries. Additional sources of information may be available locally and regionally.

Mortality data

UK The ONS is the main source of mortality data in England and Wales (see Table 3B.1).

UK Additional information is collected about deaths that result from road traffic collisions (see Table 3B.2).

Morbidity data

UK Information on morbidity in the United Kingdom comes from the following:

- **Primary care**: Limited information is collected on optometry, pharmacy, and dental services, mainly for payment purposes. More information is available on general practice consultations and prescribing (see Table 3B.3 and Section 3B.6).
- **Secondary care** databases (see Table 3B.5).
- **Health surveys.**
- Condition-specific **registers** and datasets (see Section 3B.5).

Primary care

For many years, PCTs in several parts of England used to extract and analyse general practice data to improve patient care and highlight areas of

Table 3B.1 Death certificates and death registration data

Attribute	Description
Information	Underlying and participatory causes of death (entered by a medical practitioner on the certificate) Additional information includes the following: • Date and place of death • Name, date and place of birth, and occupation of the deceased • Details of any spouse or civil partner • Usual address
Collection, coding, and analysis	Deaths must be registered within 5 days by a relative or friend of the deceased at a registry office (8 days in Scotland) It is a statutory duty for death to be registered before a funeral can occur Register information is stored at the district level Cause of death is coded by the ONS using ICD-10 Data are published annually by the ONS at the national level and local authority level
Uses	Analysis of trends and comparisons between areas Health needs analysis for serious conditions Calculation of life expectancy (see Section 3A.6)
Strengths	Complete and timely Relatively accurate Coding accuracy tends to be good because deaths are coded centrally by the ONS
Weakness	Cause of death often less accurate for older patients with several co-morbidities Problems comparing different years may arise if different ICD classifications are used, such as the shift from ICD-9 to ICD-10 in January 2001 (see Section 3B.3) Risk of bias in social class measures due to occupational advancement (see Section 3B.2)

unwarranted variation. Starting in 2013 [1], the Health and Social Care Information Centre will begin receiving GP data from practices across England, including those practices participating in the GP Extraction Service (GPES). One of the initial uses of the data will be to support practice payments through the Calculating Quality Reporting Services (CQRS) system (see Tables 3B.3 and 3B.4).

Secondary care

See Table 3B.5.

Surveys

Surveys are an important source of information for public health specialists. Some of the most relevant surveys are the Integrated Household Survey, the Health Survey for England, and its Scottish, Welsh, and Northern Irish equivalents.

Integrated Household Survey

UK This survey is comprised of the **Labour Force Survey**, the **General Lifestyle Survey**, the **Living Cost and Food Survey**, the **English Housing Survey,** and the **Life Opportunities Survey.** Conducted annually by the ONS, it covers approximately 200,000 households. The survey generates data about economic activity, education, smoking and alcohol use, illnesses, and consultations with health professionals.

Table 3B.2 Police road accidents data: 'STATS19'

Attribute	Description
Information	Injury or death due to road traffic collisions
Collection, coding, an analysis	All reported road collisions[a] involving personal injury are recorded at the time of the accident on the STATS19 form Police process the STATS19 data and send the information to the Department for Transport, which adds the information to the national road casualty database Both the police and the Department for Transport validate the information received
Uses	Indications of mortality from incidents occurring on roads Can link to A&E data on deaths from road traffic collisions
Strengths	Contains more detailed information about each incident and the types of vehicles involved than the information recorded by A&E May include incidents that did not present to health services
Weaknesses	Not all collisions are reported to the police Morbidity may be rated differently by the police and the health service

[a] Note that the term 'road traffic collisions' is preferred, since accidents have connotations of non-preventability.

Table 3B.3 Primary care data at aggregate level: CQRS system

Attribute	Description
Description	CQRS replaced the Quality Management and Analysis System (QMAS) in 2013 and is primarily designed to calculate payments Collects data on GP practices to calculate achievement and payments based on 1. The Quality and Outcomes Framework (QOF), which consists of 146 evidence-based indicators categorised into four domains: a. **Clinical** (including hypertension, asthma, diabetes, CHD, mental health) b. **Organisational** (including records, practice management issues) c. **Patient experience** (assessed through surveys and consultation length) d. Additional services 2. Nationally commissioned enhanced services 3. Locally commissioned services CQRS also collects data on how CCGs are performing against outcome indicators
Collection, coding, and analysis	Extracts from a general practice may be sent to CQRS via the General Practice Extraction Service (GPES) or via other electronic means Payments are linked to evidence-based indicators through the QOF CQRS is accessible online to staff working in public health departments
Uses	Paying general practices according to the services delivered and the degree to which certain milestones are met Registers provide an indication of disease prevalence CQRS is helpful when planning new primary care or referral services

(continued)

Table 3B.3 (*Continued*) Primary care data at aggregate level: CQRS system

Attribute	Description
Strengths	Many conditions are treated almost exclusively in primary care The link to payment provides an incentive for improving the quality and comprehensiveness of information recorded in general practice QOF scores provide an indicator of the quality of clinical care provided in a practice Relatively complete since most people are registered with a GP
Weaknesses	Accuracy is dependent on the coding and currency of the GP CQRS was designed primarily for payment, not for performance management Cannot use QOF scores to compare practices on performance because different list sizes and different population characteristics may affect QOF scores QOF is voluntary, although most practices have chosen to participate

Source: Health and Social Care Information Centre, Calculating Quality Reporting Service (CQRS), Accessed online July 24, 2014 at http://www.connectingforhealth.nhs.uk/systemsandservices/cqrs.

Table 3B.4 Clinical practice research datalink (CPRD)

Information	The CPRD system collates data from primary care and secondary care sources including the following: • Data from GP electronic patient records • HES • Mortality data • Primary and secondary care prescribing data • Disease registers
Collection, coding, and analysis	Data are coded differently in each of the previous sources; however, all of the data may be linked using the NHS number as the unique identifier
Uses	Pseudonymous data are made available to academic, pharmaceutical, and biotech organisations for research purposes
Strengths	Linked data from multiple sources for large numbers of patients Longitudinal primary care data are available Primary care data include lifestyle information (e.g. smoking, alcohol intake)
Weaknesses	Many data sources are incomplete (e.g. fewer than 500 GP practices are currently included) Data are currently only accessible to public health departments for a fee

Source: The Clinical Practice Research Datalink, Accessed online July 24, 2014 at http://www.cprd.com/intro.asp.

Health Survey for England

ENG Covering around 6000 households, this survey is conducted annually by the National Centre for Social Research and University College London. The survey involves an **interview** and an **examination** by a nurse to measure the respondent's height, weight, blood pressure, etc. There is a set of core questions (e.g. alcohol and smoking) plus a specific focus each year (e.g. cardiovascular disease, older people, sexual health).

Table 3B.5 HES

Attribute	Description
Information	Information is recorded about all NHS inpatient admissions, including the following: • Personal (name, NHS number, date of birth, ethnicity, postcode) • Administrative (start and end dates of the stay, hospital, ward, specialty code, waiting time) • Clinical (diagnosis, interventions, and procedures) A limited amount of information is also recorded for each outpatient visit and A&E attendance
Collection, coding, and analysis	Hospital episodes are coded locally by hospital coders (not clinicians) using the ICD-10 and OPCS-4 classifications of interventions and procedures, respectively Collected as part of monthly mandatory information submission by hospitals Sent to the Secondary Uses Service (SUS), which provides trusted organisations with access to the data for non-clinical uses (e.g. public health, commissioning) The data are then cleaned and collated, and then published in the HES database as a nationally available extract
Uses	Payment from commissioner to providers Analysis of hospital usage, waiting times Development of predictive risk models Assessment of the quality and outcomes of care, performance management by commissioners, and inspection by the CQC Estimation of health need for conditions that are typically managed in secondary care
Strengths	Generally complete (hospitals must submit the information if they are to be paid) Timely (information is submitted monthly and made available monthly, quarterly, and yearly from HES) Mortality data can be linked to HES databases to generate statistics that link episodes to outcomes at the individual level
Weaknesses	Accuracy dependent on quality of the clinical coders (very variable) Variable completeness Relates to episodes, not patients (therefore, may overestimate need if one patient has several episodes) Only useful for conditions that are generally admitted to hospital Only includes NHS data (not procedures that are paid for privately)

Scottish Health Survey

SCOT The Scottish Health Survey aims to collect data on both lifestyle and health status. It is most useful at a national level, as the numbers in individual health boards are small. The survey involves interviewing over 9000 adults and children each year. It provides data on cardiovascular disease and the related risk factors, including smoking, alcohol, diet, physical activity, and obesity. Information on general health, mental health, and dental health are also included. The design detail has varied from year to year although it always includes a personal interview.

Welsh Health Survey

WA The Welsh Health Survey (WHS) was first conducted in 1995 and was repeated in 1998 and 2003–2005. Since 2007, it has become an annual programme. In 1995 and 1998, these surveys were only targeted at adults but since then have covered children and adults. The WHS is a postal survey designed to provide a picture of health of the people of Wales, including the way the NHS is used and areas where services could be improved. The 2003–2005 survey included a 15-min face-to-face questionnaire. Results from the 2003–2005 survey were not directly comparable with those from the previous surveys because of differences in the questionnaires and the ways in which the survey was designed and conducted. Annual surveys since 2007 have used similar methods and questionnaires to the 2003–2005 survey.

In addition to demographic data, the content of the Welsh Health Surveys since 2003–2005 includes the following:

- General health status (SF-36)
- A range of reported illnesses and other conditions (such as eyesight or hearing difficulty)
- Reported lifestyle behaviours (including smoking, drinking, fruit and vegetable consumption, physical activity, and BMI)
- Reported use of a range of health services [4]

Northern Ireland Health Survey

NI The Northern Ireland Health Surveys have replaced the Health and Social Wellbeing Surveys that were conducted in 1997, 2001, and 2005/2006. Health surveys are now conducted every year, and they are designed to yield a representative sample of all adults aged 16 and over living in Northern Ireland.

The questionnaire consists of a household interview, which is followed by an individual interview with each person in the household aged 16 and above. The individual interview consists of core modules and modules that may recur on a regular cycle. Core items include accommodation, tenure, employment status, educational qualifications, family information, smoking and drinking, and health and ill health. Noncore items include physical activity and sexual health. Physical measurements are now limited to height and weight, although blood pressure and cholesterol were measured in the 1997 survey.

In addition to the socio-demographic details, the questionnaire covers the following:

- Lifestyle habits, including use of sunbeds and sexual health
- General health, long-standing illness
- Common chronic diseases and conditions
- Stressful life event, possible mental health problems, and mental well-being
- Informal care and the lifestyle of carers
- Characteristics of the people whom carers are looking after

Sources of information about communicable diseases

Communicable disease information is collected and collated in a number of ways and is used for the detection of emerging outbreaks, service planning, and evaluation. For example, the **GUMCAD** collects individual patient-level data on sexually transmitted infection diagnoses and tests from a range of sexual health services and GUM clinics. The data are reported to Public Health England.

Section 2G.2 covers surveillance and routine reporting of communicable diseases. See also Section 3B.5 (disease registers).

International data sources

International sources of health-related data are described in Table 3B.6.

Table 3B.6 International data sources

Data source	Details
WHO databases	WHO regional departments maintain databases of health statistics, such as the European Health for All Database (HFA-DB), which collates statistics on demographics, health, risk factors, and health services from countries within the WHO European region. This database allows international comparisons to be made and enables geographical mapping
Global Burden of Disease Study	The original Global Burden of Disease Study (GBD 1990) was commissioned by the World Bank to compare the burden of disease and risk factors around the world. As well as comparing mortality, a new measure was established to compare disease burden: DALYs (see Section 4D.5). From 2000 onwards, WHO produced updates to the study, and in 2010, a second major study was conducted (GBD 2010)
Eurostat	Eurostat is the statistical office of the EU and provides a broad range of statistics, which are divided into the following themes: • General and regional statistics (mainly geographical data) • Economy and finance • Population and social conditions • Industry, trade, and services • Agriculture and fisheries • International trade • Transport • Environment and energy • Science and technology Eurostat datasets include morbidity data, mortality data, and the EU Statistics on Income and Living Conditions (EU-SILC)
INDEPTH network [5]	The International Network for the Demographic Evaluation of Populations and Their Health (INDEPTH) is a network of sentinel sites in low- and middle-income countries. It was set up in 1998 in recognition of the lack of reliable population-based data in these countries. Data are collected on births, migration, deaths, causes of death, and other disease-related data
Demographic and Health Surveys (DHS)	Funded by the US Agency for International Development (USAID), these are nationally representative household surveys conducted in developing countries. Data are collected on fertility, reproductive health, maternal health, child health, immunisation, nutrition, HIV/AIDS status, and malaria

3B.2 Biases and artefacts in population data

Potential sources of bias and artefact should always be borne in mind when working with population data.

Biases

A bias is a systematic error (see Section 1A.14). Biases can affect population data in a number of ways, including through selection bias, biased list sizes, and status inflation.

Selection bias

Selection bias is frequently affecting routine survey data through participation (or 'response') bias, even in surveys that aim to be complete (e.g. national census), where certain groups are often under-represented (see Section 3A.1).

List size

UK GP practices sometimes overestimate their list of registered patients by delaying or failing to remove from their lists people who have died or moved away from the practice. This tendency leads to a systematic error regarding the estimated population size and structure. As a consequence, this type of bias can lead to an underestimate of service provision (e.g. in terms of vaccine uptake).

Status inflation

UK There is a tendency for people to inflate the socio-economic status of deceased people when registering a death or completing surveys. Known as 'occupational advancement', this phenomenon biases the population structure with regard to social class.

Artefacts

Artefacts in population data are caused by spurious differences between an observed population characteristic and the true underlying characteristic. Artefacts may hinder accurate comparisons from being drawn between areas or when studying trends over time. Adjusting for artefacts requires an understanding of how the data are collected and the potential sources of inaccuracy, bias, and confounding. Important artefacts relate to changes in classification systems, changes to survey questions, and changes in geographical subdivisions.

Changes in classification

UK In January 2001, the ONS replaced International Classification of Diseases (ICD)-9 with ICD-10 (see Section 3B.3). This change caused an artefact in mortality data when comparing deaths before and after this date.

Changes to questions or possible responses

UK Census ethnicity information codes changed between 1991 and 2001, when for the first time people were allowed to identify their ethnicity as 'mixed'. This change complicates the drawing of comparisons between the two censuses.

Change in geographical subdivisions

UK In 2001, small area divisions in the United Kingdom were changed from electoral wards to SOAs.

3B.3 International classification of diseases

The ICD and other methods of classification of disease and medical care.

The ICD belongs to the WHO Family of International Classifications (see Box 3B.1), the purpose of which is to provide a common language for health-related topics.

> **Box 3B.1** WHO family of international classifications
>
> - ICD
> - ICF
> - International Classification of Health Interventions (ICHI)

Between them, these classifications enable the consistent collection, analysis, and presentation of data, which enables comparisons to be drawn over time and between populations. In particular, the classifications allow the following:

- Analysis of population health
- Monitoring of disease frequency
- Classification of death certificates and hospital records
- Mortality and morbidity statistics to be collated using a common framework

ICD is primarily an international standard classification for **mortality statistics** and contains a

Table 3B.7 ICD-10 disease codes

Code	Contents
A00–B99	Certain infectious and parasitic diseases
C00–D48	Neoplasms
D50–D89	Diseases of the blood and blood-forming organs and certain disorders involving the immune mechanism
E00–E90	Endocrine, nutritional, and metabolic diseases
F00–F99	Mental and behavioural disorders
G00–G99	Diseases of the nervous system
H00–H59	Diseases of the eye and adnexa
H60–H95	Diseases of the ear and mastoid process
I00–I99	Diseases of the circulatory system
J00–J99	Diseases of the respiratory system
K00–K93	Diseases of the digestive system
L00–L99	Diseases of the skin and subcutaneous tissue
M00–M99	Diseases of the musculoskeletal system and connective tissue
N00–N99	Diseases of the genitourinary system
O00–O99	Pregnancy, childbirth, and the puerperium
P00–P96	Certain conditions originating in the perinatal period
Q00–Q99	Congenital malformations, deformations, and chromosomal abnormalities
S00–T98	Injury, poisoning, and certain other consequences of external causes
Z00–Z99	Factors influencing health status and contact with health services
U00–U99	Codes for special purposes

standard format for death certification. Its history dates back to the 1850s (*International List of Causes of Death*), and since 1948, it has been administered by the WHO.

Diseases mentioned on the death certificate are translated into codes, which may range from A00 ('cholera') to Z99.9 ('dependence on unspecified enabling machine and device'). See Table 3B.7. By applying the coding rules contained in the ICD, which prioritise and consolidate codes, a single cause of death will be selected.

The ICD is revised every 10–20 years. The WHO advises that it is problematical to translate between the codes of one revision to another. Deaths occurring during the bridging period should be dual-coded according to the old and new revisions so that comparisons may be made.

WHO member states began using the 10th revision (ICD-10) in 1994, a revision that contains twice as many codes as ICD-9. A clinically modified version of ICD-9 (ICD-9-CM) contains more precise details for describing mortality as opposed to morbidity. Although ICD-10-CM has now been written, at the time of writing, ICD-9-CM remains the standard for reporting morbidity. The next version, ICD-11 [6], is due to be published in 2015.

ICD-10

ICD-10 was the first revision of the classification to adopt alphanumeric codes and hence to face the

Box 3B.2 Examples of ICD-10 codes

M60	Myositis
J85.2	Abscess of lung without pneumonia
M11.9	Crystal arthropathy, unspecified

potential of confusion between zero and letter O and between one and the letter l). The codes used in ICD-10 range between three and seven characters in length, with a decimal after the third character if the code is four characters or longer (see Box 3B.2).

All codes for injuries (range S00-T98) must have a corresponding external cause code (range V01-Y98).

Neoplasms are coded by morphology and site codes. Code U is reserved for emerging diseases and for future use; for example, SARS is coded U04.

Diagnosis-related groups and healthcare resource group

Diagnosis-related group (DRG) is an American system to classify hospital cases into one of approximately 500 groups that are expected to require similar hospital resource use. DRGs are based on ICD diagnoses, together with procedures, age, sex, and the presence of complications or co-morbidities.

UK In the United Kingdom, the analogous healthcare resource group (HRG) is the unit of currency for commissioning and paying for health services.

3B.4 Measurements of health status

Rates and ratios used to measure health status, including geographical, occupational, and socio-economic position and other socio-demographic variations.

Common rates and ratios used to measure health status at a population level are described elsewhere (see Table 3B.8). Each of these measures can be stratified by other variables in order to make comparisons across geographical, occupational, and socio-economic groupings.

Table 3B.8 Measures of health status

Type of measure	Reference
Mortality indices	Section 1A.1
Fertility indices	Section 1A.1
Life expectancy	Section 3A.7
Measures of disease burden (YLL, DALYs, QALYs)	Sections 1A.6, 1A.7, and 4D.5

3B.5 Routine notification and registration systems

Routine notification and registration systems for births, deaths, and specific diseases, including cancer and other morbidity registers.

Registration of births and deaths

Registration of deaths is covered in Section 3A.1.

Registration of births

Registration of births, including stillbirths, is a legal requirement in the United Kingdom. It must be done within 42 days of the birth, usually at the maternity unit before discharge or sometimes at a register office.

The following information is recorded:

- Place and date of the birth
- Name, surname, and sex of the baby
- Parents' names, surnames, and address(es)
- Places and dates of parents' birth
- Date of parents' marriage or civil partnership
- Parents' jobs
- Mother's maiden surname

Disease registers

Diseases registers contain details of all cases of the disease within a defined population (Table 3B.9). They often contain more extensive and reliable data on the disease than other data sources (e.g. date of diagnosis, treatment, survival).

ENG Examples of national and regional registers in England include the following:

- Cancer
- Child abuse
- Industrial diseases
- Congenital abnormalities

Cancer registers are discussed in further detail in Table 3B.10. There are local registers too (e.g. disease registers within a GP practice).

Table 3B.9 Advantages and disadvantages of information collated by registries

Advantages	Disadvantages
• Often almost complete • Standardised/systematic method for assigning categories (e.g. stage of cancer) • Detailed • Can often be used to calculate incidence, prevalence, and mortality	• Time lag until information available • Expensive to maintain the register • Difficult to assess completeness • Difficult to achieve completeness if voluntary • Can only be used for conditions where the diagnosis is very reliable

Table 3B.10 Regional cancer registers for every new diagnosis of cancer

Attribute	Description
Information recorded	Personal identifiers (needed in order to eliminate duplicates) Socio-economic characteristics Disease status (cancer type, stage) Treatment Outcomes
Collection, coding, and analysis	Sources for collection of information include cancer centres, treatment centres, hospices, private hospitals, cancer screening programmes, other cancer registers, general practices, nursing homes, and death certificates Cancers are coded using a system common to all the registries in the United Kingdom The ONS collates, analyses, and publishes data from the registers
Uses	Monitoring trends of incidence and survival for different cancers Comparing the epidemiology and quality of care in different areas of the United Kingdom

3B.6 Prescribing data and pharmacovigilance

Pharmacoepidemiology, including use of prescribing and pharmacy sales data; pharmacovigilance.

Prescribing data records information about the volumes, costs, and types of drugs prescribed and dispensed. These data can be useful for both **managerial** and **clinical** reasons, including the following:

- Cost containment—Prescription costs are rising; money spent on prescriptions means that less is available for other areas of healthcare.
- Monitoring adherence to guidelines (e.g. NICE).
- Detecting aberrant or inappropriate clinical performance (e.g. controlled drug prescriptions, use of antibiotics).
- Identification of adverse drug effects.
- Addressing local priorities (e.g. reduction of heart disease through prescribing drugs such as statins).
- Performance-related incentive payments (e.g. prescribing elements of QOF—see Section 3B.1).

Challenges

While prescribing data in England are currently accessible at a GP practice level and are useful for measuring costs and intra-practice variation, it is more difficult to measure the quality of prescribing at the individual level. Information on why a drug was prescribed or for whom it was prescribed is not yet available, and currently information can only be obtained through the laborious process of auditing individual patient records.

Sources of data

ENG Sources of prescribing data include prescribing analysis and cost (PACT) and ePACT, although there are plans to incorporate prescribing data into a richer national database incorporating primary care and secondary care data.

PACT

PACT data provide GPs and other prescribers with regular, reliable information about their NHS prescribing habits and costs. The information is based on prescriptions dispensed by pharmacists.

ePACT

This is an electronic system for pharmaceutical and prescribing advisors. It allows real-time, online analysis of the previous 5 years of prescribing data held on the NHS Prescribing Database. The data available include the following:

- Budgets and expenditure forecasts
- Costs and volumes of prescribing
- Prescribing totals by prescriber at all *British National Formulary* (BNF) levels
- Prescribing from the nurse and extended nurse formularies
- Patient list sizes
- Low-income scheme index scores for practices (released in May 2004)
- Average daily quantities and defined daily doses (DDDs)

Measuring prescribing activity

Various units are used for measuring the volume and cost of prescribed drugs (see Table 3B.11).

Prescribing units

Prescribing costs can vary across different organisations because of different prescribing practices, but also because of the features of the local population. As a result, it is not valid simply to use an average cost per patient as a measure of prescribing spend. In England, **prescribing units (PUs)** have been developed to take account of the fact that older patients have a greater need of medication. This allows comparisons of prescribing costs across areas with different age structures in their populations. Since 1983, PUs have been further refined into

ASTRO-PUs (age, sex, and temporary resident originated PUs): Take account of a wider range of demographic factors other than age in comparisons of prescribing or resource allocation decisions.

Table 3B.11 Units used for measuring prescribing volumes and costs

Unit	Description
Item	This is the number of prescription items listed on a prescription form. While easy to measure, caution is needed regarding repeat prescriptions. For example, a GP who writes monthly prescriptions will appear to prescribe more than a GP who prescribes quarterly—even though the total amount of drug is identical
Quantity	Number of tablets or millilitres, milligrams, etc. Strength of active ingredients: stronger active ingredients may require fewer milligrams for the same number of tablets Note that caution is needed regarding potency (e.g. fewer milligrams of one type of statin are needed to achieve a particular drop in blood cholesterol compared with another)
Net ingredient cost	This is the basic price of a drug. It can be used to measure the volume of similarly priced groups of drugs at equivalent doses. However, where there is a large price difference, it is not an accurate measure of use
Actual cost	This is calculated by taking the basic price of the prescription items, deducting the *National Average Discount*, and then adding an allowance for the container. Actual cost is used in Prescribing Monitoring Documents (PMDs)
Defined daily dose	These are based on maintenance doses and are not suitable for one-off doses. Note that the DDD is not the recommended dose nor is it necessarily a dose that a patient could practically receive. For example, simvastatin has a DDD of 15 mg but is available only in 10 or 20 mg tablets
Defined daily quantity	This is an England-specific system developed by the Prescribing Support Unit (PSU) and is equivalent to the DDD

STAR-PUs (specific therapeutic group age–sex weightings-related PUs): Units specific to different therapeutic areas which also take into account demographic factors.

Measuring adherence

The terms concordance, compliance, and adherence are sometimes used interchangeably to reflect the degree to which a patient takes the medicines they were prescribed. Horne and colleagues [7] provide definitions summarised in Table 3B.12.

Compliance may be calculated from a pharmacy database using the following:

- Medication possession ratio (MPR): Ratio of days of medication supplied to days in a time interval)
- Proportion of days covered (PDC): Number of days covered over a time interval)

The PDC differs from MPR in that it counts the current supply of medication before starting the next refill. Some authors believe that compliance may be overestimated by simply summing the number of days' supply because patients typically refill their medication before completing their current supply [8].

Pharmacovigilance

Pharmacovigilance is the study of how to detect, assess, understand, and prevent the adverse effects of medicines. In particular, it involves reducing the harms associated with side effects and effects resulting from the long-term use of a medication by using the processes described in Table 3B.13.

Table 3B.12 Terminology to describe medication use: Adherence, compliance, and concordance

Concept	Definition
Compliance	Extent to which the patient's behaviour matches the prescriber's recommendations Use of the term is declining because it implies a lack of patient involvement
Adherence	The extent to which the patient's behaviour matches agreed recommendations from the prescriber Adherence develops the definition of compliance by emphasising the need for agreement between the prescriber and the patient
Concordance	Extent to which the prescriber and patient agree on therapeutic decisions that incorporate their respective views Relatively new term, used predominantly in the United Kingdom

Table 3B.13 Processes involved in pharmacovigilance

Process	Description
Monitoring	Monitoring the use of medicines in everyday practice to identify previously unrecognised adverse effects or changes in the patterns of adverse effects
Risk assessment	Assessing the risks and benefits of medicines in order to determine what action, if any, is needed to improve their safety
Information provision	Providing information to healthcare professionals and patients to optimise safe and effective use of medicines
Measuring	Assessing the impact of any action taken

Information sources used for pharmacovigilance

A range of different national and international systems is used for pharmacovigilance, including the following:

- Spontaneous adverse drug reaction (ADR) reporting schemes, such as the **yellow card** and **black triangle** systems (see the following discussion)
- Clinical and epidemiological studies in the worldwide medical literature
- Information from pharmaceutical companies
- Information from worldwide regulatory authorities
- Morbidity and mortality databases

Information derived from any of these sources may

- Identify unexpected side effects
- Indicate that certain side effects occur more commonly than was previously believed
- Reveal that certain patient groups are more susceptible to particular problems than others

Such findings can lead to changes in the marketing authorisation of the medicine, including

- Restrictions in use
- Changes in the dose of the medicine
- Introduction of specific warnings about side effects in the product information

Yellow card scheme

UK The Medicines and Healthcare Products Regulatory Authority (MHRA) runs the United Kingdom's spontaneous adverse drug reaction reporting scheme, called the Yellow Card Scheme. Yellow cards are distributed to healthcare professionals, for example, as an appendix to the BNF. Through these cards, the MHRA receives reports of suspected adverse drug reactions from health professionals and patients.

Black triangle scheme

UK New medicines and vaccines are labelled with a black triangle symbol (▾) in the BNF and on all product information and advertisements. Health professionals are urged to report **any** suspected adverse reactions that might involve one of these products. For established medicines that are not marked with a black triangle, health professionals should report only **serious** or **unusual** suspected adverse reactions.

Risk minimisation

Occasionally, where the risks of a medicine are found to outweigh the benefits, the drug or even an entire drug class may be removed from the market. More commonly, the risk of a side effect may be avoided or reduced by the following:

- Including **warnings** in the product information or on the package labelling
- Restricting the indications for use of a medicine
- Changing the legal status of a medicine (e.g. by switching from pharmacy to prescription only)

Communication with healthcare professionals and patients

UK The MHRA communicates with healthcare professionals and patients to warn about adverse effects and to provide feedback of information. It does this through the following:

- **Patient Information Leaflets** (PILs) and **Summaries of Product Characteristics** (SPCs), which are updated when new safety issues are identified
- Urgent warnings about drug hazards via letters to all doctors and pharmacists
- MHRA and CSM regular drug safety bulletin, *'Current Problems in Pharmacovigilance'*, sent to doctors and pharmacists
- Fact sheets about major safety issues for both healthcare professionals and patients
- Safety alerts on the MHRA website

3B.7 Data linkage

Data linkage within and across datasets.

Data linkage is the process of matching information in one data source with information in another.

Methods

The simplest way to link two datasets is to use a unique identifier present in both datasets. In England, the NHS number is increasingly being used to link different health data sources (see Box 3B.3). An alternative is the National Insurance number, which is now issued at birth.

Where a unique identifier is not available in both datasets, other information such as patient name, date of birth, and postcode may be used (see Section 3A.2 and Boxes 3B.3 and 3B.4). However, this approach may lead to problems when such data are recorded in different ways or where there are errors. Other more complicated methods may be used in these instances, for example, fuzzy matching or probability matching, whereby several fields from each datasets are checked in order to match records based on similarities.

Uses

By linking two databases, public health specialists can derive useful extra information and conduct additional analyses, such as the following:

- Linking HES databases to mortality data in order to determine the outcomes of hospital activity
- Linking primary care data and secondary care data to study care pathways
- Linking healthcare data and educational data to examine associations between education and health

Limitations

There are a number of limitations that must be considered prior to linking two data sources, such as the following:

- Difficulties linking data where no unique identifier exists.
- Difficulties linking historical data.
- Inconsistencies in styles and coding methods across datasets.
- May lead to data becoming identifiable (so-called **jigsaw attack**).
- Patients may have only consented for data to have been collected for a specific purpose.

Examples of data linkage

See Boxes 3B.4 through 3B.6, for examples of how data linkage may be used to improve public health.

Box 3B.3 Oxford Record Linkage Study

One of the earliest record linkage studies was the Oxford Record Linkage Study (ORLS), which started in 1963. The ORLS consists of computerised abstracts of records of all types of hospital inpatient care and records of births and deaths in the Oxford region. When data collection ceased in 1999, all patient identifiers were removed from the database. The dataset includes 10 million records relating to over 5 million people.

Box 3B.4 ENG Linkage in the NHS—*Connecting for health*

Connecting for health was a national programme for improving the information technology of the NHS to ensure that the appropriate information was available to any clinician regardless of geography. One of its aims was to ensure that patients no longer had to be asked the same information every time they saw a different health professional. *Connecting for Health* involved the development of several information systems, each containing patient information. The intention was to link these in order to provide a complete record (see also Box 3C.5).

Box 3B.5 AUS Data linkage in Australia

All Australian states and territories have data linkage units, which link health and other related data at the person level using secure, privacy-preserving methods. In addition, the Population Health Research Network is developing Australia's first national data linkage network.

Sources: Secure Unified Research Environment, Australian health data linkage units, Accessed online July 24, 2014 at https://www.sure.org.au/resources/australian-health-data-linkage-units; Population Health Research Network, Accessed online July 24, 2014 at http://www.phrn.org.au/.

Box 3B.6 SCOT Data linkage in Scotland

In Scotland, ISD holds two main linked datasets, the SMR linked dataset and the maternity and neonatal linked dataset, which allow analyses to be conducted ranging from simple patient-based counts to complex epidemiological and survival analyses.

SMR linked dataset

This dataset includes all hospital discharge records submitted between 1980 to the present day from non-obstetric specialties, as well as cancer and death registration records (SMR01, SMR04, SMR06 and GROS deaths records).

Maternity and neonatal linked dataset

This dataset brings together the obstetric histories of mothers delivering in Scotland over the past 25 years and links this with morbidity and mortality outcomes relating to their offspring. This linked dataset also has been used to produce a system which monitors and reports the incidence of congenital anomalies across Scotland (SMR02, SMR11, Scottish birth record, stillbirth, and neonatal deaths records).

ISD also regularly produces linkages that include two other datasets, namely, the Scottish Health Survey and the Scottish Longitudinal Study.

Scottish health survey

The Scottish Health Survey provides a detailed picture of the health of the Scottish population in private households. ISD holds a minimum linked dataset (the Scottish Health Survey and the SMR linked dataset).

Scottish longitudinal study

A large-scale linkage study created from a variety of administrative data, including data from the 1991 and 2001 censuses, vital events (births, deaths, marriages, etc.) and migration data (see http://www.lscs.ac.uk/sls/).

Source: ISD Scotland, Medical Record Linkage, ISD, NHS National Services Scotland, 2010. Available from: http://www.isdscotland.org/Products-and-Services/Medical-Record-Linkage/Linked-Data/.

3C

Applications of Health Services Information

Health service information is used in a variety of ways to improve health. It is used by commissioners planning, purchasing, and evaluating health services; by researchers and public health specialists for epidemiological analysis; and by regulators and auditors to identify unusual or substandard care. This chapter describes how the types of information described in Section 1 and elsewhere in Section 3 may usefully be linked for such purposes. The strengths and limitations of health service data are considered, together with some of the technologies used for their manipulation.

3C.1 Use of information for health service planning and evaluation

Health information is essential for health service planning and evaluation. Without it, services would be unresponsive to changes in circumstances, and it would be difficult or impossible to make meaningful predictions or to increase efficiency through analysis.

Information for healthcare planning

Data can be used to assess changes in health, and in healthcare, over time. These trends can then be used to help forecast demand for services in the future (see Table 3C.1).

Routine data sources

ENG See also Sections 1A.1 and 3B.1.

A large number of population measures can be obtained from routinely collected data. Several such indices are published annually by the DH and the Health and Social Care Information **Centre**, with the statistics made available at national, regional, and local levels. Some of the principal sources of **data** used for health services planning are summarised in Table 3C.2 and are described in greater depth in Section 3B.1.

Performance management

Performance management indicators are used to identify whether services are delivering against a dimension agreed to be of importance for that service. In particular, these indicators are useful to commissioners and managers for highlighting inadequate performance or potential problems with service delivery. Where problems are identified, more detailed work is usually required to investigate the issue and identify the underlying causes.

For further details, see Sections 5C.3 and 5E.

Table 3C.1 Information required to plan healthcare services

Planning step	Details
1. Healthcare **needs**	The identification of health needs and priorities involves epidemiological, qualitative, and comparative methods to describe the health problems of a population These needs can be **absolute** (e.g. quantifying the numbers of people with a particular condition, dying of that condition, receiving treatment) or **comparative** (e.g. inequalities in health outcomes, access to health services) **Population trends** (e.g. age distribution, relative deprivation) will affect the population's needs, and these can also be monitored from routine data (see Section 1C.1)
2. Healthcare **priorities**	The next step of the process is to **determine priorities** based on the most effective potential use of resources This analysis is achieved by reviewing **routinely collected data**, both national and local, conducting a search of the published and grey **literature**, establishing current best practice as defined in national guidelines, and considering the impact of **workforce** trends
3. Healthcare **review**	This step begins with a description of the **existing service**, in terms of its utilisation and distribution An analysis is then undertaken of the **differences** between the population's needs and the existing services in order to identify deficient and superfluous services

Table 3C.2 ENG + WA Examples of healthcare

Measure	Example
Mortality	ONS data from death certificates
Serious morbidity	HES data Cancer registers
Minor morbidity	GP consultation rates
General health	Census (from 2011 for self-reported, long-standing illness)
Deprivation	Indices of multiple deprivation
Demographics	Census (age, sex, ethnicity)

Health service evaluation

Health service evaluation is covered in greater detail in Sections 1A.9 and 1C.5

Routinely collected health service data may be used to evaluate health services. Health service activity may be assessed in terms of both **process** and **outcome** measures. Health service evaluations typically consider a number of dimensions. The **impact** and **cost** of services are almost always evaluated. However, service quality should also be assessed through an analysis of **acceptability** to service users, **access** to care, and the impact of the service on **health inequalities**.

An example of how health service evaluations can be conducted using routine data is shown in Box 3C.1.

Evaluations may be **formative** or **summative**: see Table 3C.3.

Box 3C.1 Summative evaluation using routinely collected data: Does the use of Marie Curie Nursing Services affect patients' place of death and their hospital use at the end of life?

The Nuffield Trust evaluated the impact of Marie Curie services on patient outcomes and service use, using only routine hospital and social care data. The study addressed two questions:

1. Were people who received this type of care more likely to die at home?
2. Did the service reduce unplanned hospital use?

The researchers conducted an observational study, using the pseudonymous records of 30,000 patients who received Marie Curie services, which were compared with the pseudonymous records of **matched controls** (i.e. people with similar demographic and morbidity characteristics but who did not receive any Marie Curie services).

The researchers found that a greater proportion of the people who received Marie Curie services died at home compared with controls (76.7% versus 34.9%) and also that their use of all forms of hospital care was lower compared to the controls

This type of evaluation was completed in a comparatively short period of time (months as opposed to the years that would have been required for a randomised controlled study) and did not require any additional data to be collected

Source: Nuffield Trust, 2012, The impact of the Marie Curie Nursing Service on place of death and hospital use at the end of life. Accessed online July 24, 2014 at http://www.nuffieldtrust.org.uk/sites/files/nuffield/publication/121114_marie_curie_summary-final_0.pdf.

Table 3C.3 Formative and summative evaluations and the use of routine data

Type of evaluation	Description	Example using routine data
Formative	Assesses whether a problem is occurring while the activities are **being developed**	Weekly reporting of QOF data by general practices to improve performance (e.g. by reporting back data regularly on children not immunised, practices can identify children that missed their appointments and re-invite them or identify where immunisation not correctly recorded and update the system)
Summative	This focuses on the impact and the effectiveness of an **established** programme	Evaluation of the effectiveness of a bowel screening programme to detect early tumours using information from cancer registries about the stage of cancer at diagnosis

3C.2 Specification and uses of information systems

An information system is a process in which raw data are transformed into meaningful information (see Figure 3C.1). This process begins with an organisational activity to generate the input, followed by data transmission, storage, and manipulation involving IT and ultimately the decisions and changes that are made according to the output.

Specification of information systems

The specification of an information system is the set of requirements agreed between the user and the developer of the system. In modern information systems, information creation and processing require a high level of engagement of all users during the developmental stages.

Uses of information systems

Information technology is used in the delivery of care both for primary purposes (e.g. recording clinical information and delivering guidance to clinicians) and for secondary purposes (e.g. for planning, analysing, and regulating healthcare). See Table 3C.4.

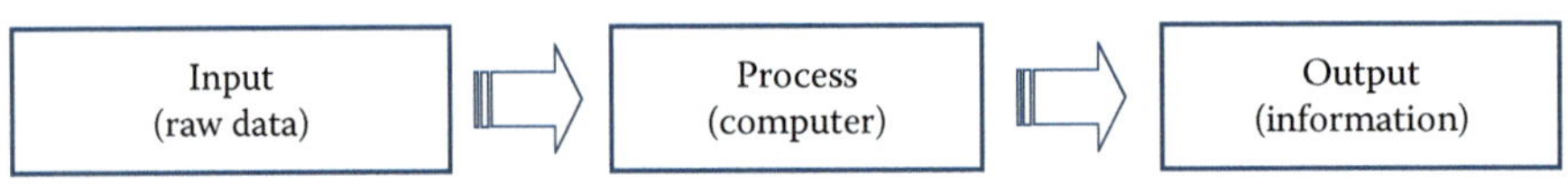

Figure 3C.1 Simple diagram of an information system.

Table 3C.4 Uses of information systems

Type of use	Description
Clinical information	Ensuring that healthcare professionals have access to the relevant clinical information about their patients (e.g. clinical notes, laboratory results, radiology images, prescriptions)
Clinical guidance	Providing healthcare professionals with online access to current relevant guidance and evidence about effective treatments
Aggregation	Analysing aggregate data for the purposes of monitoring quality, planning new services, and supporting research activity
Security	Ensuring that confidential information is not lost, destroyed, misappropriated, or corrupted
Exchange	Exchanging information securely and rapidly
Linkage	Linking different types of data from multiple sources to facilitate research
Analysis	Analysing, displaying, reporting, and mapping data
Regulation	Ensuring that data conform to national standards, including clinical terminology

3C.3 Common measures of health service provision and usage

Health service **provision** refers to the supply of healthcare (buildings, staff, services), while **access** refers to the ability of patients to utilise healthcare (opening hours, demand, capacity, travel times, language, and cultural barriers). Health service usage is a complex product of provision and access and is affected by a population's need for health services. The concepts of **use** and **need** are explored in relation to equity in Sections 1C.11 and 4C.1.

Measures of health service provision

A range of indicators may be used to assess the provision of primary and secondary care services (see Table 3C.5).

Measures of health service usage

Measures of health service use can be valuable in assessing the quality and appropriateness of healthcare. Indicators of health service utilisation in primary and secondary care are shown in Table 3C.6. See also Section 1C.3.

Examples of service usage information in England are shown in Box 3C.2.

Table 3C.5 Indicators of service provision

Primary care	Secondary care
GPs, practice nurses, community midwives, etc., per 1000 population	Consultants per 1000 population Beds per 1000 population
Practice list size per GP Average distance to nearest health centre	Average distance to nearest specialist centre (e.g. nearest dialysis unit)
Waiting times for GP appointments	Waiting list for elective surgery

Table 3C.6 Indicators of health service utilisation

Primary care	Secondary care
Consultations per patient Secondary and tertiary care referral rates	Hospital episodes • Emergency or scheduled/elective • Outpatient appointments or inpatient stays • Readmission rates
Time spent with practitioner	Length of stay
General practice list sizes	Bed occupancy
Prescriptions: • Number of items • Cost • Type of medication	No comparable data
Preventive health services: • Screening uptake rates • Scheduled immunisation uptake rates	No comparable data

Box 3C.2 ENG Practice profiles: Service usage information to improve the quality of primary care

The Network of Public Health Observatories produces summaries on GP practice populations and the performance of the practice spanning a number of domains. These summaries allow different practices in a local area to be compared with each other based on their performance

The indicators reported in these summaries include the following:

- Characteristics of patients that may affect their use of primary care services
- Indicators that may be affected by GP clinical behaviour
- Prevalence of different diseases
- Secondary care use

The website enables these data to be presented in various ways and compared against local and national benchmarks, as well as peer practices matched according to deprivation decile.

Source: Public Health England, National General Practice Profiles, Accessed online July 24, 2014 at http://www.apho.org.uk/PracProf/.

3C.4 Mathematical modelling in health service planning

The uses of mathematical modelling techniques in health service planning.

Modelling is the process of analysing and simplifying complex, real-world situations using mathematics. This process enables observations to be analysed using statistical or other analysis so that they can then be used to predict events or to provide solutions. A feedback process allows the model to be refined iteratively. See Figure 3C.2.

Limitations of models

The usefulness of a model may be constrained by the following:

- The availability of data
- The quality of data
- Incorrect assumptions incorporated into the model or the statistical analysis
- The use of inappropriate or flawed techniques

Advantages of mathematical modelling

Used properly, mathematical modelling can assist in healthcare planning by

- Supporting the decision-making process
- Dealing with complexity (both complex organisations and complex activities)
- Creating alternative scenarios
- Modelling an issue at any level of detail
- Creating short-term, medium-term, and long-term plans

Uses of mathematical models

Models have a wide range of uses in public health, including the following:

- Modelling the costs and benefits of different interventions as part of an economic evaluation (see Section 4D.5)
- Depicting different possible outcomes and their probabilities in order to aid decision-making (both clinical and managerial decisions)
- Modelling communicable disease outbreaks
- Predicting future trends in diseases based on past trends and other variables
- Predictive risk modelling (e.g. to predict increases in service demand—see the following discussion)

Predictive risk modelling

Predictive risk modelling is a technique that has been used in the financial and banking

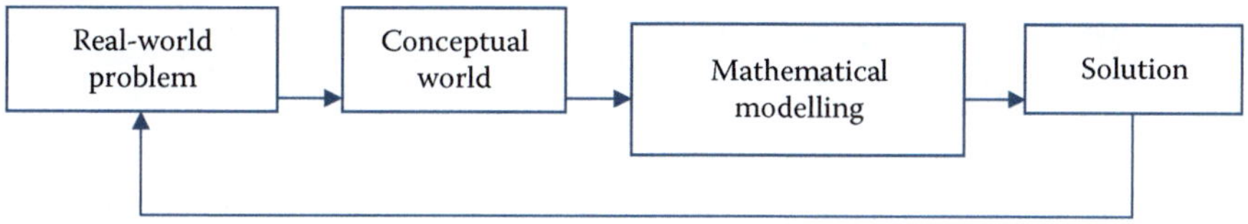

Figure 3C.2 Simple concept of mathematical modelling. (Courtesy of Professor E. Carson and Dr A. Roudsari, Centre for Health Informatics School of Informatics, City University, London, UK.)

sectors for many years and has more recently been applied to healthcare. Predictive modelling involves analysing linked, pseudonymous historical data to determine the relationship between a range of independent ('predictor') variables and a dependent ('outcome') variable of interest. The dependent variable is typically a **Triple Fail** event (i.e. an event that is a marker of suboptimal care, is costly, and is unpleasant to the patient). Examples of such events include unplanned hospital admissions and readmissions, nursing home admissions, and non-accidental injury in children.

Predictive models may be built using a range of techniques including **multiple regression, decision-tree analysis**, and **neural networks**. Once the algorithm has been built, it is used to process dependent variables in contemporary data in order to make predictions about the future. There are several prerequisites to implementing a predictive risk modelling programme (see Table 3C.7). An example of such a programme is shown in Box 3C.3.

Table 3C.7 Prerequisites to implementing a health intervention based on predictive risk modelling

Prerequisites	
Sufficient volumes and breadth of **historical data** must be available to build the algorithm The data sources must be **routinely available** and frequently updated It must be possible to **link** these data sources	Algorithm
There must be an adverse, costly, and unpleasant **outcome recorded** within one of the data sources An **efficacious intervention** must be available to mitigate the risk of the adverse outcome to be predicted The intervention must be **cost-effective**, considering the positive predictive value of the algorithm for chosen level of risk	Intervention

Box 3C.3 ENG Example: Predictive risk algorithms

In 2005, the NHS has commissioned the King's Fund and partners to develop a series of algorithms that predict which people in a population are at highest risk of future unplanned hospital admissions. Advance predictions are needed because of the rapid turnover of the group of patients who are frequently admitted to hospital.

The developers used several years' worth of linked, pseudonymous historical data to build the algorithms [14]. The data sources included inpatient, outpatient, A&E, and GP practice data. These were linked using encrypted NHS numbers, and the outcome variable chosen was an unplanned hospital admission in the next 12 months. The algorithms allow GPs to rank their population in terms of risk of unplanned hospitalisation, and an 'upstream' intervention (e.g. case management by a community matron or admission to a *virtual ward*) is offered to the patients at highest risk.

Analogous models have since been developed to predict the risk of starting intensive social care [15] and the risk of readmission to hospital within 30 days of discharge [16].

3C.5 Indices of needs for and outcome of services

An index summarises a set of data, which might be derived from multiple sources, in order to **rank** an organisation or area according to a **particular characteristic**. Indices may be used to describe various aspects of a health service, including health service **needs** and **outcomes**.

Indices of health service needs

In order to establish the needs for a health service, a broad range of indices should be collated, based on a variety of quantitative and qualitative data. These indices should then be analysed, as part of an HNA (see Section 4C.1). Examples of the types of indices that are helpful for establishing health service needs are outlined in Table 3C.8

Service outcome indices

Some indices used to describe different healthcare services are listed in Table 3C.9.

Output indices

The outputs of a health service may be weighted in a number of ways.

Table 3C.8 Examples of indices related to health needs

Index	Description
Health Poverty Index (HPI)	Collates data on three domains in order to highlight health inequalities according to geographical areas or ethnic groups. These domains are as follows: • **Root causes** (e.g. education, income, social capital) • **Intervening factors** (e.g. lifestyle, effective preventative healthcare) • **Situation of health** (e.g. premature mortality, access to secondary care)
Mental Illness Needs Index (MINI)	Aims to predict mental health needs at a small area level using past admissions as well as indicators of deprivation, overcrowding, and unemployment and underemployment
IMD	Scores the level of deprivation in an area (lower SOA level) based on income, employment, health, education, barriers to housing and services, crime, and the living environment (see Section 1C.4) [17]

Table 3C.9 Examples of indices related to healthcare services

Type of index	Description
Output index	How much of each service is being produced (e.g. number of patients treated)
Welfare index	Value to final users (e.g. degree of pain reduction)
Performance management index	How the services are being produced (e.g. extent to which doctors use appropriate treatment)
Composite index	Synthesis of the previous three indices. With multiple services, weights are added to each service, often combining indicators that are measured in non-comparable units

Ideal value-weighted output index

This index has two fundamental features:

1. A value attached to each output that reflects its **relative contribution** to health outcomes
2. The values of **other important characteristics** of healthcare (such as the process of care delivery)

A lack of health outcome data often makes the calculation of this index unfeasible.

Cost-weighted activity/output index

This index weighs separate activities or outputs according to the costs of providing them. Decision-makers who use this index are therefore equating the costs with the benefits of the service provided. There are many arguments for and against this assumption:

- Some commentators might argue that doctors do, or should do, whatever is best for their patient regardless of the cost.
- Others may argue that such decisions should be made in a more explicit way, based on cost-benefit analyses.

Performance management indices

Some features of an ideal performance index are listed in Table 3C.10, and an example is given in Box 3C.4.

Composite indices

Composite indices of healthcare performance are constructed by aggregating several underlying individual performance measures. They are used worldwide to rank healthcare organisations or systems (see Box 3C.4). They are designed to be easy to interpret and present the 'big picture'. However, it is important to pay attention to methodological issues in their construction; otherwise, misleading conclusions may be drawn.

Table 3C.10 Features of an ideal performance index

Fit for purpose	Choice of index should depend on the issue being addressed
Patient well-being	A welfare index is required to measure the patient experience
Local information	Performance indices are required at a very local level (e.g. at the level of a GP practice, hospital ward, or hospital department)

Box 3C.4 Example: The World Health Report 2000—*Health systems: improving performance*

In this report, the WHO ranked the overall health system performance of the world's healthcare systems according to an index composed of five dimensions:

1. Overall population health
2. Health inequalities
3. Health system responsiveness
4. Distribution of responsiveness
5. Distribution of financial burden for the health system

France was ranked top and Sierra Leone bottom. The UK was ranked 18th; Ireland 19th; Australia came 32nd; the United States 37th; New Zealand 41st; and South Africa 175th.

Source: Reproduced from World Health Organisation, World health report 2013: Research for universal health coverage, Accessed online July 24, 2014 at www.who.int/whr/en.

3C.6 Issues with routine health information

Strengths, uses, interpretation, and limitations of routine health information.

Routine data are derived from automated or semi-automated, ongoing, data collection systems. They include large local and national databases associated with health and social services. Data are collected irrespective of the procedure or outcome. Examples include HES, deaths, births, statutory notifications of infectious diseases, and cancer registry data.

Uses of routine data

The uses of routine data are summarised in Table 3C.11.

Strengths and weaknesses of routine data

Some of the principal strengths and weaknesses of routine data are summarised in Table 3C.12.

Improving routine data

To avoid waste and to maximise the use of resources, it is important to improve the reliability, validity, and completeness of routine data (see Table 3C.13). There should therefore be a good reason to **begin** or to **stop** collecting each item of data.

Table 3C.11 Uses of routine data

Type of use	Examples
Assessment of **burden**	Incidence/prevalence of a disease or risk factor Mortality Disease severity Health needs
Drawing **comparisons**	Time trends Benchmarking against other areas Comparisons within population subgroups (including inequalities) Identifying unwarranted variation
Health services	Assessing current provision Planning Commissioning Service improvement
Research and **evaluation**	Service evaluation Research Clinical audit Performance management

Table 3C.12 Strengths and weaknesses of routine data

Strengths	Weaknesses
Readily available Low cost Often relatively up to date Large population coverage Collection usually spans a significant time period Breadth and diversity to explore unexpected avenues Useful for initial assessment: provides baseline data on expected levels of health/disease	**Incompleteness** • Statutory returns do not guarantee completeness (e.g. even meningococcal septicaemia is only 70% notified) • Poor levels of ethnicity coding **Bias** • If healthcare providers that submit data are systematically different from providers that do not, then the collated data may be biased • Political interference may bias what data are collected or not collected and how they are presented Poor collation, presentation, and analysis More information on processes than on health status, patient experience, and outcomes Lack of uniformity in data structures, coding systems, and definitions Desired data may not be available at the required geographical level

Table 3C.13 Ways of improving the quality of routine data

Method	Details
Computerised data collation and analysis	Improves the accuracy and timeliness of the data
Feedback	Giving feedback to data providers about their data and its quality is a virtuous circle
Presentation	Data should be presented in a variety of ways which are meaningful to policymakers, media, professionals, and the public
Training	Training the coders and clinicians who are responsible for data entry, in the use of standard definitions, terminology, etc.

3C.7 Information technology and healthcare provision

Use of information technology in the processing and analysis of health service information and in support of the provision of healthcare.

Some important features of electronic communication are as follows:

- Faster and more varied methods for communicating (e.g. email, videoconferencing, and mobile telecommunications)
- Near-instant access to vast amounts of information (e.g. through the Internet)
- Emergence of new forms of inequality (the so-called **digital divide**)

For public health specialists, therefore, information and communications technology (ICT) presents both opportunities and new challenges. Information underpins the following:

- Assessment of health **needs**
- Development of health **strategies**
- Monitoring of **progress**

Better communication technology offers opportunities to improve the patient experience (e.g. remote consultations) and the sharing and dissemination of knowledge between patients and all professionals and organisations involved in improving the health of the public. New technologies can offer public health practitioners rapid access to the following:

- Data (from international comparative data down to local and individual-level data)
- Networks of healthcare professionals (e.g. managed public health networks)
- The public's views on health service development (e.g. sentiment analysis of social network data)
- Practice guidance (e.g. electronic libraries of evidence, peer-reviewed research, and practice guidance such as Cochrane and NICE)

Health informatics

The field of health informatics is concerned with the application of information technology to the acquisition, processing, interpreting, storage, transmission, and retrieval of health and healthcare-related data. Its underlying purpose is to facilitate and improve healthcare delivery, education, management, and research.

Health informatics tools include computers, clinical guidelines, diagnostic and monitoring equipment, and information and communication systems. In practice, health informatics may be broadly divided into the following:

- Public health informatics
- Clinical informatics (including nursing informatics, dental informatics)
- Bioinformatics and pharmacoinformatics

Applications

The uses of informatics within healthcare are expanding rapidly. Current applications include the following:

- Patient monitoring
- Clinical care
- GISs used in public health surveillance
- Integrating data sources for improved decision-making
- Electronic health records
- Remote consultations

An example of a large-scale information technology project in England is described in Box 3C.5.

Box 3C.5 ENG NHS Connecting for Health

'Connecting for Health' was formed in 2005 with the responsibility for delivering the NHS National Programme for IT. Initially, this was planned to be one of the world's largest IT systems; however, escalating costs meant that many aspects of the programme were ultimately abandoned.

Aspects that were completed include the following:

- Emergency care summaries (summary care records)
- Electronic prescription service
- NHS number
- NHS mail
- Picture and Archiving Communications Systems (PACS) for radiological images
- Choose and Book (electronic appointment booking system)

3C.8 Principles of information governance

Information governance involves ensuring that the collection, storage, processing, and sharing of information within an organisation adheres to legal standards and best practice guidelines. Healthcare organisations are responsible for ensuring that staff regularly complete information governance training.

Areas covered include the following [19]:

- Data protection and confidentiality
- Information security
- Information quality
- Health and care records management
- Corporate information

Laws and standards

ENG A range of standards and laws relating to information governance by healthcare organisations include the following [20]:

- The Data Protection Act 1998
- The Freedom of Information Act 2000
- The common law duty of confidence
- The international information security standard (ISO/IEC 27002: 2005)
- The NHS Care Record Guarantee for England
- The Confidentiality NHS Code of Practice
- The Social Care Record Guarantee for England

Data protection

UK Currently, in the United Kingdom, the confidentiality of patients' information is protected by the Data Protection Act 1998. This contains eight principles, which state that the data must be

1. **Processed** fairly and lawfully
2. **Obtained** and used only for specified and lawful purposes
3. **Adequate**, relevant, and not excessive
4. **Accurate** and, where necessary, kept up to date
5. Kept for no longer than necessary
6. **Processed** in accordance with the individual's rights (as defined)
7. Kept **secure**
8. **Transferred** only to countries that offer adequate data protection

IRE Similar principles apply in Ireland through the Data Protection Acts of 1988 and 2003. The Data Protection Commissioner provides information and guidance and ensures compliance with the legislation by the keepers of personal data. Responsibility rests with data controllers (i.e. the official who decides what information is to be collected or stored, to what use it is put, and when it should be deleted or altered). Data controllers in public bodies and organisations specified in the 1988 Act (such as banks, insurance companies, and those who keep personal data of a sensitive nature) are required to register with the commissioner.

Data protection requirements in the United Kingdom and Ireland may well change as a result of the EU Data Protection Directive (2012) [21,22], which seeks to harmonise data protection regulations across the EU. Once the directive is agreed, European member states will need to incorporate the directive into national law.

AUS Current privacy legislation in Australia provides for sensitive information about an individual to be collected without that individual's consent only when all three of the following criteria are met:

1. The information is necessary for research relevant to public health, or the compilation or analysis of public health statistics, or the management or monitoring of a health service.
2. The purpose cannot be served by collection of non-identified information.
3. It is impractical to seek the consent of individuals.

Australian states and territories have their own legislation, which gives protection to people whose work requires them to deal with identified information (e.g. cancer registry staff, communicable disease control officers).

NZ In New Zealand, the main legislation and codes covering the privacy of personal information are as follows:

- The **Privacy Commissioners Act 1991** which established the office of privacy commissioner and the legal requirement for data matching.
- The **Privacy of Information Act 1993** which focuses on good personal information handling practices and applies to almost every person, business, and organisation in New Zealand. It includes 12 information privacy principles covering collection, holding, use and disclosure of personal information, and the use of unique identifiers. The act also gives the privacy commissioner the power to issue codes of practice, specifies complaints mechanisms, and specifies rules governing data matching.
- The **Health Information Privacy Code 1994** which specifies a code of practice for the health sector regarding the collection, use, holding and disclosure of personal health information (i.e. that relates to identifiable individuals), access to health information, and the assignment of unique identifiers. For the health sector, this code takes the place of the information privacy principles in the act. It applies to all levels of the health system from large institutions to sole practitioners.

Caldicott guardianship

WA The original Caldicott report, published in 1997, found that compliance with data protection statutes was variable. As a result, the DH in England and the Welsh government established a register of Caldicott guardians. Every NHS and social care institution must appoint a senior member of staff to take responsibility for protecting patient-identifiable information.

The other Caldicott recommendations [23] were that NHS organisations should

- Develop **protocols** to manage the sharing of patient information with other institutions
- Permit access to patient information only to employees who **need to know** that specific information
- Review and **justify** all uses of patient information
- Instil a **culture** of data protection through training, database design, etc.

Similar arrangements for protection of patient confidentiality exist in Scotland.

Electronic data storage

UK The main information security standards that apply across the United Kingdom are BS7799 and IEC 61508 [24].

BS7799

Part 1 of this British standard, known as the *'Code of Practice for Information Security Management'*, provides guidance on **best practices** in information security management. Part 2, the *'Specification for Information Security Management Systems'*, is the **standard** against which an organisation's security management systems are assessed and certified. It has since been revised and now exists in the form of ISO/IEC 27001:2005.

IEC 61508

This standard of the **International Electrotechnical Commission** contains requirements for ensuring that computer systems are designed, operated, and maintained in ways that have sufficient integrity. Section 3 sets out the requirements on computer suppliers for new equipment.

Confidentiality

Given that healthcare workers often have access to personal information, one of the most relevant areas of clinical governance is confidentiality. The Caldicott principles provide guidelines as to how confidential data should be managed:

1. Justify the purpose(s) of using confidential information.
2. Only use it when absolutely necessary.
3. Use the minimum that is required.
4. Access should be on a strict need-to-know basis.
5. Everyone must understand his or her responsibilities.
6. Understand and comply with the law.

References

1. Health and Social Care Information Centre. General practice extraction service. Accessed online July 24, 2014 at http://www.ic.nhs.uk/gpes.
2. Health and Social Care Information Centre. Calculating Quality Reporting Service (CQRS). Accessed online July 24, 2014 at http://www.connectingforhealth.nhs.uk/systemsandservices/cqrs.
3. The Clinical Practice Research Datalink. Accessed online July 24, 2014 at http://www.cprd.com/intro.asp.
4. Welsh Government. Welsh health survey. Accessed online July 24, 2014 at http://www.wales.gov.uk/topics/statistics/theme/health-survey/?lang=en.
5. Sankoh, O. and Byass, P. (2012) The INDEPTH Network: Filling vital gaps in global epidemiology. *Int J Epidemiol* 41(3), 579–588. http://ije.oxfordjournals.org/content/41/3/579.full.pdf+html.
6. World Health Organisation. The international classification of disease 11th revision due by 2017. Accessed online July 24, 2014 at http://www.who.int/classifications/icd/revision/en/index.html.
7. Horne, R., Weinman, J., Barber, N., Elliott, R., and Morgan, M. (2005) Concordance, adherence and compliance in medicine taking. NCCSDO. Accessed online August 16, 2014 at http://www.nets.nihr.ac.uk.
8. Scott Leslie R. (n.d.) Calculating medication compliance, adherence, and persistence in administrative pharmacy claims databases. Accessed online August 16, 2014 at www.wuss.org.
9. Secure Unified Research Environment. Australian health data linkage units. Accessed online July 24, 2014 at https://www.sure.org.au/resources/australian-health-data-linkage-units.
10. Population Health Research Network. Accessed online July 24, 2014 at http://www.phrn.org.au/.
11. ISD Scotland, Medical Record Linkage, ISD, NHS National Services Scotland (2010) Available from: http://www.isdscotland.org/Products-and-Services/Medical-Record-Linkage/Linked-Data/.
12. Nuffield Trust (2012). The impact of the Marie Curie Nursing Service on place of death and hospital use at the end of life. Accessed online July 24, 2014 at http://www.nuffieldtrust.org.uk/sites/files/nuffield/publication/121114_marie_curie_summary-final_0.pdf.
13. Public Health England. National General Practice Profiles. Accessed online July 24, 2014 at http://www.apho.org.uk/PracProf/.
14. Billings, J., Dixon, J., Mijanovich, T., and Wennberg, D. (2006) Case finding for patients at risk of readmission to hospital: Development of algorithm to identify high risk patients. *BMJ* 333(7563), 327.
15. Bardsley, M., Billings, J., Dixon, J., Georghiou, T., Lewis, G.H., and Steventon, A. (2011) Predicting who will use intensive social care: Case finding tools based on linked health and social care data. *Age Ageing* 40(2), 265–270.

16. Billings, J., Blunt, I., Steventon, A., Georghiou, T., Lewis, G., and Bardsley, M. (2012) Development of a predictive model to identify inpatients at risk of readmission within 30 days of discharge (PARR-30). *BMJ Open* 2(4).

17. Data.gov.uk. English Indices of Deprivation 2010. Accessed online July 24, 2014 http://data.gov.uk/dataset/index-of-multiple-deprivation.

18. World Health Organisation. World health report 2013: Research for universal health coverage. Accessed online July 24, 2014 at www.who.int/whr/en.

19. Health and Social Care Information Centre. Information governance. Accessed online July 24, 2014 at http://systems.hscic.gov.uk/infogov.

20. http://www.connectingforhealth.nhs.uk/systemsandservices/infogov/igfaqs.

21. Saracci, R., Olsen, J., Seniori-Costantini, A., and West, R. (2012) Epidemiology and the planned new Data Protection Directive of the European Union: A symposium report. *Publ Health*, 126(3), 253–255. http://www.sciencedirect.com/science/article/pii/S003335061100401X.

22. Wikipedia. The data protection directive. Accessed online July 24, 2014 at http://en.wikipedia.org/wiki/Data_Protection_Directive; International Epidemiology Association. A new EU directive for data protection in Europe. Accessed online July 24, 2014 at http://ieaweb.org/2010/12/a-new-eudirective-for-data-protection-in-europe/.

23. Walker, P. (1999) Protecting and using patient information: A manual for Caldicott Guardians. London, UK: Department of Health. Available online at www.dh.gov.uk/assetRoot/04/06/81/36/04068136.pdf.

24. Knott, L. (2006) Patient UK: Records and computers. www.patient.co.uk/showdoc/40000769.

Section 4

MEDICAL SOCIOLOGY, SOCIAL POLICY, AND HEALTH ECONOMICS

Public health is concerned with generating and using high-quality evidence to formulate credible health advice. However, both lay and professional behaviours often diverge from scientific evidence or professional guidance.

Two disciplines help explain what people actually do and why. **Sociology** describes the rules and processes of groups such as communities, cultures, and organisations. **Economics** provides insight into how decisions are made in a world with scarce resources and infinite needs.

Section 4 explores different concepts of health and the factors that underlie the ways in which people seek and use healthcare. The distinctions between equity and equality are discussed, together with their relevance to health policy. Finally, the section on health economics provides the background and core principles of the discipline, which should provide public health specialists with the insight needed to lobby effectively for more equitable and cost-effective healthcare provision.

4A

Health and Illness

Concepts of health, well-being, and illness and the aetiology of illness.

Achieving health and well-being in the population is the primary goal for public health specialists, yet the definition of these concepts is contested. Similarly, people's reaction to illness varies between cultures. Aside from providing a number of definitions of health and illness, this chapter also discusses some preconceptions of health and illness including the norms and behaviours that are tacitly expected of people who are ill (the **sick role** and the **social role** of illness) as well as society's treatment of people that do not conform to those expectations (**deviance** and **stigma**). Finally, the chapter considers how personal characteristics and a person's position in society affect whether and how they seek help for their symptoms.

4A.1 Human behaviour

The theoretical perspectives and methods of inquiry of the sciences concerned with human behaviour.

The social sciences aim to understand the attitudes, motivations, and behaviours of human social behaviour and why these change over time. Society is a group of interacting people who share a geographical region, a sense of common identity or a common culture. As such, it is more than an aggregate of individuals. The social sciences encompass the fields of study listed in Table 4A.1.

These disciplines are of importance to public health because they can help explain:

- Individual behaviour
- Behaviour of groups within a population
- Behaviour of healthcare organisations

Data from social research may be **quantitative** (numerical data) or **qualitative** (textual or pictorial

Table 4A.1 Disciplines concerned with human behaviour

Discipline	Description
Psychology	Study of individuals' mental processes and behaviour.
Sociology	Study of social processes and interactions in societies, groups, and institutions. Sociology recognises that people in societies and groups may behave in ways that differ from the behaviour of individuals.
Anthropology	Study of human cultures (**Note:** This discipline is also called sociocultural anthropology to distinguish it from biological anthropology, which is the study of evolution).
History	Recording and interpretation of past events.

data), although in practice, most social research considers both types.

Theoretical perspectives

Before describing major theoretical perspectives used in the social sciences, it is helpful to understand some relevant terminology (see Table 4A.2).

Classically, there are three major theoretical perspectives in sociology:

- Structural functionalism
- Social conflict
- Interpretivism (or 'symbolic interactionism')

Table 4A.2 Terminology used in the social sciences

Concept	Description
Epistemology	The study of **knowledge**: its origin, nature, methods, and limits. Epistemology is concerned with what it means to be '*true*' or '*false*'; what constitutes valid '*information*'; and whether information is absolute or relative. Constructivism and positivism (see succeeding text) are at opposite ends of the epistemological spectrum.
Theoretical perspective	The philosophical stance that informs the research design and methodology. It also shapes the focus or the approach to the phenomenon or object being studied.
Methodology	The strategy behind the **choice of methods** to answer a study's research questions.
Ontology	The study of the nature of **being**. Ontology considers whether facts are constructed in people's minds or whether they exist in an external world.
Reflexivity	This position acknowledges that the process of observation affects the environment under study. Reflexivity is explicitly considered in research that takes a **constructivist** stance (e.g. anthropology). In contrast, studies taking a **positivist** perspective seldom acknowledge the impact of the researchers except in seeking to minimise differences between individual researchers (e.g. by standardising data collection instruments).

Structural functionalism

This approach views society as an **objective reality** in which the different components are interdependent and work together to promote stability. There are individual roles that adapt to the needs of society. Important sociologists who adopted this perspective include Talcott Parsons (see Section 4A.2) and Emile Durkheim (see Section 4A.3).

Functionalism is closely linked to **positivism**, which was founded by the French sociologist Auguste Comte (1978–1857) [1]. Social scientists who advocate positivism tend to value the scientific method. They believe that the social world can be studied in the same way as the material world in that hypotheses can be tested according to observable facts. Positivists often employ a quantitative approach.

Social conflict

Founded by Karl Marx, this perspective (also called Marxist) focuses on the **competition for resources** and material production to generate wealth as the major goal of society. This perspective leads to industrialisation and the establishment of different social classes. Industrialisation may affect health in a number of ways (e.g. occupational health, environmental pollution, the effects of industrial products on health) and may have a profound impact on health inequalities.

Interpretivism

This perspective focuses on individual or **small-scale social interactions**, including behaviours and communication, and how this influences the way that people interpret society subjectively. Labelling is an important aspect of this perspective. For example, a person's identity may be influenced by a label such as a diagnosis, and certain labels can lead to stigmatisation (see Sections 4A.4 and 4A.5).

A related epistemological stance is **constructivism**. This philosophy rejects the idea that there is one knowable truth waiting to be discovered. Instead, it is based on the premise that our understanding of the world is constructed by reflecting on our experiences. Each of us generates our own *'rules'* and *'mental models'* which we use to make sense of our experiences.

Methods

Studies of human behaviour may involve the use of quantitative or qualitative methods.

Quantitative methods

See also Sections 1A.25 to 1A.29.

These methods are used to answer questions such as *'How many?'* and *'What proportion?'* Examples are

- Questionnaires
- Surveys (face-to-face or telephone)
- Routine data sources (e.g. mortality data)

As with all quantitative research, three potential causes of error should always be considered, namely

- Chance
- Bias
- Confounding

Qualitative research

See also Section 1D.

Qualitative methods are used to answer questions about *'How?'* and *'Why?'* Methods include ethnography, interviews, focus groups, and case studies (see Table 4A.3).

Box 4A.1 illustrates how these epistemological theoretical perspectives can lead to different types of research and conclusions.

Table 4A.3 Qualitative methods

Qualitative method	Description
Ethnography	In anthropological research, the investigator studies a group's behaviour in great detail, often by living among them for a prolonged period of time through participant or non-participant observation.
Interviews	Interview can either be **semi-structured** (loose set of questions using a topic guide) or **in-depth** interview (where the respondent or the interviewee's responses guides the conversation).
Focus groups	The researcher brings together a group of 6–10 people and uses a range of techniques to explore the group's opinions. The **deliberations** of the focus group shape the views expressed and are considered part of the data collected.
Case studies	Multiple data collection methods are used to generate a rounded picture of a **bounded system** (i.e. an organisation fixed in place and time, such as a particular GP surgery implementing a new service). Case studies can include collection of quantitative and qualitative data.

Box 4A.1 Participant observation of euthanasia

To understand patients' decisions regarding euthanasia, the anthropologist Robert Pool conducted a participant observation study of a clinic in the Netherlands. While he initially felt 'invisible' in clinic meetings, he noticed that his name began appearing in patients' notes and sometimes his opinion was sought because he had spent significant time with patients. Therefore, through observation, Pool had affected his environment (**reflexivity**).

Several months after he left the clinic, Pool returned to interview some key members of staff. When he asked them about the number of patients considering euthanasia, towards the start of the interviews, the clinicians could remember few cases. Over the course of the interview, however, the clinicians remembered more cases.

From Pool's reflections on his research, it is possible to identify how different *epistemological* stances might have led to different methods and conclusions. A **positivist** perspective might have focused on quantifying the number of euthanasia cases, leading to the use of quantitative methods (e.g. administering a questionnaire). In contrast, a **constructivist** perspective would have explicitly considered how the estimate of cases was a reflection partly of the clinicians' recall, but also of their interpretations of the conversations they had with patients, and on the impact of the researcher in prompting this recall.

Source: Pool, R. and Geissler, W., Chapter 5: Interpreting and explaining sickness, in *Medical Anthropology*, Understanding Public Health Series, OUP, Maidenhead, UK, 2005.

4A.2 Illness as a social role

People with symptoms are not automatically patients. They become patients (or are defined by health professionals as such) because they choose to seek healthcare.

Sickness, illness, and disease

The terms sickness, illness, and disease are used interchangeably and may often co-occur; however, their meanings are distinct:

- **Sickness** covers both illness and disease.
- **Illness** refers to a patient's subjective experience of mental and physical sensations or states.
- **Diseases** are the abnormalities in form and function of organs and body systems that clinicians diagnose and treat.

According to Cassell (1976), 'Illness is what the patient feels when he goes to the doctor, disease is what he has on the way home' [2, p. 53].

For more on people's decisions to become patients, see Section 4A.8 and Section 4B.5.

The concept of illness as a social role introduces the notion that people who feel ill and those who care for and treat them behave in ways that are related to society's implicit ideas of what it means to be sick. The American sociologist **Talcott Parsons** described this as 'the sick role'.

Sick role

Parsons [3] wrote that people who are ill have certain rights and responsibilities that work together in the interest of society (see Box 4A.2). These rights and responsibilities are all both **temporary** and **universal**.

Some of the strengths and weaknesses associated with this approach are listed in Box 4A.3. An example of its use is presented in Box 4A.4.

Box 4A.2 The sick role

Rights of sick people	Responsibilities of sick people
Exemption from blame for having their illness	Duty to seek medical assistance
Exemption from normal responsibilities such as work	Duty to want to get better

Box 4A.3 Strengths and weakness of the sick role as a model

Strengths	Weaknesses
Applies well to **acute** infections (e.g. cold, flu)	Applies less well to conditions where • Individuals can be 'blamed' for their 'illness' (e.g. obesity, STIs) • There is no need for individuals to be exempted from normal duties (e.g. well controlled diabetes or asthma) • Medical assistance is not always perceived as being 'helpful' (e.g. one of the symptoms of schizophrenia is a lack of insight into the condition and therefore the recognition that treatment is needed) • A duty to 'want to get better' is part of the sick role (e.g. people with a high BMI)

Box 4A.4 Example: The sick role in a New Guinea village

Gilbert Lewis's ethnographic descriptions of sickness in a New Guinea society highlight the variations in the ways that different cultures treat people with sickness. In his account, both Western medical approaches and local rituals were used to attempt to cure a sick man. As part of the latter approach, the source of his illness was sought from his previous behaviour (fights, disputes, etc.) and spiritual cures were attempted, including placing crucifixes around the bed and conducting a Malyi ceremony. Many of these behaviours contrasted with the Western ideas of the sick role but they emphasise how a 'sick role' is not confined to Western cultures.

Source: Reproduced from Lewis, G., A *Failure of Treatment*, 2000 by permission of Oxford University Press.

Table 4A.4 Patient-centred versus doctor-centred characteristics

Characteristic	Patient centred	Doctor centred
Nomenclature	Patient, consumer, expert.	Patient.
Decision-making responsibility	Shared.	Doctor-led.
Patient's role	Self-care, active monitoring of condition, source of expertise (cf. Expert Patient Programme).	Passive recipient of care.
Written communication	Patient's notes are routinely available to patients. Correspondence between medical professionals is routinely copied to patients.	Patient's notes and correspondence are not shared with patients.
Consultation style	• Listening • Reflecting • Probing • Silence • Facilitating • Interpreting	Active (doctor)/passive (patient).

Doctor–patient role

Doctors often face a conflict between acting in their patients' best interests and serving the wider interests of society. For example, if a doctor saw a patient who worked as a lorry driver and the patient reported having had a blackout, then the doctor would be obliged to inform the *Driver and Vehicle Licensing Authority (DVLA)* in Great Britain, or similar agencies in other countries, thereby jeopardising the driver's livelihood.

Scambler [5] describes the traditional doctor–patient role as being **paternalistically doctor centred**, but in recent years, there has been a shift in some countries towards more **patient-centred** care (see Table 4A.4).

It is increasingly being recognised that patients and professionals each have their own area of knowledge and expertise and that both parties benefit from working together.

The National Health Service (NHS) has promoted such cooperation by means of the **Expert Patients Programme** (http://www.expertpatients.co.uk), which provides short courses. These courses are mainly facilitated by people with long-term conditions and are designed to empower patients by promoting self-management and encouraging shared decision-making between patients and their healthcare professionals.

See also Chapter 2I.5 and Chapter 5E.2.

4A.3 Concepts of health and well-being

Although good health is sought almost universally by human beings and is prerequisite for well-being, the definition of health is far from being universally agreed [6].

The way in which health is defined can be an important influence on health policy and on health promotion strategies. Table 4A.5 summarises some important definitions of health, including the widely used WHO definition, which:

- Explicitly links health with **well-being**
- Conceptualises health as a **positive aspiration**, not merely the absence of disease

Table 4A.5 Concepts of health

Agency	Year	Definition	Strengths	Limitations
WHO [7]	1948	'a state of complete physical, mental and social well-being and not merely the absence of disease or infirmity'	Simple, widespread appeal across cultures Conceptualises health as a human right, which requires social and physical resources Influential in shaping health policy beyond merely the absence of disease	Leaves 'most of us unhealthy most of the time' [8] Contributes to medicalisation of society (see also Sections 4A.7 and 4A.8) Not objective or measurable
Ottawa charter	1986	'a resource for everyday life, not the objective of living' (adaptation of WHO definition)		
Canguilhem [9]	1943	'the ability to adapt to one's environment'	More appropriate for the current public health burden of chronic illness Enables individuals to define their own health needs	Overly individualistic, takes little or no account of the constraints or opportunities of the sociopolitical systems in which people are embedded Reactive to events and changes in health status, with little scope to promote health as a human right
Huber et al. [6]	2011	'the ability to adapt and to self manage'		

Similarly, there is debate about what constitutes **well-being** [10]. For example, the Well-Being Institute at the University of Cambridge defines well-being as the 'positive and sustainable characteristics which enable individuals and organisations to thrive and flourish'. Other authors question whether well-being is indeed something that can be researched to uncover its essential nature, and argue that well-being is a social and cultural construct that is interesting because of what it tells us about a society and a culture.

See also Chapter 1C.7 and 2H2.

4A.4 Concepts of primary and secondary deviance

Becker [11] first described **deviance** as a behaviour that is seen as being **unacceptable within a particular culture**.

Labelling theory and deviance

People who deviate from the norm are **labelled** as being abnormal in some way. However, note that behaviour that is seen as being perfectly acceptable in one culture may be regarded as unacceptable in another [5]. On being recognised as such, deviant behaviour may be subject to **sanctions**, **punishment**, **correction**, or **treatment**.

In medicine, deviance has implications with regard to the labelling of organic and psychiatric disease. Parsons [3] considered illness as a form of deviance where the doctor is an agent of social control (i.e. the doctor **restricts** access to the sick role by labelling people as either sick or healthy).

Table 4A.6 Types of deviance

Type of deviance	Description	Example
Primary	Relates to the deviant **behaviour** before labelling has occurred By itself, this behaviour may only have minor implications for the individual.	Experiencing hallucinations and delusional thinking
Secondary	Relates to the individual's **status** once they have been publically labelled as deviant. The label may then become a 'self-fulfilling prophecy' and reinforce the deviant behaviour. This labelling tends to have greater implications for the individual than the behaviour itself in terms of their social role and self-esteem.	Schizophrenic

Box 4A.5 Example: Combating drug taking and deviant behaviour through drug rehabilitation requirements

The use of illicit drugs is a prime example of deviant behaviour in Western societies. Drug use is often linked to a range of other deviant behaviours (such as stealing and prostitution) that can result in contact with the criminal justice system. However, drug use is also recognised in many Western cultures as an addiction and as such may be regarded as an illness.

In England, the programme of Drug Rehabilitation Requirements (DRR) explicitly links this deviant behaviour with the sick role. People who are arrested and have a history of taking illicit drugs may be offered treatment and rehabilitation for their drug use in an attempt to break the cycle of drugs and crime. Participants' attendance is closely monitored and in certain circumstances they can be *required* to attend. In this way, DRRs serve as an alternative to prison, which was the traditional way of dealing with deviant behaviour.

For more information on DRRs, see: http://www.hiwecanhelp.com/your-rights/criminal-justice/DRR.aspx.

Primary and secondary deviance

Lemert [12] differentiated between **primary** and **secondary** deviance (see Table 4A.6).

As shown in Box 4A.5, the treatment of illicit drug use illustrates how behaviour defined by society as being deviant may be sanctioned to some extent through its recognition by society as an illness.

4A.5 Stigma and how to tackle it

A stigma is a mark of disgrace or infamy. The American sociologist Erving Goffman [13] defined stigma as

> *An attribute that is deeply discrediting within a particular social interaction.*

This underlines two features of stigma: that it is an **undesirable characteristic** in a **particular context** (i.e. in a particular time and society). For example, in the 1950s in England, knowledge that a person was born outside of marriage would have been considered shameful, but in

Box 4A.6 Examples of stigmatised diseases

- Leprosy
- Psychiatric illnesses
- Epilepsy
- HIV/AIDS
- Sexually transmitted infections

twenty-first-century England, it is considered normal. Stigmatisation often occurs as a consequence of labelling. For example, a disease label can lead to society treating an individual differently.

In the medical literature, stigma is used to describe various diseases or conditions that currently may lead to exclusion from society (see Box 4A.6).

Causes of stigma

Stigma is rooted in ingrained cultural norms. Stigma thrives on **inequalities**, **fear**, and **misinformation** (see Table 4A.7).

Table 4A.7 Definitions of stigma

Driver of stigma	Examples
Inequalities	Women (e.g. HIV-positive women in Africa). Marginalised groups (e.g. gay men, transgender people, prostitutes).
Fear	Fear of having to deal with a person having an epileptic fit.
Misinformation	There is a popular misconception that the term 'schizophrenia' means dual personality, whereas in fact schizophrenia is characterised by impaired social functioning, distorted thought, and hallucinations.

The media and certain religious groups may perpetuate these stigmas and in so doing will bolster people who are not currently in a stigmatised group.

Consequences of stigma

Stigma affects individuals and society and is manifested as either **felt stigma** or **enacted stigma** (see Table 4A.8).

Tackling stigma

The tackling of stigma benefits both stigmatised individuals and society as a whole. For example, reducing the stigma of STIs removes barriers to diagnosis for people with genitourinary symptoms. In turn, the early treatment of such symptoms benefits the individual (e.g. may reduce the risk of longer-term health problems) and reduces the spread of the infection among the population.

Tackling stigma requires changes in the attitudes and behaviours of both the stigmatised person and society at large. Different ways of tackling stigma are shown in Table 4A.9.

A 'virtuous circle' may be established where positive challenges to stigma can change attitudes, leading to reduced felt stigma, which itself may reduce enacted stigma (see Figure 4A.1).

Table 4A.8 Manifestations of felt stigma and enacted stigma

Felt stigma	Enacted stigma
Shame and guilt Self-stigmatisation Depression Unwillingness to speak up Withdrawal from society	Loss of job Compulsory testing Violence Quarantine Denial of health services

Table 4A.9 Strategies to address stigma

Measure	Description	Example
Education	Public education by means of challenging negative stereotypes and raising awareness of illness.	World AIDS Day initiatives.
Language	Challenging the language that is used to describe illness.	Promoting the term 'person with schizophrenia' instead of 'schizophrenic' because the illness does not define a person's entire identity.
Public acknowledgement of diagnosis	Public acknowledgement of illness by celebrities.	In 1985, Rock Hudson publicly declared that he was gay and that he was dying from AIDS.
Public acknowledgement of exposure to disease	Public campaigns sanctioning discussion of potentially embarrassing symptoms or deviant risk factors.	England: 'Sex: Worth talking about' campaign [14] increased young people's awareness of sexual health and where to seek help. Australia: annual 'join the bowel movement' campaign encourages people to talk about embarrassing signs and symptoms.
Treatment	Advances in the management of illness.	Newer antipsychotic therapies that do not produce Parkinsonian symptoms help reduce the visible marks of illnesses such as schizophrenia.
Legislation	Certain manifestations of stigma can be outlawed.	The UK's Equality Act 2010 provides a legal framework for safeguarding the rights of people with 'protected characteristics' including disability and gender reassignment.

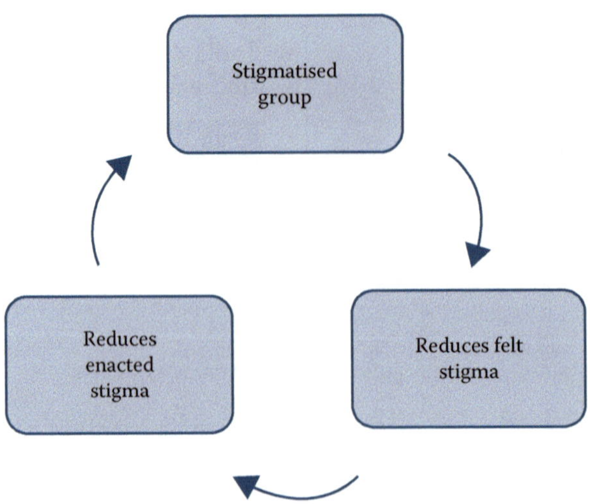

Figure 4A.1 A virtuous circle to challenge stigma.

4A.6 Impairment, disability, and handicap

In 1980, the WHO International Classification of Impairment, Disabilities, and Handicap (ICIDH) defined impairment, disability, and handicap as distinct but interrelated concepts; see Table 4A.10.

In 2001, ICIDH was replaced by the ICF (see Table 1C.11).

Measuring disability

In hospital settings, the Barthel index of **Activities of Daily Living** (ADL) score is widely used to assess disability. Using this scale, a patient's independence is assessed according to 10 domains (see Figure 4A.2).

The index, which is scored out of 20, describes the level of support that will typically be required by a patient. For example, a patient scoring 10 will require a maximal package of home care, while patients with scores above 10 will usually need residential or nursing home care.

Measuring handicap

Various tools exist for assessing handicap, including

- **Rankin scale** (used in stroke research)
- Hearing Handicap Inventory
- **London Handicap Scale** (domains include mobility, physical independence, occupation, social functioning, and economic self-sufficiency)

Social model of disability

In contrast to the aforementioned indices, the **social model** of disability considers how society disables people with physical impairments through a variety of barriers. Such barriers may be **environmental** (e.g. no wheel ramps at entrances to buildings) or **cultural** (e.g. patronising attitudes towards people with impairments).

ENG In England [15], the Office for Disability explicitly adopts the social model of disability to support government departments to consider disabilities when developing policy.

Bowels	Transfer
Bladder	Toilet use
Feeding	Walking
Grooming	Stairs
Dressing	Bathing

Figure 4A.2 Ten domains of the Barthel ADL index.

Table 4A.10 WHO international classification of impairment, disabilities and handicap

	Impairment	Disability	Handicap
Definition	A loss or abnormality of a body function (anatomical, physiological, or psychological)	An inability or restricted ability to perform an activity (in the normal human range)	A disadvantage due to impairment or disability that limits the role of an individual
Description	Malfunctioning body parts or systems	Activities a person cannot do	Social sequelae of impairment or disability
Example	Bilateral above-knee amputations	Unable to walk: wheelchair bound	Difficulties in accessing workplace, unable to mingle while socialising in bars

4A.7 Social and structural iatrogenesis

In his book *Medical Nemesis*, Ivan Illich [16] introduced the concept of **iatrogenesis**, which is a disease caused by medicine. He described three ways in which medicine can cause illness: **clinical**, **social**, and **structural**.

Clinical iatrogenesis

Medical treatment sometimes worsens the original illness or creates a new illness. Examples include

- Adverse drug reactions
- Diabetogenic drugs (e.g. steroids or certain combinations of antihypertensive drugs)
- Nosocomial infections (i.e. hospital acquired)

Social iatrogenesis

This concept describes the way in which widespread health service provision may encourage 'overmedicalisation' and can lead to people feeling less healthy even when normal (see Table 4A.11).

The rise of social iatrogenesis is reflected by the growing proportion of the GDP that is spent by many countries on certain aspects of healthcare.

Structural iatrogenesis

Structural iatrogenesis is the impact that the medical profession has on a population. As a result of increasing reliance upon medicine, the public has lost its traditional ways of coping with illness, death, pain, and misfortune. As Illich put it,

> *The so-called health professionals have an even deeper, structurally health-denying effect insofar as they destroy the potential of people to deal with their human weakness, vulnerability and uniqueness in a personal and autonomous way.*
>
> Illich [16, p. 26]

Table 4A.11 Examples of social iatrogenesis

Aspect of life	Medicalisation
Normal childbirth	Caesarean sections on demand
Ageing	Cosmetic surgery
Unruly children	Attention deficit/hyperactivity disorder

4A.8 Role of medicine in society

The role of medicine has been described as being

> *To cure sometimes, to heal often and to comfort always. (Variously attributed to Hippocrates, to a fifteenth-century French proverb, and to Sir William Osler)*

In particular, the role of biomedicine (i.e. branch of medical science that applies biological and physiological principles to clinical practice) has become an increasingly dominant, although sometimes questioned, part of Western society.

Expanding boundaries of medicine

Healthcare professionals and professional organisations are now routinely involved in areas of life that were previously outside the scope of medicine. Key examples of the role of medicine in areas previously not in the preserve of healthcare are

- Childbirth
- Euthanasia
- Abortion

Challenges to the role of medicine

The place of medicine in Western society is not undisputed. Some of the areas where it is frequently challenged are shown in Table 4A.12.

Table 4A.12 Challenges to the role of medicine

Issue	Details
Clinical iatrogenesis	Well-publicised accounts of side-effects and poor outcomes as a result of medical care have led some commentators to question the dominant role of medicine in society (see Section 4A.6).
Anti-psychiatry	Psychiatry has been challenged more than other medical disciplines. Many commentators, but especially RD Laing in the 1960s, have questioned the whole notion of mental illness. In Western societies, however, psychiatry remains the dominant model of care for mental ill health.
Internet access to health information and services	Consumer access to health information and services via the Internet has mushroomed and is removing the public's absolute dependence on the opinions of doctors. Medical opinion becomes only one of many sources of information, and in an increasing number of situations, treatments and diagnostic tests can be obtained without medical sanction.
Complementary and alternative healthcare	Other approaches to treating illness are available, and many such treatments are growing in popularity.

4A.9 Social patterns of illness

Explanations for various social patterns and experiences of illness including differences of gender, ethnicity, employment status, age, and social stratification.

Subjective (i.e. experienced) health differs markedly from measures of disease. According to the Health Survey for England, approximately 1% of the population regards itself as being in *'very bad health'*, with the proportion being correlated to age. A study by Scambler [5] found that a typical person experiences symptoms of illness approximately one day in three. However, only on about 6% of occasions will the person consult a health professional and in that sense become a patient. Whether a person seeks medical advice or not is determined by a number of triggers, including:

- Presence of a concomitant crisis
- Sanctioning by others
- Interference with normal activity
- Temporising deadlines

Some explanations for the varying patterns of illness seen between different social groups include:

- **Biology** and genetics
- **Behaviour** (i.e. differences in health seeking or risk taking between groups)
- **Social** circumstances (e.g. disproportionate effects of poverty on health)
- **Artefact** (i.e. the categories used to distinguish between social groups are in themselves problematic)

Gender

Clearly, certain diseases affect **only** men (e.g. prostate cancer) or women (e.g. endometriosis). Other diseases are **commoner** in men (e.g. renal calculi) or in women (e.g. gallstones). Furthermore, differing **behavioural patterns** also affect patterns of morbidity and mortality (e.g. dangerous driving commoner in men). Although life expectancy is lower for men, women report more ill health, which is thought to be partly due to different **reporting behaviours** between the sexes.

Ethnicity

Certain diseases are more or less common in different ethnic groups. Reasons include **genetic differences** (e.g. highest prevalence of sickle cell trait in people from sub-Saharan Africa) and **social factors** including:

- **Poverty**: In the United Kingdom, some minority ethnic groups are less affluent than White British
- **Migration**: Loss of social capital (see Section 4A.10); healthy migrant effect (see Section 4A.11)
- **Behaviour**: Differing patterns of smoking, diet, etc.
- **Access** to health services
- **Racism** (affects health through increased stress and social isolation)

As with any form of discrimination, racism may be direct or indirect:

- **Direct discrimination** occurs when someone treats another person less favourably than they would a person from a different group.
- **Indirect discrimination** occurs when rules, systems, or procedures have different effects on people from a particular group.

Employment status

Employment that is fulfilling and secure provides not only **material resources** for individuals and their families but also **psychological benefits** and **social support**. In contrast, a summary by the

Health Development Agency (now part of NICE) underlined the effects of unemployment on:

- **Physical health**: Unemployment is associated with mortality (greater suicide rates and increased cardiovascular mortality)
- **Mental health**: People who are unemployed or who have insecure employment are more prone to common mental disorders such as depression

The relationship between unemployment and health is complex. In some circumstances, health problems may be a factor in losing a job, while in others the loss of work may precipitate health problems.

Age

Clearly, there are different patterns of mortality at different ages; however, people's experiences of health services and illness also vary with age. For example, surveys indicate that older people are generally more positive about the standard of care that they have received than younger people. However, there are also examples of inequalities in healthcare access by age: for example, poorer survival from cancer in older people may be due to under-treatment compared with younger people [17].

Social class

Social class gradients in health occur at every age and for all major causes of death.

In the United Kingdom, the Black Report [18] found that despite general improvements in health and prosperity, there were still pronounced disparities in health and illness across the social classes. The report was written by the Department of Health's Research Working Group on Inequalities in Health and was led by **Sir Douglas Black**. It suggested four possible explanations for the observed differences in health (see Box 4A.7). The government's response to the report is discussed in Section 4C.10.

An example of the relationship between occupation and health is shown in Box 4A.8.

Box 4A.7 Black Report: Possible explanations for health inequalities

Explanation	Details
Artefact	The association between social class and health is an artefact of the way in which these concepts are measured.
Social selection	Health determines social class through the process of health-related social mobility (i.e. people that are ill are more likely to **drift** down the social gradient).
Behavioural and cultural	Social class determines health through differences in health-damaging or health-promoting behaviours (e.g. the association between lower socio-economic status and smoking).
Materialistic	Social class determines health through differences in the material circumstances of life (cf. Whitehall studies). Such phenomena may be direct (e.g. poor housing leading to cold and damp) or indirect (e.g. social capital or through psychosocial mechanisms).

Box 4A.8 Example: Occupation and health—Whitehall studies I and II

The first Whitehall cohort study (**Whitehall I**) examined mortality rates over 10 years among male British civil servants aged 20–64 in the 1960s and 1970s. This study revealed some marked differences in health between different employment grades. For example,

- Men in the lowest grade (messengers, doorkeepers, etc.) had a threefold higher **mortality** rate than men in the highest grade (administrators)
- Blood pressure at work was associated with **job stress**, including 'lack of skill utilisation', 'tension', and 'lack of clarity' in tasks. The rise in blood pressure from the lowest to the highest job-stress score was much larger among low-grade men than among upper-grade men. Blood pressure at home, on the other hand, was not related to job-stress level

A second longitudinal study of British civil servants (**Whitehall II**) started in the 1980s and focused on occupational effects on health and disease. The study involved around 10,000 men and women aged 35–55 in the London offices of 20 civil service departments, and many people in the cohort are still being followed up. The study found that employment grade was strongly associated with **work control**. Lack of control in the job was related to long spells of absence and an increased risk of cardiovascular disease.

Source: Reproduced from www.workhealth.org/projects/pwhiteabs.html.

4A.10 Social factors in the aetiology of disease

Role of social, cultural, psychological, and family relationship factors in the aetiology of illness and disease.

See also Section 4A.9.

As seen in Sections 2H.2 and 4A.9, there are many determinants of health outside traditional biological aetiological models, including **social factors**, **cultural factors**, **psychological factors**, and **family relationships**. Furthermore, each of these factors may influence how individuals interpret the aetiology of illness and disease.

Social factors

There are many social factors that influence health. Some of the key factors were described by Wilkinson and Marmot [19] and include:

- Social gradient
- Stress
- Early life influences
- Social exclusion
- Work
- Unemployment
- Social support
- Addiction
- Food
- Transport

Social support protects against the health impacts of stressful life events and reduces the risk of mental illness. Major socio-economic changes have been associated with significant health effects (e.g. both the collapse of the Soviet Union in the 1990s and the financial crisis in the late 2000s were associated with increased suicide rates).

Cultural factors

Cultural factors may influence beliefs about the aetiology of illness, including lay concepts of what causes illness (e.g. 'it runs in the family').

Psychological factors

The Whitehall II study (Box 4A.8) identified two key aspects of stress at work that are associated with physical and mental illness:

- Effort/reward imbalance
- Demand/control imbalance

Difficult jobs, where the worker has little autonomy over what they do, are associated with higher rates of stress and ill health.

Family relationships

Family provides a source of social support and acts as a buffer to stressors.

4A.11 Social capital and social epidemiology

Although social capital and social epidemiology were both first described in the mid-twentieth century, academic interest in the two concepts only began in earnest in the early 1990s. The concepts are now widely regarded as being important and meaningful across the social sciences.

Social capital

Social capital attributes a value to the social networks in which individuals live. These networks provide **norms** (i.e. defined limits of acceptable behaviour) and **sanctions** when these bounds are crossed (e.g. social exclusion, gossip, stigma). Social capital functions in two ways:

- **Bonding**: social capital strengthens the links between members of families and tight-knit communities, thereby providing social support
- **Bridging**: social capital strengthens the links with members outside the group (i.e. 'networking')

Social capital can be considered at the **micro** (individual), **meso** (community), and **macro** (national) levels. At all three levels, it is positively correlated with economic affluence, low crime, educational attainment, and good health. The WHO regards social networks as a determinant of health, and it advocates the provision of social support to improve health outcomes through increased social capital.

Social epidemiology

Social epidemiology is the study of the social determinants of the distribution of disease within a population. Multilevel analysis is used to determine the extent to which an individual's health is shaped by **micro** (individual), **meso** (household/small area), and **macro** (large area) characteristics.

Macro-level epidemiological factors may be **compositional** (e.g. prevalence of childhood poverty) or **contextual** (e.g. population density), with the latter being irreducible to the individual.

Social epidemiology may involve:

- **Surveillance** (i.e. monitoring of health inequalities)
- Aetiological **investigation** (i.e. determining the social explanations for the causes of ill health, such as socio-economic status, behaviour, and social support)
- Designing and evaluating **interventions** to reduce social inequalities in health

4B

Healthcare

Most of the discourse concerning healthcare focuses on formal health systems and the role of professionals as healthcare providers. This chapter begins by widening the concept of healthcare to encompass other kinds of care, including self-help and complementary practices. This chapter also considers the social roles and characteristics of healthcare providers. For example, hospitals, as the archetypal providers of healthcare, are considered in terms of their potential to constrain the actions of individuals. We also consider how professional status was created and is maintained, and we examine some situations where conflicts in professional roles may arise.

4B.1 Different approaches to healthcare

Different approaches to healthcare: including self-care, family care, community care, self-help groups.

The term **clinical iceberg** was used by Last [20] to describe the finding that professional health services treat only a very small fraction of the total burden of ill health. It has been estimated that a typical adult experiences some sort of somatic symptom once every 3–6 days [21]. Assuming that some of these symptoms will require a degree of healthcare, it is likely that the bulk of healthcare occurs in the so-called **informal sector** because patients in Britain visit only their GP approximately four or five times a year on average.

Some implications of the clinical iceberg for public health specialists are the following:

- If health service activity data alone are used, they will underestimate the burden of ill health in society. Therefore, an understanding of how care is provided outside health services is required.
- The value of conventional health services may be enhanced by recognising more explicitly the value of different approaches (e.g. that there are situations where alternatives are more appropriate).
- Self-care (taking care of oneself without professional assistance or oversight) is the commonest form of healthcare.

Acute illnesses

For a new symptom, such as a cough, a person may typically instigate his or her own management plan. For example, they may plan to wait and see what happens, unless:

- The symptom changes (e.g. the cough becomes productive) or
- The symptom persists beyond a time limit (e.g. beyond the end of the week)

Table 4B.1 Classes of medications and their restrictions

Class of medication	Abbreviation	Restriction	Example
Controlled drug	CD	Can be dispensed only with a detailed prescription. Stored in locked cupboard; closely monitored.	Diamorphine
Prescription-only medication	POM	Can be dispensed only with a prescription.	Flucloxacillin
Pharmacy list	P	Can be sold only under the supervision of a pharmacist.	Ranitidine
General sales list	GSL	Available on open shelves (e.g. in supermarkets).	Ibuprofen
Traditional herbal registration	THR	Availability [22,22a] may be restricted for certain herbs (e.g. as prescription only) but most are available on open shelves.	St. John's wort, Arnica
Vitamins and supplements		Classed as foods or food supplements and regulated under the Food Safety Act. Range of vitamins and supplements restricted by EU legislation. Available for sale on open shelves, e.g. in supermarkets.	Fish oils, vitamin C

In these circumstances, the person may choose to consult another person (e.g. a family member or a GP) or else try an over-the-counter remedy (e.g. cough mixture).

Remedies can be **orthodox** or **complementary/alternative** (see succeeding text). Orthodox medicines in the United Kingdom can be accessed without consulting a clinician for a prescription if they are listed on the pharmacy (P) or general sales list (GSL). Different restrictions apply to these lists in terms of which items may be sold and in what quantities (e.g. 32 tablets of paracetamol on the P list and 16 tablets on the GSL list). See Table 4B.1.

Long-term conditions

Self-care accounts for the vast majority of treatment of any long-term medical condition. For example, the Department of Health has calculated that a typical patient with diabetes has 3 hours of contact time with professionals per year and will therefore perform self-care for the remaining 8757 hours (see www.dh.gov.uk/assetRoot/04/10/17/02/04101702.pdf).

The population of people with a long-term condition is often represented as a triangle called the **Kaiser pyramid** (Figure 4B.1). This diagram depicts the large number of patients at the base of the triangle who have straightforward conditions, rising up through the triangle to smaller and smaller numbers toward the top of the triangle with increasingly complex disease. The proportion of self-care undertaken by patients tends to vary with the complexity of their condition (see Figure 4B.1).

Formal approaches to support self-care are now being adopted more widely by health systems (see Table 4B.2). When achieved in collaboration with professionals, such care is sometimes referred to as **shared care**.

Complementary and alternative therapies

Complementary and alternative treatments may be defined as a group of diverse medical and healthcare systems, practices, and products that are not generally considered part of conventional medicine. Increasingly, complementary practitioners share many of the attributes of healthcare professionals (see Section 4B.3). Complementary therapies range

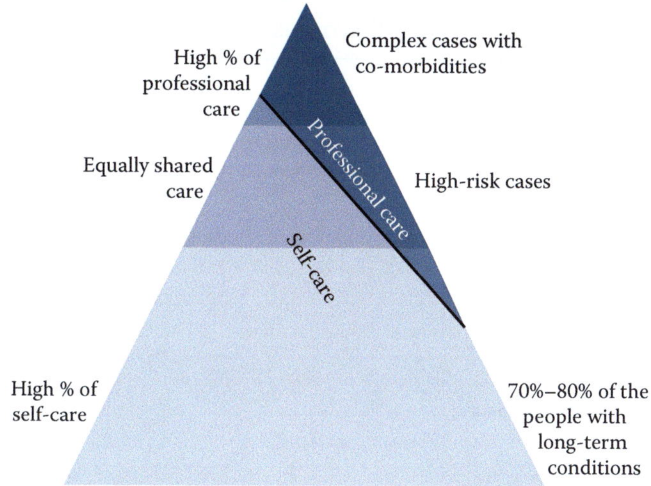

Figure 4B.1 Proportion of self-care in relation to the complexity of long-term conditions.

Table 4B.2 Approaches used to health systems to promote self-care

Approach	Details
Telehealth	These are tele-monitoring systems that allow remote exchange of information about patients' vital signs (e.g. blood pressure, glucose) and thereby connect people in their own homes with health professionals. Through the use of these technologies, patients may not need to visit health services for ongoing monitoring. Healthcare professionals can contact patients if readings become abnormally high or low. Notes: The impact of telehealth on health services is controversial, as is its cost-effectiveness. In certain countries (e.g. Canada), the term telehealth is used to describe audiovisual technologies used for remote consultations.
Extra-care housing	Extra-care housing is a type of adapted housing facility that is designed to support older people with high levels of need to live at home.
Training patients in self-management	Examples include • The Expert Patient Programme (see Section 4A.1) • DAFNE (Dose Adjustment For Normal Eating) [23], which trains adults to manage type 1 diabetes by estimating the amount of carbohydrate in each meal and then injecting the appropriate dose of insulin

in their complexity and in the degree to which they can be self-administered (see Box 4B.1).

The use of complementary therapies can differ somewhat from conventional medicine (also known as Western or **allopathic** medicine). Their uses are not restricted to the treatment of specific health complaints, but they may also be used by healthy people maintaining and promoting their well-being.

Research by the Food Standards Agency (FSA) from 2008 found that [22]:

- Thirty-one percent of people surveyed in the United Kingdom took a vitamin, mineral, or dietary supplement frequently.

Box 4B.1 Examples of complementary therapies

Home-made:

- Honey and lemon in hot water for a cold
- Avocado pulp as a skin moisturiser

Commercial:

- Ginseng for energy
- St. John's wort to combat depression

Self-administered practices:

- Meditation

Therapies delivered by a practitioner:

- Massage
- Acupuncture

- Women and people in higher social classes were more likely to report taking supplements than men or people in lower social classes.
- Nearly half of the people taking vitamins or supplements had never looked up information or received medical advice about what they should or should not take to protect or improve their health.

Family care

Friedson [25] described how people tend to discuss medical issues with their family, friends, or colleagues before seeking professional advice. This **lay referral system** is used for:

- Interpreting symptoms
- Reassurance
- Seeking advice about a remedy
- Seeking about referral to another lay person or to a professional

Where lay culture and professional culture differ, a ladder of consultations typically begins with the nuclear family, through progressively more distant and authoritative lay people, until a professional is reached. In contrast, where lay and professional cultures are more alike, patients typically take a great deal of time trying to treat themselves, and then go directly from self-treatment to consulting a doctor.

Community care

As well as forming an important part of the lay referral system, the term *community care* has taken specific meanings in different countries.

In Britain, the National Health Service and Community Care Act [26] led to a large-scale relocation of people with mental illness from large psychiatric hospitals into small local hostels or sheltered housing.

In Australia, the term relates to a joint Commonwealth, State and Territory initiative in which frail older people and people with disabilities are given funding to support themselves in continuing to live in the community.

In South Africa, the term is typically applied to mean home-based care and support for people living with HIV/AIDS.

In Ireland, the term includes public health nursing, home help, and out-of-hospital physiotherapy, occupational therapy, chiropody service, day care, and respite care service.

Self-help groups

Self-help groups now exist for almost every conceivable medical condition from achondroplasia to XXY syndrome. Typically these societies exist to:

- Provide information to patients and their carers through leaflets, help lines, and websites
- Put people in touch with others who are affected with that condition
- Raise funds in order to commission research into the condition
- Lobby government and clinicians

The rise in self-help groups in recent times is attributed to a general desire by patients to take more responsibility for their own health. As treatment options become more complex, and time with clinicians more limited, self-help groups have filled the gap between professionals' availability and the demand for disease-related information and support. The expansion of self-help communities has been facilitated by the rise of the Internet and e-mail. Note that certain self-help groups may receive considerable funds from pharmaceutical companies and other sources.

4B.2 Hospitals as social institutions

There are various ways in which hospitals may act as a social institution and thereby help shape the cultures and practices of their local community. In other words, hospitals are not only a centre for treatment but, rather, they may serve other positive and negative roles in society (see Table 4B.3).

As a responsible corporate citizen (see Box 4B.2), the NHS can engage in a range of processes with wide-ranging potential benefits, covering transport, procurement, facilities management, employment and skills, community engagement, and new buildings.

Goffman [13] defined **total institutions** as places where people are isolated from society over a period of time and lead life in an enclosed environment that is administered in a formal fashion. He went on to consider the effects of institutionalisation on social relationships in the outside world, the ways in which people adapt to and become attached to the institution, and the complicit role of medicine in this process (see Box 4B.3).

Table 4B.3 Influences of hospitals on society

Type of influence	Role in society	Details
Positive	Employer	Employer of clinical and non-clinical staff, including technicians, caterers, porters, builders, and secretaries. Health services are often one of the largest employers in a local area.
	Purchasers	Purchaser of healthcare-related products, such as drugs and medical equipment, and other goods (e.g. food and drink for patients, visitors, and staff).
	Community resource	Hospital resources can be important for the local community, where rooms in the hospital building are used for public meetings, hospital sports, catering, arts facilities, etc.
	Research facility	Medical research, such as clinical trials, are often conducted in a hospital setting with inpatients or outpatients as participants.
	Education and training facility	Undergraduate and postgraduate training of clinical staff frequently takes place in hospitals, including the training of doctors, physiotherapists, nurses, and occupational therapists.
Negative	Polluter	Travel to and from the hospital by staff, patients, and visitors adds significantly to congestion; hospital waste has an impact on carbon emissions.
	Isolation or exclusion	In general, hospitals serve as a means of separating people from the rest of society until they are healthy. At its extreme, patients with infectious diseases are isolated from other patients, visitors, and staff.

Box 4B.2 ENG Example: NHS as a corporate citizen

As a consumer, the NHS spends around £20 billion a year on goods and services, including £500 million on food. Spending this money strategically by only buying what is needed could cut costs. Seeking innovative, lower impact products and services could also

- Reduce the NHS carbon footprint
- Support local economies
- Ensure employees in supplier companies are treated fairly

Source: The Sustainable Development Unit website. Accessed online July 20, 2014 at http://www.sduhealth.org.uk/delivery/evaluate.aspx.

Box 4B.3 Erving Goffman: Asylums

Goffman used **participant observation** to study the inner workings of an American psychiatric hospital. Working as a hospital porter, he observed the effects of institutionalisation—notably the staid behaviour patterns of both staff and patients.

Goffman found that institutionalised patients were apathetic and became progressively less able to make decisions and care for themselves. Methods have subsequently been developed for avoiding these negative effects, including the following:

- Providing **information** to patients prior to treatment
- Promoting mobility and **self-care** while in hospital
- Pre-discharge **planning** and education
- Reducing length of stay
- Providing more care in the **community**

4B.3 Professions

Professions, professionalisation, and professional conflicts.

See also Section 5E.3.

The three original professions—clergy, medicine, and law—are characterised by the following traits:

- Specialist area of **knowledge**
- A professional **association**
- Ethical code
- Control over **certification** or licensing

Medicine is often used as a model for the study of professions. In contrast, the status of nursing as a profession has been controversial and has taken much longer to establish.

Professions

Writing in the 1950s, **Talcott Parsons** described various aspects of the medical profession and its effects on patients:

- A clearly defined **knowledge base** that is highly developed, theoretical, and specialised
- Patients expected to defer to doctors' **authority**
- Self-governing and **self-policing**
- Potential to **exploit power** over patients for financial gain
- A commitment to **public service** and ethics
- **Protection** for patients against exploitation

In the 1960s, nursing was often described as a 'semi-profession' because it lacked the powers of self-regulation and a specialised body of knowledge.

Professionalisation

Many sociologists have studied the emergence of the professional status in medicine. Professionalisation tends to involve establishing the following:

- Acceptable **qualifications** (e.g. in medicine, Larson [27] argues that the introduction of a university-based medical degree improved the credibility of the profession)
- A professional **body** (e.g. General Medical Council) to oversee the conduct of members of the profession
- Occupational **closure** (where there is no entry from outsiders, amateurs, or the unqualified)

Successful professionalisation protects members of an occupation from external control; acquires specialised knowledge, monopoly, and autonomy for the profession; and ensures that the profession is guided by a code of professional ethics.

Professional conflicts

Parsons' functionalist account of how medicine works as a profession has since been challenged, in part because sociologists began to question whether the espoused principles of altruism, etc., actually reflected doctors' behaviour. For example, feminist critiques of the medical profession focused on the gendered nature of the profession:

- In the 1970s, professions (such as medicine) were largely **populated by men.**
- Professions seemed to espouse **'traditional masculine' values** (technical expertise, rationality, etc.).
- Entrance to the profession favoured men over women.

The medical profession is currently prone to conflicts in a number of areas:

- With **nursing and allied health professions** regarding disputes over professional boundaries
- With complementary practitioners over recognition
- With **managers** regarding issues of professional autonomy and self-control
- With **patient groups** regarding issues of consumerism and paternalism
- With the **government** over terms and conditions of employment, regulation, and health service policy

4B.4 Clinical autonomy

Role of clinical autonomy in the provision of healthcare.

As discussed in Section 4B.3, **autonomy** is a key attribute of any profession. Autonomy refers to control over terms and conditions of work, whereas **clinical autonomy** refers specifically to the control of the profession over the content and delivery of healthcare.

In the 1960s, 1970s, and 1980s, sociology focused largely on how the medical profession had achieved its autonomy. Since the 1990s, the focus has shifted towards the growth of and challenges to autonomy in other professions allied to

Table 4B.4 Factors that may restrict the autonomy of clinical professions

Balancing factor	Description
Management	The role of management in setting clinical priorities and **monitoring standards** of care (see Chapter 5E.2).
Costs	Since all healthcare decisions are spending decisions, **cost containment** is necessary to safeguard resources, either implicitly or explicitly. Explicit cost containment rules can limit clinicians' capacity to make decisions based on the characteristics of the individual patient.
Guidelines	Some clinicians argue that the proliferation of guidelines and protocols has undermined the role of clinical judgement from medicine. Alternatively, Armstrong [28] argues that **evidence-based medicine** is the medical profession's best response to falling public trust in clinical practice.
Revalidation	Both **external assessment** and **revalidation** open doctors' practice to greater scrutiny and to scrutiny from those outside the profession (see also Chapter 5A.11).
Competition	In a private healthcare system, **consumer satisfaction** is required in order for a provider or insurer to remain viable.

medicine (e.g. physiotherapy). Levels of autonomy for all clinical professions are balanced by various factors (see Table 4B.4).

The structure of healthcare systems is often balanced such that there is a trade-off between clinical autonomy, financial autonomy, and control over terms and conditions of work.

4B.5 Illness behaviour

Behaviour in response to illness and treatments.

Section 4A covers many of the factors affecting when and why people seek help when they feel unwell and how they behave when they are diagnosed with a disease. Some of the factors explored below apply both to people with symptoms and to clinical professionals.

Factors that influence illness behaviour

Mechanic [29] identified ten variables that influence illness behaviour:

1. **Visibility** of symptoms and signs
2. Perceived **seriousness** (by the patient) of the symptoms, based on perceptions of present and future probabilities of danger
3. Amount of **disruption** caused by the symptom to work, family, etc.
4. Frequency and persistence or recurrence of **symptoms**
5. **Tolerance** threshold of person exposed to symptoms
6. **Knowledge**, information, and assumptions of the evaluator
7. Basic needs leading to **denial**

8. Needs leading to **competition** with illness
9. Competing **interpretations** assigned to symptoms once recognised
10. Availability of treatment: access, cost (not only money but also emotional, such as stigma)

Cultural differences

Pilowski and Spence [30] noted some marked cultural differences between Anglo-Saxon (stoical, withdrawn) and Mediterranean groups (emotionality) in their interpretation and response to symptoms. Similarly, Zborowski [31] found that Americans of Irish origin had a matter-of-fact attitude toward pain, whereas people with an Italian or Jewish background tended to be more demanding and dependent on medical help.

Phenomenology of symptoms

Diseases that present with striking symptoms (e.g. bleeding, jaundice) are more likely to receive prompt medical attention than those that are less dramatic.

Lay referral and intervention

See also Section 4B.1

Sometimes, a lay person may intervene to initiate medical consultation, for example, on behalf of a child or by calling an ambulance for a person who is having an epileptic fit or suffering from chest pain.

4B.6 Psychology of decision-making in health behaviour

In order to improve health outcomes through greater concordance with treatment, clinicians need to understand the issues that may influence a patient's decision about whether or not to follow therapeutic recommendations (see Box 4B.4). There are a number of models and theories that attempt to offer explanations for why people behave as they do with regard to health (see Chapter 2H.7). Zola [32] proposed five 'triggers' for help seeking, shown in Figure 4B.2.

Box 4B.4 Beliefs about medication: reasons for variable adherence among patients

It is estimated that 30%–50% of medications are not taken as prescribed. Non-adherent behaviour is sometimes regarded by prescribing clinicians as the preserve of certain recalcitrant patients, or due to patients' forgetfulness, confusion, or a lack of understanding.

Research into adherence (i.e. the extent to which the patient's behaviour matches agreed recommendations from the prescriber) suggests a more nuanced picture. There does not appear to be a clear pattern of non-adherence among different socio-demographic groups or diseases. However, patients' beliefs about medicines do provide some insights: while many patients believe that their medication is necessary, they may also have concerns about the risks of side effects and dependence.

High levels of concerns about the risks of medicines often correlate with self-reported non-adherence. This finding has led some researchers to conclude that '*viewed from the patient's perspective, [non-adherence] often represents a logical response to the illness and treatment in terms of their own perceptions, experiences and priorities, including concerns about side effects and other unwelcome effects of medicines*'.

Sources: Horne, R. et al., Concordance, adherence and compliance in medicine taking, Report for the National Co-ordinating Centre for NHS Service Delivery and Organisation R & D (NCCSDO), 2005. [Online], Accessed online June 1, 2014 at http://www.nets.nihr.ac.uk/; Horne, R. and Weinman, J., *J. Psychosom. Res.*, *47*, 555, 1999.

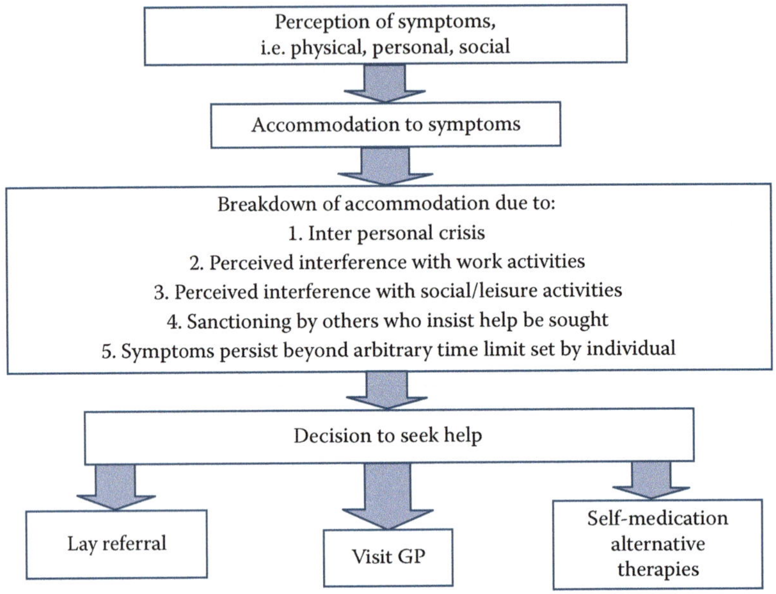

Figure 4B.2 Zola's 'triggers' for help seeking. (From Moffat, J., Help seeking and delay literature—Key insights, Cancer Research UK, 2010, Accessed online July 20, 2014 at http://www.cancerresearchuk.org/prod_consump/groups/cr_common//@nre/@hea/documents/generalcontent/cr_043179.pdf; Crinson, I., Section 4. Lay health beliefs and illness behaviour. Health knowledge website, 2007, Accessed online July 20, 2014 at http://www.healthknowledge.org.uk/public-health-textbook/medical-sociology-policy-economics/4a-concepts-health-illness/section4.)

4C

Equality, Equity, and Policy

The concepts of need and social justice are much debated since they lie at the heart of health policy in many countries. For example, one of the principles of the NHS is a commitment to **distributive justice** through the principle of equal access for equal need. Likewise, a commitment to **procedural justice** underpins the right to fair process in decision-making about rationing and prioritisation in healthcare.

This chapter begins with a description of various concepts relating to the concepts of need and social justice, and how they relate to other healthcare priorities such as efficiency. The remainder of the chapter discusses how healthcare policy is made, including the extent to which policymaking is based on the principles of social justice and equity for different population groups.

4C.1 Need and social justice

Concepts of need and social justice.

Need

Doyal and Gough [36] considered physical health as a basic, objective need, which is required by a person in order to participate in social life. However, they note that a need for *healthcare* does not automatically follow from the need for health [37].

Culyer and Wagstaff [38] provided the most influential definition of need for healthcare, namely that a need is equal to a person's **capacity to benefit** from healthcare (i.e. there is only a need for healthcare when an effective treatment exists). An individual's capacity to benefit for a particular healthcare intervention may vary according to factors such as gender, age, or illness severity as well as their adherence to the treatment and whether they engage in harmful behaviours such as smoking.

Given that the resources available to any health service are finite, the issue of determining the relative needs of patients will always be crucially important. Indeed, some authors have extended the definition of need to encompass the affordability by society for an effective treatment. In terms of allocating healthcare resources, Bradshaw [39] differentiated need into four categories: **felt** need, **expressed** need, **normative** need, and **comparative** need (see Table 4C.1).

In certain circumstances, these needs may overlap, as illustrated in the Venn diagram in Figure 4C.1.

Social justice

The term **social justice** embodies a notion of fairness that extends beyond individual rights in order to achieve a just society. The major theories of social justice were defined by Jost and Kay [40] and are set out in Table 4C.2. Social justice is used to defend a plethora of initiatives and policies emanating from across the political spectrum.

Of these concepts, **distributive justice** and **procedural justice** are of greatest relevance to equity and healthcare policy; therefore, they are described in more detail in the succeeding text.

Distributive justice

Distributive justice is sometimes used synonymously with social justice. With its focus on fairness, it considers equity through social comparison (e.g. by using relative deprivation as the basis for allocating resources).

The concept of distributive justice dates back at least to the time of Aristotle, with his view that social order is ensured by the just distribution of benefits. Three more recent interpretations of distributive justice are utilitarianism, justice as fairness, and maximising individual capabilities.

Utilitarianism

The eighteenth-century philosopher **Jeremy Bentham** expounded utilitarian philosophy. Utilitarianism stipulates that individuals and societies should make their choices with the aim of achieving the **greatest good for the greatest number**. This philosophy forms the basis for many arguments within public health but it risks marginalising and disadvantaging vulnerable and minority groups in society. An example of the application of utilitarianism is the institutionalisation of people with severe mental illness for the 'greater good' of the rest of society.

Justice as fairness

The most influential concept of social justice comes from the twentieth-century philosopher **John Rawls**. His theory of *Justice as Fairness* [41] outlined two principles for achieving a fair society, namely basic liberties as a right for everyone and the difference principle (see Box 4C.1).

Rawls proposed a model for societal decision-making named the **veil of ignorance**. In this model, people who make resource allocations should adopt a stance of ignorance regarding their personal future position in society. As Rawls put it, '…no one knows his place in society, his class position or social status; nor does he know his fortune in the distribution of natural assets and abilities, his intelligence and strength, and the like'. Since a policymaker may occupy any position in the society, it forces them to consider society from the perspective of all members, including the worst-off and best-off members.

Rawls's theory applies to all social goods, not just health and healthcare. So, in the same way that goods need to be distributed fairly across individuals within society, the resources attached to health and healthcare also need to be balanced with the requirements for other social goods (e.g. law and order).

Maximising individual capabilities

The philosopher **Amartya Sen** refined Rawls's concept to focus on making society less unjust (rather than perfectly just, which is unlikely to be achievable). Sen argues that a person's **individual capabilities** should be the primary means of achieving optimal well-being, as opposed to focusing on the possession of goods.

Procedural justice

While distributive justice is concerned with the **outcomes** of society in distributing rights and resources, procedural justice examines the **ways** in which those outcomes are reached. Procedural justice principles can be applied as a proxy for

Table 4C.1 Bradshaw's categories of need

Type of need	Alternative name	Description	Measurement
Felt need	Need for health	This concept relates to an individual's subjective experience of feeling unwell. Felt need does not necessarily relate to health service use. For example, someone with a headache may well report being in pain but seek no health service intervention.	Felt need can be measured through **surveys** (e.g. in the United Kingdom, the **census** asks about experience of illness).
Expressed need	Demand	Expressed need occurs when a patient seeks healthcare for a felt need.	**Waiting lists** can be used as a proxy measure of expressed need.
Normative need	Need for healthcare	This concept relates to a clinician's judgement of an individual's health state. A professional's assessment of whether an individual has a normative need depends not only on the patient's experience of symptoms but also on a range of other factors, such as the following: • Whether an effective treatment exists • Whether the treatment is available • Whether the patient is in a suitable state to benefit from the treatment Normative need is therefore dependent on the nature of health system and the availability of technology. Public health specialists may identify a normative need where individuals have no felt need (e.g. recommendation for weight loss in a person with a high BMI who has no wish to change their diet and lifestyle).	**Needs assessment**
Comparative need	Relative need	This concept describes the process of comparing the services available for areas with a similar prevalence of disease and similar epidemiology. If one area has a greater service provision, the other area may be said to be in relative need of health services. Comparator areas may be neighbouring boroughs or the country as a whole.	**Deprivation** and **mortality** measures may be useful for indicating a need for health but do not necessarily reflect a need for healthcare.

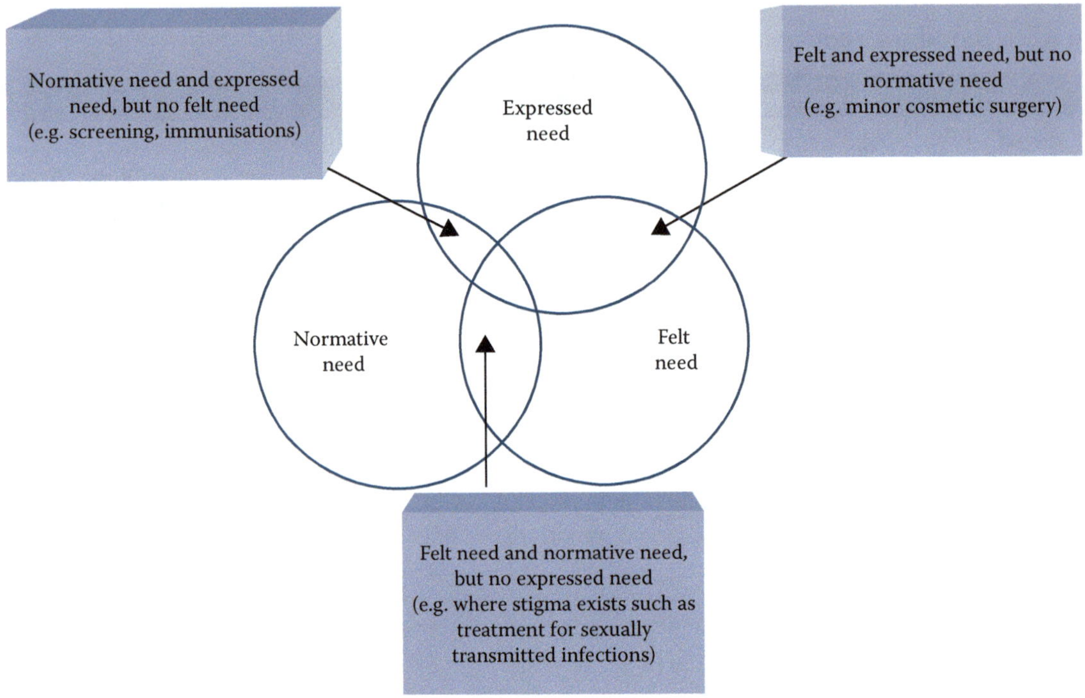

Figure 4C.1 Types of need. (Adapted from Bradshaw, J., A taxonomy of social need, in *Problems and Progress in Medical Care*, 1972, Figure 3.1 by permission of Oxford University Press.)

Table 4C.2 Major theories of social justice

Theory	Description
Distributive justice	Means of ensuring a **fair distribution** of societal goods.
Procedural justice	The way in which **decisions or agreements** are made.
Interactional justice	How people **treat each other** (moving beyond institutions and the state).
Retributive justice	How society **punishes** acts of injustice.
Restorative justice	Bringing together victims and perpetrators to **restore justice after a harm** has taken place (e.g. Truth and Reconciliation committees).

Box 4C.1 Justice as fairness

Basic liberties are a right for everyone	Restricting the individual liberties of some members of society is not justified even if it could lead to the greater good of society.
Difference principle	Resources need not be distributed equally, but social and economic inequalities should benefit those who are most disadvantaged. For example, society can agree to pay a doctor more than a cleaner because the doctor has the potential to save people's lives.

distributive justice when it is not possible to know the outcomes of a policy (e.g. as related to events that may or may not take place in the future).

Thibaut and Walker [42] argue that the most important requirement for procedural justice is **voice** (i.e. the opportunity for an individual or a community to express views about a decision). This concept is seen in health systems that enshrine public participation as a central part of service development. Leventhal et al. [43] define six other criteria that influence our perceptions of procedural justice (see Box 4C.2).

Box 4C.2 Leventhal et al. six criteria of procedural justice

For a process to be considered fair, it must

- Be **consistent**
- Be **neutral** (i.e. not biased by preconceptions or self-interest)
- Be based on **accurate information**
- Have the potential to be **corrected**
- Take account of **all parties**
- Be made **ethically**

4C.2 Priorities and rationing

In the context of healthcare, the concepts of **rationing** and **prioritisation** involve making decisions about how **finite resources are allocated.** The term rationing is often used synonymously with prioritisation. However, rationing always has a dimension of restriction, while prioritisation is required even when extra resources are available to rank various choices according to their importance.

Prioritisation frameworks are summarised in Section 4C.5.

Rationing

There are two certainties in life: death and scarcity.

Maynard [44]

In economics, the term **scarcity** refers to finite resources, which may be monetary or related to materials, equipment, or human resources. In health and healthcare, there will always be finite resources but infinite demand; therefore, a system of decision-making is required for deciding which services to provide and which not to provide.

Explicit rationing systems use transparent, consistent criteria to make entitlement decisions. Such systems are often controversial. However, rationing decisions are made every day and at every level within healthcare, ranging from:

- A GP receptionist's judgement of whether a patient should be offered an emergency appointment (based on an implicit decision of whether such an appointment is justified by the severity of the patient's symptoms); to
- National guidance recommending or limiting the use of a new healthcare technology (based on an evaluation of its cost-effectiveness)

National, organisational, and individual rationing decisions

Rationing decisions may occur at the national, organisational, or individual levels. See Table 4C.3.

Stakeholder involvement in rationing

According to the principles of procedural justice, rationing decisions are influenced by the

Table 4C.3 Levels of rationing

Level	Agency	Advantages	Disadvantages
Macro	Government or state level (e.g. NICE 'do not do' guidance, which specifies procedures of limited or no clinical effectiveness)	Saves duplication of work at local level	No scope for local decision-making or autonomy
Meso	Healthcare organisations (e.g. referral review panels to prevent or minimise unnecessary hospital use)	Can respond to local circumstances	Little scope to address individual circumstances Risk of unnecessary duplication if the similar reviews are occurring in neighbouring areas
Micro	Individual clinician (e.g. consultation duration and frequency; intensity and scope of interventions provided)	Can respond to individual circumstances	Vulnerable to inconsistencies. Lack of accountability in decision-making

Table 4C.4 Ways in which the views and experiences of stakeholders can influence rationing

Perception of outcomes	For example, if large breasts were seen as a necessity rather than an aesthetic choice, then plastic surgery for breast augmentation would be more likely to be funded.
Acquisition of opinions	Willingness-to-pay (WTP) methods for valuing benefits will reach different conclusions according to the following: An individual's **ability to pay** An individual's **likelihood of requiring** the service An individual's **likelihood of being required to pay** for the service
Position of groups in society	For example, attitudes toward older people may influence the degree of funding provided for social care, dementia treatments, etc.
Social norms	For example, given four hypothetical candidates for a heart transplant, which patient should be prioritised? A person who smokes A person who drinks excessive alcohol A person who is overweight A person who is in prison

views and experiences of decision-makers (see Table 4C.4).

For these reasons, decision-makers should consult a wide range of stakeholders, including:

- Patients
- Clinicians
- Voters
- Local and national politicians
- Healthcare managers
- Representatives of the pharmaceutical industry

Rationing criteria

In healthcare, rationing decisions generally aim to take into account the need for a service, its cost-effectiveness, and the principle of fairness (see Box 4C.3).

Box 4C.3 Rationing criteria

Need	The concept of need can apply at two levels: **Individual capacity to benefit** (see Section 4C.1) (e.g. in England most dementia drugs are currently recommended only for people with mild to moderate forms of dementia, not severe forms). **Societal** (e.g. in societies with declining birth rates, a wider range of individuals may have access to IVF treatment for infertility than in countries with rapidly growing populations).
Cost-effectiveness	By definition, this assessment only considers effective treatments. In England and Wales, for example, NICE usually considers treatments above a certain threshold cost per QALY as not being cost-effective (see Section 4D.8).
Fairness	Individuals in similar circumstances should have equal access to care; however, the process for allocating resources should also be fair (i.e. it should consider the concepts of **procedural justice**—see Section 4C.1).

4C.3 Balancing equity and efficiency

According to the principle of distributive justice, healthcare resources should be allocated **equitably**. However, in order to ensure that scarce resources are used to their greatest effect, the process of allocation should also be guided by principles of **efficiency**. A system that distributes resources equitably may require some **sacrifice** of efficiency, and vice versa. Clearly, the manifestation of equitable and efficient allocation also depends on the exact definitions used for each principle (Box 4C.4).

Concepts of efficiency

See also Section 4D.1.

Box 4C.4 Definitions

Concept	Definition
Equity	Fairness
Equality	Same for all
Efficiency	Greatest benefit achievable from a given resource

Definitions of efficiency typically relate to a utilitarian philosophical position (i.e. to achieve the greatest aggregated good across the greatest number in the whole community). For example, Donaldson et al. [45] defined efficiency in healthcare as securing the, '... greatest improvements in well-being from available resources'.

Therefore, the concept of **efficiency** within healthcare depends also on the definition of **well-being** used (see also Section 4A.3). This may be problematic because an improvement in health status does not always improve well-being. For example, offering people a choice of how they wish to be treated may in fact provide more well-being than would occur if all individuals were offered the best available treatment.

Economists describe the state of ultimate efficiency as being a **Pareto optimal** (*not to be confused with the Pareto principle [also known as the 80:20 rule] which states that for many phenomena, 80% of the consequences result from 20% of the causes*). In Pareto optimal circumstances, efficiency has reached the point where no further improvements can be made in one part of the system without disadvantaging other parts. Therefore, on a healthcare system that is not Pareto optimal, providing more resources for

Box 4C.5 Example: A hypothetical equity/efficiency alignment in the provision of universal immunisations

In order to achieve herd immunity to measles, 95% of the population need to be vaccinated. The uptake of vaccinations using a standard system (call recall, with injections given at general practices) is relatively cheap and easy to use and achieves 80% coverage of the population.

For a variety of reasons, the remaining 20% of children do not attend for immunisations offered in the standard way. Additional resources will therefore be required to encourage these groups to be vaccinated (e.g. mobile vaccination clinics, targeted health promotion, individual calls and visits). Although the unit cost of vaccinating these hard-to-reach people is much higher than the standard unit cost, it may well be more efficient to spend this money because the 95% coverage achieved will offer herd immunity to the whole population.

one part of the system may not disadvantage other parts, and so this change in resource allocation would be an efficient choice.

Concepts of equity

The two principal types of equity are **vertical** and **horizontal** equity (see Chapter 1C.11).

Conflict between efficiency and equity

An intervention is efficient if it produces the **greatest net health gains** in a population for a given budget; whereas to be **equitable,** the intervention should be **distributed fairly** within the population.

Overall improvements in health status may mask widening differences in access to healthcare between constituent groups of the population. Even when the geographical distribution of services is similar, some groups within the population will require extra resources in order to access them and thereby achieve the same health gain.

Alignment between equity and efficiency

Conflicts between equity and efficiency are sometimes reconciled by incorporating the concepts of **distributive justice** and **externalities** into the definition of well-being.

To meet the principles of distributive justice, the benefits of healthcare should be shared fairly. Therefore, an inequitable but Pareto efficient system is distributively unjust (i.e. the system benefits everyone but some people receive unfair amounts of benefit). Moreover, since the well-being of individuals is dependent both on their own health status and on the health of society as a whole, so such a system may in fact be inefficient as well as inequitable.

Externalities

An externality is a by-product of the production or consumption of goods, which is enjoyed by society in general (see Chapter 4D.1). Equitable care provides positive (i.e. beneficial) externalities and therefore improves the well-being of society. See Box 4C.5.

4C.4 Consumerism and community participation

To adhere to principles of procedural justice, individuals and communities need to play an active role in making decisions about healthcare. Biomedical models of healthcare have traditionally had connotations of a passive role for patients, whereby expert health professionals cared for patients. In contrast, the conceptualisation of patients as consumers transforms them from being **passive recipients** of care into **customers** who have the right and the capacity to choose whether and where to seek health or healthcare.

See also Section 4C.6 and Chapter 2I.5.

Consumer rights in healthcare

In the UK health system, the concepts of the *'patient as a consumer'* and *'healthcare as a product'* were introduced in the 1980s. In 1991, the Department of Health produced *'The Patients' Charter'* which set out a list of rights that individuals could expect from their healthcare services. In common with many private companies, the NHS now uses **satisfaction surveys** and **sentiment analysis** of social media feeds as key tools for assessing the quality of its provision.

Patient and consumer choice

Consumers of products have the choice of whether to consume services and, if so, where. In England, several policies to modernise the NHS have focused on providing more choice to patients. Examples include the 'Choose and Book' system, where patients can choose which hospital to use for elective care. Such policies are intended to:

- Introduce **competition** between healthcare providers
- Improve the **responsiveness** of the healthcare system to consumers' preferences
- Enhance the **efficiency** of healthcare services

Despite these initiatives, choice within healthcare is often constrained (see Table 4C.5).

Community participation

While consumerism is focused on an individual's rights, community participation is more closely aligned to the joint responsibilities to society. As such, community participation in healthcare typically involves individuals acting in the interests of other people. Two prominent models of community participation in healthcare are where community groups:

- **Support** mainstream services. For example, Volunteers for The Food Chain prepare and deliver meals to people with HIV that are designed by dieticians to meet the specific dietary needs of such people.
- **Replace** mainstream services. For example, women's health collectives were established in the 1970s in the United States and Canada to address concerns that women's needs were 'often ignored, underrepresented and trivialised' in mainstream services. Run by and for women, they provide information and healthcare services to women.
- **Participate** in running mainstream healthcare services (see Box 4C.6).

See Chapter 2I.5.

Table 4C.5 Constraints in choice within healthcare

Type of constraint	Description
Healthcare gatekeeping	Where patients are obliged to see a GP (or another **gatekeeper**) in order to access specialist healthcare services.
Urgency of treatment	In circumstances of acute healthcare need (e.g. following a road traffic collision), individuals may not have the choice of *whether* to accept healthcare leave alone *where* to seek services.
Disempowerment	Individuals who are **unwell** in hospital may not feel empowered to question decisions that they would have challenged if well or on familiar territory. In a small minority of circumstances (e.g. under a section of the Mental Health Act), this freedom to challenge decisions is suspended.
Information asymmetry	Patients may depend on clinicians to advise them about the **complexities** of the management of their conditions. While growing access to the Internet has meant that some consumers have an abundance of information available to them, this differential may potentially widen inequalities. For example, older people and people on low incomes may be less likely to have Internet access.

Box 4C.6 Example: NHS Foundation Hospitals—Community participation in running healthcare

In England, NHS Foundation Trusts (FTs) have different regulatory and financial arrangements from other NHS Trusts. It is of note that they were established as **public benefit corporations**, meaning that they have a **board of governors** (comprised of patients, staff, and members of the public) who have responsibilities regarding the appointment of the trust's chair, non-executive directors, and chief executive. The board of governors also has the right to be consulted on the trust's strategic direction.

In addition, FTs are required to **recruit members** (i.e. people living or working in their local community who want to be informed about the management of the trust). In this respect, FTs have the potential to bring true community participation to the hospital system.

In its early evaluation of FTs, the King's Fund found that they had attracted a large membership, with over half a million people being members of the first wave of FTs; however, it was unclear to what extent these members were representative of their local populations. With a few notable exceptions, the evaluation concluded that, ***'so far there is little compelling evidence that members or governors have made a significant impact on the management of foundation trusts'.***

Sources: Reproduced from Lewis, R. et al., *Social Enterprise and Community Based Care: Is There a Future for Mutually-Owned Organizations in Community and Primary Care?* King's Fund, London, U.K, 2006; Foundation Trust Network, *New Voices, New Accountabilities: A Guide to Wider Governance in Foundation Trusts*, Foundation Trust Network, London, UK, 2005, Available online at www.nhsconfed.org/ftn.

4C.5 Prioritisation frameworks and equity of service provision

See also Section 4C.2 and Chapter 5F.

International frameworks

Sabik and Lie [48] compared how eight countries approached explicit priority setting. Countries approached the issue differently based on their most pressing problem. For example, long waiting lists in Norway, cost pressures in Oregon, and the so-called postcode lottery in England. The authors distinguished two types of approach (see Table 4C.6).

The practice-based approaches were implemented to a greater degree than were the principle-based approaches. However, the authors noted that the

Table 4C.6 Priority-setting approaches

Approach	Description	Examples
Outlining principles	This approach starts by defining some abstract principles that will be used to guide priority-setting decisions. This approach was taken in Norway, the Netherlands, Sweden, and Denmark. Social justice principles featured in some of the countries' defining principles, but not in all.	Sweden had criteria based on need and solidarity; Denmark's criteria included both equal human worth and social and geographical equity.
Defining practices	This approach starts by defining some priorities, often by selecting and adapting an existing list of priorities. General principles emerge through reflecting on the priority process. This approach was taken in Israel, New Zealand, England (establishment of NICE), and the US State of Oregon.	Equity was a core principle by which New Zealand's decisions were made (alongside acceptability, effectiveness, and efficiency).

priority-setting exercises had not solved the problems that led to their creation (e.g. waiting lists were still a problem in Norway).

Local frameworks

ENG While the creation of NICE was a national approach to prioritisation, local areas also need their own approach to making prioritisation decisions for their population. The Yorkshire and the Humber Public Health Observatory reviewed a range of prioritisation frameworks being used in the NHS and considered the extent to which three approaches considered equity, among other factors (see Table 4C.7).

Table 4C.7 Prioritisation frameworks

	Programme budgeting and marginal analysis (PBMA)	Save to invest	Multi-criteria decision analysis (MCDA)
Focus	Makes decisions on the allocation of funding between and within healthcare resource groups	Commissioning of hospital care across different procedures	Ranks the relative priority of selected preventive health interventions
Description of the method	Panel convened to • Decide locally relevant decision-making criteria • Review current activity and expenditure • Identify areas for growth and maintenance and areas to cut • Consult with stakeholders at all stages	List of procedures drawn from a survey of NHS commissioners Effectiveness of the procedures reviewed Informed value judgements used to estimate minimum and maximum levels of reduction in volume that may be possible Estimates of savings determined from Hospital Episode Statistics and tariff data	Online tool that ranks interventions according to five criteria: • Affordability • Certainty (evidence of effectiveness) • Cost-effectiveness (cost per QALY) • Reach (% population likely to be reached) • Inequality (disadvantaged versus whole population)
Geography	National and local	Local and GP practice	National and local
Do the criteria include Evidence base	Depends on the criteria chosen by the marginal analysis panel	Yes	Yes
Efficiency		Cost-effective alternatives considered	Yes (cost per QALY)
Equity		Yes (main aim is to reduce the 3–4-fold variation in hospital admissions)	Yes
How to handle uncertainty or conflict between criteria?	Sensitivity analysis	Minimum and maximum savings for each PCT calculated	Weighting for each criterion informed by a discrete choice experiment

4C.6 Public access to information

By providing the public with access to healthcare information, it may be possible to improve individuals' **understanding of health and disease** and make services more accountable. For example, by making information more accessible on patients' rights and the availability and quality of services, patients are better able to decide where to seek care when given a choice. Increasingly, patients are being offered access to information about their own healthcare. For example, in the NHS, patients now have a right to see the information recorded in their medical records.

Understanding of health and disease

The Internet has transformed the way in which many people access health information. According to the National Consumer Council it has

> *The potential to result in a much more active patient and more balanced relationship with health professionals.*
>
> Sihota and Lennard [49]

However, alongside this explosion in the availability of information, public health specialists should keep the following issues in mind:

- Variable **quality** of information available on the Internet
- Varying degrees of **applicability** to any individual patient
- Different levels of **health literacy** regarding technical terminology
- Potential to worsen health **inequalities** because of varying access to the Internet and different levels of health literacy

Making information accessible

About services and rights: The Freedom of Information Act

UK The Freedom of Information Act [50] applies in England, Wales, and Northern Ireland, and there is a similar act in Scotland. The act applies to all ***'public authorities'***, including:

- Central and local government
- NHS bodies
- Schools, colleges, and universities
- Police
- Many other non-departmental public bodies, committees, and advisory bodies

The act requires public authorities to specify the kinds of information that they publish, how such information is made available, and whether it is available free of charge or upon payment. In addition, the act gives any person the legal right to ask for, and be given, any information held by a public authority (although certain exceptions apply). Public authorities must provide the information requested within 20 working days. Information can be withheld to protect various interests that are allowed for by the act, in which case an explanation should be provided stating why the information was withheld.

A person requesting information may be asked to pay a small amount to cover costs such as photocopying or postage. If the public authority thinks that it will cost it more than a set amount to find the information and prepare it for release, then it can turn down the request. This amount is known as an **appropriate limit** and is currently set at £600 for central government or £450 for other public authorities.

About individuals: The Data Protection Act

UK When people ask for information that a public body holds about themselves, the request is handled under the Data Protection Act rather than under the Freedom of Information Act. There are slightly different rights under the two acts, with different fees and different timeframes being applicable.

NZ Under the Official Information Act [51], any person can request government agencies (e.g. ministers, departments, local authorities) to release information. This information must be made available unless there is a good reason for withholding it.

HK The main privacy law in Hong Kong is the Personal Data (Privacy) Ordinance (Cap 486), known as 'The Ordinance'. The Ordinance, which generally reflects the OECD guidelines for the Protection of Privacy and Trans-border Flows of Personal Data [52], has been in force since December 1996. The purpose of the ordinance is to protect individuals' right to privacy by regulating the handling of personal data in Hong Kong. It applies to any person or organisation, both public and private, that collects, holds, processes, or uses personal data. It is currently under review and its main focus is on business practice.

The culture of sharing medical notes with patients is less well developed in Hong Kong than in other countries such as the United Kingdom.

4C.7 User and carer involvement

User and carer involvement in service planning.

See also Section 4C.4 and Chapter 2I.5.

Since the 1980s, governments across Western Europe and North America have encouraged patients to contribute to the planning and development of health services. In England and Wales, the involvement of patients is seen as a key strategy for improving the quality of healthcare. In particular, such involvement tends to lead to more **accessible** and **acceptable** health services.

Policy initiatives to promote user involvement

UK The United Kingdom has a long history of patient and public involvement in policy initiatives in both health and social care (Department of Health 1999). Table 4C.8 lists the organisations with prime responsibility for public and patient involvement across the United Kingdom.

Table 4C.8 UK organisations with responsibility for public and patient involvement

Country	Organisation	Description
England	**HealthWatch [54]**	A national organisation with local offices in each local authority area
Scotland	**Scottish Health Council**	A national body, part of Quality Improvement Scotland, with local offices in each health board area
Wales	**Community Health Councils**	One council for each of the eight health boards
Northern Ireland	**Patient Client Council**	Five local offices (one for each of the health and social care trust areas)

Source: Hartree, N. and Tidy, C., Monitoring the NHS, 2014, Accessed online July 20, 2014 at http://www.patient.co.uk/doctor/Monitoring-the-NHS-Local-Involvement-Networks-(LINks).htm.

4C.8 Power, interests, and ideology

Appreciation of concepts of power, interests, and ideology.

See Chapter 5D.4.

Policy changes are heavily influenced by power relationships within and between different groups of people.

Power

Power is the capacity to make something happen. It often involves making other people and organisations do things that they would not otherwise have done. French and Raven [55] identified six types of power (see Box 4C.7).

By recognising which individuals have which types of power, public health specialists can identify which people need to be influenced in order to secure support for a particular policy. This type of analysis can also be used to identify and to counter different negative sources of power. Finally, it can help identify which sources of power an individual is underusing.

Interests

See Chapter 5B.2.

Ideology

A political ideology describes a belief of how power should be **allocated** and to what **ends** it should be used. Such an ideology can be a construct of political thought, and it often defines different political parties and their policies.

Box 4C.8 groups some common ideologies into themes, but note that one ideology may belong to several groups and that related ideologies often overlap. For this reason, modern political parties often subscribe to a combination of ideologies. Note also that the meanings of political labels differ between countries.

Box 4C.7 French and Raven [55] types of power

Type of power	Description
• Resource	Also known as **reward power**, a person with this type of power has control of resources (e.g. budgets, people) and therefore has the power to reward people with promotion or funds.
• Position	By virtue of holding a particular job within an organisation, the **post-holder** is entitled to the rights and privileges associated with that role.
• Coercive	The type of power that comes from the ability to **punish** (e.g. through the withdrawal of privileges or the imposition of penalties).
• Personal	Also known as **charisma**. This power resides in the personality of the person.
• Expert	This type of power vested in a person because of their acknowledged **expertise**. A public health specialist has a degree of expert power.
• Negative	This power is the capacity to **stop** things from happening to prevent something from even being discussed.

Box 4C.8 Types of ideology

Class struggle	Collectivity	Ethnicity	Religion
Socialism	Socialism	Nationalism	Christian-based ideologies
Communism	Religious socialism	Fascism	Christian anarchism
Marxism	Christian socialism	Nazism	Hindu-based ideologies
Leninism	Democratic socialism	Neo-Nazism	Hindu nationalism
Stalinism	Communism	Racism, racialism	Islam-based ideologies
Neo-Marxism	Religious communism		Islamism, Muslim fundamentalism
	Marxism		Jewish-based ideologies
			Religious Zionism

4C.9 Inequalities in health and access to healthcare

Inequalities in health (e.g. by region, ethnicity, socio-economic position, or gender) and in access to healthcare, including their causes.

Inequalities in health can arise or become manifest for many interrelated reasons. As a first step, it is important to consider if these observed effects are in fact real or if in fact they could be interpreted in a different way. Bartley [56] used four models to explain health inequalities (see Table 4C.9).

Table 4C.10 gives an indication of where in the rest of the book to find further discussion on these factors and ways to address them. Three examples are given to illustrate principles underlying the inequalities.

The Black Report (see Box 4C.9) found that income fundamentally influences health and that this influence lies **outside** the scope of the healthcare system. A number of studies have since been published that investigated the issue in more detail and provided potential solutions (see Table 4C.11).

Boxes 4C.10 and 4C.11 give examples of ethnic and geographic inequalities.

Table 4C.9 Bartley's explanations of health inequalities

Type of factor	Description
Individual factors	Individual health behaviours such as smoking, diet, and exercise.
Materialist	Living in deprived conditions places people at risk of ill health (e.g. through poor housing or poor access to services).
Psychosocial	The effects of social circumstances may cause psychological effects, which in turn cause physiological effects.
Life course	The effect of social circumstances is cumulative and there are certain critical periods that affect later life. Therefore, adults in affluent circumstances who experienced deprivation as a child may have poorer health in later life.

Table 4C.10 Signposting to other sections on inequalities in health in the book

Types of cause		Reference
Measurement and interpretation	Extent to which ill health manifests as disease.	4A.8 Explanations for various social patterns and experiences of illness.
		4B.5 Behaviour in response to illness and treatments.
	Artefact.	Observed inequalities are not real, just a feature of the way factors are measured (Box 4C.9).
	Health affects social circumstances not the other way around.	Box 4C.9.
Individual behavioural factors	Health behaviours (variations in diet, exercise, smoking, and drinking).	2E Health and social behaviour.
	Exposure to harmful or protective environmental factors.	2F.1 Environmental determinants of disease.
Materialist (access to resources) and psychosocial factors	Access to appropriate healthcare	1C.10 Equity in healthcare.
	Effect of socio-economic position on environmental exposures and health behaviours.	2I.2 Pre-determinants of health.
		2I.5 Concept of deprivation and its effect on health of children and adults.
		Effect of socio-economic circumstances on ethnic inequalities in health (Box 4C.10).
		Regional differences in health (Box 4C.11).
Life-course factors		2A.

Box 4C.9 UK The Black report

The Black report [18] was commissioned by the Labour government in the late 1970s but was published after the Conservative party came to power in 1979. The incoming government attempted to suppress the publication of the report (although the endeavour backfired) as it did not support its findings.

Black and colleagues noted a **social class gradient** in both **morbidity** and **mortality** that was

- Present at every age
- Present for all major diseases
- Increasing over time

The authors listed four possible explanations for the gradient that they observed, namely

1. Statistical artefact—the way that social class is measured
2. Social selection—the ill become poorer
3. Behavioural factors—direct impact of nutrition, etc.
4. Indirect impact of deprivation—effect on physical health is mediated by psychology

Table 4C.11 Solutions to inequality proposed by key studies

Study	Proposal
Benzeval [57]	Improve **physical environment** Address **socio-economic factors** (income and employment) Promote healthier **lifestyles** Improve **access** to **services**
Acheson inquiry [58]	Evaluated government policies regarding health inequalities Focus on policies affecting health of **families and children** Reduce inequalities in **income** and improve **housing** standards
Saving lives: Our Healthier Nation [59]	Prominence given to health inequalities and four priority areas: • Cardiovascular disease • Accidents • Cancer • Mental health
Wanless reports	Three reports: 2002—made the **economic case** for public health 2004—securing good health for the **whole population** 2006—**funding** of social care for older people
Marmot report [60]	Policy objectives: 1. Give every child the best **start in life** 2. Enable all children, young people, and adults to maximise their capabilities and **take control** over their lives 3. Create **fair employment** and good work for all 4. Ensure a healthy **standard of living** for all 5. Create and develop healthy and sustainable **places and communities** 6. Strengthen the role and impact of **ill-health prevention** 7. See also Chapter 5D

Box 4C.10 To understand ethnic inequalities on health, take account of social inequalities

Nazroo and Karlsen [61] conducted a series of studies exploring ethnicity and ethnic inequalities in health. As shown in the figure, some of the differences in health status can be accounted for by variations in socio-economic factors. In addition, the authors concluded that ethnic identity is a complex concept that is inadequately captured simply by recording a person's country of origin.

Box 4C.11 North–south divide in health experience in England

The Office for National Statistics Regional trends [62] show that for many health indicators, health is worse for people living in the North of England (Yorkshire and the Humber, North West, and the North East) compared with people living in the South (South East, London, and South West).

There is no clear explanation for these inequalities in health. The trends are consistent over time and across a range of health indicators, suggesting that measurement error is unlikely to be the cause. There are clear social differences between regions (deprivation is generally higher in the North than in the South); therefore, **materialist** and **psychosocial** explanations are plausible. Likewise, several conditions that do not follow the usual social gradient pattern, such as breast cancer incidence, are not higher in the North.

4C.10 Health and social effects of migration

If properly managed, migration can bring considerable financial and cultural benefits to both individuals and countries. However, mismanaged migration and human trafficking represent significant health risks.

The UN's **International Organization for Migration** estimates that [63] 3.1% of the world's population are migrants, which is the highest proportion recorded in world history. This figure has remained relatively stable over the last 10 years but the proportion varies greatly between countries. The main reasons for migration are listed in Table 4C.12.

A distinction is made between **voluntary** and **forced** migrants (see Table 4C.13).

Classification of migrants

Migration is the permanent relocation of people between one country and another (see Box 4C.12).

Migrants may be classified as **documented** or **undocumented,** depending on whether the state authorities in the host or transit country have authorised residence and employment. Undocumented migrants (sometimes inappropriately referred to

Table 4C.12 Reasons for migration

Reason	Description
Economic liberalisation	Increases in trade and globalisation lead to increased demands for skilled labour—especially in the IT, financial, and hospitality sectors.
Economic decline	Counter to what might be expected, temporary economic recessions tend not to lead to a downturn in migration.
Demographic changes	Most developed countries have populations that are expected to shrink and to become older over the course of the coming decades. The young, growing populations of developing countries may serve to counter this '*population time bomb*'.
Transnational migration	These are migrants who shuttle between multiple homes and maintain links with more than one country. Such people are said to live in '*transnational migration space*'. This growing phenomenon is facilitated by dual citizenship and multiple voting rights.
Conflict	There is no end in sight for wars and political upheaval.

Table 4C.13 Voluntary versus forced migration

Reasons for voluntary migration	Reasons for forced migration
Employment	War and conflict
Study	Industrial, environmental, or natural disasters
Rejoin family members	Famine
Retirement	Development projects (e.g. dams)

Box 4C.12 Types of migration

Type of migration	Alternative name	Definition	Rate
Emigration	Out-migration	Process of people leaving one country on a permanent or semi-permanent basis	Number of people departing from a country per 1000 of its population per annum
Immigration	In-migration	Process of people entering a country to take up residence	Number of people arriving per 1000 of the population of the receiving country per annum

Table 4C.14 Asylum seekers and refugees

Type of person	Definition
Asylum seeker	Person who requests sanctuary in a destination country on grounds of having escaped persecution in the country of origin.
Convention refugee	Person recognised by the destination country as having a '*well-founded fear of being persecuted for reasons of race, religion, nationality, membership of a particular social group, or political opinion, is outside the country of his nationality, and is unable to, or owing to such fear, is unwilling to avail himself of the protection of that country*'. Such a person is accorded the full rights of the 1951 UN Convention on Refugees.
Quota refugee	Person who is granted limited refugee status by the destination country before leaving the country of origin, usually as part of an agreement by which the destination country agrees to take a finite group of refugees over a short period of time.

as *'illegal immigrants'*) are people who have either entered a host country without legal authorisation or overstayed their period of temporary, authorised entry. Table 4C.14 sets out the difference between **asylum seekers**, **convention refugees,** and **quota refugees**.

Health and social effects

Migration has profound social effects and can also have significant health implications, both positive and negative. The **healthy migrant effect** refers to the phenomenon that the people with the capacity to migrate tend to be the healthiest—and often the most socially advantaged—members of the country of origin.

On the other hand, migration is an important social determinant of health. It is often associated with poorer social status in the destination country, where first-generation migrants tend to work in jobs that are lower paid, have lower status,

Table 4C.15 Factors affecting the health of migrants

Factor	Effects on health
Reason for migration	Forced migration is likely to be associated with poorer health and social conditions than planned, voluntary migrations.
Rights of the migrant	While documented migrants have greater rights than undocumented migrants, language barriers and lack of knowledge of the host country's systems can prevent people from accessing services to which they have a right.
Geography	Contextual factors, such as similarities between the country of origin and the destination country.
Generic	Factors affecting health and social circumstances in all communities (e.g. age, gender, socio-economic position, and ethnicity). These factors may have particular effects on certain migrant populations. For example, women from certain countries of origin may have restricted access to services such as healthcare (e.g. cervical screening) in their country of destination because of the societal and cultural attitudes in their host country.

and are more dangerous. At the extreme, undocumented migrants and victims of human trafficking may be in positions of exploitation and abuse.

The effects of migration are impossible to generalise. They vary according to the factors listed in Table 4C.15.

It is important to recognise that our understanding of the health needs of migrant populations is limited by inadequate data. Routinely collected data rarely capture a person's country of origin, so it is difficult to know what proportion of a community are migrants and the extent to which migrants are using health services. Moreover, communication between health systems, healthcare workers, and migrant communities is often inadequate. As a result, migrants may have problems accessing services (due to lack of knowledge about what is available or concerns about their rights/treatment if they do access them) and healthcare systems may be ill prepared to respond to migrants' needs appropriately.

First-generation migrants often retain patterns of disease from their country of origin. For example, stomach cancer (which has a high prevalence in Japan and China due to diets that are rich in smoked, salted, and pickled foods) is common among first-generation Japanese and Chinese immigrants to the United States. However, the incidence is much lower among the migrants' descendants who adopt the lifestyle practices of the destination country.

The European Observatory on Health Systems and Policy [64] reported that migrant populations across Europe tend to have the following:

- Increased risk of communicable disease, occupational diseases, and poor mental health
- Increased risk of maternal and child health problems and lower use of antenatal care services
- Lower use of screening but similar or higher use of primary and specialist services
- Decreased risk of cancers but variable risk of cardiovascular diseases

People who have been subject to forced migration are at particular risk of the phenomena listed in Table 4C.16.

Migration also has implications for non-migrants both in the country of origin and in the destination country (see Table 4C.17).

Table 4C.16 Risks to people subjected to forced migration

Risk	Description
Epidemics	Poor sanitation and overcrowding in refugee camps.
Sexual violence	Sexual violence and STIs: due to rape and assault as weapons of war.
PTSD	Post-traumatic stress disorder is highly prevalent among asylum seekers and refugees.
Risks in transit	For example, a group of Chinese migrants was asphyxiated while being trafficked in a cargo container on board a ship crossing the English Channel in 2000.
Hostility on arrival	On arrival in the destination country, migrants often experience poor living conditions, a lack of social integration, stigma, and open xenophobic hostility.

Table 4C.17 Effects of migration on countries

Original country	Drain of healthcare workers from low and middle-income countries to high-income countries risks destabilising local provision of services. Loss of highly skilled people, especially new graduates, places financial and human resources pressures, which are partly compensated for by **remittances** (the term for the portion of migrants' wages that is sent back to the country of origin).
Destination country	Allows the host country to address shortages of individuals with specific skills and knowledge. Source of income generation (overseas students are worth an estimated £8bn to the UK economy [65]). Change to demographic profile (the Office for National Statistics estimates from the 2010 census that 25% of births in the United Kingdom were to women not born in the country). Possible risk to the health of the population (rationale for TB screening at points of entry for migrants from certain countries). Drain on state resources (e.g. education, healthcare, law and order).

Source: Adapted and supplemented from WHO, *International Migration, Health and Human Rights*, Health & Human Rights Publication Series, Issue No. 4, WHO, Geneva, Switzerland, 2003.

4C.11 Health effects of international trade

Greater openness in international trade has the potential for both positive and negative effects on health and healthcare. The WHO works with the World Trade Organization and other organisations on addressing both the direct and indirect effects of trade on health [67].

Circumstances where greater trade openness has or could have direct implications on health include the availability of **medical technologies**, **infection risks**, and **food safety** (see Table 4C.18).

The indirect effects of increased trade on health mainly occur through impacts on economic and environmental determinants. These factors have great relevance to the concepts of distributive and procedural justice described in Section 4C.1 (Table 4C.19).

Table 4C.18 Direct impacts of international trade on health

Factor	Impact on health
Medical technologies	By influencing **trade tariffs** or **patent restrictions**, it may be possible for countries to gain access to drugs and other health technologies at more affordable prices. Mechanisms such as the Trade Related Aspects of Intellectual Property Rights (TRIPS) Agreement have been used in an attempt to improve access to HIV drugs in sub-Saharan African countries.
Infection risks	Infectious diseases may be transported within traded goods or by means of an infected tradesperson.
Food safety	Countries can restrain trade in a foodstuff on the grounds of health (e.g. if there is a credible risk of exposure to zoonotic diseases or to toxins).

Table 4C.19 Positive and negative effects of trade on distributive and procedural justice

Positives	Negatives
More equitable distribution of resources if more countries can trade	Unequal negotiating power between nations may lead to unfair trade agreements.
Greater competition and reduced prices	Global environmental consequences of transporting goods across greater distances. Reduced capacity to monitor and influence conditions of producers. Exacerbate health inequalities through the effects of migration (see Section 4C.10).

4C.12 Global influences on health and social policy

When the United Nations was formed in 1945, member states agreed to work together to promote the *'economic and social advancement of all peoples'*. More than 60 years later, the health of the world population is still under threat from environmental and political crises, and income and health inequalities continue to rise between the richest and poorest nations.

Health promotion

At an international level, cooperation to promote health may be of particular value through

- The exchange of ideas and mutual learning
- Pooling of resources
- Joint action

Social policy

The field of international social policy compares the welfare provision found in different countries, ranging from the Nordic **welfare model** of comprehensive provision at one extreme to the scantier provision available in other countries.

UK In Britain, the Welfare State was established following the **Beveridge Report** [68], which identified five **giant evils** in society, namely

1. Squalor
2. Ignorance
3. Want
4. Idleness
5. Disease

By creating the welfare state (i.e. a series of policies designed to support people with financial, health, or social needs), the government acknowledged its responsibility to care for the population *'from the cradle to the grave'*.

International social policy also addresses the potential impact of **globalisation** on the welfare state and the influential roles played by **international actors** such as the International Monetary Fund, the United Nations, the World Bank, and the World Trade Organization.

4C.13 Critical analysis of investment in health programmes in general and in global initiatives

Critical analysis of investment in health improvement, and the part played by economic development and global organisations.

Challenges to evaluating health improvement investment

Although health promotion interventions have the potential to reduce future healthcare costs by avoiding disease, the evidence for this return on investment is equivocal. Even where a health promotion programme is demonstrably successful (e.g. stop-smoking programmes), the overall cost to the state from a population with higher longevity may outweigh the savings from lost productivity and acute illness.

It is therefore important to remember that the objective of health promotion is not to save money but to **reduce morbidity and mortality**. Health promotion programmes should be assessed, along with other healthcare or social care programmes, using the methods of economic evaluation and cost-effectiveness analysis (CEA) described in Section 4D.

Hale [69] identified a number of potential reasons why the use of economic analysis may be problematic in the context of health promotion interventions, including the following:

- Health promotion programmes have **multiple objectives**.
- Clients are essentially healthy at the time and so the benefits are **broader** than simply gains in health status.
- QALYs do not capture the **full range of benefits** from health promotion interventions.
- **RCTs** are needed to confirm that any observed utility benefits were caused by the intervention; however, these are difficult to conduct in the field of health promotion because of the timeframes involved.
- Economic evaluations of health promotion interventions are highly dependent on the rate or rates of **discounting** applied.

Economic development and global organisations

Overseas aid has increased in recent years and is set to increase further. According to the Institute of Fiscal Studies [70], 16 European countries, including the United Kingdom [70], have committed to reaching a target of spending 0.7% of gross national income on overseas development assistance by 2015. Of this figure, approximately 15%–20% is spent directly on healthcare, and the majority of overseas aid is spent on the wider determinants of health (e.g. education, water, social services, government, and civil society).

McCoy et al. [71] summarised the global funding landscape according to three functions:

- **Providing** (the need to raise or generate global health funds)
- **Managing** (the management or pooling of global health funds as well as mechanisms for channelling funds to recipients)
- **Spending** (the expenditure and consumption of global health finance)

However, investment in economic development and global organisations is often compromised by the following:

- 'Chaotic' global health landscape (as described by McCoy and others).
- Plethora of agencies involved (including the rising number of private and non-governmental organisations). This complexity makes coordination and accountability difficult.
- Inadequate systems for tracking and monitoring global health financing, so it is not known how much money is spent on global funding.

In the United Kingdom, DfID reviewed its aid policies in 2011 in an attempt to address these problems and to respond to the changing circumstances of recipient countries. DfID agreed to spend its resources in fewer countries and to channel funds through fewer **managing agencies**. Decisions about where and what to fund have sought to balance [71] 'need' in terms of i**ndicators of health burden** (e.g. poverty) with 'need' in terms of **capacity to effect change** (e.g. barriers being corruption and mismanagement at a local level).

4D

Health Economics

Economics is based on the notion that we live in a world of **scarcity** where there are infinite demands but only finite resources (i.e. demand will always exceed supply). This chapter considers how these finite resources can best be allocated to address the public's demand for health and for healthcare. It describes a range of techniques used by health economists, including **economic evaluation**, and the role of economics in policymaking and public health.

4D.1 Health economics

Principles of health economics (including the notions of scarcity, supply and demand, marginal analysis, distinctions between need and demand, opportunity cost, discounting, time horizons, margins, efficiency, and equity).

Economics is the social science of how goods and services are produced, distributed, and consumed; it is traditionally divided into **microeconomics** and **macroeconomics** (see Table 4D.1).

An axiom in healthcare is that **demand exceeds supply**. The amount of resources that could potentially be spent on healthcare is infinite; therefore, the resources that are actually available for healthcare will always be relatively **scarce**. As a result, **choices** must be made over how to spend the healthcare budget. Health economics is the science of making these decisions (i.e. how best to employ scarce resources that have alternative uses). The discipline is divided into **positive** and **normative** economics (see Box 4D.1).

Scarcity

Healthcare can be regarded as a **production process** that uses a number of **inputs** to produce **outputs**. The inputs or **factors of production** are divided into four categories (see Table 4D.2).

It can be seen that none of these resources is infinite. The term **scarcity** is used where more of a resource is wanted than is available. Under these circumstances, every choice that is made involves a **sacrifice**, since the same resource cannot subsequently be used for anything else. This sacrifice is called the **opportunity cost** and it represents the benefits that are forgone. Opportunity cost is a fundamental concept of health economics.

Table 4D.1 Types of economics

Field of economics	Unit of interest	Topics covered
Microeconomics	Elements **within the economy**	Individuals Households Firms Buyers Sellers Markets
Macroeconomics	**Entire economy**	Unemployment Inflation Economic growth Monetary policy (interest rates, the money supply, etc.) Fiscal policy (public spending, tax, etc.)

Box 4D.1 Positive and normative economics

Type of health economics	Topics covered
Positive	How **markets** work How **interventions** affect outcomes
Normative	What should be **produced** What **resources** to use How to distribute goods

Table 4D.2 Factors of production

Inputs	Description
Land	Physical resources of the **planet**, including mineral deposits
Capital	Resources **created by humans** to aid production, such as tools, machinery, and factories
Labour	Human resources, in the sense of people as **workers**
Enterprise	Human resource of **organising** the other three factors to produce goods and services

Opportunity cost

The opportunity cost is the **benefit forgone** by not using resources for their **next best alternative** use. In economics, a calculation of the opportunity cost is often used to value benefits of a service. For example, the opportunity cost may be quantified as the health benefits (in terms of life years saved, QALYs gained, etc.) that could have been achieved had the money been spent on the next best alternative intervention or healthcare programme.

Opportunity cost can be calculated directly by means of **CEA** or **cost–utility analysis (CUA)** (see Chapter 1C.14).

Need and demand

Economists draw a distinction between **need** and **demand** (see Table 4D.3). Where need is not identified, it is not expressed, and it is therefore not a demand. Moreover, the healthcare demanded does not represent all healthcare needs. See Figure 4D.1.

Demand in healthcare

As in Section 4C, where a distinction was made between the need for health and the need for healthcare, the demand for health should be distinguished from the demand for healthcare. The demand for healthcare is a **derived demand**. In other words, although healthcare may be unpleasant in its own right, it is still demanded because of its potential to improve health. Health, however, is affected not only by healthcare but also by many other factors. Indeed, healthcare may not always lead to an improvement in health.

The demand for healthcare may be quantified in terms of:

- Bed occupancy
- Consultation rates
- Waiting lists

Rising demand

In developed countries, the demand for healthcare is rising for several reasons, including:

- Demographics (ageing population)
- Innovation (technology)

Table 4D.3 Distinction between need and demand

	Need	Demand
Definition	A capacity to benefit from healthcare	A request for healthcare The amount of a good or service that consumers are willing and able to purchase at a given price
Description	The three types of need are • Expressed need • Felt need • Normative need (see Section 4C.1 for details)	Must be expressed by people by one of the following: • Attending the place where the service is offered • Waiting for the service • Paying for the service

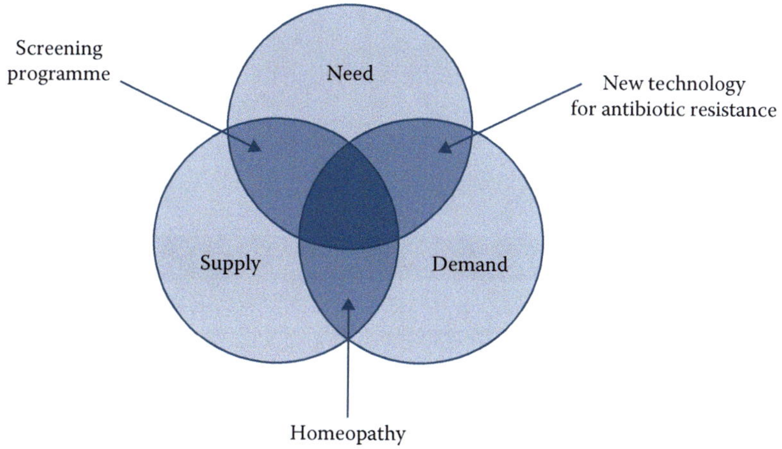

Figure 4D.1 Need, supply, and demand.

- Lifestyle (harmful factors such as smoking and excessive alcohol use)
- Information (educated consumers)
- Rising standards of living (quality-of-life expectations)

Determinants of demand

According to economic theory, demand is determined by four factors, namely **price**, **income**, **preferences,** and **alternatives** (see Table 4D.4).

Substitutes and complements

The demand for one good may be related to the demand for another. Substitutes and complements are related goods, where a **change in price of one good affects the demand for the other**. See Table 4D.5.

Demand curve

Normally, when the price of a good falls, consumers are willing to buy more of it. As a result, the demand curve slopes downwards (i.e. a reduction in price leads to more of the good being supplied). See Figure 4D.2.

Table 4D.4 Four factors that determine demand according to economic theory

Factor	Description
1. Price of health/healthcare	When user fees are introduced to healthcare systems (e.g. a charge to see a doctor or a prescription charge), then demand falls. This is known as price **elasticity** of demand. In England, certain people, such as children and pregnant women, are exempt from prescription charges in order to ensure that their demand for health is not affected by the price of healthcare.
2. Individuals' income	Studies have shown that the introduction of user fees reduces demand disproportionately in people on lower incomes (i.e. their demand is more **income elastic** compared to people with higher incomes).
3. Tastes and preferences	Different people place different values on different lifestyle factors. People also place different values on the benefits of healthcare: some people are more likely to seek healthcare for particular symptoms than others. For example, a person may choose to trade off the unhealthy effects of a takeaway meal against the convenience of not having to cook.
4. Price and availability of complements and substitutes	Substitutes for healthcare may include other types of healthcare (e.g. complementary medicine). Some people who use these services may choose not to use conventional healthcare. Other people (e.g. people who place a particularly high priority on health) may use both types of healthcare.

Table 4D.5 Substitutes and complements

	Definition	Example
Substitutes	Products where an increase in the price of one of good causes an **increase** in demand for the other good	Two different brands of the same vaccine
Complements	Products where an increase in the price of one good causes a **decrease** in demand for the other good	Needles and syringes

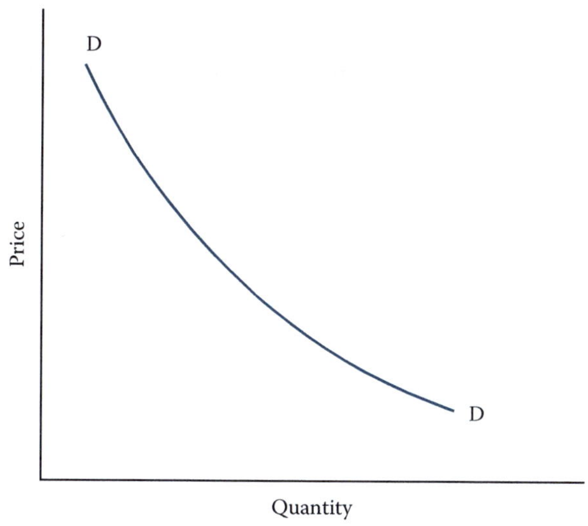

Figure 4D.2 Demand curve.

All things being equal,* a change in price leads to a **movement along the curve**, whereas a change in certain other factors leads to a **shift of the curve** (i.e. the curve itself moves). See Table 4D.6.

Price elasticity of demand

The price elasticity of demand is a measure of how sensitive the demand for a particular good is to changes in price. It is calculated using the following formula:

$$\text{Price elasticity of demand (PED)} = \frac{\text{Percentage change in quantity demanded}}{\text{Percentage change in price}}$$

By convention, PED is then transformed into the absolute value (i.e. the + or – sign is removed) prior to interpretation. Note that the absolute value is written using two vertical lines (e.g. $|-0.5| = 0.5$). Table 4D.7 shows the meaning of different absolute values of the price elasticity of demand.

Table 4D.6 Phenomena affecting the demand curve

Phenomenon	Resulting effect	Change seen on the demand curve
Fall in price	More product is demanded.	Movement **rightwards along** the **demand** curve
Rise in price	Less product is demanded.	Movement **leftwards along** the **demand** curve
Falls in income	Purchasers not willing to pay as much.	**Leftward shift** of the **demand** curve
Increased population Increased income Changes in taste (e.g. as a result of advertising)	Purchasers willing to pay more.	**Rightward shift** of the **demand** curve

Table 4D.7 Price elasticity of demand

Absolute value of PED	Definition	Characteristic
|PED| > 1	Price elastic	Large response in demand to changes in price.
|PED| = 1	Unit elasticity	Response in demand is proportionate to changes in price.
|PED| < 1	Price inelastic	Small response in demand to changes in price.
|PED| = 0	Perfectly inelastic	No response in demand to changes price.

* Note that economists often use the Latin term *ceteris paribus* for 'all things being equal' or 'all other things being held constant'.

Table 4D.8 Price elasticity of income

Value of IED	Definition	Characteristic
IED > 1	Luxury goods	Disproportionately large amounts of the good are demanded as incomes **rise**.
IED > 0	Normal goods	The amount of the goods demanded changes in line with income (as would be expected from demand curve).
IED < 0	Inferior goods	Larger amounts of the good are demanded as incomes **fall**.

Income elasticity of demand

The income elasticity of demand is a measure of how sensitive the demand for a particular good is to changes in income. It is calculated using the following formula:

$$\text{Income elasticity of demand (IED)} = \frac{\text{Percentage change in quantity demanded}}{\text{Percentage change in income}}$$

Table 4D.8 shows the meaning of different absolute values of the price elasticity of income.

Supply

Supply is the amount of a good or service that producers are willing and able to sell at a given price. It is determined by:

- The **price** of the good
- The **cost** of producing the good (e.g. raw materials, labour)
- Prices of related goods
- The number of other suppliers

The supply of healthcare is the care that is made available; it is the capacity of services to meet need. Healthcare supply may be quantified in terms of:

- Staffing (e.g. whole-time-equivalent consultants, nurses)
- Beds
- Equipment
- Budget

Supply curve

If a product sells at a low price, then producers will be disinclined to make large amounts of it. If the price rises, then producers will make more of the product and therefore the **supply curve** (S) **slopes upwards**. See Figure 4D.3.

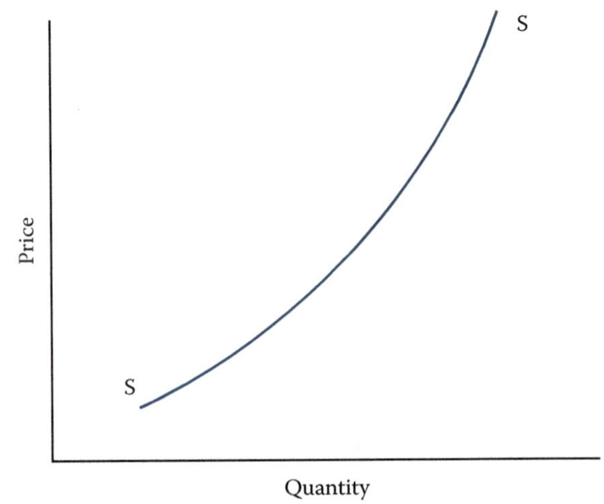

Figure 4D.3 Supply curve.

A change in price, *ceteris paribus*, results in movement along the supply curve. A change in any other factor, *ceteris paribus*, results in a shift of the supply curve (e.g. an increase in labour supply leads to a rightwards shift) (Table 4D.9).

Markets

A market is a location (physical or virtual) where consumers and suppliers **trade** goods or services.

Market equilibrium

The price of a good reaches **equilibrium** at the **intersection** of the **supply curve** and the **demand curve**. If the price is set higher than this point, then producers will want to produce more of the good. However, when the price is set higher, there will be fewer consumers willing to pay for the good thereby returning the price back to the equilibrium point. See Figure 4D.4.

Table 4D.9 Phenomena affecting the supply curve

Phenomenon	Resulting effect	Change seen on the supply curve
Rise in price	More product is supplied.	Movement **rightwards along** the **supply** curve
Fall in price	Less product is supplied.	Movement **leftwards along** the **supply** curve
More land More labour New technology available Price of inputs falls	Producers find it easier to produce the product.	Rightward shift of the **supply** curve
Less land Less labour Price of inputs rises	Producers find it more difficult to produce the product.	Leftward shift of the **supply** curve

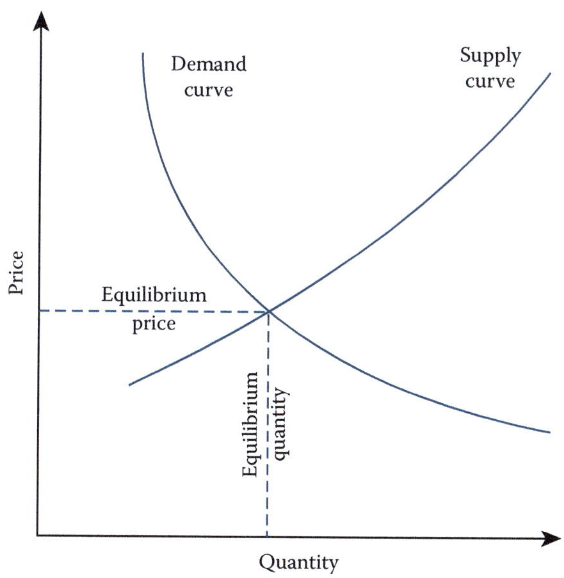

Figure 4D.4 Supply and demand curves.

Perfectly competitive markets

It is a principle of economics that in a perfect market, the **supply and demand of a good are determined independently** (i.e. **producers** determine the **supply** of a good and **purchasers** determine its **demand**). The price of a good rises or falls until the amount supplied equals the amount demanded (i.e. equilibrium is reached).

Another fundamental principle of economics is that **demand will equal supply in a perfect market**. While neither health nor healthcare is a perfect market, certain aspects of the concepts of supply and demand do remain applicable.

In the real world, there are no perfectly competitive markets; however, there are several approximations, including the market for horse betting. A perfect market would have a range of characteristics, including **atomicity**, **homogeneity**, and **free entry** (see Box 4D.2).

In a perfect market, the producers are **price-takers** (i.e. the market sets the price). Under such circumstances, producers produce goods at the lowest possible cost in the long run, and they earn only **normal profits**. If producers do not operate in a price-taking way and, instead, if they have the ability to influence the price of a good or the total quantity of the good that is produced, then the market is said to have **failed**.

Note:

- A normal profit is the same profit that could be achieved in the best alternative business. This type of profit contrasts with an **economic profit**, which is revenue additional to the normal profit.
- The **long run** is defined as the timeframe in which firms can enter or exit the market and in which they can change their capital (e.g. build an extra operating theatre).

Box 4D.2 Characteristics of a free market

Feature	Description
Atomicity	Many buyers and many sellers.
Homogeneity	Identical products.
Free entry	Sellers are free to join and leave the market.
Equal access	Production technology is available equally to all sellers.
Perfect information	All buyers and all sellers know the products and prices of all sellers.
No externalities	An externality is a benefit or disbenefit to someone other than the purchaser (e.g. an externality of an immunisation programme is herd immunity).

Causes of market failure in healthcare

A market may fail if any of the conditions listed in Box 4D.2 are not met. The principal causes of market failure are listed in Box 4D.3 and include the production of **externalities**, **public goods**, and **merit goods**.

Agency

As will be seen in the section on markets in the succeeding text, a key characteristic of a perfect market is that each consumer has perfect knowledge about the goods on offer. One of the many reasons why healthcare is an imperfect market is that consumers lack perfect knowledge about the complexities of healthcare. Instead, they rely on **agents** such as doctors and dentists to inform them what services they need. For example, patients with angina only receive angioplasty if their cardiologist thinks that they will benefit from the procedure.

Perfect agents (like perfect markets) do not exist, because a perfect agent would have to strike a perfect balance between all of the following conflicting priorities:

- **Health status** of an individual patient
- **Preferences** of an individual patient
- **Utility** to society

Moreover, agents may sometimes be motivated by other factors, such as their own self-interest.

Supplier-induced demand

Supplier-induced demand occurs when agents act in their own interests, recommending more healthcare than is necessary (i.e. more healthcare than a perfect agent would recommend). For example, a dentist might recommend a dental filling that was not strictly necessary in order to earn the fee for performing the procedure.

This phenomenon can be difficult to identify because only price equilibrium points can be observed. For example, if the costs of dentistry increased and the demand for dental services decreased, then it is difficult to say whether the demand decreased to the extent that would be expected in the absence of supplier-induced demand. However, if the cost of a dental consultation increased when more practitioners entered the market, then the market would be demonstrably abnormal, and supplier-induced demand would have been detected.

Supplier-reduced demand

In contexts where the supply of healthcare is particularly scarce, **supplier-reduced demand** may be seen. Here, an agent may not recommend a particular healthcare intervention, whereas a perfect agent would have done so in the same circumstances. To an observer, it would appear that it was less demand for a service than was in fact the case.

Rather than seeking to demonstrate and punish supplier-reduced demand, policymakers can design contracts to eradicate the phenomenon (e.g. by linking payment to quality indicators).

Box 4D.3 Causes of market failure

Cause of market failure	Description
Externality	This is a **side effect** of the product that is **not traded** on the market (e.g. herd immunity as a side effect of immunisation is an externality). Externalities may be beneficial (termed **positive externalities**) or harmful (**negative externalities**).
Public goods	These goods are *extreme* examples of an externality, such as a health promotion poster campaign. Public goods are characterised by • **Non-rivalness** (when one person reads a poster, other people do not suffer) • **Non-excludability** (it is impossible to stop a person from reading the poster)
Market control	A properly functioning market relies on many buyers and many sellers. Therefore, a market may fail if there is a • **Monopoly (single producer)** • **Oligopoly (few producers)** • **Monopsony (single purchaser)** • **Oligopsony (few purchasers)**
Imperfect information	**Agency**: patients do not normally have perfect knowledge of healthcare; therefore, they rely on doctors and other clinicians as their agents (see later text). **Uncertainty**: patients are unable to predict their demand (e.g. when they will need trauma care). **Moral hazard** (in systems such as the NHS, there is no price to consumer at the time of use). **Adverse selection** (in systems such as the commercial health insurance market in the United States, people at low risk of illness tend to opt out of paying for health insurance).
Merit goods	Belief that certain goods, such as health services, are special in some way.

Margins

Choices made by consumers often result in small increases or decreases in the demand for one product relative to another. These fluctuations are known as marginal changes, where the margin is defined as the **incremental variation in inputs that is required to have a corresponding variation on outputs**. See Box 4D.4.

The process of **marginal analysis** involves examining the effect of small changes on the existing pattern of expenditure. Such analyses can help identify the following:

- Where additional resources should be targeted
- Where reductions should be made if expenditure has to be cut
- How resources can be reallocated to achieve an overall gain in benefit with no overall change in expenditure (see Box 4D.5)

Economies and diseconomies of scale

The average cost curve for the production of a good tends to fall as more of the good is produced, but

Box 4D.4 Margins

Concept	Definition
Marginal cost	Cost of producing one extra unit of service. This cost will reflect any **stepped costs** that are encountered (such as having to open an additional operating theatre because the capacity of the existing theatres has been exceeded).
Marginal benefit	Benefit derived from one extra produced unit.

Box 4D.5 Example: Targeting a screening programme

A small-scale screening programme targeted at the high-risk groups may show a low cost per case detected.

However, expansion of the programme will entail screening progressively lower risk groups or screening more frequently. The number of screens required to detect each additional positive case will rise, increasing the cost per case detected.

Source: Reproduced from Cohen, D., *BMJ*, 309, 781, 1994.

then reaches a nadir beyond which the cost tends to rise. In other words, the curve is U-shaped (see Figure 4D.5; Cost curve for the production of a good.). This phenomenon occurs because as more of a good is produced, the average cost falls due to more efficient use of the inputs; however, a point is reached where **diseconomies of scale** begin to feature. These diseconomies may be caused by the following:

- Difficulties in managing an organisation that is so large that it is **unwieldy**
- Diseconomies of **scope,** where it becomes increasingly costly to reach remote areas of the country

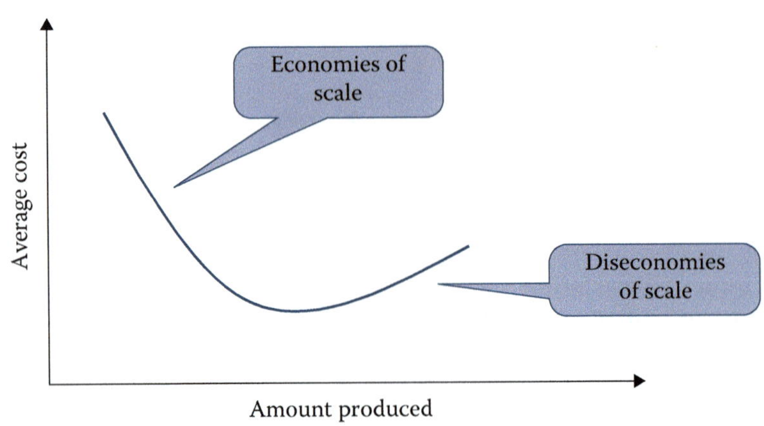

Figure 4D.5 Cost curve for the production of a good.

Box 4D.6 Types of efficiency

Type of efficiency	Definition
Technical efficiency	Maximum output for given **inputs** (or minimal **inputs** needed for a given output).
Economic efficiency	Maximum output for a given **expenditure** (or minimal **costs** needed for a given output).
Allocative efficiency	Set the level of production such that **marginal benefit is greater than the marginal cost** (i.e. produce goods that consumers value more than their cost to produce).

Efficiency

See Section 4C.3 for a comparison of equity, equality, and efficiency.

Efficiency is a measure how much of a good is being achieved from the available resources. It can be considered in three ways: **technical** efficiency, **economic** efficiency, and **allocative** efficiency. These concepts are described in the succeeding text and are defined in Box 4D.6.

Technical efficiency

Technical efficiency addresses the issue of using **given resources** to **maximum advantage**. An intervention is technically efficient if the same (or greater) outcome could not be produced with less of one type of input. For example, consider the treatment of osteoporosis using alendronate: if a 10 mg daily dose is as effective as a 20 mg dose, then the lower dose is more technically efficient.

Economic efficiency

Economic efficiency refers to the maximisation of outcomes for a given cost, or the minimisation of costs for a given outcome. Consider, for example, a policy of changing from maternal age screening to biochemical screening for Down's syndrome. If the sum of the costs of the new biochemical screening programme is less than (or the same as) the cost of the maternal age programme, and outcomes are equal (or better), then the biochemical programme is economically efficient in relation to the maternal age programme.

Allocative efficiency

Allocative efficiency is the achievement of the best possible combination of healthcare programmes to maximise the health of society. The concept of allocative efficiency takes account not only the **productive** efficiency with which healthcare resources are used to produce health outcomes (i.e. technical and economic efficiency) but also the efficiency with which these outcomes are **distributed** among the community. Allocative efficiency is achieved when resources are allocated so as to **maximise the welfare** of the community. Given that there will always be scarcity, a decision-making system is required that determines how much is provided of different kinds of healthcare. There are three decision-making options: the free market, the command system, and the mixed system (Box 4D.7).

Equity

Section 4C.3 compares equity and efficiency.

In economics, equity is the concept of fairness. Equity may be **vertical** or **horizontal** (see Chapter 1C.10). An example of where equitable principles align with efficiency is provided in Box 4D.8.

Discounting

Discounting is a method used in economics to deal with the phenomenon of **positive time preference**, which is the human nature of preferring benefits to be realised now and for costs to be borne at a later date. Positive time preference

Box 4D.7 Decision making options

Decision-making option	Description
Free market	Healthcare resources are allocated according to consumers' purchasing behaviour.
Command system	Planning is used to allocate healthcare according to some pre-determined criterion, such as 'need.'
Mixed system	Combines elements of the free market with elements of the command model.

Box 4D.8 Example: Equity versus efficiency in cervical screening

The NHS policy on cervical cancer screening has been primarily based on maximising coverage through the use of financial incentives on GPs. However, high-risk women have tended to have lower participation rates, particularly in socio-economically disadvantaged groups. Researchers have calculated that the screening programme could have achieved the same cost-effectiveness in terms of cancers avoided with less extensive but more equitable coverage.

Source: Reproduced from Sassi, F. et al., *BMJ*, 323, 762, 2001.

occurs because the future is uncertain; therefore, it is logical to want benefits earlier and costs later. However, many public health interventions, such as stop-smoking campaigns, are costly today but will not realise their benefits of a reduction in lung cancer deaths until many years into the future. Positive time preference can be adjusted for in calculations of costs and benefits using a **discounting rate** whose magnitude reflects the strength of the time preference. Discount rates vary widely but are typically between 0% and 6%. Note that the discount rate for benefits is particularly controversial and that the discount rate used in a calculation need not be the same for costs and benefits.

Using the discount rate, the present cost is calculated by adjusting the cost in a future year by the discount factor.

$$\textbf{Present cost} = (\textbf{Cost in year } n) \times (\textbf{Discount factor})$$

where

$$\text{Discount factor} = \frac{1}{n(1+r)}$$

and r = discount rate; n = years.

Because of the large impact of discounting on public health interventions, sensitivity analyses should always include a range of discount rates for both costs and benefits (see Section 4D.5).

Special features of healthcare

Economics is a core discipline within public health. However, economists regard healthcare as a special case for several reasons, including **imperfect markets** and **agency**. Other reasons, such as **immediacy**, **uncertainty**, and **necessity**, will be explored later in this chapter. See Box 4D.9.

Box 4D.9 Distinguishing features of healthcare

Distinguishing feature of healthcare	Description
Supply and demand	Demand and supply are not truly independent in healthcare.
Imperfect markets	All healthcare systems (but especially those that are publicly funded) are imperfect markets.
Immediacy	Life and death decisions often need to be made with very short timescales.
Agency	The nature of healthcare that people need, especially when they are critically ill, is largely specified by healthcare providers.
Uncertainty	Illness is often unpredictable.
Necessity	Healthcare is an unavoidable commodity.

4D.2 Assessing performance

See also Chapter 1C.9.

The performance of an allocation system may be assessed in terms of its **efficiency** (including its **Pareto efficiency**) and its **equity** (see Section 4C.3). In contrast, the performance of a healthcare system may be assessed in terms of the benefits it generates per unit of expenditure. This process is known as **economic analysis** (see Section 4D.5).

The WHO advises that when assessing the performance of a healthcare system, a range of dimensions should be assessed, including efficiency, resource use, and feedback (see Box 4D.10).

Box 4D.10 Dimensions for assessing a healthcare system (WHO)

Aspect of a healthcare system	Description
Social goals	Measuring the contribution of the health system to socially desirable goals
Resource use	Measuring the resources used to achieve health outcomes
Efficiency	Estimating the efficiency with which the resources are used to achieve health outcomes
Review	Evaluating how the system influences health outcomes and efficiency
Feedback	Designing and implementing policies to improve outcomes and efficiency, and monitoring their effect

4D.3 Financial resource allocation

Financial resource allocation involves transferring funds from purchasers to providers in order to meet healthcare objectives. The allocation process can be used to promote:

- Equity
- Changes in activity
- Efficiency

Expenditure by a health service may broadly be divided into **recurrent** and **capital** spending (see Box 4D.11).

NHS funding

ENG In England, the vast majority of funding for the NHS comes from general taxation and national insurance contributions, with the remainder coming from patient charges (e.g. prescription charges and dental charges). Recurrent revenue allocations to PCTs cover hospital and community health services, prescribing, primary medical services, and HIV/AIDS. See Figure 4D.6.

The method for allocating NHS funding in England changed in 2013. Before then, the Department of Health made allocations to PCTs based primarily on a national weighted capitation formula together with a number of additional factors (see Figure 4D.6 and Table 4D.10).

In 2013, the commissioning system changed. Instead of PCTs commissioning services, services began being commissioned by CCGs, the NHS Commissioning Board, Public Health England, and local authorities. Accordingly, the resource allocation has changed significantly (see Figure 4D.7) [75].

SCOT + NT + WA The UK government allocates central funding to Northern Ireland, Scotland, and Wales for services that are the responsibility of their devolved legislatures including healthcare. Such funds are allocated according to the **Barnett formula** and represent about 80% of public spending in these countries. The Barnett formula has been in use since the late 1970s although it in fact has no statutory basis. The parliament or assembly in each country decides how to spend its block of funds, including what proportion to spend on healthcare and other services.

Box 4D.11 Types of expenditure

Type of expenditure	Definition	Examples
Capital	Expenditure results in acquiring or enhancing an asset (i.e. property that has value and could be sold to meet commitments or debts)	Buildings, equipment
Recurrent	Expenditure that does not result in acquiring or enhancing an asset	Staff, drugs, consumables

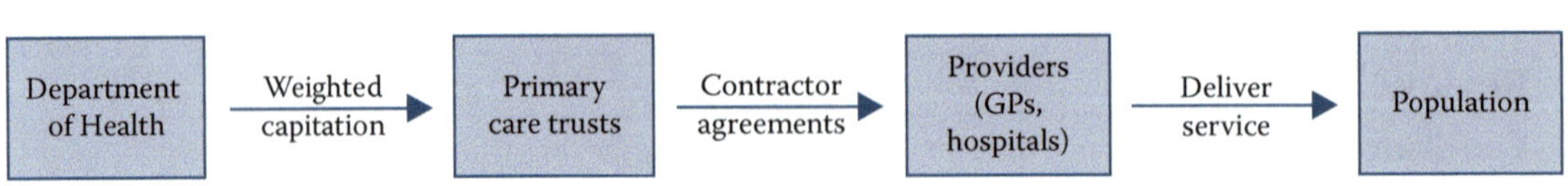
Department of Health
Weighted capitation
Primary care trusts
Contractor agreements
Providers (GPs, hospitals)
Deliver service
Population

Figure 4D.6 The allocation of funds prior to 2013. (From Department of Health, *NHS Allocations*, Department of Health, London, UK, 2006, Available online at: www.dh.gov.uk.)

Table 4D.10 Funding of PCTs prior to 2013

Allocation factor	Description
Weighted capitation	Formula for allocating resources to PCTs based on: • Size and age distribution of the population • Additional need • Unavoidable geographical variations in the cost of providing services (the so-called market forces factor)
Recurrent baseline	The previous year's actual allocation, plus any adjustments made in-year.
Distance from target	The difference between the weighted capitation and the recurrent baseline.
Pace of change policy	This determined the level of extra resources allocated to PCTs that were below their weighted capitation target. The pace of change policy was decided by ministers for each allocation funding round.

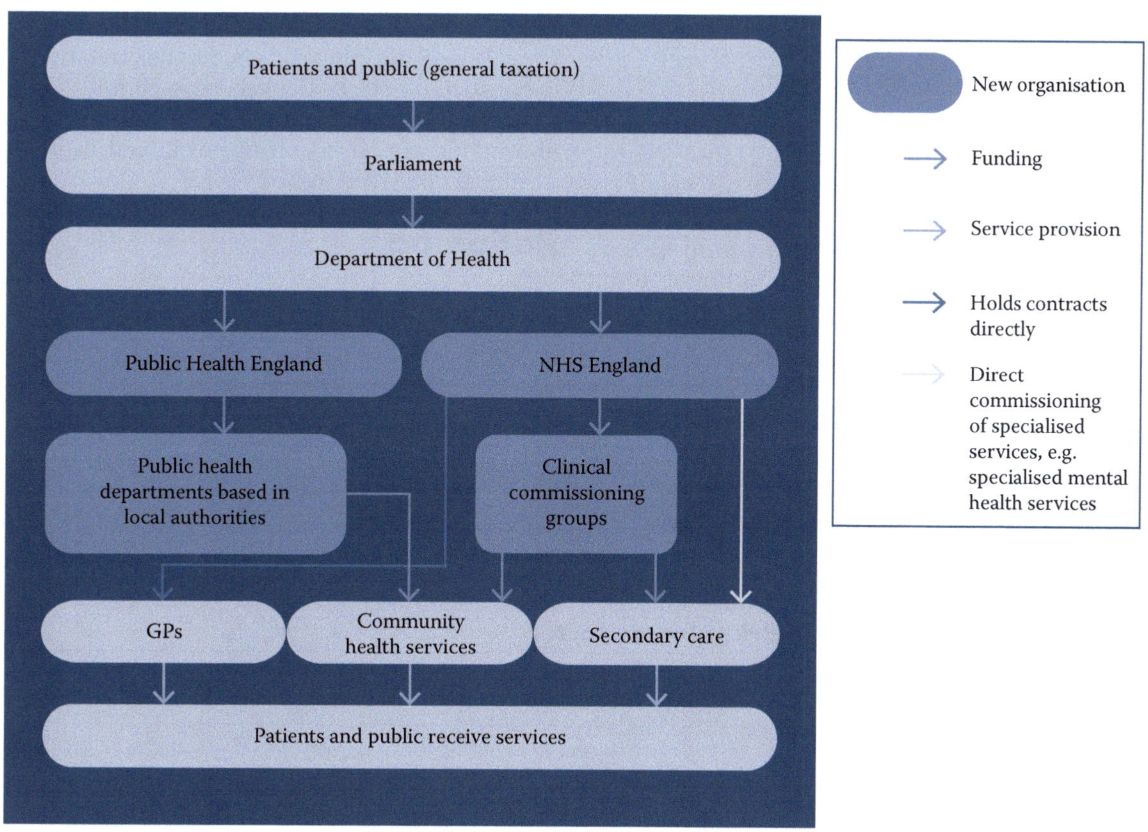

Figure 4D.7 ENG Funding of healthcare since April 2013.

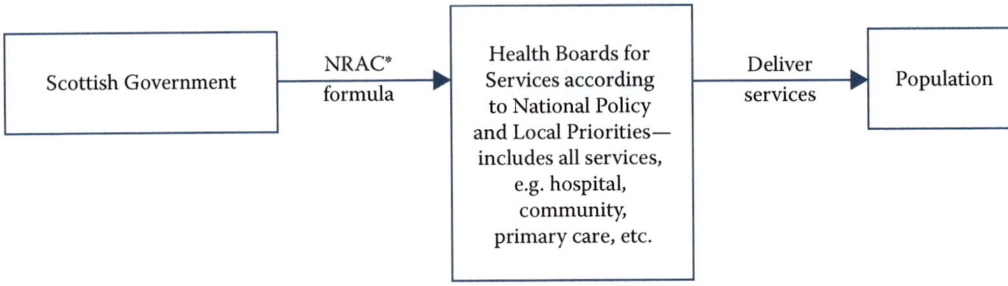

Figure 4D.8 The allocation of funds within Scotland. *NRAC, National Resource Allocation Committee.

SCOT In contrast to England, there is no purchaser/provider system in Scotland. The Scottish Government allocates funds to health boards, which provide healthcare services within their area. Where necessary, funding flows between different health boards in order to pay for specialist tertiary care. The Scottish Government allocates funds within Scotland on the basis of the National Resource Allocation Committee (NRAC) formula (see Figure 4D.8).

WA The Welsh Assembly decided to move toward allocating resources to LHBs according to a new needs-based system informed by the Welsh Index of Multiple Deprivation (see Chapter 1C.8). However, the transition to this new system involved allocating additional funds to underfunded areas rather than by moving funds away from relatively overfunded areas (such as North Wales) to relatively underfunded areas (such as Southeast Wales). This approach was adopted for political reasons and has slowed the pace of change. LHBs are, in turn, expected to allocate their resources to reflect local needs rather than based on demand [76].

NI In Northern Ireland, the Health and Social Care Board allocates funds for health and personal social services between five commissioning groups, covering nine programmes of care. These allocations are based on the weighted capitation formulae described in Box 4D.12.

Rationing

See Section 4C.2.

Box 4D.12 Funding allocation methods

Weighted capitation	PCTs receive their share of resources calculated according to: • Size and age distribution of the population • Additional need • Unavoidable geographical variations in the cost of providing services (called the **market forces factor**)
Recurrent baseline	This is the previous year's actual allocation, plus any adjustments made in-year
Distance from target	This is the difference between the weighted capitation and the recurrent baseline
Pace of change policy	This determines the level of extra resources that are allocated to PCTs that are below their weighted capitation target. The pace of change policy is decided by ministers for each allocation funding round

4D.4 Healthcare systems and incentives

Systems of health and social care and the role of incentives to achieve desired endpoints.

Various methods are used around the globe to fund health and social care ranging from private health insurance to public funding. There are also numerous ways in which these health systems pay providers of health services. Each of these systems has different methods for incentivising providers.

Health system funding

The principal methods of healthcare funding are private insurance, social insurance, and public funding (see Table 4D.11).

Payment of providers

See also Chapter 5F.2.

The main methods of paying healthcare providers are by **salary**, **fee-for service**, or **capitation** (see Table 4D.12).

Financial incentives

Financial incentives may be used to encourage or discourage certain behaviours by providers (e.g. the provision of particular services) and patients (e.g. the uptake of particular services).

UK As part of the UK government's public service modernisation agenda, explicit financial incentives were introduced with the aim of improving the efficiency and quality of the NHS in England (see Table 4D.13).

Social care

Social care covers a wide range of services that support people with ADL and particularly focuses on the groups shown in Table 4D.14.

Around 70% of the social care budget for England is spent on adult community care services, especially for older people, people with physical or learning disabilities, and people with mental illness. Many of these people pay for their own social care, with the remainder receiving financial assistance from the state either through **welfare benefits** or through social services funding. Some people who require social care are given **direct payments** that provide them with the freedom to budget and purchase their own care rather than having it arranged by the local authority.

Integrated care

In response to problems of fragmentation in care, efforts have been made in many areas to improve the integration of care, including the so-called **horizontal integration** between medical treatment and social care. Such integration requires health and social care organisations to work together to deliver flexible services that are tailored to allow people to live independent lives.

See Chapter 5B for more details of integrated care.

Monitoring performance

See Chapter 5E for systems of monitoring performance of health and social care providers.

ENG The Care Quality Commission provides independent assessments of the quality and performance of health and social care commissioners and providers on behalf of the government and the public.

WA The Care and Social Services Inspectorate for Wales is the body that regulates, inspects, and enforces health and social care regulations. Although technically part of the Welsh Government, it operates as independent body. The inspectorate regulates care homes and children's homes, as well as domiciliary and day care services, nursing agencies, fostering and adoption agencies, boarding, and special schools. The regulations and standards for social care are set by the Welsh Government.

The performance of healthcare providers in Wales, both NHS and private, is monitored by the Healthcare Inspectorate Wales. This is another arm

Table 4D.11 Healthcare funding systems

Method	Description	Advantages	Disadvantages
Private health insurance	Individuals purchase insurance by paying monthly premiums. Private insurance may be provided by or through a person's employer.	• May incentivise insurers to compete on the basis of cost, quality, and customer services. • May incentivise providers to compete on the basis of quality and cost so that insurers choose to fund their services.	• Adverse selection: people who know they are at low risk of ill health will not want pay premiums that are priced for people at higher risk. As a result, fewer low-risk people enter the risk pool, so a risk of the risk pool increases and premiums rise. Solutions include community rating (i.e. setting the same premiums for all persons living in a given territory) or compulsory insurance (where low-risk people subsidise higher-risk people). • Providers may compete based on their perceived quality rather than actual quality. • Generally leads to an inefficient system.
Social insurance	A social insurance fund is created from the contributions made by employees, employers and government. The fund is used to pay for the healthcare of employees and their dependents.	• Generally lower cost than private insurance. • The government is a strong partner and can influence costs.	• Only provides insurance for people who are employed and another government scheme is required for people who are not covered.
Public funding	Funded mainly through taxation. May be supplemented by some user charges (e.g. prescription charges). Providers may be public (e.g. NHS Trusts) or private (e.g. private hospitals providing NHS-funded care).	• Normally lower cost. • Government can influence costs.	• May result in less competitive pressure if services are publicly provided.

Table 4D.12 Payment of providers and associated incentives

Payment method	Effect of incentive
Salary	Restricts the number of patients seen and the services provided
Fee-for-service	Increases the number of patients seen and the services provided Increases the use of more expensive services
Capitation/block contract	Increases number of patients on a patient list, especially healthy patients Reduces the number of patient contacts and the services provided

Table 4D.13 Incentives to improve the quality and efficiency of healthcare

Financial incentive system	Description
Quality and outcomes framework	In England, general practices been offered incentives to improve the quality of their provision. The quality and outcomes framework (QOF) is a voluntary system of financial incentives aimed at improving quality within the General Medical Services (GMS) contract for GPs.
Payment by results	Providers are paid for providing intervention based on the national average cost of delivering that Healthcare Resource Group. Providers are therefore incentivised to increase provision and reduce costs below this fixed average payment. Note that the term Payment by Results is somewhat of a misnomer: a better term might be Payment by Activity.
Delayed discharge	The publication *Delivering the NHS Plan* requires local authorities to use some of their resources to reduce the number of people who remain in hospital after being deemed medically fit to be discharged. A failure on the part of the local authority to make appropriate alternative provision available to patients may result in hospitals charging social care departments for the cost keeping people in hospital unnecessarily.
Readmissions	NHS trusts are held accountable for the cost of unplanned readmissions occurring within 30 days of discharge. This incentive is aimed at ensuring that patients are not transferred prematurely and improving the quality of post-discharge care.
Vaccinations	A fee-for-service incentive is used to encourage providers to deliver certain items of service to patients. An example is the fee received by GP practices for administering vaccinations.
Case mix	Case-mix payments adjust payment according illness severity. For example, the UK health economy uses different HRGs as the units of charging for services (e.g. inguinal hernia repair with or without complication). HRGs are based on the average cost of a patient treated with that diagnosis; therefore, providers have an incentive to deliver care costing no more than the fixed payment of that HRG.

Table 4D.14 Principal groups of people may require social care

Group	Examples of services provided
Older people	Residential care homes, nursing homes, home carers, meals-on-wheels, day centres, lunch clubs
Disabilities	Adaptations, carers, and other services for people with physical disabilities or learning disabilities
Mental health	Ranging from support for people with mild mental illness, up to exercising legal powers for compulsory admission to mental health hospitals
Ex-offenders	People leaving prison may need help with resettlement, especially if they have drug or alcohol problems
Families	Particularly where children have special needs such as a disability
Child protection	Including monitoring of children at risk of non-accidental injury
Children in care	Fostering, accommodation in children's homes, and adoption

of Welsh Government that operates as an independent body. The inspectorate monitors organisations against published Standards for Health Services in Wales. In addition to reviewing LHBs and NHS Trusts in Wales, the inspectorate also monitors private healthcare facilities and armed forces healthcare in Wales. Other issues coming under the inspectorate's remit include controlled drugs, deprivation of liberty, and monitoring of the Mental Health Act.

4D.5 Economic appraisal

Techniques of economic appraisal include: economic evaluation, option appraisal, cost-effectiveness analysis and modelling and valuing health.

Economic evaluation

In healthcare, markets are highly imperfect; therefore, it is inefficient to use market forces as the only incentives. Before other incentives can be deployed, encourage the use of particular interventions; we first need to know which interventions are most effective so we know which interventions to incentivise. The process of **economic evaluation** (also called **economic appraisal**) involves comparing the **costs** and **consequences** of two or more alternative treatments. For example, an economic evaluation may be used to compare the costs and benefits associated with switching from one vaccination programme to another.

Option appraisal

An option appraisal is the process of determining and comparing different options for meeting an objective. An option appraisal generally involves comparing two or more **new** options rather than comparing a new option against a current service. Option appraisal normally includes an economic appraisal as well as an assessment of factors such as **affordability**, **achievability**, and **impact**.

Types of economic evaluation:

The most commonly used types of economic evaluation are:

- cost-benefit analysis (CBA)
- cost effectiveness analysis (CEA)
- cost utility analysis (CUA)

See Table 4D.15. Note that all of these methods measure costs in terms of money but differ in the way that they value outcomes.

Table 4D.15 Types of economic evaluation

	CBA	CEA	CUA
Description	Involves calculating costs and benefits of an intervention in monetary terms and calculating the difference between the two	Compares the cost of different interventions that aim to achieve the same type of outcome	Measures outcomes in terms of QALYs or DALYs to enable comparisons to be made across different disease areas
Valuation of costs	Monetary	Monetary	Monetary
Valuation of outcomes (consequences)	Monetary	Clinical (e.g. cases of malaria averted, mmHg of blood pressure reduced)	QALYs or DALYs
Result	Net benefit (i.e. outcomes minus costs)	ICER	ICER
Advantages	Can compare the value of different interventions across different sectors of the economy (i.e. not simply the health sector); therefore, examines allocative efficiency also	Useful for comparing different interventions for the same disease or issue (i.e. for assessing economic and technical efficiency)	Can compare interventions for different medical conditions; therefore allows some assessment of allocative efficiency
Disadvantages	Requires a monetary value to be placed on life and/or health, which is difficult	Cannot be used to compare across different diseases areas or conditions. For example, interventions aimed at increasing life years gained cannot be directly compared with interventions aimed at improving the quality of life	Cannot be used to compare with interventions from other, non-health, sectors of the economy

Note: The terms CEA and CUA are often used interchangeably.

Other types of economic evaluation are **CMA** and **CCA**.

- Cost-minimisation analysis (CMA)
  - A type of CEA where the effect of each intervention on the consequences is the same (i.e. this analysis simply assesses how the costs of two or more interventions differ from each other).
  - For example, treatment A and treatment B both prevent 100 strokes per year. Using a CMA, the cheaper option would be chosen.
- Cost–consequence analysis (CCA)
  - In this type of analysis, the different consequences of each option are simply listed, rather than attempting to express the consequences using the same units.
  - CCA is therefore a **disaggregated** approach because the costs and consequences are not combined into a single indicator such as the net benefit or the incremental cost-effectiveness ratio (ICER).
  - In England and Wales, NICE allows CCA to be used for assessing public health interventions.

Cost-effectiveness

Figure 4D.9 illustrates how the results of a CEA or a CUA may be plotted in one of four quadrants based on a comparison of a new intervention versus an old intervention.

In the top left and the bottom right quadrants of the diagram, one of the interventions **dominates** and therefore the decision is obvious. However, in the bottom-left and the top-right quadrants, **trade-offs** are required. Often, when a new intervention is assessed, the results of an economic evaluation place it in the top-right quadrant (i.e. it is more effective than the old treatment but also more expensive). In these circumstances, calculating the ICER is helpful for assessing how the additional cost compares with the additional benefit.

Incremental cost-effectiveness ratio

The ICER for a therapeutic intervention or treatment is the ratio of the change in costs to the incremental benefits.

$$\text{ICER} = \frac{\text{Total cost of new intervention} - \text{Total cost of old intervention}}{\text{Outcome of new intervention} - \text{Outcome of old intervention}}$$

The outcome of a CUA is usually expressed in QALYs; therefore, the ICER is expressed as the cost per QALY. The ICER indicates the cost-effectiveness of one intervention or treatment relative to another; however, health must still be valued and so decisions will still need to be made about the affordability of an intervention. For example, a **threshold** may be set, below which any new intervention will generally be accepted. The NICE does not publish a fixed threshold; however, in general, treatments with an ICER below £20,000 to 30,000/QALY are likely to be accepted. This threshold can be represented as a **cost-effectiveness plane** on the cost-effectiveness diagram (see Figure 4D.10).

Note: NICE also considers other factors such as the opinions of professionals and patient groups.

Framing an economic evaluation

When critically appraising an economic evaluation, some of the key points to consider are the **design**, the **target population**, the **perspective** from which the evaluation was conducted, and the **time horizon** used (see Table 4D.16).

Costs

The choice of which costs to include in an economic evaluation primarily depends on

- The **perspective** (i.e. the viewpoint from which the costs and benefits are regarded)
- The **timeframe** for the evaluation

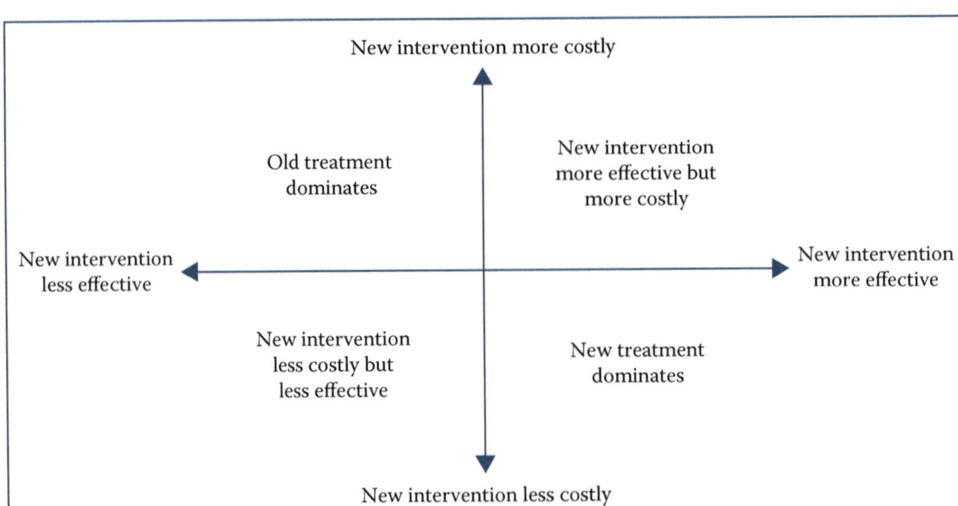

Figure 4D.9 Possible outcomes of CEA/CUA.

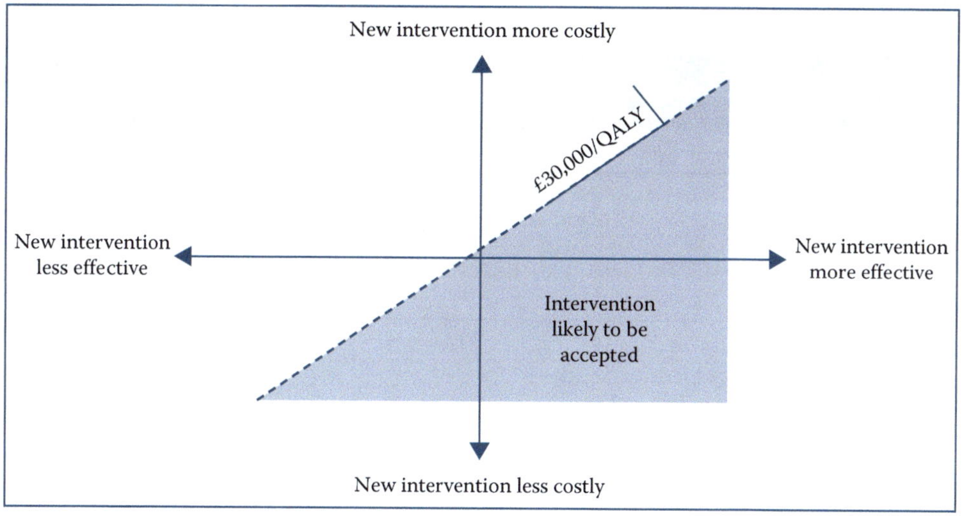

Figure 4D.10 Cost-effectiveness plane.

The costs of the alternative interventions are then calculated. Depending on the perspective adopted and the timeframe chosen, different costs may or may not need to be included. Potential costs include

- Costs to other government agencies (e.g. social care department)
- Costs from a loss of productivity
- Costs to the patient's family
- Out-of-pocket costs to the patient
- Future costs

Costs may be classified as shown in Table 4D.17.

Valuing resources

The use of resources may be evaluated by using **micro** (bottom-up) or **macro** (top-down) approaches. Values are typically derived either from an RCT (where the interventions represent different arms of the trial) or using some form of economic modelling (see succeeding text). The analysis should take account of **opportunity costs**, should take a **long-run** economic perspective, and should be adjusted for **discounting** (see Table 4D.18).

Health outcomes

There are two aspects to assessing health outcomes or benefits:

1. Measuring health
2. Placing a value on different measures of health or health states (which may be monetary or non-monetary)

Researchers may value a health state **directly** (e.g. by asking somebody with HIV to value their current health on a rating scale). Alternatively, the health state could first be measured (e.g. using the EQ5D instrument) and then assigning a preassigned value obtained beforehand from surveys offered to wider samples.

The type of health outcome measured depends on the type of economic evaluation being used:

- CBA—monetary terms
- CEA—morbidity measure (e.g. peak expiratory flow) with no value assigned
- CUA—non-monetary terms (e.g. QALYs or DALYs)

Measuring health

There are various types of health measures that may be used for measuring health, including

- Mortality (deaths averted or life years gained)
- Morbidity (prevalence, incidence, or clinical measures such as x-ray findings or blood test results)
- Disease-specific measures (profiles or indices, such as the results of a COPD questionnaire)
- Generic health measures (profiles or indices such as the Nottingham Health Profile, WHOQOL, SF-36, EQ5D); see Box 4D.13

Table 4D.16 Appraising an economic evaluation

Aspect for consideration	Details
Objectives	• For example, adding to the evidence base or making a specific decision.
Audience	• Who will be using the information? For example, the government, a managed care organisation, WHO, pharmaceutical companies, non-governmental organisations.
Type of evaluation	• CBA, CEA, CUA, etc.
Perspective	• Affects which costs and outcomes are included. Usually, one of the following perspective is adopted: • Societal perspective (the broadest perspective, which considers all of the costs and benefits regardless of who pays for/receives them) • Health service's perspective • Patient's perspective
Target population	• Group of patients for whom the intervention is intended. • May also identify subgroups for separate analysis (i.e. subgroups for whom costs/benefits differ).
Boundaries	• Many interventions have spill-over effects (i.e. other people are affected), which need to be considered. For example, a stop-smoking intervention offered to mothers may improved the health of children as well as the mother due to a reduction in passive smoking; HIV interventions may lead to reduced transmission as well as an improvement in the patient; dementia interventions may have a positive impact on carers. • Boundaries on the types of health outcomes considered (e.g. physical, mental).
Time horizon	• The time horizon should extend far enough into the future to capture all of the important outcomes and costs (e.g. lifetime horizon). • The difficulty is that data tend to be only available for a limited period, beyond which the parameters will need to be modelled. The further into the future, the less accurate these models tend to be. • The discount rate or rates applied, if any (see Section 4D.1).
Defining the intervention	• The definition should be clear—'who?' 'does what?' 'to whom?' 'where?' and 'how often?'
Comparator(s)	• If resources were unlimited, the ideal scenario would be to compare all possible interventions; generally, however, this is not feasible. • The most relevant comparison is usually the current practice, although this can sometimes be difficult to define. • Note that the current practice may not be efficient; therefore, sometimes the best available alternative or a do-nothing option are used.
Cost data	• (See main text)
Outcome data	• (See main text)

Table 4D.16 (*Continued*) Appraising an economic evaluation

Aspect for consideration	Details
Design	• RCT (piggyback studies) where healthcare utilisation data are collected during an RCT and used to assess costs. However, this approach may only include the costs and benefits seen during the trial period. Moreover, the costs and benefits seen under trial conditions may not be generalisable. • Modelling studies (where decision analytic models are populated with data from a wide variety of sources—see later text). • Combination studies: Most economic evaluations use a combination of RCT and modelling Fox-Rushby and Cairns [77].

Table 4D.17 Types of costs used in an economic evaluation

Type of cost	Description
Direct	Costs incurred exclusively for that output (e.g. disposable surgical equipment)
Indirect	Costs shared across several outputs (e.g. and autoclave that sterilises equipment for several operation)
Overhead	Costs shared across the entire organisation (e.g. communications department)
Tangible	Costs that can readily be measured in currency terms and with certainty
Intangible	Costs that are difficult to measure in currency terms (e.g. psychological costs associated with illness or treatment, such as pain and suffering)
Fixed	Costs that do not vary with the volume level of activity
Variable	Costs that vary in proportion to the quantity produced

Table 4D.18 Types of cost used when valuing resources

Type of cost	Description
Opportunity costs	It is the **opportunity cost** that should always be considered when valuing resources (i.e. the forgone value of the next-best use of the resources).
Long-run costs	Costs should be assessed from the **long-run** perspective (i.e. where all inputs, including capital inputs such as buildings, can be altered freely). In the long run, the average cost is equal to the marginal cost.
Discounted costs	Costs should be adjusted for human time preference by means of **discounting** (see Section 4D.1).
Marginal cost	Cost of producing one extra unit of service, reflecting any **stepped costs** that are encountered.

Box 4D.13 EuroQol eQ-5d

The EuroQol eQ-5d is a standardised instrument for measuring the health outcomes used in an economic evaluation. It is based on five dimensions:

1. Mobility
2. Self-care
3. Usual activities
4. Pain/discomfort
5. Anxiety/discomfort

Each dimension is scored out of 3 (there is also a version that scores out of 5) to give a final score (e.g. 2-1-1-1-2).

Monetary valuation of health

Monetary valuation is used in CBA. It has a number of advantages, including the following:

- Outcomes can be **compared directly** to costs to give a net benefit (easier than considering whether the cost per unit of outcome represents good value for money).
- **Non-health outcomes** can also be included (e.g. impact on family income).
- Comparisons can be made with interventions used in **other sectors** of the economy (e.g. education or transport).

The principal approaches to valuing life in monetary terms are the **human capital**, **revealed preference**, and **stated preferences** methods (see Table 4D.19).

Non-monetary valuation of health

Because of the difficulties involved in placing a monetary value on life and health, non-monetary valuations are often preferred. Both QALYs and DALYs are calculated using non-monetary methods and may be used in CUA.

Quality-adjusted life years

Economists use **utility** as an expression of an individual's preference for a particular health status or health outcome. A commonly used unit of utility is the QALY, which combines the **quality** and **duration** of life gained from an intervention as a **single measure**. In the United Kingdom, for example, the NICE collects evidence on the cost per QALY produced by the treatments that it appraises.

$$\text{QALY} = \text{Utility value in a health state} \times \text{Years of life in that state}$$

The benefit of a health intervention is the **gain** in QALYs that it produces. Normally, utility values range between 0 (= death) and 1 (= perfect health); however, negative values (i.e. worse than death) may also potentially be used.

For example, 2 years in perfect health followed by 3 years in a health state with utility value of 0.6 would be 3.8 QALYs:

$$(2\times1)+(3\times0.6)=3.8$$

As we have seen, there are two principal approaches to calculating utility values:

1. Providing scenarios of a disease state and valuing the disease state directly.
2. Using a health measure (e.g. EQ5D) to score a disease state. Each score will then be allocated to a preassigned utility value that was determined using a general population sample. Note that different countries may have different value sets.

The second of these methods is used more often than the first, because it is less time-consuming. There are multiple ways of assigning utility values, including the use of **rating scales, time trade-off, standard gamble,** and **person trade-off** (see Table 4D.20). The value of a QALY therefore depends on the method used. Ideally, the method should be based on **preferences** and should have **interval properties**.

Table 4D.19 Approaches to valuing life in monetary terms

	Approach	Advantages	Limitations
Human capital	The expected value of the individual's productivity is calculated (both market and household 'non-market' productivity), and then adjusted for the individual's life expectancy. May use wage as an indicator of productivity.	Objective	Identifying changes in productivity may not be easy. The value of children, older people, and unemployed people appears lower than the value of working-age males. Does not reflect how much society is willing to pay for treatment. Improvements in health are only valued for their improvement in productivity.
Revealed preference (Hedonic wage)	Individuals' preferences regarding the value of a health risk or benefit gain are traded against income (e.g. British soldiers' pay is greater than other comparable public sector posts because soldiers face substantial risks during their service life).	Based on actual consumer choices (indicates actual WTP for items such as airbags, smoke alarms, etc.) Provides insight into an individual's valuation of their own life	Focused on immediate accidental deaths as opposed to deaths due to chronic exposures (e.g. asbestos) Biased toward males of working age. Ignores imperfect labour markets (i.e. no knowledge of risks, few job options). Limited generalisability: people who undertake risky jobs are unlikely to be representative of the general population.
Stated preferences	Individuals are asked what they would choose given different hypothetical situations. Different methods may be used, including: • **Contingent valuation** where an attempt is made to elicit a person's maximum WTP to avoid a risk or to improve health • **Discrete choice** experiments where a person is asked to choose between different interventions based on cost	• Measures the strength of preference • Can be applied to any intervention	• Stated preference may not reflect reality. • Requires large and costly surveys. • Issues with validity, reliability, and bias (people may state different preferences from those that they actually hold).

Table 4D.20 Methods for calculating QALYs

Method	Description	Problem
Rating scales	Subjects are asked to attribute values between 0 and 1 to a series of health states. With visual analogue scales, respondents place a mark on a 10 cm line that represents death at one end and full health at the other.	Doubtful interval properties
Time trade-off	Respondents are asked how many years of life with the disease they are willing to give up for one year of full health.	Influenced by time preference (cf. discounting)
Standard gamble	Respondents imagine that they have the disease and are asked to gamble on taking a hypothetical treatment that will either fully cure the disease or kill them. The treatment has a probability (p) of full cure and a probability ($1 - p$) of death, and p is varied between 0 and 1.	Biased by respondents' attitude to risk
Person trade-off	Subjects are asked to imagine groups of patients with a severe disease (X) and a mild disease (Y). They are then told to imagine that there is a cure for both diseases and sufficient funds to pay for the cure of one patient with severe disease X or the cure of several patients with mild disease Y. Subjects are asked whether they would cure one person in health state X or (n) people in health state Y, where the value of (n) is varied until the subject is indifferent between the two alternatives.	May be affected by factors other than the health state alone

Two key issues in determining value preferences are the following (see Box 4D.14):

- **Who** is consulted
- **How** they are asked

Disability adjusted life years

As with QALYs, DALYs combine life expectancy and morbidity into a single indicator:

$$\text{DALY} = \text{YLL} + \text{YLD}\,(\times\,\text{Age weighting and discounting at } 3\%)$$

where

YLL is the years of life lost (usually up to the age of 75)
= (75 – Average age of death from the condition) × Number of deaths from the condition

and

YLD is the years lived with disability
= Number of cases × Disability weight × Average length lived in that disease state

The benefit of a health intervention is the number of DALYs averted (i.e. the lower the number of DALYs, the better).

Unlike QALYs, for which a number of methods may be used to calculate utility values and the utility value may vary depending on the population surveyed, disability weights for DALYs were derived using a group of **12 experts** who assigned disability weights using the person trade-off method during the Global Burden of Disease Study. This exercise was initially undertaken for 22 conditions but several hundred other diseases have since been assigned disability weights based on these initial conditions.

Table 4D.21 compares DALYs with QALYs, and Table 4D.22 sets out some of the advantages and disadvantages of each measure.

Economic modelling

Economic evaluations may sometimes be based on a single RCT; however, there are often several

Box 4D.14 Issues determining how value preferences to generate QALYs are determined

Issue	Description
Who	There is evidence that the value of a QALY changes radically depending on who makes the value judgement. However, it remains controversial whether the people consulted should be health professionals, the general public, or patients who have experience of the particular medical condition or treatment in question.
How	Five main approaches are used to derive quality-of-life weightings (see later text). Note, however, that the **chronicity** of the hypothetical illness influences valuations, as does the **way in which questions are asked**. Since responses are given to imagined situations, they may not accurately reflect real life.

Table 4D.21 Characteristics of DALYs

Similarities with QALYs	Differences from QALYs
Combine morbidity and mortality into a single dimension	Measure **disease burden** (rather than **quality of life**)
Similar methods used for calculating morbidity weightings (e.g. standard gamble)	Are **age weighted** (i.e. more weight is afforded to productive years and childhood is valued less than early adult life) Are **discounted** at 3% (discounting varies with QALYs)

Table 4D.22 Advantages and disadvantages of QALYs and DALYs

	Advantages	Disadvantages
QALYs	Combine quality of life and mortality Allow comparisons of health outcomes across different medical specialties Can be specific to the population of interest therefore more valid	QALYs may not be equal and therefore may not be comparable (calculation depends on who and how asked). Not weighted. Therefore, no consideration given to whether some QALYs are worth more than others (e.g. depending on age, productivity, deservingness, and family circumstances). May not be generalisable to countries where measures such as the EQ5D have not been tested.
DALYs	Combine morbidity and mortality Good for international comparisons Good for previously neglected areas such as mental health Discounting used	Based on 'expert' rather than population opinions (controversial weightings that may not be relevant everywhere). Age weighting may be criticised as being discriminatory (e.g. should childhood be valued less than adult life?). Requires good data on disease morbidity and mortality for the country in question.

Box 4D.15 Decision trees

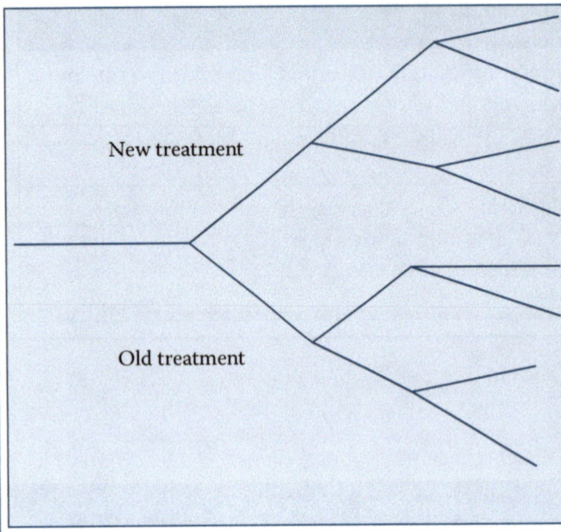

The first division of the tree represents the old and the new treatments. The next branch shows the potential outcomes for each treatment (either unproblematic or adverse events). Subsequent branches show potential consequences of those side effects (such as recovery or death).

A probability is assigned for each branching point (except for the initial division into old and new treatments).

Each final branch is assigned a cost (in £) and a benefit (in QALY). For the old treatment, the sum of the costs and benefits are added together, multiplied by the probability of each branch. The same is done for all the branches of the new treatment. The ICER then represents the incremental costs and benefits of moving from the old to the new treatment.

different sources of information available on treatment effect, costs, benefits, disease progression, etc. Therefore, modelling processes may be used to combine such data. A model is a simplification of the real world where only the most important components considered. Models have a number of advantages, including the ability to

- Link information from various sources
- Extrapolate beyond the data observed in an RCT
- Generalise to other settings
- Simulate head-to-head comparisons that have not been conducted in reality

The two most commonly used models in economic evaluation are **decision trees** and **Markov models** (see Boxes 4D.15 and 4D.16).

While good models are explicit and transparent, their validity remains questionable because they could easily be manipulated by slightly changing one parameter. This problem of **parameter uncertainty** can be addressed by conducting a **sensitivity analysis** in which different parameters are varied across their range of plausible values to assess the effect on the ICER. Parameters can be altered one at a time (**one-way sensitivity analysis**) or simultaneously (**multi-way sensitivity analysis** and **probabilistic sensitivity analysis**).

Sensitivity analysis

When data are collected or assumptions are made within an economic evaluation, uncertainty inevitably arises regarding the accuracy of these parameters or of the models themselves. See Table 4D.23.

This uncertainty leads in turn to uncertainty about the final cost-effectiveness estimate. The impact of this uncertainty should be assessed with a sensitivity analysis, of which there are two types: **deterministic** sensitivity analysis and **probabilistic** sensitivity analysis (see Table 4D.24).

Box 4D.16 Markov modelling

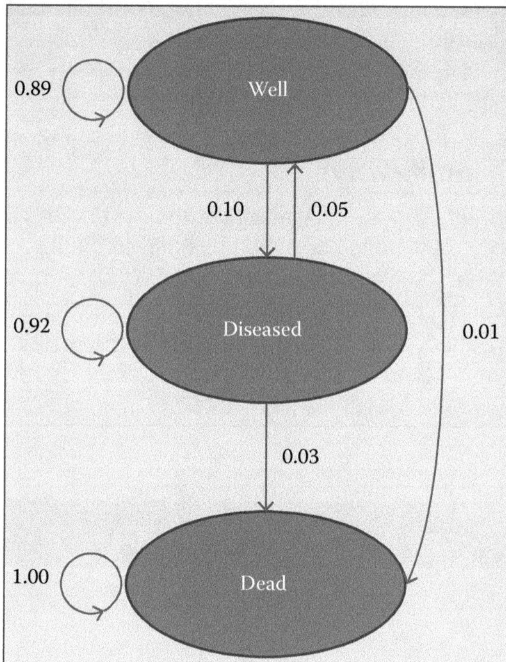

Markov models are useful for analysing **chronic diseases**.

Each circle represents a health state (e.g. well, diseased, dead).

Individuals move from state to state over the time of a cycle (e.g. 1 year) according to a set of **transition probabilities** (numbers in blue). Different treatments will have different transition probabilities and different costs. Costs and utility values can be assigned to each disease state.

The model is then run with a hypothetical cohort population for a defined time horizon (e.g. 20 years, or until the whole cohort has died). Costs and outcomes for each treatment option are then calculated based on this simulation, and an ICER is calculated to compare the two options.

The Markov model incorporates **time** (by having cycles) and facilitates modelling **repeat events**.

Some limitations of Markov models:

- It is difficult to include interactions between patients (hence a limitation in their use without modification for infectious diseases).
- They are 'memory-less' (the model ignores how long a patient has been in a disease state, which could affect transition probabilities).
- As with all models, Markov models rely on the accuracy and availability of the data on which they were built.

Table 4D.23 Types of uncertainty in economic evaluation

Type of uncertainty	Description
Methodological uncertainty	Uncertainty in the methodological approach (e.g. which perspective is most appropriate).
Parameter uncertainty	Unexplained variation, sampling variation, and random variation may lead to different possible values for parameters (e.g. represented by the confidence interval around a treatment effect).
Model structure uncertainty	Uncertainty about the assumptions within the model.
Heterogeneity	Different subgroups with different parameters (e.g. the intervention may be more effective in females than in males).
Generalisability	Uncertainty about whether the results apply in other contexts.

Table 4D.24 Types of sensitivity analysis

Type of sensitivity analysis	Description
Deterministic	Involves modelling different plausible parameter values and model assumptions to assess how varying them affects the ICER (e.g. varying the discount factor and time horizon). Parameters may be varied one at a time (**one-way**) or several parameters may be altered simultaneously (**multi-way**).
Probabilistic	Incorporates parameter uncertainty into the model by defining parameters as **distributions** (rather than point estimates) and then sampling from the distribution in a cohort simulation. This method can consider variation across all parameters simultaneously. The result of a probabilistic sensitivity analysis is a **Cost-Effectiveness Acceptability Curve** (CEAC), which displays the probability of an intervention being cost-effective at different threshold **WTP** values.

4D.6 Marginal analysis

See Section 4D.1.

4D.7 Decision analysis

Decision analysis is a process that involves

- Division of a problem into simpler, manageable components
- Detailed examination of each component
- Formation of components into a logical sequence so as to identify the best solution

All options are first identified and listed, together with the **probability** and **utility** of each possible outcome (see Box 4D.17).

Box 4D.17 Example: Decision analysis

For a particular disease there is a

- Standard treatment, which results in either cure or death
- New treatment, which results in cure or death or disability

A decision tree is constructed to illustrate these possibilities. Note that the branches emanating from each node are mutually exclusive and that the probabilities at each branch must therefore add up to 1.

The probabilities of each outcome in a chance node are included, and utilities are assigned to every possible outcome using a common scale (i.e. a value between 0 and 1).

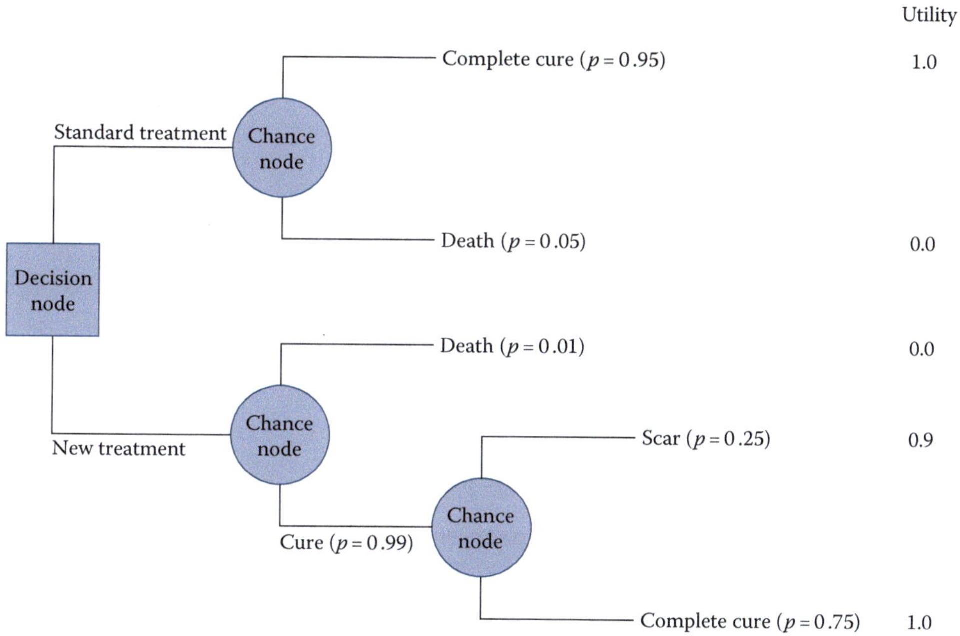

For each treatment, the sum of the utilities for each possible outcome is multiplied by its probability.

Standard treatment = (0.95 × 1.0) + (0.05 × 0.0) = **0.95**

New treatment = (0.01 × 0.0) + (0.99 × 0.25 × 0.9) + (0.99 × 0.75 × 1.0) = **0.966**

The option with the higher overall utility is chosen (in this case, the new treatment). Finally, a sensitivity analysis is conducted in which each probability and utility is varied within a confidence interval to test the robustness of conclusions.

Source: Reproduced from Jefferson, T. et al., *Elementary Economic Evaluation in Health Care*, 2nd edn., BMJ Books, London, UK, 2000.

4D.8 Economic evaluation and priority setting

Role of economic evaluation and priority setting in healthcare decision-making, including the cost-effectiveness of public health, and public health interventions and involvement.

See Section 4C.5 for priority-setting frameworks including programme budgeting and marginal analysis (PBMA).

Both CUAs and CBAs allow interventions with disparate outcomes to be compared on the same scale. Such interventions might include public health initiatives that tackle the risk factors for multiple diseases (e.g. smoking and obesity) and the wider determinants of health. Since the benefits of public health interventions may not be realised for decades, the principle of **discounting** becomes particularly important (see Section 4D.1).

Economic evaluation

UK In England and Wales, NICE provides priority-setting advice using economic evaluations as part of their **health technology appraisals**. These also study the medical, ethical, and social implications of new health technologies and are used to help inform policy.

The process of economic evaluation consists of **identifying** then **critically appraising** and **synthesising** the evidence, so that recommendations of cost-effectiveness (expressed as cost per QALY) can be made (see Table 4D.25).

Public health interventions

Public health activities may be **direct** or **indirect** (see Table 4D.26).

When evaluating a public health intervention, NICE follows the process shown in Table 4D.27.

Table 4D.25 Economic evaluation process

Type of evidence	Description
Identification of evidence	A search of the published and unpublished evidence is performed using economics search filters. Both qualitative and quantitative studies are sought from the published literature and the grey literature.
Critical appraisal	The quality of individual studies is appraised according to the hierarchy of evidence (see Chapter 1C.5), where RCTs (or cluster RCTs for community interventions) are particularly highly valued.
Synthesis of evidence	Assessment of applicability, construction of evidence tables, meta-analysis, and summaries of the evidence in the form of evidence statements.

Table 4D.26 Types of public health activity

Type of public health activity	Examples
Direct	Stop-smoking services Obesity clinics Health promotion posters
Indirect	Creation of parks and open spaces Restrictions on advertising fast foods

Table 4D.27 NICE process for evaluating a public health intervention

Stage	Description
Background work	Topics for evaluation are set by ministers. Stakeholders are identified who will scrutinise and validate the evaluation process. Quality assurance arrangements are put in place.
Preliminary work	The scope of the evaluation is determined (i.e. definition, settings, population, exclusion criteria). A preliminary literature search is conducted.
Detailed work	Key questions are set and an analytical framework is constructed. A review of the evidence is conducted (selection of studies, quality assessment, evidence of implementation). The evidence is synthesised in the form of **evidence statements**.

NICE uses a discount rate of 3.5% for both costs and benefits in its analyses and adopts the following economic perspectives: NHS, society, and the individual.

For each question addressed by the evaluation, an evidence statement is presented that documents both the **strength** of the evidence (i.e. its quality, quantity, and appropriateness) and its **applicability** to the target population. NICE rates the strength of evidence according to the scale shown in Chapter 1C.5.

For example, a hypothetical evidence statement might be

A body of 2+ evidence of efficacy offers consistent findings about the impact of pogo sticks on weight loss. The evidence is directly applicable to the target population in terms of ethnicity, age and gender.

Cost–consequence analysis

Because of the complexities of public health interventions, NICE sometimes uses a **cost–consequence** approach in addition to CEA. This technique enables non-quantifiable outcomes, such as distributive justice, to be considered in an explicit way (see Section 4C.1). It presents a table of the lifetime impact of the new treatment on individuals or groups of individuals in terms of

- Resource use (both healthcare and productivity losses)
- Health outcomes (symptoms, life expectancy, and quality of life [QoL])

References

1. Fletcher, R. (2013) Auguste Comte. Encyclopedia Britannica. Accessed online July 20, 2014 at http://www.britannica.com/EBchecked/topic/130750/Auguste-Comte.
2. Pool, R. and Geissler, W. (eds.) (2005) Chapter 5: Interpreting and explaining sickness. In: *Medical Anthropology*. Understanding Public Health Series. Maidenhead, UK: OUP.
3. Parsons, T. (1951) *The Social System*. New York: Free Press.
4. Lewis, G. (2000) *A Failure of Treatment*. Oxford, UK: Oxford University Press.
5. Scambler, G. (ed.) (1997) *Sociology as Applied to Medicine* (4th edn.). London, UK: Saunders.
6. Huber, M., Knottnerus, J.A., Green, L. et al. (2011) How should we define health? *BMJ* 343, d416.
7. WHO (2013) Preamble to the Constitution of the World Health Organization. *International Health Conference*, New York, June 19–22, 1946.

8. Smith (2009) Quoted in: Godlee, F. (2011) What is health? *BMJ* 343, d4817.
9. No Authors (2009) *The Normal and the Pathological*. Quoted in: What is health? The ability to adapt (Editorial). *Lancet*, 373, 781. doi:10.1016/S0140-6736(09)60456-6.
10. Ereaut, G. and Whiting, R. (2008) What do we mean by 'wellbeing'? And why might it matter? Research Report DCSF-RW073. Linguistic Landscapes. Accessed online June 1, 2014 https://www.gov.uk/government/uploads/system/uploads/attachment_data/file/222254/DCSF-RW073.pdf.
11. Becker, H.S. (1963) *Outsiders: Studies in the Sociology of Deviance*. New York: Free Press.
12. Lemert, E.M. (1967) *Human Deviance, Social Problems, and Social Control*. Englewood Cliffs, NJ: Prentice-Hall.
13. Goffman, E. (1963) *Stigma: Notes on the Management of Spoiled Identity*. London, UK: Prentice-Hall.
14. Department of Health (2011) 'Worth Talking About' Campaign Evaluation 2010/2011. COI Management Summary on behalf of the Department of Health [Online]. Accessed online June 1, 2014 http://www.nhs.uk/sexualhealth-professional/Documents/Worth_Talking_About_post_wave_campaign_evaluation_2010.pdf?wt.mc_id=21103.
15. Office for Disability Issues webpages. Accessed online July 20, 2014 at http://odi.dwp.gov.uk/about-the-odi/index.phphttp://odi.dwp.gov.uk/about-the-odi/index.php.
16. Illich, I. (1975) *Medical Nemesis: The Expropriation of Health*. London, UK: Marian Boyars.
17. Macmillan (2012) Improving cancer treatment, assessment and support for older people. http://www.macmillan.org.uk/Aboutus/Healthandsocialcareprofessionals/Macmillansprogrammesandservices/Improvingservicesforolderpeople/ProjectImprovingcancertreatment, assessmentandsupportforolder-people.aspx.
18. Black, D., Morris, J.N., Smith, C. et al. (1980) Inequalities in health: Report of a research working group (Black Report). London, UK: Department of Health and Social Security. Available online at www.sochealth.co.uk/history/black.htm.
19. Wilkinson, R. and Marmot, M. (2003) *Social Determinants of Health: The Solid Facts* (2nd edn.). Copenhagen, Denmark: WHO. Available online at: www.euro.who.int/document/e81384.pdf. A short, readable summary providing evidence of the health implications of social, cultural and economic circumstances.
20. Last, J.M. (1963) The iceberg: 'Completing the clinical picture' in general practice. *Lancet* 2, 28–31.
21. Barsky, A.J. and Borus, J.F. (1995) Somatization and medicalization in the era of managed care. *JAMA* 274, 1931–1934.
22. McHugh, S. and Moon, N. (2008) Consumer consumption of vitamin and mineral food. GfK Social Research. Consumer consumption of vitamin and mineral food supplements. Commissioned by: The Food Standards Agency/Central Office for Information. Accessed online July 20, 2014 at http://www.foodbase.org.uk//admintools/reportdocuments/472-1-841_viminsup-consumer.pdf.
22a. NHS Choices (2011) Supplements—Who needs them? A Behind the Headlines report. Accessed online July 20, 2014 at http://www.nhs.uk/news/2011/05May/Documents/BtH_supplements.pdf.
23. Dose Adjustment For Normal Eating (DAFNE) Website (for Type 1 Diabetes). Accessed online July 20, 2014 at http://www.dafne.uk.com/.
24. The Sustainable Development Unit website. Accessed online July 20, 2014 at http://www.sduhealth.org.uk/delivery/evaluate.aspx.
25. Friedson, E. (1959) Specialties without roots: the utilization of new services. *Hum Organ* 18, 112–116.
26. National Health Service and Community Care Act (1990) NHS and Community Care Act 1990. London, UK: HMSO.
27. Larson, M.S. (1977) *The Rise of Professionalism: A Sociological Analysis*. Berkeley, CA: University of California Press.
28. Armstrong, D. (2002) Clinical autonomy, individual and collective: The problem of changing doctors' behaviour. *Soc Sci Med* 55, 1771–1777.
29. Mechanic, D. (1968) *Medical Sociology*. New York: Free Press.
30. Pilowski, I. and Spence, N.D. (1977) Ethnicity and illness behaviour. *Psychol Med* 7, 447–452.
31. Zborowski, M. (1952) Cultural components in response to pain. *J Soc Issues* 8, 16–30.
32. Zola, I.K. (1973) Pathways to the doctor—From person to patient. *Soc Sci Med* 7, 677–689.
33. Horne, R. Weinman, J., Barber, N., Elliott, R., and Morgan, M. (2005) Concordance, adherence and compliance in medicine taking. Report for the

National Co-ordinating Centre for NHS Service Delivery and Organisation R & D (NCCSDO). [Online]. Accessed online June 1, 2014 at http://www.nets.nihr.ac.uk/.

34. Horne, R. and Weinman, J. (1999) Patients' beliefs about prescribed medicines and their role in adherence to treatment in chronic physical illness. *J Psychosom Res* 47(6), 555–567.

35. Moffat, J. Help seeking and delay literature—Key insights. Cancer Research UK, 2010. Accessed online July 20, 2014 at http://www.cancerresearchuk.org/prod_consump/groups/cr_common//@nre/@hea/documents/generalcontent/cr_043179.pdf.

35a. Crinson, I. (2007) Section 4. Lay health beliefs and illness behaviour. Health knowledge website. Accessed online July 20, 2014 at http://www.healthknowledge.org.uk/public-health-textbook/medical-sociology-policy-economics/4a-concepts-health-illness/section4.

36. Doyal, L. and Gough, I.R. (1991) *A Theory of Human Need*. New York: The Guilford Press.

37. Burt, J. (2010) Equity, need and access in health care: A mixed methods investigation of specialist palliative care use in relation to age, PhD thesis. UCL, London, UK, Chapter 2, pp. 23–67.

38. Culyer, A.J. and Wagstaff, A. (1995) Need, equity and equality in health and health care. Discussion Paper 95. Centre for Health Economics, University of York. [Online]. Accessed June 1, 2014 https://www.york.ac.uk/media/che/documents/papers/discussionpapers/CHE%20Discussion%20Paper%2095.pdf.

39. Bradshaw, J.R. (1972) The taxonomy of social need. In: McLachlan, G. (ed.) *Problems and Progress in Medical Care*. Oxford, UK: Oxford University Press, pp. 69–82.

40. Jost, J.T. and Kay, A.C. (2010) Social justice: History, theory, and research. In Fiske, S.T., Gilbert, D., and Lindzey, G. (eds.) *Handbook of Social Psychology* (5th edn.), Vol. 2. Hoboken, NJ: Wiley, pp. 1122–1165.

41. Rawls, J. (1985) Justice as fairness: Political not metaphysical. *Philos Publ Aff* 14, 223–251. [Online]. Accessed online June 1, 2014 at http://links.jstor.org/sici?sici=0048-3915%28198522%2914%3A3%3C223%3AJAFPNM%3E2.0.CO%3B2-0.

42. Thibaut, J.W. and Walker, L. (1975) *Procedural Justice: A Psychological Analysis*. Hillsdale, NJ: L. Erlbaum Associates.

43. Leventhal, G.S., Karuza, J., and Fry, W.R. (1980) Beyond fairness: A theory of allocation preferences. In Mikula, G. (ed.) *Justice and Social Interaction*. New York: Springer-Verlag, pp. 167–218.

44. Maynard, A. (2001) Economic-based medicine: an evolving paradigm. *J Roy Coll Phys Edinb* 31(Suppl 9), 16–7.

45. Donaldson, C., Gerard, K., Mitton, C. et al. (2004) *Economics of Health Care Financing: The Visible Hand*. Basingstoke, UK: Palgrave MacMillan.

46. Lewis, R., Hunt, P., and Carson, D. (2006) *Social Enterprise and Community Based Care: Is There a Future for Mutually-Owned Organizations in Community and Primary Care?* London, UK: King's Fund.

47. Foundation Trust Network (2005) *New Voices, New Accountabilities: A Guide to Wider Governance in Foundation Trusts*. London, UK: Foundation Trust Network. Available online at www.nhsconfed.org/ftn.

48. Sabik, L.M. and Lie, R.K. (2008) Priority setting in health care: Lessons from the experiences of eight countries. *Int J Equity Health* 7, 4. doi:10.1186/1475-9276-7-4. http://www.equityhealthj.com/content/7/1/4.

49. Sihota, S. and Lennard, L. (2004) *Health Literacy: Being Able to Make the Most of Health*. London, UK: National Consumer Council. Available online at www.ncc.org.uk/nccpdf/poldocs/NCC064_health_literacy.pdf.

50. The Freedom of Information Act (2000) Accessed online June 1, 2014 at http://www.legislation.gov.uk/ukpga/2000/36/contents.

51. The Official Information Act (1982) Accessed online June 1, 2014 at http://www.legislation.govt.nz/act/public/1982/0156/latest/DLM64785.html.

52. OECD (1980, updated 2013) OECD Guidelines on the protection of privacy and trans-border flows of personal data. Accessed online June 1, 2014 at http://www.oecd.org/internet/ieconomy/oecdguidelinesontheprotectionofprivacyandtransborderflowsofpersonaldata.htm.

53. Hartree, N. and Tidy, C. (2014) Monitoring the NHS. Accessed online July 20, 2014 at http://www.patient.co.uk/doctor/Monitoring-the-NHS-Local-Involvement-Networks-(LINks).htm.

54. Health Watch website. Accessed online July 20, 2014 at http://www.healthwatch.co.uk/about-us.

55. French, J.R.P. and Raven, B.H. (1960) The bases of social power. In: Cartwright, D. and Zander, A. (eds.) *Group Dynamics*. New York: Harper and Row.

56. Bartley, M. (2004) *Health Inequality: An Introduction to Concepts, Theories and Methods*. Cambridge, UK: Polity Press.
57. Benzeval, M. (1995) *Tackling Inequalities in Health*. London, UK: King's Fund.
58. Acheson, D. (1998) Independent inquiry into inequalities in health report. London, UK: TSO. Available online at www.archive.official-documents.co.uk/document/doh/ih/ih.htm.
59. Department of Health (1999) *Saving Lives: Our Healthier Nation*. London, UK: The Stationery Office. Available online at www.archive.official-documents.co.uk/document/cm43/4386/4386.htm.
60. Marmot. M., Allen, J., Goldblatt, P., Boyce, T., McNeish, D., Grady, M., and Geddes, I. (2010) Fair Society, Healthy Lives. The Marmot Review. Accessed online August 16, 2014 at www.instituteofhealthequity.org.
61. Nazroo, J.Y. and Karlsen, S. (2001) Research findings 10. Ethnic inequalities in health: Social class, racism and identity ESRC. www.lancs.ac.uk/fass/apsocsci/hvp/pdf/fd10.pdf.
62. Ellis, A. and Fry, R. (2010) Regional health inequalities in England. Office for National Statistics. Accessed online June 1, 2014 at http://www.ons.gov.uk/ons/rel/regional-trends/regional-trends/index.html.
63. United Nations, Department of Economic and Social Affairs, Population Division (2009) Trends in International Migrant Stock: The 2008 revision (United Nations database, POP/DB/MIG/Stock/Rev.2008). Accessed online July 20, 2014 at http://esa.un.org/migration/p2k0data.asp.
64. Rechel, B., Mladovsky, P., Devillé, W., Rijks, B., Petrova-Benedict, R., and McKee, M. (eds.) (2011) Migration and health in the European Union. The European Observatory on Health Systems and Policy. Accessed online June 1, 2014 at http://www.euro.who.int/en/about-us/partners/observatory.
65. Branagh, E. (2012) David Cameron warned on foreign student policy. The Independent. Accessed online July 20, 2014 at http://www.independent.co.uk/news/education/education-news/david-cameron-warned-on-foreign-student-policy-7803672.html.
66. WHO (2003) *International Migration, Health and Human Rights*. Health & Human Rights Publication Series, Issue No. 4. Geneva, Switzerland: WHO.
67. Drager, N. (1999) Making trade work for public health. *BMJ* 319, 1214. Accessed online July 20, 2014 at http://www.who.int/trade/en/Drager_Making_Trade_Work_for_the_Public_Health_1999.pdf.
68. Beveridge, W. (1942) Social insurance and allied services. Policy. Accessed online June 1, 2014 at http://www.sochealth.co.uk/resources/public-health-and-wellbeing/beveridge-report/.
69. Hale, J. (2000) What contribution can health economics make to health promotion. *Health Promot Int* 15, 341–348.
70. Fitzsimons, E., Rogger, D., and Stoye, G. (2012) Chapter 7. UK development aid. In: *The IFS Green Budget: February 2012*. Institute of Fiscal Studies. Accessed online June 1, 2014 at http://www.ifs.org.uk/budgets/gb2012/12chap7.pdf.
71. McCoy, D., Chand, S., and Sridhar, D. (2009) Global health funding: How much, where it comes from and where it goes. *Health Pol Plann* 24(6), 407–417. doi:10.1093/Heapol/Czp026. Accessed online July 20, 2014 at http://heapol.oxfordjournals.org/content/24/6/407/F1.expansion.html.
72. Cohen, D. (1994) Marginal analysis in practice: An alternative to needs assessment for contracting health care. *BMJ* 309, 781–784.
73. Sassi, F., Le Grand, J., and Archard, L. (2001) Equity versus efficiency: A dilemma for the NHS. *BMJ* 323, 762–763.
74. Department of Health (2006) *NHS Allocations*. London, UK: Department of Health. Available online at www.dh.gov.uk.
75. Holder, R. and Thorlby, R. (2013) The new NHS in England: Structure and accountabilities. The Nuffield Trust. Accessed online July 20, 2014 at http://www.nuffieldtrust.org.uk/talks/slideshows/new-structure-nhs-england.
76. Gibbons, B. (2005) Publication of Professor Townsend's Final Report Inequalities in Health: The Welsh Dimension 2002–2005. Accessed online July 20, 2014 at http://wales.gov.uk/.
77. Fox-Rushby, J. and Cairns, J. (2005) *Economic Evaluation*. Maidenhead, UK: Open University Press.
78. Jefferson, T., Demicheli, V., and Mugford, M. (2000) *Elementary Economic Evaluation in Health Care* (2nd edn.). London, UK: BMJ Books.

Section 5

ORGANISATION AND MANAGEMENT OF HEALTHCARE AND HEALTHCARE PROGRAMMES

Management is not limited to managers. Every member of an organisation has some managerial role. At its simplest level, this may involve controlling your own time and resources; at its most complex, it includes directing multiple projects, staff, and budgets.

Section 5 covers the major theories of management science, from working with people to managing finances. The challenges and benefits of working in teams are discussed, together with an overview of ways to motivate individuals. To enable a team to function optimally, an understanding of personalities is needed, especially the different ways that people think and how they function when working together. At a higher level, organisational structure and culture can contribute to a health system's success or failure in meeting its goals. Understanding organisations, how they function (and more importantly, why they fail), is therefore fundamental to implement change in health systems. However, to be successful, public health professionals also need to work across organisational boundaries and interact with a wide range of professional and lay groups. To do so, they must recognise the different professional roles and cultures that exist in health and non-health organisations.

Change is an essential part of any health service provision. As new technologies, diseases, and different political priorities emerge, healthcare must evolve and transform to meet the needs of its population. So, robust strategies are needed to manage change carefully.

Finally, healthcare systems exist in a world with finite resources. Public health practitioners will be all too aware of constraints on resources and how this affects the capacity of organisations to provide healthcare. A basic understanding of financial and managerial accounting is therefore invaluable when establishing and maintaining the provision of health services.

5A

Understanding Individuals, Teams/Groups, and Their Development

When things are going well, the benefits of working with others are clear. Colleagues help stimulate ideas and can promote enthusiasm, enjoyment, interest, increased productivity, and a greater sense of reward. However, there are also times when working with other people leads to conflict, stifles creativity, and impedes the progress of a project.

Public health practitioners frequently find themselves working with people from different professional groups, often across organisational boundaries. Knowledge of management principles, team dynamics, and interactions between professions is therefore vital for understanding how groups function. It can also offer ways to analyse and address conflict and to modify our own attitudes and practices accordingly.

5A.1 Individuals, groups, and team dynamics

Motivation, creativity, and innovation in individuals and its relationship to group and team dynamics.

People function differently when working alone as opposed to working in groups. Individual performance is covered in other sections of the book (motivation is covered in Section 5C.1, creativity and innovation in Section 5A.2, and personal effectiveness in Section 5A.4). Here, we focus on group work, which at best may result in outcomes that individuals working alone could never have produced. However, it is important to consider the **composition**, **dynamics,** and **leadership** of a group to ensure that its members are motivated to work together as productively as possible.

Groups may be convened **formally** in order to perform a specific task or **informally** by individuals on the basis of a common interest. Various definitions of groups and teams exist, but what many definitions have in common is that these are groups with a degree of **mutual accountability**.

Team dynamics

Within a group, individuals may adopt one or more roles, as determined by a compromise between

- How an individual wants to behave
- How other group members expect them to behave
- The group's task

Belbin [1] described eight roles that should be represented by members of a *team if it is to perform effectively. These team roles can be used to identify strengths and weaknesses in a team environment, and an understanding of the different roles can help improve team dynamics. These positions can be remembered with the mnemonic ICE FIRST: see Table 5A.1. Belbin [2] later added a ninth role of *specialist*, that is, a person with a high level of skill in one particular discipline. Note that a team member may fulfil multiple roles.

Groups can be motivated by means of the following:

- **Feedback** to remind the team members of the importance of their group's task, together with their individual roles within it.
- **Leadership**: a good leader develops team spirit and elicits a high level of commitment from team members.

Team development

Tuckman [3] described a four-stage process through which newly formed teams typically progress and develop: see Box 5A.1. A fifth stage, **adjourning**, was added in 1975, which refers to the disbanding of the team after its task has been completed. The model is significant because it recognises that groups do not start off fully formed and functioning [4].

Table 5A.1 Belbin's eight roles for an effective team

Implementer/ company worker	Make things happen High degree of self-discipline Deliver on time
Coordinator/chair	Default chairperson Step back to see the big picture
Evaluator/monitor	Fair and even-handed observers and judges of what is going on Can become almost machine like May have difficulty inspiring themselves or others to be passionate about their work
Finisher/completer	Perfectionists Strong sense of duty Complete painstaking and unpleasant tasks if they believe that this will improve quality May frustrate their team mates
Innovator/plant	Come up with unusual and innovative solutions to problems
Resource investigator	Vigorously pursue contacts and opportunities Excellent networkers Tend to lose momentum towards the end of a project
Shaper	Eager individuals that provoke their team into action May be insensitive to the feelings and perceptions of others
Team worker	Ensure that everyone in the working group is getting along Good listener and diplomat Talented at smoothing over conflicts

Box 5A.1 Tuckman's stages of team development [3]

Forming	Tasks and rules are established. Resources are acquired. Reliance is placed on the leader.
Storming	Internal conflict. Members resist the task emotionally.
Norming	Conflict is settled. Cooperation develops. Views are exchanged. Norms (i.e. new standards) are developed.
Performing	Teamwork is achieved. Flexible roles are developed. Solutions are found and implemented.

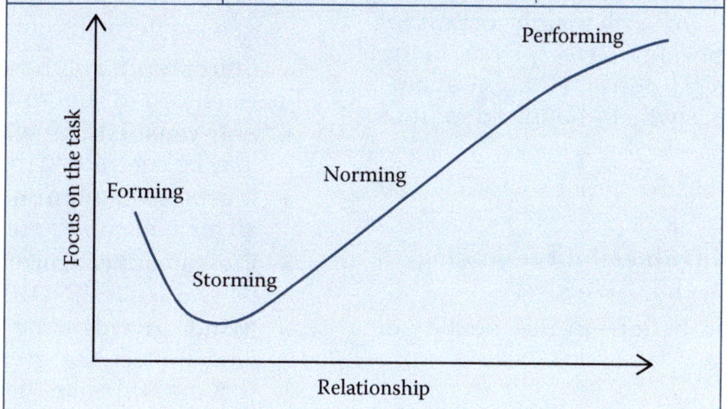

Teamwork and successful teams

Handy [5] argued that the ideal team does not only achieve **formal** goals (i.e. those set by its organisation) but also accomplishes **informal goals** such satisfying its members' psychosocial needs [6]. Handy described the ideal team as having the traits listed in Box 5A.2.

See Section 5C.3 for methods of evaluating the performance of teams and team members (e.g. 360° feedback).

Poor teamwork

While good teamwork can be a key factor in ensuring the success of a project or task, there are several pitfalls that can lead to poor teamwork and project failure, including

- Conflicts
- Criticism of individuals rather than ideas
- Domination and poor listening by team members
- Lack of commitment, absenteeism, and presenteeism
- Disregard for deadlines
- Too much conformity leading to **groupthink**

Groupthink

This phenomenon occurs in teams when a desire to reach consensus causes critical appraisal and the thorough discussion of ideas to

Box 5A.2 Handy's traits of ideal teams (1978)

Organisation	Common purpose. Clearly defined task. Clear team objective.
Members	Members have specific expertise. Members know their roles.
Teamwork	Members support each other. Members complement each other in skills and personalities. Members are committed to accomplishing the task.
Leadership	Leader who coordinates and takes responsibility.

be superseded. Although conflict can be detrimental to teamwork, productive conflict over ideas is important for enhancing creativity and preventing important factors from being missed. Irving Janis [7] described eight symptoms of groupthink, which he divided into three categories:

1. Overestimation of the group's power and morality
   - Illusions of **invulnerability**—leading to over-optimism and risk-taking
   - **Unquestioned belief**—in the morality of group decisions
2. Closed-mindedness
   - Collective **rationalisation**—of warnings that are deemed contrary to the group
   - **Stereotyping** of those outside the group
3. Pressure towards uniformity
   - **Self-censorship**—withholding ideas that may be contrary to the group
   - Illusions of **unanimity**—false belief that all team members are in agreement
   - Pressure for **conformity**—placed on members who question the group's ideas
   - **Mind guards**—self-appointed members who protect the group from information that may threaten the group

5A.2 Creativity and innovation

Barriers to, and stimulation of, creativity and innovation (e.g. by brainstorming).

Creativity is one of the key strengths that public health professionals can bring to their working environment. Because it focuses on the 'bigger picture', the public health viewpoint is well placed for challenging established practices in positive ways.

Stimulation of creativity

The following techniques have all been used by successful organisations to stimulate creativity and innovation among staff:

Brainstorming (a method for promoting creativity in which team members *'think out loud'* in order to solve a problem. The process is conducted in a noncritical atmosphere that is conducive to independent thought and discussion)

Suggestion boxes (to enable staff to voice new ideas anonymously)

Team away-days (offsite meetings attended by team members)

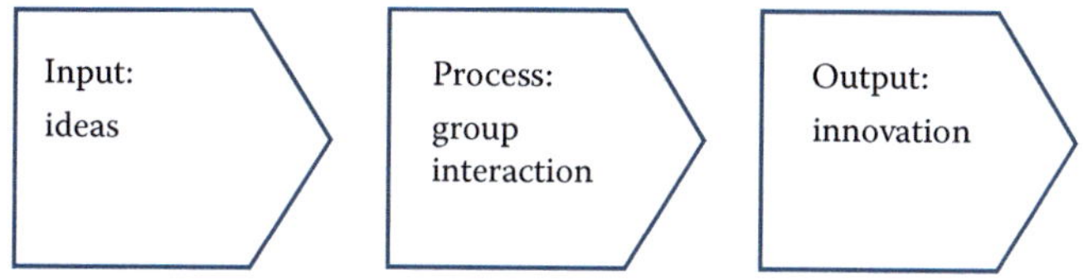

Figure 5A.1 Sequence for creativity.

Mind mapping (a visual method to illustrate ideas and their interconnections)
Reward (prizes for innovative ideas)

Innovation

Amabile [8] argued that creativity in companies requires three components:

- **Motivation** (especially intrinsic motivation, i.e. satisfying your own needs—see also 5C.1)
- **Expertise** (technical, procedural, and intellectual knowledge)
- **Flexible thinking** (how flexibly and imaginatively people approach problems)

Creativity itself can be thought of as a three-step sequence consisting of an **input**, a **process**, and an **output**: see Figure 5A.1.

Diffusion of innovations

Rogers [9] described five factors that increase the likelihood that ideas will spread rapidly, namely,

1. Relatively **advantageous**
2. **Compatible** with existing systems
3. **Simple**
4. Amenable to being **trialled**
5. **Visibly** more efficacious

His model of diffusion (1995, 5A.13) described how people adopt new innovations.

Dearing [10] argued that practitioners should also consider the potential of new programmes to be scaled up and disseminated. For example, in England, the government introduced a number of measures aimed at increasing the 'pace and scale' at which innovations are diffused. These include [11]

- Establishing academic health science networks, to **link research with healthcare** delivery
- Expanding the role of NICE to produce **implementation guidance** alongside its healthcare technology appraisals
- Developing a web portal to **share innovative practices** with patients and the public

Barriers to creativity and innovation

The following factors can hamper innovation:

- Uncertainty
- Overfamiliarity
- Fear of change
- Team conflict
- Groupthink (see the 'Poor team work' section)

5A.3 Inter-professional learning

Learning with individuals from differing professional backgrounds.

Several developments in health systems have led to an increased focus on inter-professional education:

- Changing populations (e.g. increasing recognition of multiple morbidities among patients)
- Changing professional boundaries and requirements for clinical practice
- Changing healthcare structures
- Emphasis within healthcare on multi-professional teams and clinical networks

Inter-professional learning is more than simply large, didactic teaching sessions or training sessions with people from other professional groups. Rather, it should involve small-group sessions that enable students to learn *'with, from and about one another'* [12].

ENG In England, inter-professional education has gained increasing momentum since early commitments in the *NHS Plan* [13]. The Bristol Royal Infirmary Inquiry (a high-profile inquiry into excess mortality at a paediatric cardiac unit from 2001) highlighted the fact that patients were being cared for by distinct groups of health professionals and that collaboration and inter-professional teamwork were poorly organised. The inquiry report made a number of recommendations to promote inter-professional learning, arguing that these measures should start as early as possible during clinical training in order to reduce ***'damaging intertribal rivalries'*** in the health service.

The DH's [14] strategy to promote inter-professional learning, *Working Together—Learning Together* (see www.dh.gov.uk), included a commitment to include inter-professional learning during

- Education and training for all health professionals
- Undergraduate and pre-registration programmes
- Continuing professional education
- Practice placements

The department has since supported and funded a number of initiatives, both nationally and locally.

In England, Scotland and Wales, the speciality of public health is itself an example of an inter-professional discipline. In the past, although there was a formal route for doctors to train in public health, the expertise and input of other professional groups was not always recognised or regulated. Now, individuals from a range of non-medical backgrounds can enter the same formal specialist training programmes with medics and non-medics following a **common recruitment process and training programme** to become registered public health consultants, subject to professional regulation and revalidation (see Section 5A.10).

UK See Box 5A.3.

There are several potential advantages and disadvantages of moving away from single profession towards more inter-professional education: see Box 5A.4. Note, however, that there is currently little evidence that inter-professional learning produces the anticipated advantages. This is partly due to the **long lead time** for evaluating the impact of pre-registration professional learning (e.g. there is 10–12 years before medical students will be practising consultants).

Box 5A.3 Example: Expansion of the public health workforce beyond medicine

Many disciplines are involved in delivering public health. In the past, a formal route for doctors to train in public health existed but the expertise of other professional groups was not always recognised or regulated.

Public health in the UK has changed in recent years to enable individuals from a range of non-medical backgrounds to enter formal specialist training programmes. Both medics and non-medics follow a **common recruitment process and training programme** to become public health consultants.

Once they have completed training, doctors remain registered with the General Medical Council. A new organisation, the UK Public Health Register, has been developed to maintain a register of non-medical public health professionals who have completed specialist training or have been assessed through a portfolio of work as competent to work as a public health consultant.

Source: Reproduced from *The UK Voluntary Register for Public Health Specialists*: www.publichealthregister.org.uk/index.asp; Faculty of Public Health: www.fph.org.uk.

Box 5A.4 Potential advantages and disadvantages of inter-professional learning

Potential advantages	Potential disadvantages
Improves **communication** between different professions Reduces the formation of **professional *'silos'*** **Promotes clinical debate** by increasing awareness of **different professional perspectives** Improves **teamwork** through enhanced appreciation of the roles of other staff Improves **patient care** by ensuring that care is centred on the patient rather than on professional structures Enhances **capacity** by expanding clinical roles as required by the situation and needs of the team	Undermine **peer support** by reducing traditional professional networks **Costly** to reconfigure training and education programmes

5A.4 Personal management skills

Personal management skills (e.g. managing time, stress, difficult people, meetings).

Effective managers need skills not only in managing people and projects but also in managing their own resources. Many of the skills needed to manage other people are the same skills required to manage ourselves, namely, understanding ourselves and others, as well as the ability to plan, delegate, organise, direct, and control.

Self-awareness

Being personally effective relies on having insight into your own working style, learning preferences, and relationships with others. Formal mechanisms to raise self-awareness include annual **appraisal** as well as special tools and questionnaires such as the **Myers–Briggs Type Indicator**. Less formal approaches include **reflective practice** and **action learning** activities.

Time management

Time management is a key component of self-management. Time can be managed by

- Prioritisation (e.g. into long-, middle-, and short-term plans; see Figure 5A.2)
- Organising offices, workstations, and desks to reduce distractions
- Managing paperwork and e-mails systematically
- Delegation

Covey [15] identified a set of **seven habits** that were associated with efficient time management, namely,

1. Being **proactive** (controlling your own environment and deciding on the best response to different stimuli and changing conditions)
2. Beginning with the **end in mind** (considering your own aims and focusing on meeting these so as to avoid distractions)
3. Putting **first things first** (prioritising tasks in order of importance, not urgency)
4. Thinking **win–win** (assuming success should be good for everyone and avoiding a confrontational approach)
5. Seeking first to **understand**, then to be understood
6. **Synergising** (recognising the value of other people's contributions)
7. **Sharpening** the saw (taking time out)

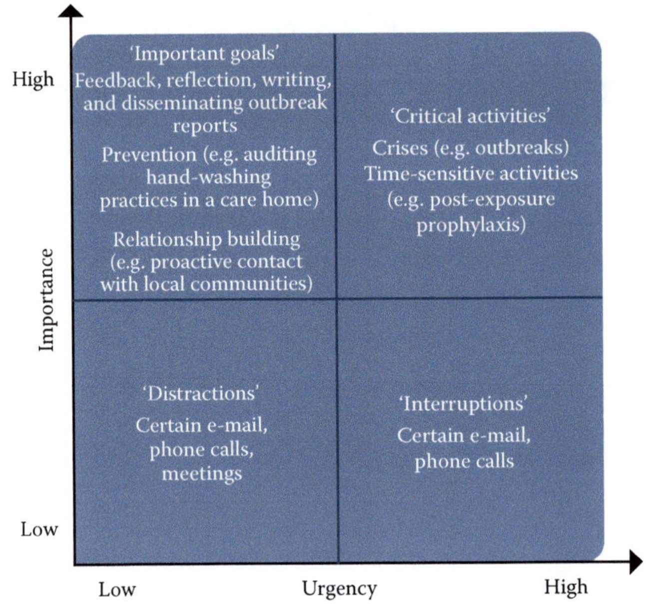

Figure 5A.2 The time management matrix and examples of activities that may fall into each quadrant, as applied to a health protection practitioner. (Ascribed to Covey but adapted by many others.)

Stress management

Several factors can cause stress, including increased **competition**, **job security, achievement of demanding objectives,** and **rapid change**. Methods of dealing with stress include

- Recognising the **symptoms** of stress in yourself and others
- Understanding the **factors** that cause stress
- Applying a range of **strategies** to avoid, reduce, and manage stress

Difficult people

Difficult relationships with other people can arise due to the reasons listed in Table 5A.2.

See also Section 5A.9 for strategies to manage conflict and Section 5A.8 for negotiating skills.

Meetings

Well-run meetings can reduce stress, save time, and improve the effectiveness of an organisation. They tend to have the following features:

- Carefully **planned** with a realistic and succinct agenda.

Table 5A.2 Causes of difficult relationships with colleagues

Difficult situations	Situations such as radical organisational change, threats to employment, or professional roles can call cause friction between colleagues. A good manager seeks to mitigate the effect of these situations on personal relationships and team productivity by carefully using **communication skills** to improve the delivery of unpleasant or bad news.
Personality clashes	By recognising **personality types**, especially your own personality characteristics, it is possible to identify the people with whom you are likely to clash and to develop strategies for dealing with them.
Inappropriate behaviour	Mechanisms such as **appraisal** (see Section 5A.11) and **feedback** (see Section 5A.5) should be used appropriately to manage inappropriate behaviours or poor performance.

Table 5A.3 Effective behaviours before, during, and after meetings

Stage	Strategies and behaviours

Before	• Consider your **own aims**—What is your opening position, your ideal result, and your fallback position?
	• Conduct some background research on the **other attendees**—What are their aims likely to be? How might you be able to influence them?
	• Sell the **benefits**—Avoid focusing on your proposal, rather how it will benefit them.
	• Build the **relationship**
	• When setting up your own meeting, consider
	  • Timing (giving adequate notice)
	  • Venue
	  • Agenda (distribute this in good time)

During	• Listen first—to gauge the mood of the meeting. • Use words carefully—use appropriate language for other meeting attendees. • Realise when you have achieved your objectives—stop arguing beyond this point. • Use summary statements or 'sound bites' to help put across a message. • Read papers before, not during, a meeting.
After	• Follow through with any promises you have made or tasks you have been assigned. • Send out minutes with action points that were decided upon.

Source: Adapted from Jessop, E., *Oxford Handbook of Public Health Practice*, 2006, Chapter 7.2 by permission of Oxford University Press.

- Well chaired.
- High **participation** before the meeting.
- Participants are **aware of the contribution** that the meeting will make to the managerial process of the organisation.

Jessop [16] described several strategies and behaviours that should be adopted by public health professionals before, during and after a meeting. See Table 5A.3.

5A.5 Effective manager

An effective manager has a high degree of personal effectiveness (see Section 5A.4) and can help improve the quality and productivity of an organisation by means of delegation, feedback, and listening.

Delegation

See Section 5A.6.

Feedback

Feedback is crucial for the regulation of any system. It is the process whereby elements of its output are returned to its input so as to regulate further output. Likewise, the feedback that a manager provides to an employee influences the performance of that employee.

The way in which feedback is delivered is pivotal, and managers need to practise giving feedback, especially since this is an activity that many managers actively avoid. A good manager will provide feedback only on **specific**, **observable behaviours** and will ensure that the feedback is provided **non-confrontationally** in order to promote **realistic** behaviour changes—perhaps as part of Iles's [17] **'criticism sandwich'** (good news, bad news, more good news).

Listening

Iles [17] argues that the success of organisations can be assessed by the speed with which bad news travel upwards through the management hierarchy. One way to ensure that the senior management team is kept informed of developments is to use the technique of **management by wandering around** (MBWA). Developed at the Hewlett–Packard Corporation, managers employing MBWA set aside time in their diaries each week to walk through their departments and engage in impromptu discussions. Although very simple (it has been described as the *'technology of obvious'*), MBWA can be extremely effective, particularly at times when an organisation is facing financial difficulties or reorganisation.

During their walk, managers should

- **Listen** to what employees are saying
- **Explain** organisational policy face to face with employees
- Be prepared to offer on-the-spot **assistance** to employees

5A.6 Principles of leadership and delegation

There are countless definitions of leadership but most encompass the notion that a leader influences others to follow. Different models of leadership are described in detail in Section 5C.1.

Although related, leadership and management are typically regarded as separate concepts.

See Section 5C.1.4.

Leadership

Leadership requires the development and communication of a shared vision to colleagues in order to achieve constructive change. Kotter [18] identifies processes associated with successful leadership:

1. **Establishing direction**
2. **Aligning people**
3. **Motivating and inspiring**

Successful leaders are able to foster an environment within their organisation that encourages

- Appropriate **risk-taking**
- Recognition and **reward** of success
- **Empowerment** that allows other leaders to emerge

The principal aim of a manager is to maximise the output of the organisation through

- Controlling
- Leading
- Organising
- Planning
- Staffing

(mnemonic = CLOPS)

Delegation

Delegation is a key skill of an effective manager. It is the process of assigning authority and responsibility for a specific activity to another person. While a manager may delegate tasks, the ultimate responsibility for these tasks cannot be delegated.

As well as its most obvious benefit of sharing the burden of work, delegation can serve other purposes, such as

- Reinforcing the role of leaders through **promoting involvement**
- **Developing skills** in team members

However, many managers struggle to delegate successfully, fearing that a job will not be done properly by anyone else. Iles [17] describes three rules that the effective manager should follow when delegating any task:

- The manager must be confident that the employee **understands** the task.
- The employee and manager must both be confident that the employee has the **skills** and **resources** necessary for the task.
- The manager must provide **feedback** to the employee.

Delegation of goals

Drucker [19] described the technique of **management by objectives** (MBO) where managers delegate **goals** rather than tasks. Employees are set a target to meet but are free to choose the tactics and strategies that they will use to accomplish it. MBO has the following advantages:

- Managers avoid becoming so engrossed in day-to-day events that they lose sight of the organisation's objectives.
- All employees participate in the strategic planning process.
- The organisation's performance can be readily measured against defined objectives.

5A.7 Effective communication

Principles, theories, and methods of effective communication (written and oral) in general, and in a management context.

See also Sections 2H.9 and 6C.

In a managerial context, the functions of communication within an organisation relate to

- **Production** (direction, coordination, and control of activities)
- **Innovation** (stimulation of change and development of new ideas)
- **Maintenance** (preservation of the values and relationships that bind the organisation)

Communication methods

Communication methods vary depending on the purpose of the message. In addition to formal, planned communication activities, communication also occurs in unstructured or tacit ways (e.g. through the body language of employees). Internal and external communication activities serve different purposes and often involve different media. Both, however, may be equally important. (See Table 5A.4.)

Persuasive communication

Monroe's *Motivated Sequence* [20] described five steps for making persuasive speeches or presentations, which are as follows:

1. Get **attention**—This may be through an emotive story, a shocking example, or a dramatic statistic.
2. **Establish the need**—Provide evidence for the extent of the problem and demonstrate its importance.
3. **Satisfy the need**—Provide a detailed description of a viable solution to the problem, summarising at the end.
4. **Visualise** the future—Describe what will happen if nothing is done.
5. **Action**—Provide the audience with specific actions that you want them to take, this may be to meet again to discuss plans.

A similar ('4 Ps') structure has been proposed for blog writers:

1. **Promise**—Explain to the reader why it is worth their while reading on.
2. **Picture**—Paint a picture of the issue using anecdote.
3. **Proof**—Provide statistics and other evidence to back your argument.
4. **Push**—Inspire the reader to do something different.

Table 5A.4 Dimensions of communication in a management context

Dimension	Quality	Description
Formality	Formal	Communications that are routed through a so-called *official channel* (e.g. a written memorandum from a chief executive to the directors of an organisation).
	Informal	Information passed among colleagues in an unstructured way (e.g. a chat in a shared office space or over coffee).
Direction	Diagonal	No obvious line of authority exists through which the information may be communicated.
	Vertical	This is the principal channel by which details of strategies, policies, and tactics permeate from decision-makers down to the frontline—and also by which news from the frontline is fed back (see Section 5A.5).
Method	Verbal	Verbal communication may be spoken or written.
	Oral	Oral forms of verbal communication include speaking to another person **remotely** (telephone, videoconference, etc.) or **face to face** (discussion, debate, interview, presentation, or meeting).
	Written	Written verbal communication may be **one to one** (e-mail, letters, faxes) and **one to many** (e.g. notices, bulletins, newsletters, Tannoy, websites, blogs, and social networking sites such as Twitter). Written communication is required as evidence in certain circumstances (e.g. research ethics).
	Nonverbal	There are no words involved (e.g. eye contact, body language, sign language). People express visual cues through their gestures and appearance (e.g. clothing, hair style, makeup). Organisations also convey impressions through nonverbal means (e.g. branding designs, maintenance of buildings and office space).

5A.8 Principles of negotiation and influencing

Because they typically lack resources and position power (see Section 4C.9), public health practitioners must often rely on other people to achieve their aims. This relies on an ability to influence others. The processes of negotiating and influencing both involve considering a situation from multiple points of view.

Negotiation

Negotiation is the skill of resolving situations where two parties have conflicting desires. A negotiator investigates the situation with the aim of finding a solution that is acceptable to both sides. The most effective negotiating style will depend on the situation; it is influenced by the desire to meet your own needs and those of the other party.

In Table 5A.5, Fisher and Ury's four fundamental principles of negotiation [21] are described.

Different styles of negotiation are shown in Figure 5A.3.

Influence

To **influence** is to mobilise resources that modify the behaviours of others, which can be achieved by means of

- **Conformity** (changing social norms leads to changes in individual behaviour)
- **Compliance** (a request for a change in behaviour)
- **Obedience** (an order to change behaviour)

According to Covey [15], every person has a **circle of concern** (i.e. a range of issues in which the person has emotional involvement) and a smaller **circle**

Table 5A.5 Fisher and Ury's four fundamental principles of negotiation

Principle	Description
1. Separate the people from the problem	People problems tend to relate to perception, emotion, and communication. Agree on a common framing of the problem first and ensure both groups are talking to each other.
2. Focus on interests, not positions	Interests represent what people really want or need, positions are what are adopted in order to achieve this, i.e. people or organisations may adopt an extreme position just to counter opponents.
3. Invent options for mutual gain	The outcome needn't be win for one party, lose for another (see Figure 5A.3).
4. Insist on objective criteria	Use third-party precedents or guidance to understand what is 'fair' or accepted in a given situation.

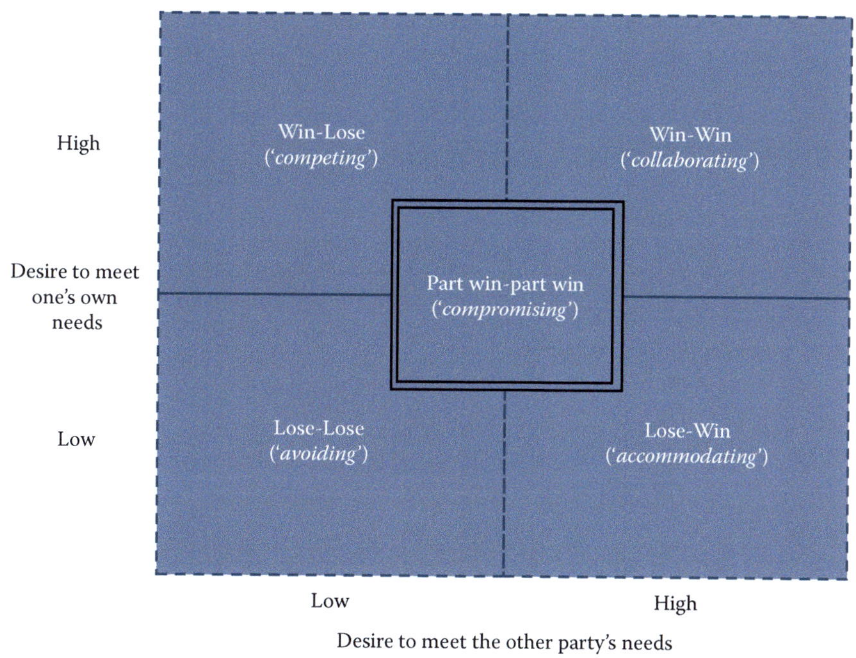

Figure 5A.3 Different negotiating styles. (From Forsyth, D.R., *Group Dynamics*, 5th edn., Brooks/Cole, Pacific Grove, CA, 2009.)

of influence (i.e. a smaller range of issues that the person has the power to alter): see Figure 5A.4.

People who are **proactive** concentrate their efforts on their circle of influence—thereby enlarging it and thus becoming more powerful. In contrast, **reactive** people focus their attention on their circle of concern—to the detriment of their circle of influence.

Public health advocacy

Advocacy is a field within public health that seeks to develop and shape public opinion in a strategic way. Public health advocates use whatever media and methods are most effective in accomplishing this goal. Even when the underlying message is not contentious (e.g. improving road safety), the

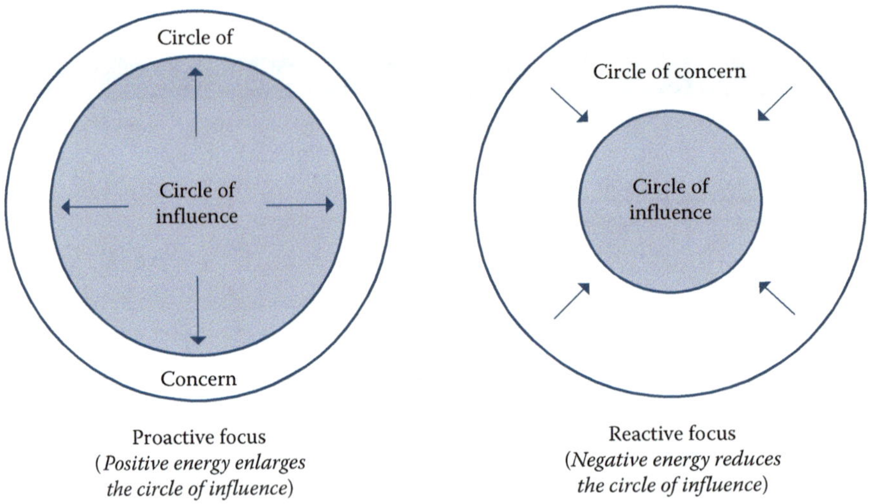

Figure 5A.4 Circles of concern versus circles of influence. (From Covey, S.R., *The 7 Habits of Highly Effective People*, Simon & Schuster, Inc., New York, 1989, http://www.cut-the-knot.org/manifesto/ctk.shtml.)

means used by public health advocates often are (e.g. graphic television adverts designed to shock the audience).

Chapman [23] identified the following 10 steps that should be addressed when acting as a public health advocate:

1. Identify the **public health objectives**
2. Attempt to find a **win–win outcome**
3. Identify the key **decision-makers** and how they can be influenced
4. Identify the **strengths and weaknesses** of both sides of the argument
5. Set out the **media objectives**
6. Choose how to **frame** the key issue
7. Identify **symbols** and 'word pictures' to illustrate the argument
8. Compose ***'sound bites'***
9. **Personalise** the topic by addressing the issue from the perspective of the ordinary citizen
10. **Mobilise** large numbers of sympathisers rapidly

5A.9 Power and authority

Theoretical and practical aspects of power and authority, role and conflict.

Power is the ability to make choices or influence outcomes (see Section 4C.9) while authority can be seen as the right to make decisions and issue orders. According to Weber [24], authority manifests itself in three ways: see Box 5A.5.

Role

Belbin proposed that people fulfil four different types of role:

1. **Team** (the distinct ways in which people behave and **relate to others** in a team; see 5A1.1)
2. **Functional** (**duties and processes** according to professional title, e.g. surgeon, nurse)
3. **Professional** (the **qualifications**, knowledge, and skills brought by an individual)
4. **Work** (the **tasks and responsibilities** undertaken by each person in the project)

Box 5A.5 Manifestations of authority

Type of authority	Description	Example
Traditional authority	Authority is derived from preserved **customs**.	Medical Royal Colleges
Charismatic authority	Authority comes from the **personality** and **leadership** qualities of the individual. These inspire obedience and loyalty from others.	Nelson Mandela, Adolf Hitler (**Note:** Charisma is not always a force for good)
Rational–legal authority	Authority is derived from powers that are **bureaucratically** and **legally** attached to certain positions.	Chief Medical Officer

Source: Weber, M. *The Three Types of Legitimate Rule* (translation). Quoted in: *Tripartite classification of authority*. Wikipedia website at en.wikipedia.org/wiki/Tripartite_classification_of_authority. University of California, Berkeley, CA, 1958.

Conflict

Differences of opinion may result in conflict. These can provide a healthy creative tension and prevent groupthink (see Section 5A.1.1) but can threaten the success of a project. The three principal methods for avoiding conflict are

1. **Negotiation** (discussion aimed at reaching an agreement: see Section 5A.7)
2. **Mediation** (a form of negotiation that is led by an impartial third party)
3. **Arbitration** (a form of mediation where the two parties agree to be bound by the decision of the impartial third party)

Unresolvable conflicts between two or more parties are more likely to occur where their goals are not aligned or when resources are scarce or threatened. When conflict does occur, it may be prevented from escalating further by the following conflict–resolution principles:

- Mutual respect
- Identification of shared values
- Honesty
- Shared objectives
- Combating disinformation

5A.10 Changing behaviour

Behaviour change in individuals and organisations.

One of the hallmarks of health systems is that they are characterised by almost continuous change. These transformations encompass innovations in practice, structural reconfigurations, and evolution in the population and its health needs (see Section 5C.2). In order to adapt to this perpetually changing environment, healthcare professionals and public health practitioners must be prepared adapt their behaviour and to embrace the opportunities that change may bring.

Binney and Williams [25] described different 'types' of attitude that people may have towards change: see Box 5A.6.

Adopting change

Rogers [9] developed the *'diffusion'* model to explain how people generally move towards change: see Figure 5A.5. In addition, Section 5C.2 covers the frameworks for managing change.

Box 5A.6 Attitudes to change

Missionaries	Pleased to embrace change—they adopt it, adapt to it rapidly, and actively encourage others to do so.
Believers	Understand the merits of the changes and believe in them—but are a little more cautious since they can see both the benefits and the risks involved.
People who pay lip service	Acknowledge that change is probably necessary but typically are not active in supporting or adopting it.
Hiders and refugees	Ignore or try to hide from the change—often through fear or lack of interest.
Members of the underground resistance	Actively try to block the changes.
Honest opponents	Declare their resistance—they openly challenge the need for change.
Emigrants	Simply *leave*, wanting nothing to do with the changes, preferring to seek their employment elsewhere.

Source: Binney, G. and Williams, C., *Leaning into the Future: Changing the Way People Change Organizations*, Nicholas Brealey Publishing Ltd., London, UK, 1995.

Innovators	First to embrace change.
Early adopters	Part of the first sizeable 'wave' of people who take up change, innovation—many of them becoming committed disciples of the change.
Early majority	Typically they have 'watched and waited' before either seeing the benefits or summoning the confidence to take up the change themselves.
Late majority	Follow in due course—they are less change-oriented, are slower to respond, and need more convincing.
Laggards	Those who show little or no interest, do not want to 'get involved'.

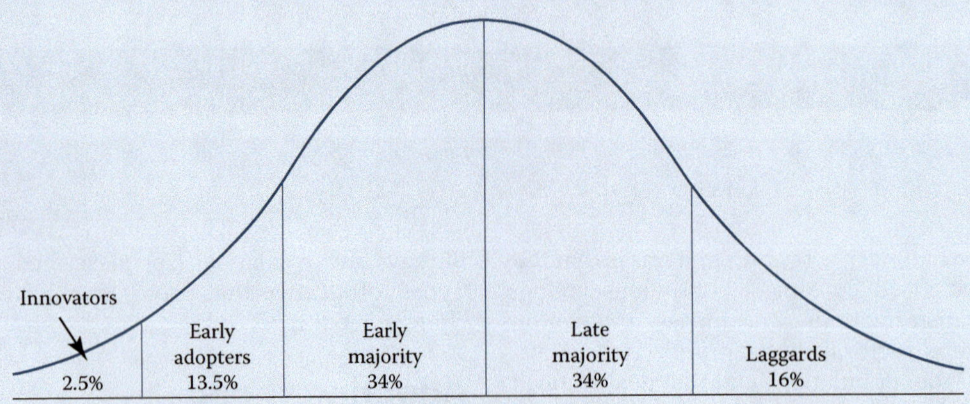

Figure 5A.5 Adoption curve. (Reproduced from Rogers, E., *Diffusion of Innovation*, 4th edn., Free Press, New York, 1995. http://www.southtees.nhs.uk/Improvement%20Alliance/spread/background.htm.)

Table 5A.6 Summary of theories for changing behaviour in an organisational context

Theory	Focus	Key concepts
Social learning theory	Behaviour is explained via a three-way, 'dynamic reciprocal' theory in which personal factors, environmental influences, and behaviour continually interact.	• Behaviour capability • Reciprocal determinism • Expectations • Self-efficacy • Observational learning • Reinforcement
Organisational change theory	Concerns processes and strategies for increasing the chances that healthy policies and programmes will be adopted and maintained in formal organisations.	• Problem definition (awareness stage) • Initiation of action (adoption stage) • Implementation of change • Institutionalisation of change
Diffusion of innovations theory	Addresses how new ideas, products, and social practices spread within a society or from one society to another.	See earlier (adopting change, p 533, diffusion of innovations Section 5A.2) Characteristics that determine rate of change include • Relative advantage • Compatibility • Complexity • Trialability • Observability
Social constructivist theory (e.g. appreciative inquiry method)	Reality created through the language used. For example, in 'appreciative inquiry', the act of asking questions of a group influences the group to start its own inquiry and discussions, which in turn prompts change.	• **Assumption**: tangible improvements can be generated through the process of inquiry • **Approach**: focus on positives rather than problems • **Goals**: designed to influence attitudes and thinking

Altering behaviours

Several theories from the behavioural and social sciences provide a basis for understanding why people engage in certain behaviours. As well as helping to explain and predict these behaviours, the insights from these theories can also help guide the design and implementation of strategies. A summary is given in Table 5A.6 but see also the frameworks for managing change (Section 5C.2) and the frameworks for changing health behaviours (Section 2H.4).

Further reading

Ann S.-S. Appreciating the challenge of change, pp. 381–398, Chapter 22.

Helen, P. Managing people: The dynamics of teamwork, pp. 418–434, Chapter 24.

Walshe, K. and Smith, T. (eds.) (2006) *Healthcare Management*. OUP McGraw-Hill, Berkshire, UK.

Kim, J. Personal effectiveness. pp. 365–380, Chapter 21.

5B

Understanding Organisations, Their Function, and Structure

In public health practice, there are many opportunities to learn how different organisations work, for example, through liaison with different stakeholders or during organisational mergers. Both positive and negative experiences can provide valuable insights into how organisations work.

This chapter provides public health practitioners with some systematic approaches to understanding organisations, which should be of use when forming partnerships, adapting to a changing environment, and managing organisational changes.

5B.1 Organisational environments

Internal and external structures and organisational environments.

There are many definitions of an organisation but all have in common three elements: **people (covered in 5A)**, **objectives (5D)**, and **structure**.

Internal organisational environment and structure

Organisational structure is required for the allocation of responsibility, as well as for grouping different functions and decision-making. Large organisations are often classified into three main structures:

- **Divisional**: grouping based on major departments (e.g. in a local authority, divisions that are likely to be involved in public health may include HR, finance, and housing).
- **Functional**: grouping based on the service provided (e.g. in a hospital some services might include orthopaedics, general surgery, psychiatry, paediatrics).
- **Matrix**: here, different projects employ the expertise of staff from different divisional or functional groups, often under a project manager. For example, a local authority project addressing increasing rates of obesity might involve staff from public health, information/intelligence, transport, finance, leisure and education.

External organisational environments: healthcare systems

Frameworks that only conceptualise organisations as discrete entities may be inadequate for understanding the healthcare sector, where organisations never operate in isolation. Instead, a systems approach is generally more helpful. Checkland [27] defines a system as a set of elements, connected

Box 5B.1 ENG **Example: Establishing integrated cancer systems in London**

Cancer survival in England has been improving for many years but the improvement has been slowest in London, despite the fact that the capital has some of the country's best cancer centres. The 'Case for Change', a report by NHS London, found that the fragmented care system and competition between major hospitals led to poorer patient care and to delays in diagnosis. It proposed an integrated system for London, in which providers worked collaboratively to provide care. Two systems were established in 2011 to improve cancer pathways: *London Cancer* (North and North East London) and the *London Cancer Alliance* (North West, South West and South East London).

Source: Cancer services: Case for change, March 2010, http://www.londonhp.nhs.uk/wp-content/uploads/2011/03/Cancer-case-for-change.pdf; http://www.londoncancer.org/.

together, which form a whole; a system shows properties pertaining to **the whole rather than to its component parts**.

When implementing change, NHS managers are encouraged to use **systems thinking** to understand the interrelationships between and within healthcare organisations and teams (see Section 5C.2). **Systems thinking** is a set of tools that can be applied to biological entities, buildings, abstract systems, or human entities. In systems comprised of human entities, the system can be understood in different ways at different levels. For example, we might consider a local health economy as the system (e.g. a cluster of general practices that commissions mainly from a local district general hospital, which works in partnership with a local authority). This 'system' sits within a national health and social care system.

Systems can be considered

- **Open** (capable of exchanging materials, energy or information with external agencies)
- **Closed** (completely autonomous)

Effects within a system occur as a result of **feedback** (i.e. the influence of one element on another). To understand systems and how to effect change within them, Iles [29] (undated, briefing paper) describes three steps:

1. **Modelling**: familiarisation and summarising the system (may use quantitative techniques such as computational simulation modelling)
2. **Mapping**: grouping factors (e.g. categorising factors obstructing the change)
3. **Telling the 'story'**: presenting a compelling narrative for change

An example of how systems thinking is changing the configuration of health services is given in Box 5B.1 [30].

5B.2 Evaluating internal resources and organisational capabilities

There are a number of models that can be used to assess how well an organisation is positioned to achieve its intended objectives. One of these is the McKinsey 7S model, which identifies seven aspects of an organisation that need to be aligned if it is to be successful [31]. (See Figure 5B.1.)

Shared values

The shared values of an organisation are core to this model, as they are the guiding concepts shared by an organisation's members, and are central to the development of all the

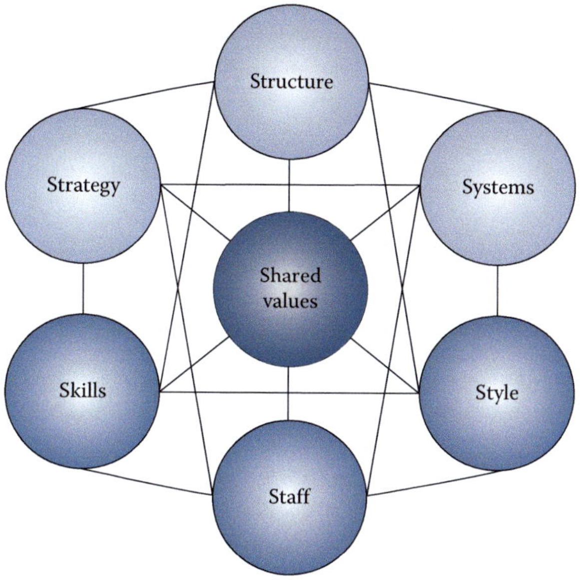

Figure 5B.1 McKinsey 7S model: Seven aspects associated with successful organisations. (From The management centre [Undated], Management thought leadership, Accessed online July 20, 2014 at http://www.managementcentre.co.uk/management-consultancy/thought-leadership).

other elements. An organisation's values may be classified as follows:

- **Ownership and finance** (typically, a distinction is made between **public** and **private sector,** although organisations such as social enterprises fit somewhere between the two).
- **Major purpose** (e.g. the primary purpose of a hospital is to provide healthcare, whereas improving health is only one part of a local authority's purpose).
- **Prime beneficiary:** organisations may primarily serve **members** (e.g. mutual societies or unions), **owners or managers** (e.g. companies), or the public (either '**public in contact**' or **clients** or the '**public at large**'). In terms of health, hospitals deliver healthcare to the public in contact, whereas the prime beneficiary of public health organisations is the public at large.

Two useful indicators of whether an organisation has shared values are the degree to which employees subscribe to the same corporate identity (private or public) and how well they articulate the **main purpose** and **prime beneficiaries** of the organisation.

Strategy

An overarching strategy typically articulates where the organisation wants to be in 5 years' time and how it is going to get there (see Section 5D).

Structure

This describes the hierarchy of, and interconnections within, an organisation. An evaluation of an organisation's structure may focus on formal arrangements (divisional, functional, or matrix—see previous discussion) or informal structures (which are influenced by personal relationships or animosities, group norms, and informal leaders.)

Systems

The systems of an organisation include its procedures, processes, and rewards. Although such 'systems' are typically defined within a single organisation, it is important also to consider the impact of processes and procedures that occur between teams and different departments.

Style

Handy [32] described four styles of organisational culture:

1. **Power**—The organisation revolves around a small group of people or a single boss.
2. **Task**—The organisation is oriented to interdisciplinary teams whose members have different skills.
3. **Role**—Employees have specific roles and responsibilities, which are allocated according to their job description.
4. **Person**—Organisations employ people who they believe are highly skilled and provide them with autonomy to approach a task however they think is best.

Staff

The numbers and types of employees working within an organisation

Skills

The capabilities of key personnel and the organisation as a whole

5B.3 Stakeholder interests

Identifying and managing internal and external stakeholder interests.

A stakeholder is a person or group that has an interest (a *'stake'*) in the outcomes of a project or organisation. This interest may stem from

Professional reasons
Personal reasons
Democratic representation
Commitment to achieving a particular outcome

Consulting stakeholders at the preliminary stages of a project tends to garner their support, and the input of stakeholders almost invariably improves the quality of a project. Stakeholder support can be helpful in securing additional resources, which in turn increases the likelihood that the project will succeed.

Stakeholder analysis

The process of **stakeholder analysis** involves the following:

- Identifying a comprehensive list of stakeholders—both internal and external.
- Assessing their degree of interest and their relative power: see Figure 5B.2.

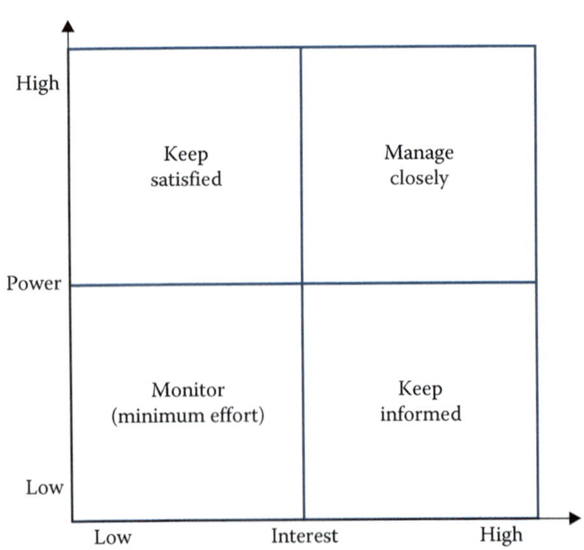

Figure 5B.2 Assessing stakeholders' degree of interest and power.

- Estimating their reaction to the project based on their perceived ideological, strategic, or financial interests in the project.

If the reaction of a particular stakeholder is unlikely to be positive, consideration can be given as to what alterations might win their support, based on the powers of **leverage** that they may potentially exert. Where winning such support is unrealistic, attention can be paid to ways in which their opposition may best be managed.

The powers held by stakeholders differ according to whether they are internal or external actors.

Internal stakeholders

Internal stakeholders, such as managers and employees, have their own interests that they will tend to pursue. For example, middle managers might seek promotion and employees may seek more favourable working conditions. All internal stakeholders possess a degree of power that they may be driven to use in order to promote or impede the implementation of a particular strategy. These powers include

- Authority (formal power through the organisational hierarchy)
- Control of strategic resources
- Threats of resignation or industrial action
- Possession of expert knowledge or skills

External stakeholders

Different external stakeholders have varying levers at their disposal. For example, central government can exert influence on organisations through taxation, government spending, legal action, regulation, and threatened changes in the law. In contrast, community and pressure groups can exert influence by

- Publicising activities that they regard as unacceptable
- Campaigning for changes in the law
- Refusing to cooperate with the organisation
- Conducting illegal actions such as sabotage

5B.4 Inter-organisational relationships

Structuring and management of inter-organisational (network) relationships, including inter-sectoral work, collaborative working practices, and partnerships.

There is growing academic and managerial interest in the field of inter-organisational relationships, such as **strategic alliances**, **joint ventures,** and **social networks**. Such arrangements have the potential to benefit organisations at both the micro and the macro levels. At a micro level, individual employees benefit from discussing professional practices with people from related fields. This additional insight may enable them to perform better at their job. At a macro level, networks could lead to innovation and efficiency gains.

Types of inter-organisational relationships

Barringer and Harrison [33] classify the principal types of inter organisational relationships as shown in Box 5B.2.

Integrated care

With a few notable exceptions, healthcare organisations rarely operate in isolation. As a result, patients often experience problems when their care is fragmented between different providers—problems such as **duplication** (where two providers deliver the same care unnecessarily) **gaps in care** (where one organisation wrongly assumes that another organisation has delivered a particular element of care) or **conflicting care** (where advice from one provider differs from that given by another). Disintegrated care is a particularly problematic for patients with complex health and social care needs.

In the health policy community, better integrated care is seen as a way of potentially achieving two goals simultaneously:

Box 5B.2 Principal types of inter-organisational relationships

Joint ventures	Two or more organisations pool a portion of their resources to form a separately owned venture. Advantages include economies of scale and of scope, as well as opportunities to innovate and to launch projects more rapidly than would otherwise be possible.
Networks	These are collections of organisations that organise joint projects by means of informal arrangements rather than legally binding contracts. Such networks often operate in a hub-and-spoke configuration, where a central organisation coordinates the others and each organisation focuses on its particular speciality.
Consortia	Organisations with a common need come together to form a new entity that satisfies that need on their behalf. For example, a group of neighbouring health authorities might form an HR consortium because it would be more costly for the individual health authorities to operate their own HR departments.
Alliances	There are arrangements between two or more organisations that establish an exchange relationship, but no new entity is formed. Such arrangements are typically informal and short term.
Interlocking directorates	An executive director of one organisation sits on the board of another organisation. Such arrangements can help spread innovation and cooperation among organisations.

- Reducing costs (by reducing wastage and preventing costly adverse outcomes such as unplanned hospital admissions)
- Improving the patient experience (especially for the increasing numbers of patients with complex, long-term health and social care needs)

Integration can occur between primary and secondary care (vertical integration) or between social care and healthcare (horizontal integration). Rosen and Ham [34] classify different levels of integration in terms of

- Macro (policy, financial, and regulatory environment)
- Meso (organisational and clinical structures and processes)
- Micro (patient interactions with different professionals and teams)

5B.5 Social networks and communities of interest

See also Section 4A.10.

Social networks

A *social network* is a group of people or organisations that are connected through social bonds. Relationships are viewed in terms of

- **Nodes** (individual actors such as family members, neighbours, friends, and colleagues)
- **Ties** (ranging from casual acquaintances to close familial ties)

In its simplest form, a social network is a map of all of the relevant ties between the nodes. These concepts may be displayed as a *social network diagram*, in which the nodes are marked as the points and the ties as interconnecting lines. The network can also be used to determine the social capital of individual actors (see Section 4A.10).

Online social networks

Social networking refers to a category of internet applications to help connect friends, colleagues, or other acquaintances using a variety of tools. These applications, known as **online social networks**, have grown rapidly. At the time of writing, the most popular social networks outside China were Facebook, Twitter, and LinkedIn.

For organisations, online social networking brings the following:

- **Opportunities** to interact with their stakeholders, including clients and patients, in new ways (e.g. through Twitter feeds and blogs) and to engage in **conversations**.
- **Challenges**: it requires a shift from largely unidirectional communication to two-way conversations. This change means that organisations need to adopt different communication styles, typified by faster responses, shorter messages, and more informal language.
- **Risks**: there is greater potential for the spread of inaccurate information on health and exposure to harmful social norms and practices.

Dunbar's number

The maximum size of a person's social network is consistently found to be around 150 people [35]. Known as **Dunbar's number**, this represents the maximum number of individuals with whom any one person can maintain stable relationships. The number was calculated using a regression equation based on data from 38 primate genera and is thought to be determined by characteristics of the neocortex. Therefore, while [36] sites such as Facebook may appear to increase the size of a person's social networks, research suggests that in reality, people still interact meaningfully with fewer than 150 people.

Communities of interest

Communities of interest are groups of people with a common concern who may not necessarily be linked in terms of their location, profession, socio-economic circumstance, or other characteristics. Members of such a community are often scattered across a country or across the globe, and they come from many walks of life. Communities of interest have flourished with improved access to the internet. They offer members the opportunity to engage in discourse and critical thinking about topics from the perspective of their common interest. They may also be important communities for healthcare providers and commissioners to consult about service provision.

Examples of communities of interest with particular relevance to public health include:

- Older people experiencing isolation and poverty
- People with learning disabilities
- Disabled people
- Asylum seekers and refugees
- Ex-offenders
- People diagnosed with certain conditions

5B.6 External influences on organisations

Assessing the impact of political, economic, sociocultural, environmental, and other external influences.

A common framework for reviewing the opportunities and threats in an organisation's external environment is known as PESTELI. For the purposes of public health, this analysis has been extended to DEPESTELI (see Table 5B.1).

Table 5B.1 DEPESTELI framework of reviewing external influences on organisations

Demographic structures	Age, sex, ethnicity, etc., of the population
Epidemiological patterns	Prevalence and incidence of diseases and risk factors within the population
Political factors	Current government policy, taxation, likely future changes to the political landscape
Economic influences	Competition, the availability of financial resources, unemployment, labour supply, etc.
Sociological trends	Attitudes and beliefs, lifestyle choices, press attitudes
Technological innovations	Research and development activity, new approaches, methods, or equipment
Ecological factors	Interactions with the wider environment, pollution, waste management, transportation
Legislative requirements	Relevant laws affecting the organisation, healthcare legislation, employment laws, etc.
Industry analysis	Market knowledge, demand, liaison with users, etc.

Further reading

Iles, V. Systems thinking briefing paper. http://www.reallylearning.com/Free_Resources/Systems_Thinking/systems_thinking.html.

Walshe, K. and Smith, J. (eds.) (2011) *Health Care Management*. Open University Press, Berkshire, UK.

5C

Management and Change

Change is a constant feature in the healthcare sector: technology keeps advancing, organisations are restructured, and populations' needs evolve. The magnitude of such changes may range from imperceptible alterations through to wholesale transformation, and they may occur at the individual, team, or whole-system levels. Public health specialists have a key role in managing change within healthcare systems to ensure that they meet the population's needs as effectively, equitably, and efficiently as possible. This chapter describes a range of leadership models and frameworks for managing change. These may be useful both for evaluating how change has been managed in the past and for guiding current change processes.

5C.1 Management models and theories

Understand the basic management models and theories associated with motivation and leadership and change management and be able to apply them to practical situations and problems.

In a managerial context, **leadership** involves developing ideas, shaping goals, and connecting with employees at an emotional level. **Management**, in contrast, involves taking responsibility for and controlling ourselves, or our colleagues, teams, or organisations.

Motivation

Motivation is a measure of a person's drive to initiate and persist in a given behaviour. While the employees of an organisation may be highly able to perform a task, unless they are motivated, they will not dedicate their abilities fully to the job in hand. As a result, all organisations aim to promote motivation. Indeed, this is one of the fundamental roles of a manager (i.e. to complete tasks via employees).

There are several theories of workplace motivation. Two major management theorists—**Maslow** and **Hertzberg**—produced seminal theories to describe and predict what motivates individuals in their place of work. A third theorist, **McGregor**, has built on Maslow's work to propose a classification of different managers' attitudes to employees.

Maslow's hierarchy theory

The **hierarchy of human needs** is one of the most widely employed managerial theories. It states that

- Only unsatisfied needs influence human behaviour
- Human needs are ordered according to their importance and complexity
- In the long run, people are only motivated by higher-level needs after their lower-level needs have been satisfied (**pre-potency**)
- The higher a person is up the hierarchy, the more they express their individuality, humanity, and psychological health

Box 5C.1 Maslow's hierarchy of human needs

Hierarchy	Description	Work context
Self-actualisation	Instinctive human need to make the most of one's unique abilities	Promotion, opportunities for creativity/innovation
Self-esteem	Subjective appraisal of a person as intrinsically positive or negative	Job title, reviews, appraisals
Love and belonging	Affection and happiness in the workplace	Professional associations, social events, supportive manager
Safety	Absence of danger	Company pension, substantive contract
Physiology	Basic needs, such as warmth and shelter	Pay

Box 5C.2 Advantages and disadvantages of Maslow's hierarchy model

Advantages	Disadvantages
Identifies individuals who fail to progress beyond the lower levels of the hierarchy Highlights how basic problems (e.g. workplace temperature) can inhibit motivation Makes intuitive sense	Overly individualistic No allowance for altruism

See Box 5C.1.

At the higher levels of the hierarchy, respect and recognition become much more powerful motivators than financial reward. Some of the advantages and disadvantages of the hierarchy as a theory are listed in Box 5C.2.

Although Maslow stressed that not everyone experiences these needs in the order of his hierarchy, the very concept of an order of needs is disputed. For example, the need for warmth and shelter in a homeless person does not preclude them from simultaneously having strong needs for love and belonging.

Herzberg's two-factor theory

This theory, which is also known as the **motivator–hygiene theory**, contends that some workplace factors lead to **job satisfaction** while others cause dissatisfaction. Factors are therefore divided into **motivators** (which give positive satisfaction) and **hygiene factors** (which do not give positive satisfaction but whose absence causes dissatisfaction): see Box 5C.3. Managers should aim to maximise both groups.

Box 5C.3 Herzberg's two-factor theory

Motivators	Hygiene
Varied work	Good pay
Responsibility	Good working conditions
Recognition	Job security

McGregor's theory X and theory Y

Theory X and theory Y are simplified, polar extremes of managerial attitudes towards workers and their

Box 5C.4 Summary of McGregor's theory X and theory Y

Dimension	Theory X (carrot and stick)	Theory Y (integrated goals)
Employees' attitudes to work	Inherently lazy, dislike work	Work is natural, as important as rest.
Employees' attitudes to responsibility	Avoid responsibility, seek direction	Given the right conditions, employees accept and seek responsibility.
Strategies for achieving results	Coercion, threats of punishment	Seeking commitment to objectives; making maximal use of employees' capabilities.
Motivational drivers	Safety, physiology	Affiliation, self-esteem, self-actualisation (as well as safety, physiology).

intrinsic motivations. **Theory X** can be summarised as the 'carrot and stick' approach, where direction is from a **central, controlling authority**. **Theory Y**, in contrast, assumes that **organisational and individual goals are integrated**. Many management approaches tend to have theory X as their implicit basis, whereas McGregor argues that theory Y may, in fact, be more appropriate for running an organisation (Box 5C.4).

Leadership

Leadership theory has been a topic of study throughout human history, and over 100 definitions of leadership have been published. The terms 'management' and 'leadership' are sometimes used interchangeably, but Mullins ([37], p. 283) distinguishes leadership from management in the following way:

> *Management may arguably be viewed more in terms of planning, organizing, directing and controlling the activities of subordinate staff. Leadership, however, is concerned more with attention to communicating with, motivating, encouraging and involving people.*

In line with this definition, contemporary studies of leadership tend to focus on *change management* and on empowering others. See Box 5C.5.

Change management

Change can be classified in terms of its magnitude and its origin (Table 5C.1).

Change management approaches may be employed in all of the earlier types of change. Their intention is to ensure (1) that change can be effected when required and (2) that its outcomes are beneficial to the organisation and its clients (patients and the public).

In 2008, the NHS Institute for Innovation and Improvement described several industrial improvement approaches that had been adopted by the NHS to manage change. The most pertinent are listed in Box 5C.6.

Force-field analysis

Lewin's *force-field analysis* model proposes that the status quo will change whenever the driving forces are stronger than the resisting forces. Therefore, in order to implement change, driving forces need to be strengthened and/or resisting forces need to be weakened. Examples of such forces are shown in Figure 5C.1.

Formula for change

Beckhard and Gleicher's formula for change proposes that three factors are needed in order for change to occur:

1. Dissatisfaction with the status quo
2. Vision of future possibilities
3. First steps in the direction of the vision

The product of D × V × F must be greater than resistance in order for change to occur (i.e. **D** × **V** × **F** > **R**).

ADKAR model

This model focuses on the 'people' dimension of change. It proposes that staff need to go through

Box 5C.5 Theories and models of leadership

Participative theories	These models (by **Likert** and others) argue that participative styles of leadership lead to increased job satisfaction and improved performance. An example is **MBWA** (see Section 5A.5).
Contingency theories	These theories argue that the most effective leadership style depends on the context. For example, the managerial grid described by Blake can be used to determine whether a boss-centred or a subordinate-centred approach will work better.
Instrumental theories	These theories contend that a leader's behaviour patterns (e.g. participation or delegation) affect the performance of others.
Charismatic theories	These theories include inspirational and transformational leadership styles. By enthusing others, the leader raises other people's confidence in their vision and values. Charismatic leaders include people who are not appointed to authority but who assume leadership in other ways.
VMC model	In this model, leaders are seen as possessing the following qualities: **v**ision, **m**anagement skills, and **c**ommitment. The three qualities are required in different proportions depending on the task at hand (e.g. vision is relatively unimportant in accountancy).

Table 5C.1 Types of change

Magnitude	**Incremental**	Modifications, building on what has gone before
	Transformational	Radical shifts, often starting by removing what has gone before
Origin	**Spontaneous**	Arising from interactions, or in reaction to events
	Emergent	Continuous adjustments
	Deliberate	Planned, discrete changes

Box 5C.6 Change management models

Model	Description
Total quality management (or 'continuous quality improvement')	Organisational approach to improvement based on the premise that • most workers are **motivated** to perform well and that • powerful insights into problems can be obtained by means of careful **data** collection and simple statistical analysis
Business process reengineering	Organise around **processes** rather than isolated narrowly defined functions. Requires • Multi-skilled workers, not specialists • Radical change, led by senior management

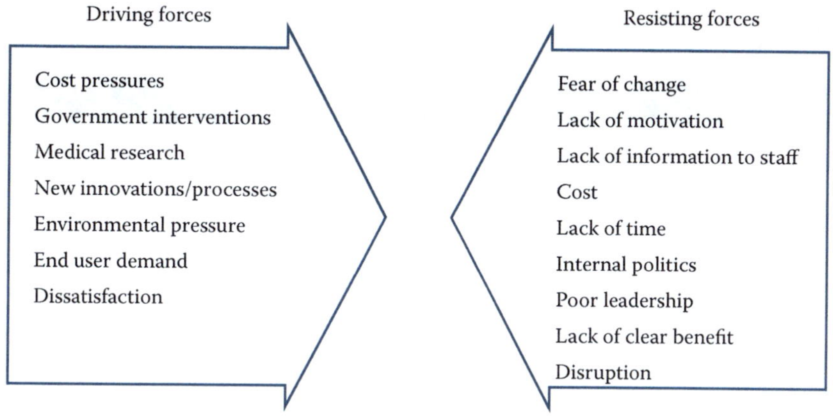

Figure 5C.1 Drivers and resistors of change.

five sequential steps in order for successful change to occur:

- **Awareness** of the need to change: this involves ensuring that staff know why change is being proposed (e.g. by dissemination of the results of a SWOT analysis via emails/newsletters/team meetings)
- **Desire** to support the change: motivation of staff by selling the benefits of change and addressing their concerns
- **Knowledge** of how to change: information and training about the change process
- **Ability** to implement the change: provision of education and training about new tasks/systems
- **Reinforcement** to sustain the change: encouraging and keeping the change in place through communication, feedback, and incentives

5C.2 Frameworks and tools for managing change

Critical evaluation of a range of principal frameworks for managing change.

One of the most commonly used tools for managing change is the *SWOT* analysis (**s**trengths, **w**eaknesses, **o**pportunities, and **t**hreats). Two other principal frameworks—*PESTELI* and *McKinsey's 7S*—can be used to support the central SWOT analysis (i.e. PESTELI and 7S can be used to ensure that each of the four components of SWOT is considered systematically and in sufficient depth).

SWOT analysis

A SWOT analysis considers positive and negative factors, both internal and external. It involves listing all of the *strengths, weaknesses, opportunities, and threats* facing the organisation or team. The analysis should focus primarily on the medium term. Some of the pros and cons of conducting a SWOT analysis are listed in Box 5C.7.

McKinsey's 7S

This analysis is described in more detail in Section 5B.1. It systematically identifies the strengths and weaknesses of the organisation and thus can be used to feed into a SWOT analysis. It is particularly useful for assessing internal factors that influence the performance of a team or organisation.

In healthcare, the 7S schema is often used to assess how changing one 'S' might impact on another 'S'.

PESTELI analysis

This tool, which is described further in Section 5B.6, is used to identify potential external opportunities

Box 5C.7 Pros and cons of a SWOT analysis

Strengths	Weaknesses
Most widely used tool by UK businesses Considers both internal and external factors Simple, can be done quickly No (low) cost	Review of its use found that it generated lists of factors that were Too long Too general Often meaningless Often not put into practice Too focused on processes rather than outcomes

and threats in order to identify the internal changes required to address contextual changes.

Other change management tools

Some further examples of change management tools are listed in Table 5C.2 Note that the ways in which change management tools are used vary greatly. In addition, the context in which they are applied has a major influence on their success. As a result, evaluating the success of these tools can be problematic.

Organisational development

In this approach, it is the **alteration** of employees' on-the-job behaviour that is seen as key to achieving wider organisational change. Interventions are used to prompt desired behaviours; these can

Table 5C.2 Further examples of change management tools

Quality improvement tools/approaches	Description
Theory of constraints	Every organisation or system has at least one constraint (i.e. a factor limiting its achievement of greater success). By identifying the constraint, organisations can focus on the area where change will be required to improve performance.
6 sigma	This process starts by defining the level of quality required. It then seeks to reduce variations in the quality of outputs by undertaking a thorough ('root–cause') analysis of problems causing variation using tools such as process mapping.
Lean	Made famous by its application in Toyota, this process is characterised by • Focused on **cutting out waste** from processes • **Describing** processes in great detail, so that areas of ambiguity and difficulty can be identified early • Viewing work as series of rapid **experiments**, where any aspects that do not function are rapidly reviewed, changed, and evaluated • Encouraging people at all levels of the organisation to **initiate** change
Plan-do-study-act (PDSA)	Developed by Deming [39] (see [38]), this approach to continuous improvement is widely used in healthcare. Many small PDSA cycles can lead to widespread improvement (see Schonn model Figure 5C.2).

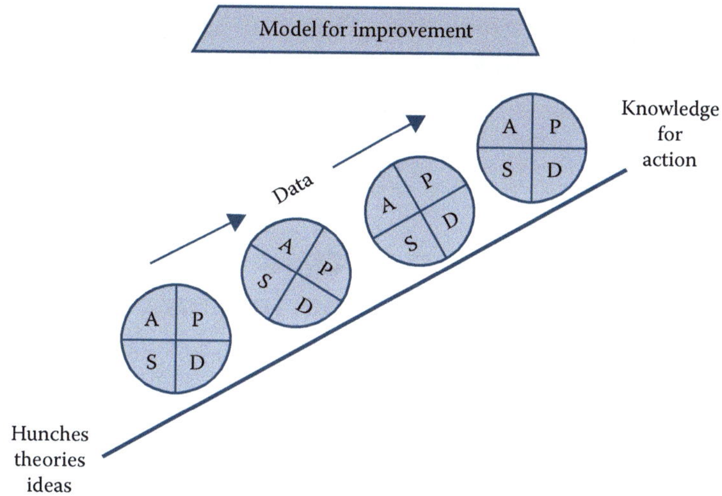

Figure 5C.2 Schonn's PDSA model for improvement over time. (From Boaden, R. et al., *Quality Improvement: Theory and Practice*, NHS Institute for Innovation and Improvement, Coventry, UK, Accessed online March 23, 2014 at http://www.lj.se/info_files/infosida32905/quality_improvement_nhs.pdf, 2008.)

be targeted at the individual, group, or organisational level. They include changes in

Technology
Physical setting
Goals and targets

Change management summary

A number of change management theories, models, and tools have been covered in Sections 5A, 5B, and 5C. These are summarised in Table 5C.3.

Table 5C.3 Stages of change management

Stages of change management	Approaches	Section
Current situation	McKinsey's 7S DEPESTELI Stakeholder analysis	5C.2 5B.6 5B.3
Need for change	SWOT analysis Developing a vision Theory of constraints, 6 sigma, Lean (**Note:** Also include implementation steps)	5C.2 5D.6 5C.2
Drivers and resistors of change	Force-field analysis Formula for change	5C.2 5C.1
Communicating a vision	Promotion of the change Leadership theories	5A.8 5C.1
Implementation	Diffusion of innovation PDSA Staff (motivation theories, ADKAR)	5A.2 5C.2 5C.1
Monitoring and evaluation	Evaluation of the effects of the change	1C.5

5C.3 Performance management [40]

An understanding of the issues underpinning the design and implementation of performance management against goals and objectives.

The process of *performance management* ensures that the aims of an organisation, department, or individual staff member are being achieved effectively and efficiently. It should be

Integrated (i.e. the organisation's goals are reflected HR policies and in the goals that individuals and teams are set)

Strategic (i.e. it should address broad, long-term issues, and goals)

For performance management to be successful, organisations need to develop a culture in which employees and teams take **responsibility** for their own contributions. The key steps involved are summarised in Box 5C.8.

Objectives and performance standards

Performance management involves translating the goals of an organisation into a set of objectives, which may be expressed as

Targets to be met (e.g. achieving financial balance by the end of the financial year)

Tasks to be completed by specified dates (e.g. by January 2004, 98% of patients are to spend under 4 hours waiting in the emergency department)

Ongoing targets, called **performance standards** (e.g. maintaining the intraoperative wound rate below a certain value)

Box 5C.8 Key steps of performance maintenance

Performance management step	Description
Identifying areas of best practice	Highlighting what works well within the organisation (and should be built upon) and outside the organisation (and should be followed).
Goal setting	Managers define their expectations and set strategic goals at the organisational, departmental, and individual levels.
Agreement of a developmental plan	Plans are agreed between managers and teams or individuals.
Continuous monitoring and improvement	Contemporaneous feedback and formal reviews are undertaken.
Strategic focus	Organisation, team, and individual activities are linked to the overall organisational strategy.

Table 5C.4 Objectives and target-setting methods

Method	Description
Key performance indicators (KPIs)	These are specific targets used by organisations to measure progress towards organisational goals, to assess performance against a national benchmark, or to make comparisons with other organisations. Examples of KPIs are risk-adjusted hospital length of stay, mortality rates, readmission rates, etc.
Balanced scorecard	This is a framework for translating an organisation's mission and strategy into a set of performance measures covering different perspectives. The perspectives in a health organisation may include clinical outcomes, patient views, financial performance, and HR/staffing.
Performance measures sheets	This approach is used to ensure that any performance measures being used are still relevant. The process involves checking • The purpose of the measure • How it relates to the organisation's objectives • How it is calculated • The source of data used in the calculations • What actions are taken on the basis of the results
Four-column matrix	This approach helps teams to link their projects to an organisation's aims. Four aspects are reviewed: 1. Established project aims 2. Established project measures 3. How the project links to the organisation's wider aims 4. How the project measures are linked to the organisation's performance measures
Benchmarking	This approach explicitly compares organisations on the same metrics to each other. Analogous approaches are league tables and rankings.

Objectives should be *SMART*, that is, they should be

Specific
Measurable
Achievable
Realistic
Timescale set for completion

Regular performance monitoring can provide a clear picture of how well an organisation is achieving its main strategic goals and indicate areas where there is potential for improvement. Several methods for assisting this process are described in Table 5C.4.

Design and implementation

Performance management is a **cyclical process** rather than an isolated event. The cycle is difficult to implement well because it requires the engagement of all members of an organisation, particularly line managers. Evidence suggests that performance management is **well regarded** by employees and managers alike, especially insofar as it emphasises personal development. However, performance-rating schemes often involve considerable amounts of **bureaucracy**, which can be very time-consuming. Implementation of performance management requires

- **Training** of managers and employees (especially initially)
- Clarification of the **definition** of 'performance'
- Understanding the organisation's **performance culture**

- Stressing the **personal benefits** to individual employees of participation in the process
- Remembering that performance management is a **tool** for line managers whose success depends on their ability to use it effectively

Further reading

Boaden, R., Harvey, G., Moxham, C., and Proudlove, N. (2008) *Quality Improvement: Theory and Practice in Healthcare*. NHS Institute for Innovation and Improvement.

5D

Policy and Strategy Development and Implementation

Public health specialists may be involved in organisational planning in a range of different settings. This process may include influencing **policies** and developing a **strategy** in order to transfer these policies into action. There are many difficulties involved in policy development and implementation; therefore, a sound understanding of the underlying theories and techniques is essential.

This chapter also summarises approaches to **health service development**, **planning**, **organisation**, and **funding** (all of which are instrumental to service delivery) and how these approaches differ internationally.

5D.1 Differences between policy and strategy and the impact of policies on health

According to Goodwin [42] **policy** refers to 'goals and objectives', whereas **strategy** 'determines how those goals and objectives are to be implemented'. See Table 5D.1.

Brownson et al. [43] note that policy change has had a major impact on public health, citing examples of seat belt laws and regulations governing permissible workplace exposures. They recommended using appropriate metrics to measure these changes, noting that the appropriate metrics may need to be non-traditional health measures (e.g. taxation, polling data).

5D.8 covers frameworks for evaluating a policy change.

Table 5D.1 Differences between policy and strategy

	Policy	Strategy
Definition	A vision composed of goals and objectives (i.e. an overarching course of action)	How a policy will be implemented (i.e. a framework for achieving the vision)
Scope	General principles of an organisation	Key steps needed for a policy to be implemented
Example [44]	EU health policy • Protecting people from health threats and disease • Promoting healthy lifestyles • Helping national authorities in the EU cooperate on health issues	EU health strategy for the 5-year period (2008–2013) Fostering good health in an ageing Europe: • Health promotion measures for older people, the workforce, children, and young people • Actions on tobacco, nutrition, alcohol, mental health, and other broader environmental and socio-economic factors • New guidelines on cancer screening and a communication of rare diseases • Follow-up of communication on organ donation and transplantation Protecting citizens from health threats • Strengthen surveillance and response • Health aspects of adaptation to climate change Supporting dynamic health systems and new technologies • Community framework for safe high-quality and efficient health services • Support for managing innovation in health systems • Support implementation of e-health solutions

5D.2 Principles underpinning the development of policy options and the strategy for their delivery

The principles underpinning policy development are, to some extent, dependent on the policy under consideration and the organisations involved. Table 5D.2 provides a list of policymaking principles.

Policy delivery

The steps involved in policy delivery include setting an agenda, formulating a policy, implementing the policy, and evaluating it (see Table 5D.3).

Table 5D.2 Policymaking principles

Principle	Description
Develop clear, shared goals	Define what the policy is designed to achieve. Achieving policy goals often requires multiple departments or organisations to work together.
Involve stakeholders	Consider the needs and experience of the individuals, families, groups, and businesses likely to be **affected by the policy**. Consult **outside experts** and the people who will **implement** the policy early in the process.
Avoid unnecessary burdens	Appraise of the likely **benefits and costs** of the policy. Seek to minimise the **cumulative burden** of policy implementation.
Look to the future and outside	Plan for **contingencies** by considering what developments and changes on the horizon might affect the policy's implementation. **Learn lessons** from other countries and settings.
Learn from experience	Use **evidence** and **research** to understand the problems and how to address them. Consider policymaking as a **continuous** learning process, not as a series of one-off initiatives. Use **pilots** to encourage and test innovations. **Evaluate** the policy by seeking feedback from the people who implemented it and act on the lessons learnt.

Source: Adapted from HM Government, Modernising government, The Stationery Office, March 1999.

Table 5D.3 Steps involved in delivering a policy

Step	Details
1. Agenda setting	This step generally follows on from some form of **problem** or other pressure leading to the need for a change. It involves establishing some potential broad goals for a policy.
2. Policy formulation	Alternative policy proposals are reviewed and appraised, based on evidence and consultation with experts. **Health impact assessments (HIAs)** are undertaken for each option that may be undertaken. Potential barriers should be considered (see Section 5D.5). Stakeholders should be consulted (see Section 5D.3).
3. Implementation	This step involves • Interpreting the policy • Strategic organisation (putting in place the structures and resources required) • Applying the policy in practice (see Section 5D.4)
4. Evaluation	Evaluating the policy and making any necessary revisions based on the findings (see Section 5D.4).

5D.3 Stakeholder engagement in policy development including its facilitation and consideration of possible obstacles

See also 5B.3 for stakeholder interests.

Gilson et al. [46] identified three key steps involved in **stakeholder analysis** for evaluating policies and developing viable policy proposals (see Table 5D.4).

Table 5D.4 Steps involved in stakeholder analysis

Steps	Relevant questions	Possible actions
1. Identify stakeholders	• Which individuals and groups are relevant to the policy issue at hand? That is, who are the key stakeholders?	• Invite relevant stakeholders to take part in policy-forming process.

2. Determine the **current position** of each stakeholder	• Are the stakeholders likely to support the proposal, be neutral, or oppose it?
	• What is each stakeholder's **interest** in the issue?
	• What is the **ideology** of each stakeholder? Compare each stakeholder's core values of with those underpinning the proposed policy.
		• Consider **deals** or **incentives** that may bolster a stakeholder's support for the issue.
		• Consider potential or perceived effects of a policy on each stakeholder (or the group they represent) in terms of
		  • Quality of life, job satisfaction
		  • Resources (funding, staff)
		  • Reputation
		  • Power
		• **Focus arguments** on aspects of key interest to individual stakeholders (e.g. costs to budget holders).

3. Determine the relative **power** of each stakeholder	• What capacity does each stakeholder have to influence policy options?	• Consider each stakeholder's
		  • **Resources** (both tangible assets, such as access to funding, and intangible assets, such as networks and skills)
		  • **Position** (particularly in the political system)
		  • **Motivation** to exercise resources to influence policy in this area
		• **Provide resources** to individuals and groups who are supportive of a policy (e.g. provide training to community groups).
		• Attempt to **weaken** the collective power of stakeholders who oppose the policy (e.g. **highlight areas of discord** among opposers).
		• **Prioritise** engaging with representatives of organisations with the greatest interest and power to influence other stakeholders.
		• Concentrate efforts at **critical periods** (e.g. when debates or key meetings are due to occur).

Table 5D.5 Obstacles to the effective engagement of stakeholders

Obstacle	Description
Hidden agendas	Individuals may hold personal opinions that do not reflect the official positions of their organisation (e.g. if a policy change affects them personally).
Limited access	It may not be possible to meet the people with the greatest potential to influence a policy if they are too busy or cannot be engaged.
Competing priorities	Another policy issue may be higher on a stakeholder's agenda.
Ignorance	Decision-makers may be unaware of a policy, or they may not support it if they are unaware of its potential benefits.

Intelligence about stakeholders' positions, interests, and power may be obtained either

- **Directly** (through **one-to-one** meetings with individuals or **consultation events** involving the representatives of several organisations)
- **Indirectly** (by asking third parties or by analysing documentation published by a stakeholder)

Possible obstacles to engaging stakeholders are listed in Table 5D.5.

5D.4 Implementation and evaluation of policies including the relevant concepts of power, interests, and ideology

See also 4C.8 on the appreciation of concepts of power interests and ideology.

Policy implementation involves three main steps (see Table 5D.6).

Policy evaluation

The nature and scale of implementation can fundamentally change the nature of a particular policy. Glasgow et al. [47] developed the RE-AIM framework for evaluating health promotion policy.

The five aspects of this framework can be applied to other policy initiatives (see Table 5D.7).

Policy evaluation should adhere to the general principles of any evaluation (covered in Section 1C.9), but in addition, it should take account of both the **original policy** and how it was **implemented** (in terms of reach, adoption, implementation, and maintenance). These aspects of implementation are all affected by the **power**, **interests,** and **ideology** of those who interpret and implement it (see Section 5D.3).

In order to evaluate policies effectively, a number of challenges must be addressed (see Table 5D.8).

Table 5D.6 Three steps of policy implementation

Step	Description
1. Interpretation	Translating the policy into a strategy for accomplishing its goals
2. Organisation	Dividing the policy into appropriate administrative units Choosing appropriate service delivery methods based on evidence, expert opinion, and stakeholder engagement
3. Application	Committing to definitive actions with appropriate staffing, skills, and resources

Table 5D.7 RE-AIM framework for evaluating policy

Step	Description
Reach	Assessed using measures of uptake or participation among eligible individuals or groups.
Efficacy	What were the positive and negative outcomes when the policy was delivered as intended?
Adoption	What proportion of sites adopted the policy, and what was the representativeness of these sites (e.g. worksites, health departments, or communities)?
Implementation	Was the policy delivered as intended?
Maintenance	How was the policy enforced over time (once public attention has waned and incentives have stopped)?

Table 5D.8 Challenges to policy evaluation

Challenge	Description
Definition	Agree the exact **nature of the policy** and what it was intended to achieve. Note that policies rarely remain static: they tend to evolve and are influenced by implementation and context.
Resources	Allocate **sufficient resources** for evaluation. When a new policy is introduced, a budget should be agreed for evaluation so that sufficient time and expertise is available.
Timeline	Use **appropriate time horizons**: policymakers may seek the results of an evaluation during implementation or shortly after in order to decide whether to continue or change direction. However, it can take several years for policies to be fully implemented and even longer for the impacts to become evident, particularly health outcomes and unexpected consequences.
Sequencing	**Plan evaluation activities before policies are implemented** to ensure that sufficient baseline data will be collected. Designate an appropriate 'control' group in order compare the effects of the policy to a setting where the policy is not active. It is generally preferable, although not always feasible, for evaluations to be planned prospectively.

5D.5 Problems of policy implementation

Problems of policy implementation may arise for many reasons, such as

- **Direct resistance** (e.g. strikes over pay freezes or redundancies)
- **Incomplete accomplishment** of tasks, such as record keeping
- **Policy adaptations** to address variations in individual or circumstances

5D.6 Developing healthcare strategy

Strategy communication and implementation in relation to healthcare.

Healthcare strategies are medium- or long-term **action plans** that are designed to improve health or to focus on corporate priorities, such as containing healthcare costs, reducing waiting lists, or improving the recruitment and retention of staff. In order to have an impact, a strategy needs to be communicated to local stakeholders and decision-makers and implemented effectively.

Communication

In strategic communication, the following should be considered:

- Audience
- Strategic objectives
- Key message
- Media (communication channels)

Often a range of media will be employed, including press releases, annual reports, and direct communication to stakeholders (see also Section 5A.8). Strategy communication involves more than simply presenting a 'finished product'. It is insufficient for an individual or team to write a strategy document and then send it to stakeholders and decision-makers. Rather, sophisticated communication mechanisms should be used to ensure that the people responsible for delivering the strategy, as well as people who will be affected by its implementation, are appropriately involved in

- Agreeing strategic objectives
- Producing a baseline assessment of the current state of healthcare provision
- Committing resources
- Monitoring implementation and delivery

The means of communication will depend on the stage of the strategy's development and the audience being targeted. It typically includes the elements described in Table 5D.9.

Implementation

Approaches to strategy implementation include **all-out attack** and **inside-venture** and **strategic alliances** (see Box 5D.1).

Table 5D.9 Communication involved in strategy development

Stage of development	Audience and agencies	Communication methods and media
Strategy formation	Commissioners Partner organisations Experts and specialists Practitioners Service users	Working groups Surveys Focus groups Meetings
Dissemination	All stakeholders	Report publication (hard copy and on websites) Newsletters, blogs and tweets Media releases Public events
Monitoring implementation	Commissioners Scrutiny and review boards Public	Executive boards Local strategic partnerships Public reports

Box 5D.1 Approaches to strategy implementation

Implementation approach	Details
All-out attack	In this approach, all current strategic plans are abandoned and are replaced with a new strategy [48]. This tactic typically occurs when a large organisation acquires, or is merged with, another organisation.
Inside-venture approach	This method relies on the power of internal rewards and innovation [49]. Here, an organisation encourages its employees to be innovative and, where their ideas are feasible, employees are rewarded with their own project team to develop their innovation.
Strategic alliances	This tactic includes establishing **joint ventures** with other bodies, where two or more organisations go into partnership to pursue a set of agreed goals while remaining independent.

5D.7 Theories of strategic planning

Strategic planning is an activity through which an organisation addresses the major decisions that it faces. A decision is not deemed *strategic* merely by being important; rather, to be strategic, a decision or issue must

1. **Define** the institution's relationship with its environment
2. Be of importance to the **whole organisation**
3. Depend on inputs from several functional areas
4. Affect the **administration** and **operation** of the entire institution

Two theories of strategic planning are the **four-step models** and the **ranked order approach**.

Four-step model

The four-step model is commonly used in the development of strategy. Many of the management tools discussed elsewhere can be incorporated into this model (see Table 5D.10).

Ranked order approach

This approach involves defining the strategy in terms of a priority list. The following components of the strategy are first defined:

- Policies
- Plans
- Actions
- Goals
- Objectives
- Ideal state
- Strategies
- Tactics

These items are then ranked into a hierarchy, such that

- The item in a lower rank explains **how** the item immediately above it will be achieved.
- The item in a higher rank addresses **why** the item immediately below it needs to be achieved.

Table 5D.10 Four-step model to strategy development

Step	Purpose	Management tools	Section
1. Where are we now?	Analysis of the current situation	Needs assessment Benchmarking McKinsey's 7S DEPESTELI SWOT Stakeholder analysis	1C.1 5C.3 5B.1 5B.6 5C.2 5B.3 and 5D.3
2. Where do we want to get to?	Setting the future direction	Review organisational vision, aims, and objectives SMART targets	 5C.3
3. How are we going to get there?	Options appraisals and implementation of the strategy. Route map from step 1 to step 2	Results of HNA and other evaluations (e.g. economic evaluation) Review evidence Change management methods	1C.1 and 4D.5 1A.31 5C.2
4. How will we know when we have got there?	Monitoring and evaluation of the strategy	Key performance indicators PDSA Strategy evaluation	5C.3 5C.2 5D.4

In this way, the **top rank objective** (TRO) does not address 'why', and therefore—by definition—this is the crux of the strategy upon which everything else depends.

Action planning

Once a strategy has been developed, the next stage in its implementation is to write an **action plan**, which should cover the following items:

- **Name** of the strategy
- **Actions** (tangible components of what will be done)
- **Location**
- **Personnel** (including the line-management structure of the programme)
- **Timing** (the start and completion dates)
- **Resources** (staff, supplies, information, other resources)
- **Audit** (progress measurement and reporting)
- **Benefits** to the public of implementing this strategy
- Performance **rewards** (if any)
- A **risk register** (to identify risks) and **contingency plans** (to mitigate them)

5D.8 Analysis, in a theoretical context, of the effects of policies on health

Walt and colleagues [50] set out several frameworks and theories for undertaking policy analysis and evaluating health policy. They provide the structure to explore how policies originate and identify the main drivers and influences on the direction of policy and, in some cases, how these change as policies are developed and implemented.

The most prominent frameworks are described in Table 5D.11.

Table 5D.11 Key frameworks and theories used in policy analysis

Framework/ theory	Authors	Description
Stages heuristic	Lasswell [51]	Four stages 1. **Agenda setting** (only a small number of the many problems faced by societies rise to the attention of decision-makers) 2. **Formulation** (legislatures and other decision-making bodies design and enact policies) 3. **Implementation** (governments execute these policies) 4. **Evaluation** (impact is assessed) Criticised for being artificially linear.
Policy triangle	Walt and Gilson [52]	Considers the impact of **actors**, **context**, and **processes** and how these interact with the content of the policy to shape policymaking.
Multiple-streams theory	Kingdon [53]	Assumes that the following factors flow in independent streams: • **Problems** (conditions faced by a society that may or may not become identified as an issue requiring public attention) • **Policies** (the range of ideas and technical proposals to address these problems) • **Politics** (the national mood and social pressure) At points in time and place where these streams merge, windows of opportunity emerge where it is possible to change policy.
Punctuated equilibrium theory	Baumgartner and Jones [54]	Policymaking has periods of stability with minimal policy change, which are disrupted by bursts of rapid transformation. Key concepts • **Policy image** (the way in which a given problem and set of solutions are conceptualised) • **Policy venue** (the set of actors or institutions that make decisions concerning a particular issue) When a particular policy venue and image are dominant over time, the policy process will be **incremental**. When new actors and images emerge, **transformation** is possible.
Top-down and bottom-up implementation	Sabatier [55]	**Top-down** theories view policy as driven by the 'values, interests, and preferences of the governing elite'. In contrast, **bottom-up** theories recognise the effect of front line staff and 'street-level bureaucrats' in shaping policy as they interpret, adapt, and implement directives.

5D.9 Major national and global policies relevant to public health

Walt's [56] definition of health policy [57] encompasses many organisations, agencies, and directives beyond health services:

> *Health policy embraces courses of action that affect the set of institutions, organizations, services, and funding arrangements of the health care system. It goes beyond health services, however, and includes actions or intended actions by public, private and voluntary organizations that have an impact on health. [56]*

National policy areas that are likely to have an impact on health include **welfare**, **education**, **employment**, and **taxation** (see Box 5D.2 also Section 2H.11). At a global level, policies of relevance to health also include **travel**, **trade** restrictions, and **environmental** policy.

Box 5D.2 ENG The Marmot review: Strategies for reducing health inequalities

An independent review, chaired by Professor Sir Michael Marmot, was established in 2010 at the request of the Secretary of State for Health. The review was tasked with identifying the most effective, evidence-based strategies for reducing health inequalities in England.

The review's findings were published in the report 'Fair Society Healthy Lives' and recommended action on six policy objectives. Meeting these objectives will require the involvement of several government departments. The most important departments for each objective are listed within square brackets:

1. Give every child the **best start in life** [health, education]
2. Enable all children, young people, and adults to **maximise their capabilities** and have control over their lives [education, employment]
3. Create **fair employment** and good work for all [work and pensions, treasury]
4. Ensure healthy **standard of living** for all [work and pensions, treasury]
5. Create and develop healthy and sustainable **places and communities** [communities and local government; environment, food, and rural affairs]
6. Strengthen the role and impact of **ill-health prevention** [health, communities, and local government]

Source: Fair society healthy lives, *The Marmot Review*, February 2010, http://www.instituteofhealthequity.org/projects/fair-society-healthy-lives-the-marmot-review.

5D.10 Health service development and planning

The aims of health service improvement are to

- Enhance the **quality** of patient care
- Improve strategic **outcomes**
- Contribute to improved public **health**

Health service development

The health service needs to continually develop to ensure that services remain effective, evidence-based, and appropriate for local needs whilst working with budget resource constraints. Drivers of change within health services are outlined in Table 5D.12.

Health service planning

Health service planning involves translating a strategy into specific **objectives** and then choosing **methods** for achieving these objectives. The degree to which healthcare provision is planned varies between countries. However, even in the United States, which is generally regarded as a mostly unregulated health market, an element of planning exists for large, costly facilities in order to avoid wasteful overprovision.

ENG Since April 2013, detailed planning for local services in England has been the responsibility of local health and wellbeing boards (i.e. local

Table 5D.12 Drivers of change in health services

Driver	Example
Advances in technology	New drugs, equipment, procedures, screening programmes, and healthcare settings.
New information flows	Information such as the production cost per item can be used to inform clinicians of the financial impact of their decisions.
National policy pronouncements	In England and Wales, NICE makes assessments of both effectiveness and value for money.
Public perception	Rationing debate, particularly with regard to novel high-cost drugs and the so-called postcode lottery (see Section 4C.5).

Table 5D.13 Examples of specific health service planning arrangements in England

Domain	Organisation	Details
Health service provision	NHS England	NHS England provides guidance to local CCGs that sets out national expectations, priorities, and standards that should inform their contracts with providers and how services should be organised.
Information and surveillance	PHE	PHE provides health intelligence and surveillance through specialist disease registries and local health protection units.
Training [59] and workforce development	Health Education England (HEE) Local Education and Training Boards (LETBs)	HEE and the LETBs plan education and training to meet local and national needs.

Source: Green, A., *An Introduction to Health Planning for Developing Health Systems*, 2007, by permission of Oxford University Press.

authorities working with CCGs, with input from NHS England). These boards produce JSNAs and *Joint Health and Wellbeing Strategies* (JHWSs).

See Section 1C.1 for more on needs assessments.

Certain specific aspects of health service planning fall under the remit of other national and local organisations, including those listed in Table 5D.13.

5D.11 Health service funding

Methods of organising and funding health services and their relative merits, focusing particularly on international comparisons and their history.

The funding and organisation of healthcare should be arranged so as to maximise efficiency and equity. See Table 5D.14.

See also 4D.3 for more on principles of efficiency and equity applied to health service funding.

Organisation of health services

A health organisation can be described in terms of its **commissioner**, its **setting**, the way in which it is **accessed**, as well as its **financial** flows.

Commissioner

The purchaser, or commissioner, of healthcare determines which services are made available to patients.

UK In the early 1990s, NHS organisations that previously both purchased and provided health services were split. This involved the establishment of separate

- **Provider trusts** (e.g. acute hospital trusts and mental health trusts)
- **Health authorities** (Wales and England) or **health boards** (Scotland and Northern Ireland) with a role confined to the purchasing of services [in 2002–2003, this responsibility moved to PCTs (England) and LHBs (Wales), which also provided services such as district nursing and community physiotherapy. In 2013 in England, this responsibility moved mostly to CCGs].

In the mid-1990s, the UK government experimented with the concept of **fund holding general practices** in which GPs were given a budget from which to purchase services for their patients including drugs and some hospital care. A subset of fund holding practices, known as the **total purchasing pilots**, purchased all hospital and community health services for their patients. In 1999, Scotland, Northern Ireland, and Wales assumed new powers to determine how to organise the NHS in each nation. Since then, commissioning arrangements within the United Kingdom have become increasingly divergent:

ENG In England, the commissioner was traditionally the local health authority or board, acting on behalf of the government. In 2004, the

Table 5D.14 Principles of efficiency and equity applied to health service funding

Efficiency	Equity
• **Allocative efficiency** (benefits exceed the costs) • **Operational efficiency** (scarce resources used to their best advantage)	• **Financial equity** (financial burden is proportional to ability to pay) • **Equity of opportunity** (if not equity of access then equity of utilisation) • Reducing **health inequalities**

Table 5D.15 Summary of commissioning responsibilities in England since April 2013

Organisation	Health service commissioning responsibility
CCGs	Comprises general practices with board-level representation from GPs, specialist nurses, and hospital doctors, CCGs commission local health services for their registered population (e.g. A&E, elective hospital care, and mental health services)
Local authorities	Local health improvement programmes (e.g. sexual health, prevention of obesity, substance misuse)
NHS England	Specialist care and selected public health services (e.g. screening and immunisations)

government introduced **practice-based commissioning** (PBC) where GP practices had the right to identify new providers of healthcare for their patients, including in-house arrangements or other primary care providers. Under the PBC initiative, commissioning was still conducted by PCTs, with participating GP practices holding indicative budgets.

Since April 2013, commissioning has been diversified (see Table 5D.15). NHS England is directly responsible for specialist commissioning and for authorising CCGs, which commission care at a local level, supported by commissioning support units (CSUs).

WA In Wales [61], the concept of commissioning secondary care services was removed on October 1, 2009. Since then, seven LHBs commission primary care from independent contractors and provide primary care through community services and some salaried staff. The Welsh Health Specialised Services Committee commissions specialised and tertiary care from appropriate providers. In contrast to England, the commissioning of healthcare in Wales is not predicated on patient choice from a range of providers competing in a market made up of 'any willing provider'.

SCOT In Scotland [62], there is no sharp distinction between purchasers (commissioners) and providers. Instead, the [63] Scottish Government allocates a budget for healthcare to each of the 14 territorial health boards, which are responsible for planning and providing healthcare services for their local populations. This is intended to instil shared aims, common values, and clear lines of accountability while breaking down traditional barriers between primary and acute care.

Acting on behalf of NHS Scotland, the National Services Division (NSD) is responsible for commissioning and performance managing national screening programmes, specialist clinical services, and national managed clinical networks.

Internationally, commissioners include **mutual societies** (as in France) and **managed care organisations** (as in the United States).

5F covers the principles of commissioning and contracts

Healthcare setting

UK In the United Kingdom,

- **Primary health care** is mostly delivered in GP surgeries.
- **Community health services** (such as district nursing) are provided by provider trusts in England or by combined hospital and community trusts in Wales and community health partnerships in Scotland.
- **Secondary** and **tertiary care** are provided by hospitals, delivering both inpatient, day-case, and outpatient care.

EU In many continental European countries, specialists work in **town-centre offices** rather than in the outpatient departments of hospitals as occurs in the United Kingdom. **Polyclinics** also exist, where several specialists share premises and diagnostic services.

Novel healthcare settings include telephone-based services, hospital at home, and walk-in centres located in shopping streets or transport hubs.

Table 5D.16 Advantages and disadvantages of single registration

Advantages	Disadvantages
Gate keeping role **avoids over-investigation** and reduces pressure on secondary care. **Continuity** of care. **Single person** receives all correspondence and **coordinates care**.	Less consumer choice for patients. Conflict of interest: GP is caring for the individual patient and bearing in mind implications for all other patients.

Access to healthcare

UK The United Kingdom has a system of **single registration** in which members of the public are only entitled to register with a single GP. Although individuals are free to change GP at any time, they may not be registered with more than one GP concurrently. Advantages and disadvantages of single registration are listed in Table 5D.16.

GPs in the United Kingdom act as gatekeepers to elective secondary care. In contrast, members of the public in countries such as France are free to access secondary care directly. This freedom tends to be less cost-effective for the system but popular with the public.

Funding of health services

The five principal forms of funding healthcare are described in Table 5D.17. In general, funding of health services can be described as either **progressive** or **regressive**:

- **Progressive**—a tax is said to be progressive where a higher percentage of income is paid as income rises.
- **Regressive**—a regressive tax charges a lower percentage of income as income rises.

Healthcare systems that are funded through direct taxation (e.g. social insurance) tend to be more progressive than those based on direct payments or on private insurance. All healthcare funding systems have advantages and disadvantages (see in Table 5D.17). Some of the major disadvantages relate to moral hazard and adverse selection.

Moral hazard and adverse selection

Moral hazard and adverse selection are both examples of **market failure** that are caused by asymmetric information between patients and providers. See Table 5D.18.

See 4D for further details.

History of healthcare services

UK United Kingdom

Prior to the establishment of the NHS in 1948, patients in the United Kingdom generally had to pay for their own healthcare [64]. Various charitable hospitals used to operate (e.g. the Royal Free Hospital in North London) and some local councils ran hospitals for their local population; however, such provision was by no means universal. This all changed on July 5, 1948, when the Health and Housing Minister, Aneurin Bevan, founded the NHS. It was based on a cooperative that the coalminers ran in his hometown of Tredegar, South Wales, and which followed the following principles:

- Services were provided **free at the point of use**.
- Services were financed from **central taxation**.
- Everyone was eligible for care, including foreign visitors and temporary residents.

The original structure of the NHS was **tripartite**:

1. Hospital service
2. Primary care
3. Community services

In the 1950s, rising costs led to the introduction of out-of-pocket charges for prescriptions and dental treatment. To this day, these remain the major exceptions to the NHS in England being free at the point of use. In Scotland, Northern Ireland, and Wales [65], prescription charges have recently been abolished.

Other important NHS developments are summarised in Table 5D.19.

International comparisons

A brief comparison of health systems in eight countries is presented in Tables 5D.20 and 5D.21.

Table 5D.17 Health systems with their advantages and disadvantages

Funding approach	Description	Advantages	Disadvantages
Taxation	Healthcare services are funded through general taxation.	Highly efficient. Fewer inequalities. Universal coverage.	Consumer and provider moral hazard.
Social insurance	A (more-or-less) compulsory insurance system in which employers and employees contribute to a fund. The government pays contributions for people out of work.	Fewer inequalities. Universal coverage.	Consumer and provider moral hazard.
Private insurance	Insurance system in which individuals contribute to a fund. Some employers contribute to schemes for employees.	Patients have a choice of insurer.	Exacerbate inequalities because unemployed people and people with low incomes may be uninsured or underinsured. Consumer and provider moral hazard. Adverse selection.
User charges	Individuals pay for health care out-of-pocket as fees are incurred.	Contains health service demand.	Exacerbates inequalities because demand is reduced. disproportionately in lower-income groups. Demand is reduced for both effective and ineffective treatments.

Table 5D.18 Moral hazard and adverse selection

Type of market failure	Description	Consequences
Consumer moral hazard	Where the consumer does not face the full cost of a health service, there is a tendency to **overuse services** in the knowledge that the insurer (private or public) will foot the bill.	This can lead to both **overconsumption** of healthcare when ill and **underuse of preventive** healthcare services.
Provider moral hazard	This occurs where a service becomes ignorant of costs to consumers or where the remuneration system offers incentives to **over-provide care** (e.g. fee for service where the insurer always pays).	This tends to lead to the **overprovision** of elective and preventive health care services.
Adverse selection	This occurs where purchasers of health insurance are more aware of their own **personal risk** than the insurer, then people with low risk will tend not to purchase insurance—which is designed (and priced) to cover people of average risk.	The average risk level of people remaining in the risk pool will rise, as will the **cost of insurance premiums**, thereby exacerbating the problem As a result, people at low risk will be uninsured, and people at high risk will be priced out of the market.

Table 5D.19 UK Key NHS developments

Decade	Major developments
1950s	• More equitable distribution of hospitals • More medical staff • Outpatient departments established
1960s	• More equitable distribution of GPs • Primary care teams established • Shift away from large mental hospitals
1970s	• English NHS reorganised: regional health authorities established • Financial pressures mount • Public health transfers to NHS from local government
1980s	• General managers appointed • Internal market established
1990s	• Fund holding GPs purchase selected elective care services for their own patients • Hospitals become semi-autonomous trusts

2000s	• NHS policy diverges across the home nations:
	  • In England, the introduction of competition and choice lead to a plurality of providers, including NHS employees, private sector, and the third sector; public health transfers from NHS to local government.
	  • In Scotland and Wales, the concept of commissioning is removed, and NHS health services remain provided by NHS employees.

2012	Health and Social Care Acts published in the United Kingdom devolved nations. Major changes to NHS structures in England (see Figure 5D.1)

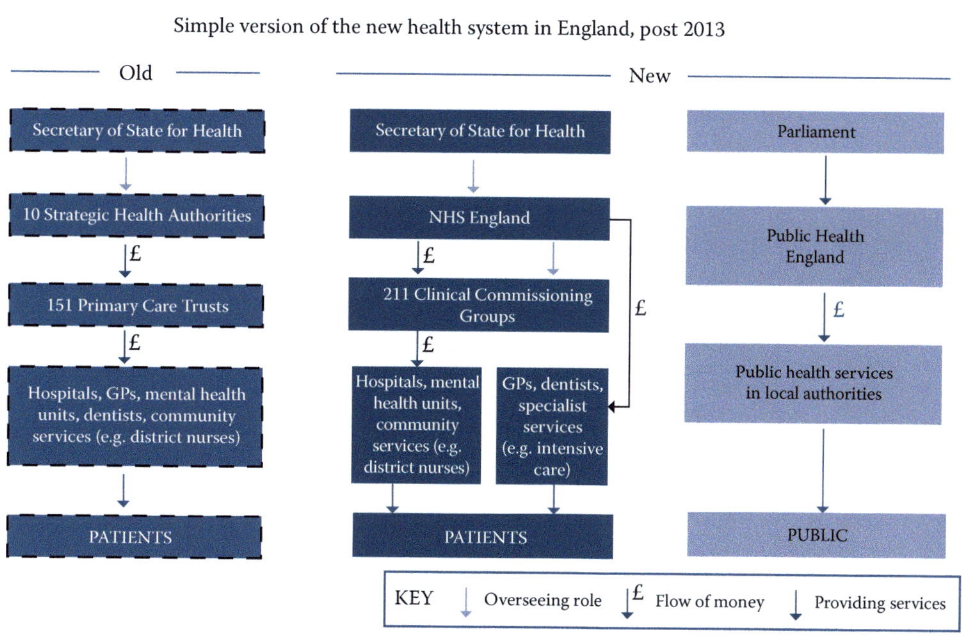

Figure 5D.1 Recent NHS changes in England.

Table 5D.20 International comparisons

<table>
<tr><th>Country</th><th>Organisation</th><th>Detail</th><th>Funding provision</th></tr>
<tr><td rowspan="3">Australia</td><td>General</td><td>Universal free healthcare to all. Complex range of providers and regulators.</td><td rowspan="3">Public health insurance system (Medicare) tax levy, which reimburses approximately 80% of healthcare fees.</td></tr>
<tr><td>Primary care</td><td>Self-employed GPs.</td></tr>
<tr><td>Secondary care</td><td>Public hospitals (70% acute beds) and private hospitals (which Medicare part subsidises).</td></tr>
<tr><td rowspan="3">Canada</td><td>General</td><td>Public funding but private providers. Provincial government and Royal Colleges regulate providers.</td><td rowspan="3">National health insurance plan (Medicare) that covers health services.</td></tr>
<tr><td>Primary care</td><td>GPs paid on fee-for-service basis.</td></tr>
<tr><td>Secondary care</td><td>Mostly not-for-profit private hospitals.</td></tr>
<tr><td rowspan="3">France</td><td>General</td><td>Health care provided by private and public hospitals and by private practitioners.</td><td rowspan="3">National health insurance system funded by tax and compulsory social insurance from employers and employees.
Most citizens have supplementary mutual insurance funds that cover cost-sharing out-of-pocket expenses.</td></tr>
<tr><td>Primary care</td><td>Open access to generalists and to specialists with no gatekeeping GPs.</td></tr>
<tr><td>Secondary care</td><td>Inpatient care provided by public and private hospitals (profit and not for profit).
Outpatient care mainly provided by private specialists in their own offices.</td></tr>
<tr><td rowspan="3">Germany</td><td>General</td><td>Over 90% covered by statutory health insurance and remainder by private insurance. Self-regulating healthcare system.</td><td rowspan="3">General taxation and social insurance fund.</td></tr>
<tr><td>Primary care</td><td>Free access to office-based doctors (generalists and specialists) with full range of diagnostics.</td></tr>
<tr><td>Secondary care</td><td>Outpatient care provided by office-based doctors, who act as gatekeepers to elective inpatient care.</td></tr>
<tr><td>United Kingdom</td><td>General</td><td>Primary care mainly but not exclusively provided by GPs. GPs act as gatekeepers to specialist services, provided in hospitals or in the community (occupational, psychological and occupational therapy). Many hospitals are publicly owned except for a few providers of private elective care.
The government is the main purchaser and provider of healthcare in Scotland, Wales, and Northern Ireland. In England, NHS care is provided by a range of providers.</td><td>General taxation.</td></tr>
</table>

Table 5D.20 (*Continued*) International comparisons

Country	Organisation	Detail	Funding provision
	Primary care	Provided by GPs, dentists, community pharmacists, and optometrists. Walk-in clinics and NHS Direct (helpline service) act as alternative forms of primary care in some countries. Commissioning arrangements vary between nations (see earlier).	
	Secondary care	Access is through emergency ambulance, referral from a GP, or self-referral to an A&E department.	
United States	General	Healthcare is mostly provided by private organisations. The government funds healthcare through four major routes: • Medicare (people aged 65+ and people with chronic kidney disease) • Medicaid (people with very low incomes) • Veterans • State Children's Health Insurance Program	Voluntary private care is funded by working-age people and their employers. Significant numbers of people are uninsured or underinsured.
	Primary care	Except in certain managed care plans, family doctors have no gatekeeper role.	
	Secondary care	Variety of private, non-profit, and public hospitals.	
New Zealand	General	Costs of medical care largely funded by the state.	General taxation revenue.
	Primary care	Primary health organisations (PHOs) employ GPs and other staff. Laboratory services and pharmaceuticals are largely provided at no cost to consumers.	Capitated funding with co-payments for working-age adults. Dental care on a fee-for-service basis.
	Secondary care	Public and private hospital systems. Private sector mainly provides elective surgical services.	Taxation. National public insurer covers costs of injury treatment. Patient charges in private system.
Hong Kong	General	A mixture of public and private. Public sector is highly subsidised, providing primary through to tertiary care services. Private sector is run as a business model, with services provided by generalists and specialists.	General taxation.
	Primary care	72% by private practitioners, 28% by public general outpatient clinics.	
	Secondary care	82% by public (hospital authority) hospitals, 18% by private hospitals.	

Table 5D.21 Major events in the history of public health

Approximate date	Event
450 BC	Hippocrates studies medicine as a discipline in itself. He • Records **clinical experiences** (e.g. obese people more prone to disease; differentiates epidemic and endemic diseases) • **Hypothesises** about disease causation (e.g. the four humours: blood, phlegm, black bile, and yellow bile)
1350 AD	City of Venice introduces **quarantine**, whereby incoming ships from ports infected with plague were required to sit at anchor for 40 days before docking.
1500	Fracastorius writes about **contagion** in the context of syphilis.
1650	Sydenham carefully describes a series of diseases and hypothesises about **miasma** (i.e. 'bad air' as the cause of disease).
1650	Gaunt analyses the bills of mortality to describe **disease patterns**.
1670	Leeuwenhoek first visualises bacteria using a **microscope**.
1800	Jenner deliberately **vaccinates** a boy with the pus from cowpox sores, thereby immunising the boy against smallpox.
1840	Chadwick notes differences in life expectancy between the **social classes**. His campaign leads to the Public Health Act 1848, which established a Central Board of Health with powers to supervise street cleaning, refuse collection, water supply and sewage disposal.
1845	Snow identifies the cause of an **outbreak** of cholera in London as infected water coming from a water pump in Soho. Snow arranges for the **handle of the broad street pump** to be removed and thereby terminates the outbreak.
1850	Farr, working as registrar general of the United Kingdom, uses **statistical analysis** as the justification for sanitary reforms.
1875	Pasteur confirmed **germ theory**, produced **artificial vaccines**, and described the process of **pasteurisation** (i.e. heat treatment of food to reduce its load of microorganisms).
1875	Koch defines four postulates that must be met to signify **disease causation** by a microorganism.
1883	Bismarck introduces **universal health insurance** in Germany (the oldest universal insurance system in Europe).
1948	Bevan establishes UK's **National Health Service** (the largest and the oldest single-payer healthcare system in the world). See Table 5D.19.
1974	Lalonde report sets out the **health field concept**: health is determined by the environment, lifestyle, biology, and healthcare. See Section 2H.2.
1977	Alma Ata WHO Assembly sets out the vision of *'Health for All by 2000'*. See Table 2H.28.
1980	The Black Report (made infamous by the failed attempt of the incoming government to suppress its publication) highlights the correlation between **social class** and infant mortality rates and life expectancy and inequalities in the use of medical services.
2000	UN Assembly agrees eight **Millennium Development Goals** to be achieved by 2015. These include halving extreme poverty, halting the spread of HIV/AIDS, and improving maternal health.

5E

Health and Social Service Quality

To achieve the best health outcomes and positive patient experiences, it is necessary to maximise the quality of health and social care services. However, quality may mean different things to different constituencies. Therefore, nationally agreed clinical guidelines may be helpful in setting common expectations about healthcare quality while allowing flexibility for variations in individual patient circumstances.

Health and social care professionals are responsible for providing high-quality services. While professional bodies use appraisal and revalidation to monitor individual performance, it is increasingly being recognised that

- Patients and the public have a legitimate role, not only in **judging** the quality of care they have received but also in **shaping** the way care should be provided in the future.
- Having the right **organisational structures** and **processes** are important for preventing errors and improving individual performance.

There is a range of different approaches to evaluating and improving the quality of services. These are covered elsewhere in the book:

Different approaches to evaluation of healthcare quality	1C.9 *Principles of evaluation, including quality assessment and quality assurance*
Frameworks and tools designed to promote quality improvement in healthcare organisations	5C.1 *Management models and theories* 5C.2 *Frameworks for managing change management*

5E.1 Principles underlying the development of clinical guidelines, clinical effectiveness and quality standards, and their application in health and social care

Principles of guideline and quality standards development

Purpose of guidelines and quality standards

ENG In England, NICE is responsible for developing clinical guidelines, service guidance, and quality standards for health and social care at a national level. In Table 5E.1, the purpose of these two types of guidance as defined by NICE is given.

Development principles

The concept of evidence-based medicine stipulates that guidelines that are based on scientific evidence should take precedence over individual clinical judgement. However, in order to be acceptable to clinicians, clinical guidelines need to be **credible** and their development must be seen to have been **accountable.** The principles underlying the development of NICE guidance (see Table 5E.2) are similar to those used in development of guidance produced by other bodies such as the Scottish Intercollegiate Guidelines Network (SIGN).

At a local level, organisations may need to adapt or develop specific guidelines. The steps to follow in this process include

1. Define the clinical issue
2. Establish a local guideline group
3. Identify existing guidelines, which may be regional or national
4. Appraise the validity of these guidelines
5. Adapt the guidelines to fit local circumstances
6. Pilot the local guidelines and identify any problems encountered
7. Establish dissemination and implementation strategies
8. Monitor the impact of the guidelines on an ongoing basis

Appraisal criteria

The *Appraisal of Guidelines for Research and Evaluation in Europe* (AGREE) instrument may be useful both for evaluating and developing guidelines (see Table 5E.3).

Table 5E.1 Purpose of clinical guidelines and quality standards

Guidance	Purpose
Clinical guidelines	• Assess how well different treatments and ways of managing a specific condition work and whether they represent good value for money. • Define the clinical care that is suitable for most patients with a specific condition.
Quality standards	• Clarify what represents high-quality care by providing measurable indicators of both process and outcomes of care. • Measure and improve the quality of care.

Source: NICE, How NICE clinical guidelines are developed: An overview for stakeholders, the public and the NHS (5th edn.), 2012, Accessed online July 20, 2014 at http://publications.nice.org.uk/how-nice-clinical-guidelines-are-developed-an-overview-for-stakeholders-the-publicand-the-nhs-pmg6f/nice-clinical-guidelines.

Table 5E.2 Principles underlying the development of NICE clinical guidelines

Attribute	Principles
Aim	Improve the quality of care for patients.
Consultation	Take account of the views of those who might be affected by the guideline, including • Healthcare and other professionals • Patients and carers • Health service managers • NHS trusts, the public • Government bodies • The healthcare industry
Use of evidence	Based on the best available research evidence and expert consensus.
Development process	Use a **standard process** and standard ways of analysing the evidence, which are respected by the NHS and other stakeholders, including patients.
Transparency	Clarify how each recommendation was agreed.
Status	Advisory rather than compulsory but should be taken into account by clinicians and other professionals when planning the care of individual patients.

Source: NICE, How NICE clinical guidelines are developed: An overview for stakeholders, the public and the NHS (5th edn.), 2012, Accessed online July 20, 2014 at http://publications.nice.org.uk/how-nice-clinical-guidelines-are-developed-an-overview-for-stakeholders-the-publicand-the-nhs-pmg6f/nice-clinical-guidelines.

Table 5E.3 The AGREE criteria for appraising clinical guidelines

Criterion	Description
Scope and purpose	Clear definitions of the guideline objective, clinical question, and group of patients to whom the guideline applies.
Stakeholder involvement	Range of professionals, together with patient involvement.
Rigour of development	Systematic appraisal of evidence, explicit consideration of benefits and risks, evidence of external review prior to publication.
Clarity and presentation	Specific, unambiguous recommendations.
Applicability	Target users clearly defined; costs and other barriers discussed. Auditing criteria outlined. Guideline piloted.
Editorial independence	Editors independent of funding body. Conflicts of interest recorded.

Application of guidelines and quality standards in health and social care

The levers for promoting the adoption and implementation of guidelines and quality standards include

- Inclusion in the annual **outcomes frameworks**, which report on **national performance** of health and social care systems and provide a means for **benchmarking** local services
- Incorporation into **contracts** between commissioners and providers, with **rewards** or **penalties** attached to performance (5F.2)
- Inclusion in **inspection and monitoring** regimes (see Figure 5E.1)
- Inclusion in organisational **performance management tools** (5C.3)

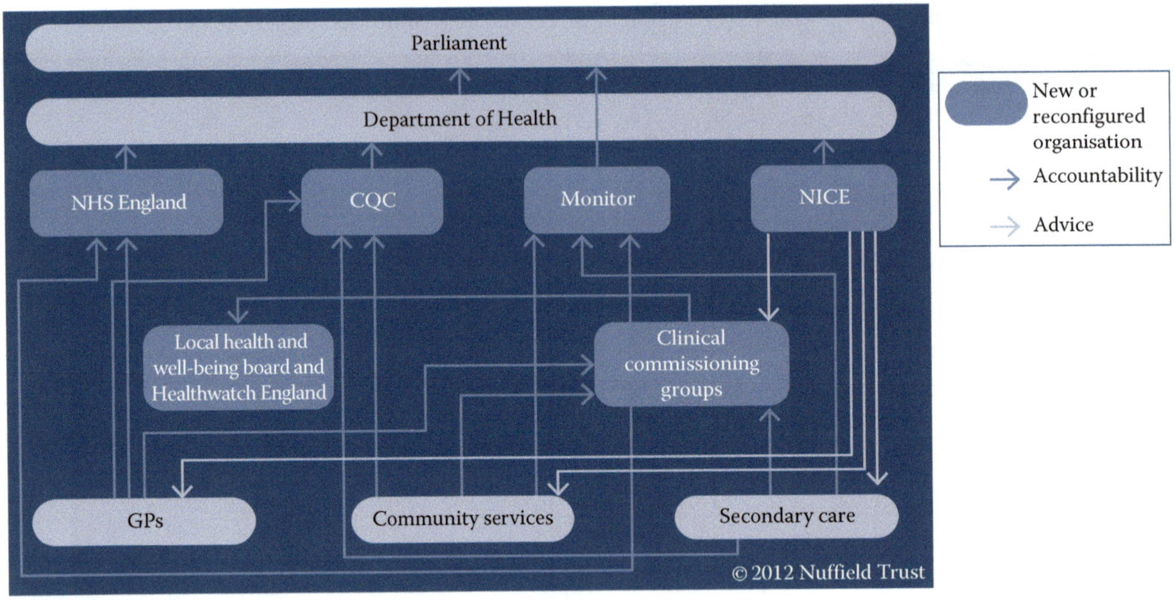

Figure 5E.1 Systems for regulating the quality of healthcare services in England. (From Holder, R. and Thorlby, R., The new NHS in England: Structure and accountabilities. The Nuffield Trust, 2013, Accessed online July 20, 2014 at http://www.nuffieldtrust.org.uk/talks/slideshows/newstructure-nhs-england.)

5E.2 Public and patient involvement in health service planning

The public can be involved in health services in a range of ways, from simply feeding back experiences of their own care to taking part in the delivery of new models of health services. Individuals can be involved as

- Consumers of healthcare or carers
- Members or leaders of community groups (e.g. minority ethnic groups)
- Representatives of groups with specific health interests (e.g. breast cancer support groups)

Consultation and involvement of the public in healthcare are described in more detail in Sections 2I.4 and 4D.7.

ENG Healthwatch [71] is the statutory organisation responsible for ensuring patient and public involvement in health service planning in England. At a national level, Healthwatch is a part of the Care Quality Commission. From April 2013, local Healthwatch organisations replaced Local Involvement Networks (LINks). Local Healthwatch groups can influence planning in a number of ways (e.g. by providing feedback to providers and clinical commissioning groups on patent and public experience of local services). In addition, a member of these local organisations sits on the local Health and Wellbeing Board.

5E.3 Professional accountability, clinical governance, performance, and appraisal

Professional accountability

Professional accountability is the principle that individuals are responsible for the quality of the service that their organisation delivers. Donaldson [72] argued that accountability for quality and outcomes is a matter both for the individual practitioner and for their employing organisation, with health organisations having a duty to provide the **culture**,

support, and **resources** needed by individual practitioners in order to deliver high-quality care.

UK Systems of professional accountability have been strengthened in many countries over the past decade.

When the NHS was first established, clinicians—particularly doctors—were held accountable for their actions solely through professional bodies. In recent years, however, clinicians have partly ceded their high degree of professional autonomy and self-regulation in favour of

- A regulatory system that involves members of the public (e.g. half of the General Medical Council's 24 members are lay people)
- Statutory oversight by the **Council for Healthcare Regulatory Excellence** (a nondepartmental public body that is funded by the DH and answerable to parliament)
- Explicit standards of accountability, such as **clinical governance**

Clinical governance

ENG In the NHS, the profile of professional standards was raised in 1998 with the introduction of **clinical governance**. The government's consultation document *A First Class Service: Quality in the new NHS* (1998) defined clinical governance as

> *A framework through which NHS organizations are accountable for continually improving the quality of their services and safeguarding high standards of care by creating an environment in which excellence in clinical care will flourish.*

The Health Act 1999 enshrined clinical governance as a statutory duty for all NHS organisations. Its introduction required a change in the culture of accountability, away from considering clinical standards the responsibility of single professional groups such as doctors, towards regarding it as the responsibility of the entire organisation, 'from the cleaners to the chief executive'.

The DH clinical governance support team outlined a diagram consisting of

- Five *'foundation stones'* of practice
- Seven *'pillars'* of clinical governance
- A *'capping stone'* of the partnership between patients and professionals

Clinical governance is based on the principle that good **systems** of clinical care improve patient outcomes. Clinical governance involves **demonstrating** that these systems and practices are in place and are working well. For example, in terms of risk management, clinical governance would require a demonstration that an incident-reporting system was working effectively.

Role of professional bodies

UK Several organisations are involved in setting and maintaining clinical standards for clinicians working in the NHS.

Organisation	Professional group	Role
General Medical Council (GMC)	Doctors (United Kingdom)	• Controls entry to national medical register of doctors and specialist registers • Sets standards for medical education and training • Takes action where standards not met
National Clinical Assessment [73] Service (NCAS)	Doctors, dentists, pharmacists (United Kingdom)	• Advisory body where concerns can be raised about professionals
Medical Royal Colleges	Doctors	Set and monitor the standards of postgraduate medical training

As well as the GMC which regulates doctors, there are eight other major professional regulatory bodies for healthcare in the United Kingdom. These include the General Dental Council (GDC), the Nursing and Midwifery Council (NMC), the Health and Care Professionals Council (HCPC), and the Royal Pharmaceutical Society of Great Britain. Each of these bodies

- Maintains **registers** of accredited professionals
- States how professional competence should be **maintained**
- Holds **hearings** when serious professional misconduct is alleged
- Is **overseen** by the Council for Healthcare Regulatory Excellence
- Will be required maintain ongoing evidence professionals' **competence** to practise

In the United Kingdom, public health specialists who do not have a medical or dental background are regulated by the **UK Public Health Register** (UKPHR). This register is analogous to the public health specialist registers of the GMC and GDC, in that its aim is to ensure high standards of public health practice and thereby protect the public. In contrast to the GMC and GDC, however, the disciplinary procedures and sanctions of the UKPHR are not underpinned by law.

Finally, **nonspecialist** public health practitioners in the United Kingdom may be regulated by a range of different professional bodies, including the UKPHR, the Chartered Institute for Environmental Health, and the NMC.

NZ The Medical Council of New Zealand requires all registered medical practitioners to participate in approved continuing professional development activities. For most practitioners, this takes the form of an approved recertification programme specific to their field of practice. Other clinicians (particularly doctors in training positions) are required to have a formal collegial relationship with a nominated peer who is working in their field. Under the *Health Practitioners Competency Assurance Act*, this system of recertification is being extended to other groups of health practitioners. In contrast, the accreditation of healthcare agencies remains voluntary, although a standardised system is provided by Quality Health New Zealand.

Changes in professional accountability

Changes in professional accountability have arisen for a number of reasons, including the

- **Publicity** of several serious untoward incidents, which prompted suggestions that current systems for accountability were inadequate
- Recognition that efforts in the 1990s to **contain healthcare costs** and reduce waiting times may have harmed clinical quality
- Changes in the **autonomy** afforded to professionals working in other fields
- Introduction of more **business practices** into health (e.g. corporate governance)

ENG In England, recommendations to modernise professional regulation followed the **Fifth Report of the Shipman Inquiry**. This was a large-scale investigation into the reasons why Dr Harold Shipman, a GP who worked near Manchester, was able to murder an estimated 250 of his patients without detection. The recommendations from this enquiry were legion, but in summary they were designed to

- **Align** organisation-wide and professional regulation systems to ensure patient safety
- **Strengthen** revalidation processes and fitness to practise
- **Support** the safe expansion in roles of professionals in regular contact with patients

Appraisal

Appraisal is a regular, nonthreatening, confidential dialogue that occurs between a manager and an employee, aimed at

- Reviewing progress towards objectives that were previously agreed
- Setting new objectives
- Identifying developmental needs

Appraisal enables employees to achieve more from their work and to develop specific competencies. Its use is now widespread within the public and private sectors (see Box 5E.1) [74].

Box 5E.1 UK Revalidation

Revalidation of doctors was introduced by the GMC in late 2012 and requires all doctors to revalidate their licence to practise every 5 years. This process involves regular appraisal during which doctors must demonstrate that they are up to date and fit to practise. Appraisal, from the GMC's *Good Medical Practice*, is based on the following principles:

- Good clinical care
- Maintaining good medical practice
- Teaching and training
- Relationships with patients
- Working with colleagues
- Probity
- Health

The first doctor to be revalidated through the system was the Chief Medical Officer Dame Sally Davies in December 2012.

In public health, the UKPHR will operate an equivalent system of revalidation for its registrants, which is also based on GMC Good Medical Practice principles.

Sources: General Medical Council revalidation website, Accessed online July 20, 2014 at http://www.gmc-uk.org/doctors/revalidation.asp; Faculty of Public Health revalidation pages, Accessed online July 20, 2014 at http://www.fph.org.uk/revalidation.

5E.4 Risk management and patient safety

Providing healthcare is a risky undertaking. There are risks of different kinds to the

- Patient
- Practitioner
- Provider
- Commissioner

Risk management involves identifying, monitoring, and minimising these risks through a range of means. In England, systems of clinical governance (see Section 5E.3) provide the framework for organisational risk management.

Risks to patients

Patients trust healthcare organisations to improve their health. However, patients are harmed in around 10% of hospital admissions [77]. Patient safety is a particular concern because

- There are risks associated with all types of healthcare
- Patients can be more vulnerable to existing hazards (e.g. many people carry MRSA in their nasopharynx, but immunocompromised patients are at substantially higher risk from infection)

Risks to patients cannot be eliminated but they can be minimised by ensuring that systems are reviewed and questioned regularly (e.g. by **critical event audits** and by learning from complaints). In England, the Chief Medical Officer chaired a working group to devise recommendations to reduce adverse events in the NHS, which led to the report *An organisation with a memory* (see Box 5E.2).

UK The **National Reporting and Learning System** (NRLS) is the system for monitoring patient safety in England. Previously a role of the National Patient Safety Agency, the NRLS transferred to the NHS Commissioning Board in 2012. In addition to the NRLS, information on incidents in the NHS comes from

- Clinical negligence claims
- Data from death registrations
- Hospital activity data
- National surveys

Box 5E.2 UK A major failure in patient safety: The Francis Inquiry into poor care in the NHS in England

The Francis Inquiry into the care provided by Mid Staffordshire NHS FT was published in February 2013. The inquiry, Chaired by Robert Francis QC, was initiated in 2005 after long-standing and serious concerns about care in the trust, including high mortality rates. At the time, poor levels of care were noticed by both patients and staff but outside bodies such as the Healthcare Commission gave the trust apparently favourable reports.

The inquiry was extremely extensive—it received information from over 900 patients and families and found

- Chronic shortages of staff and substandard levels of care
- Staff deterred from sharing their concerns
- Many patients that 'suffered horrific experiences'

Francis concluded that patients were 'routinely neglected by a Trust that was preoccupied with cost cutting, targets and processes and which lost sight of its fundamental responsibility to provide safe care'.

The report made over 200 recommendations. These included recommendations for the Department of Health, to urgently review

- The gathering and use of mortality data in the NHS
- External bodies (such as the Care Quality Commission) to restore public confidence in the system

Source: http://www.midstaffsinquiry.com/index.html

Risks to practitioners

Important elements of quality assurance include ensuring that clinicians are

- **Immunised** against infectious diseases
- Working in a **safe environment** (e.g. following COSHH regulations)
- Keeping **up to date** with current regulations and safety alerts

Risks to the organisation

Poor quality is a threat to any organisation. In addition to reducing risks to patients and practitioners, organisations can reduce their own risks by

- Ensuring high-quality **employment practice** (including locum procedures and reviews of individual and team performance)
- Providing a **safe environment** (including estates and privacy)
- Ensuring adherence to **safety standards** and established policies

Associated organisations (such as GP cooperatives, community pharmacists, and residential care homes) should be covered by clinical governance frameworks by ensuring that they agree to comply with the standards of the organisations with which they are associated.

UK In the United Kingdom, clinical governance arrangements are complemented by, and integrated with, a strong **risk management framework**. This framework includes the maintenance of **risk registers**, which were introduced after the Turnbull Committee's report on corporate governance in the wake of the financial collapse of Barings Bank. A risk register ensures that clinical governance risks feature highly the priorities of the board of directors of all NHS organisations.

Negligence

Negligence claims are now a feature of all healthcare services. They are often expensive and lengthy and are undesirable for all concerned.

ENG In England, a special health authority called the NHS Litigation Authority [79] is responsible for handling all claims made against the NHS. It analyses all claims to identify common failures and to promote organisational learning from litigation. According to the NHS Litigation Authority, there were over 8600 claims of negligence against NHS bodies in 2010–2011, costing £729 million including damages to patients and the legal costs to the NHS. The highest value claims tend to relate to maternity services.

5F

Finance, Management Accounting, and Relevant Theoretical Approaches

Good health is often described by patients as being priceless. Healthcare is indeed an expensive commodity, and it requires adequate funding both to continue existing programmes and to introduce new technologies. Public health specialists have an important role in promoting the use of efficacious, cost-effective technologies to benefit the population. A strong grasp of the following methods is therefore required: **costing, payment methods** (including contracting and commissioning), and the **auditing** of healthcare spending.

5F.1 Cost of health services

Linkages between demographic information and health service information—its public health interpretation and relationship to financial costs.

Public health specialists need to understand the cost of health services for several reasons (see Table 5F.1).

Costs are split categorised as being **direct**, **indirect,** and **overheads** (see Table 5F.2).

The process of assigning costs to health services is complicated by a number of factors, including the following:

- **Defining the service or episode of care**. For example, does hip replacement surgery consist only of the operation and the associated inpatient stay, or does it also include the pre-operative assessment and post-operative physiotherapy?
- **Apportioning the indirect costs and overheads**. In healthcare, labour accounts for upwards of two-thirds of the budget. Staff costs are categorised as indirect cost, since they are spread over many patients. Moreover, a single episode of care typically requires the input of more than one healthcare professional.
- **Case mix**. The same procedure can vary widely in its complexity depending on the patient's characteristics, including demographic factors and co-morbidities.

Health service information can be used to determine costs at an **aggregate** or at an **individual** level (see Table 5F.3). In England, NHS trusts have historically reported the costs of care at an aggregate level by considering the total cost for conducting a large number of a particular procedure. The DH collects these **reference costs** and produces **average unit costs** for each procedure, which may then be grouped into similar types of activity, known as HRGs. These HRGs have then been used to set national price tariffs in the NHS [80,81].

However, aggregate costs have some limitations. It may be difficult to **verify the accuracy** of the underlying reference costs, and it is not possible to break down costs into their constituent parts (e.g. between staff costs, drug costs, and the costs of investigations). Such information can be

Table 5F.1 Uses of healthcare cost information

Purpose	Details
Monitoring	The first stage in the process of **monitoring** and **controlling** spending is to establish accurate cost information.
Review	Cost information provides an indication of the intensity of **resource utilisation** spent on different health services. This information can then be used to **regulate** the level of activity.
Benchmarking	It may be possible to identify and address areas of abnormal spending by comparing local costs to regional and national benchmarks. This process may help identify local services that are relatively inefficient.
Quality assurance	Cost information may identify services that are relatively underfunded and may therefore potentially be delivering services of inferior **quality**.
Early warning	Cost information may sometimes serve as an early warning of **nascent public health problems** (e.g. increasing costs of child paediatric services reflecting a rise in the prevalence of childhood morbid obesity).

Table 5F.2 Different types of costs

Type of cost	Definition	Example
Direct	Costs incurred exclusively for that output	Disposable surgical equipment
Indirect	Costs shared across several outputs	Autoclave that sterilises equipment from several operations
Overheads	Costs shared across the entire organisation	Cost of the organisation's press officer

Table 5F.3 Methods of determining healthcare costs

	Aggregate	Individual level
Definition	Total costs of a procedure over a time period or within one clinical specialty	Resources used by individual patients, potentially spanning several departments
Examples	• Inpatient, A&E, or outpatient activity levels • Readmission rates • Acute bed occupancy • Referral rates per 1000 registered population • Consultation rates • Ratio of generic to patented prescriptions • Ratio of first to repeat outpatient appointments	• Procedures • Length of stay • Drugs administered/prescriptions issued • Investigations performed

Box 5F.1 ENG Example: Spend and outcome tool (SPOT)

SPOT compares expenditures with outcomes in each healthcare specialty between similar healthcare organisations. It is commissioned by NHS England and produced by Public Health England.

An example chart is shown, which compares expenditure (horizontal axis) against outcomes (vertical axis). The position of each specialty on the chart indicates which areas the organisation should prioritise or investigate: Programmes lying to the left or right of the central box should be prioritised for spending; those lying to the top or bottom may need reviewing.

In this particular example, the organisation may wish to examine healthcare expenditure and outcomes for a range of conditions (Figure 5F.1).

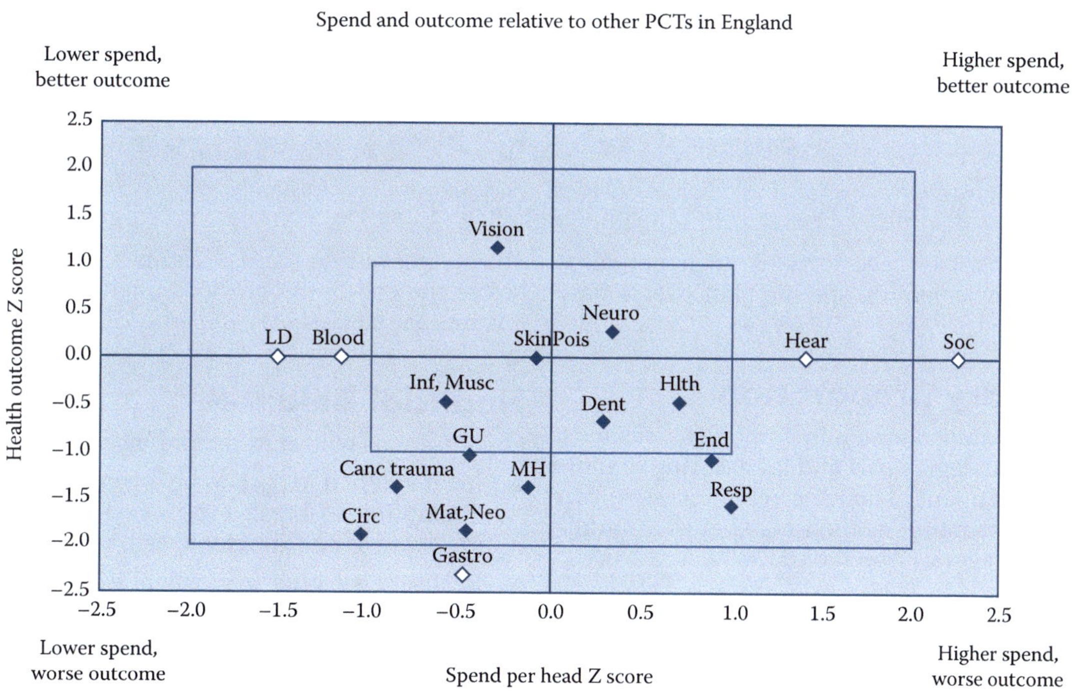

◇ No outcome indicators readily available
◆ Outcome indicators available

Programme area abbreviations

Infectious diseases	Inf	Hearing	Hear	Disorders of blood	Blood
Cancers and tumours	Canc	Circulation	Circ	Maternity	Mat
Respiratory system	Resp	Mental health	MH	Neonates	Neo
Endocrine, nutritional and metabolic	End	Dental	Dent	Neurological	Neuro
Genito urinary system	GU	GI system	Gastro	Healthy individuals	Hlth
Learning disabilities	LD	Musculoskeletal	Musc	Social care needs	Soc
Adverse effects and poisoning	Pols	Trauma and injuries	Trauma		

Figure 5F.1 PCT or CCG spend and outcome factsheets and tool (SPOT). (From Yorkshire and Humber Health Intelligence, PCT CCG Spend and Outcome Factsheets and Tool [SPOT], Public Health England, Accessed online 20 July, 2014 at http://www.yhpho.org.uk/spot.)

helpful in identifying opportunities to make **potential savings**.

As a result, systems for measuring and collecting individual patient-level costs (PLCs) data have been introduced into the English NHS since early 2000s and will in future be the preferred approach for calculating national tariffs.

Service line reporting

ENG In business terms, a service line is the natural 'business unit' of an organisation—a distinct unit with identifiable customers, products, revenues, and costs that is run as an independent business with its own income and expenditure. Service line reporting has been introduced in FTs to develop a better understanding of their operational and financial performance and in turn improve their strategic and clinical decision-making. Service line reporting measures a trust's profitability by each of its service lines rather than just at an aggregated level for the whole Trust (see Box 5F.1). It is seen as a way of enabling clinicians to become more autonomous and accountable for delivering quality and productivity [83].

5F.2 Paying for services

Budgetary preparation, financial allocation, contracts, and service commissioning.

Budgets consist of specific sums of money allocated for implementing specific plan over a particular period.

The budget setting process begins several months before the end of the previous financial year and involves the steps shown in Figure 5F.2.

Budgetary preparation

Budget preparation is an important mechanism for achieving strategic goals and for assuring organisational and financial management processes. Two types of accounting method may be used: **financial** or **managerial** (see Table 5F.4).

Budgets typically reflect an organisation's priorities. Budgets follow the financial year, which varies between countries (see Table 5F.5).

In order to ensure that budgetary decisions reflect both economic realities and remain sensitive to the strategic mission of the organisation, the preparation of a budget should involve both **financial** and **managerial** staff. There are three main approaches to budget setting, which are shown in Table 5F.6. An organisation may use different approaches depending on the service [84] under consideration.

Financial balance

Organisations will, at different times, choose to

- Incur a **deficit** in part of the organisation while attempting to break even overall (e.g. when investing in new developments)
- Realise a **surplus** (e.g. when establishing an operating reserve to guard against future cash flow shortfalls)
- Break even

ENG Government financial orders require NHS organisations to remain in continuous financial balance on every day of every year. In contrast, NHS FTs have no statutory duty to break even. They can generate and retain a surplus and can also incur a deficit, although the regulatory framework requires FTs to demonstrate financial viability over the medium term [84].

Table 5F.4 Accounting methods

Accounting method	Description
Financial	Financial accounting is a specialised field and relates to the use of accounting information for reporting to external bodies (e.g. for auditing purposes or for shareholders). Financial reports are • Created for a set time period (e.g. a financial year) • Historically factual • Predictive of the organisation's future financial situation
Managerial	Less technically complex than financial accounting, managerial accounting is primarily for use by people working within an organisation, including public health specialists. By using a combination of historical data and estimated data, managerial accounting can be used to guide decision-making relating to • Day-to-day operations • Future operations • Organisational strategies

Table 5F.5 Financial years by country

Country	Fiscal year
United Kingdom,[a] Hong Kong, Canada	1 April–31 March
Australia, New Zealand	1 July–30 June
Ireland	1 January–31 December
United States[a]	1 October–30 September

[a] In the United Kingdom, the fiscal year for personal tax affairs runs from 6 April to 5 April, and in the United States, it follows the calendar year.

Table 5F.6 Budget setting in healthcare

Approach	Description	Advantages	Disadvantages
Historical or incremental	Based on previous year's budget, adjusted for inflation and changes to services	Easy to apply Useful for services that do not change year on year	Does not facilitate innovation
Zero-based	Fresh financial plan, requires re-evaluating all services and contracts	Useful for new services	Requires significant resources to prepare
Activity-based	Budget based on a defined activity level and includes information on how the budget will vary if levels of activity change	Enables providers to be paid based on the number of treatments they deliver	Requires detailed data and understanding of activity and costing

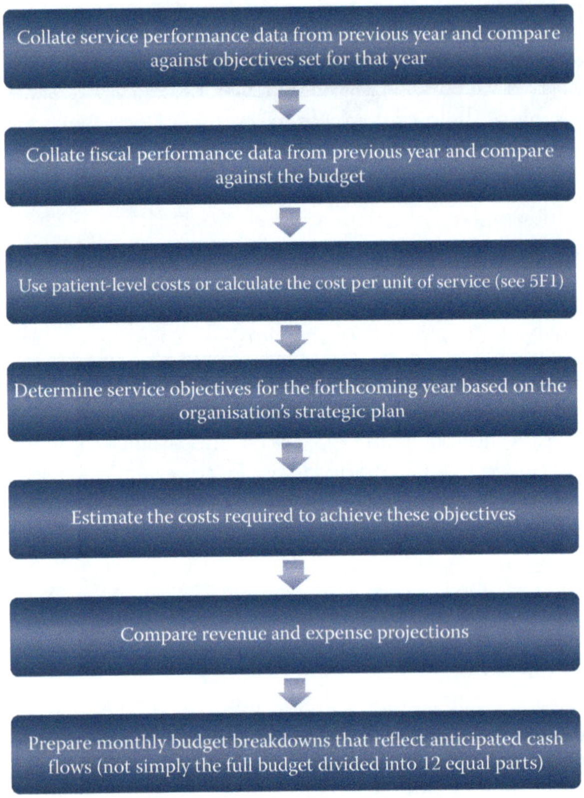

Figure 5F.2 Steps involved in setting budgets.

Financial allocation

Decisions about how to allocate financial resources within healthcare organisations may be decided using **programme budgeting marginal analysis** [85] (PBMA):

- **Programme budgeting** is a way of analysing how money has been spent across medical specialties.
- **Marginal analysis** refers to an explicit consideration of the benefits and costs of increasing or decreasing resources for a programme. It can be used to make decisions about how funding is allocated at a macro-level (between programmes) or micro-level (within programmes).

Brambleby and Fordham [86] define eight steps for undertaking PBMA (Box 5F.2).

Box 5F.2 Eight steps for PBMA

1. Choose a set of meaningful programmes
2. Identify current activity and expenditure in those programmes
3. Think of improvements
4. Weigh up incremental costs and incremental benefits and prioritise a list
5. Consult widely
6. Decide on changes
7. Effect the changes
8. Evaluate progress

Source: Brambleby, P. and Fordham R.J., What is PBMA? Evidence-based-medicine, 2003, http://www.medicine.ox.ac.uk/bandolier/painres/download/whatis/pbma.pdf.

Contracts

Contracts are agreements between two or more parties that set out what one party will do in return for specified resources. Contractual payments can be made in **advance** or in **arrears**. Charlesworth et al. [87] summarise the principal payment methods used in healthcare and how these may influence the behaviour of providers (see Table 5F.7).

ENG In the English NHS, contracts with healthcare providers are agreed as part of the commissioning process. Considerations that have the potential to affect the way that services are delivered include the following:

- **Selecting the provider**. In the English NHS, providers of care can be NHS organisations, private companies, or third-sector organisations including charities and social enterprises. The Health and Social Care Act 2012 places a duty on commissioners to select the provider on the basis that 'competition and choice of hospital provider leads to better outcomes'. Monitor regulates the selection of providers to ensure that the selection process is not anticompetitive.
- **Agreeing the price**. Prices are fixed for many procedures at a national level. Previously, this was set by the DH based on a national tariff. Beginning in 2013, Monitor and NHS England assumed the responsibility for determining prices.

Table 5F.7 Payment methods used in healthcare

Payment method	Description	Effect on provider behaviour: Advantageous	Effect on provider behaviour: Disadvantageous
Block budget	Periodic lump sum for all services provided within a defined time period. A salary may also be considered as form of block contract.	More investment in preventive care. Limits healthcare activity. Risk sharing between organisations.	Less responsive to public expectations and demand. Can result in perverse incentives.
Capitation	Risk-adjusted, periodic lump sum per enrolled patient.	More investment in preventive care. Limits healthcare activity.	Less responsive to public expectations and demand.
Resource group	Payment for services, which are grouped by similar resource levels required (e.g. by diagnostic resource groups or HRGs).	More responsive to public expectations and demand.	Less investment in non-reimbursed preventive care. Increases healthcare activity.
Fee for service (payment by results)	Payment for each item of service and patient contact.	More responsive to public expectations and demand.	Less investment in non-reimbursed preventive care Increases healthcare activity.

Source: Adapted from Charlesworth, A. et al., Reforming payment for health care in Europe to achieve better value. Nuffield Trust, London, UK, 2012, pp. 9, 15, Accessed online March 23, 2014 at http://www.nuffieldtrust.org.uk/sites/files/nuffield/publication/120823_reforming-payment-for-health-care-ineuropev2.pdf.

- Agreeing the **payment arrangements and schedules**. Payments can be made in advance or in arrears. The main arrangements used in healthcare are shown in Table 5F.7.
- Agreeing measures to **monitor and improve quality**. The QOF and the *Commissioning for Quality and Innovation* (CQUIN) [88] payment framework are examples of pay-for-performance schemes whereby a proportion of a provider's income depends on achieving quality goals.

The QOF indicators are described in Section 3B.

Healthcare organisations use contracts to ensure that they are provided with the range of goods and services they require in order to provide healthcare. A 2011 report by the National Audit Office found that the prices different hospitals paid for the same item (e.g. blankets) varied widely. The report identified savings of around £500 m that could be made through better procurement and contracting.

Commissioning of services

In the English NHS, the term **commissioning** is used to describe the processes by which a purchaser of healthcare (e.g. a Clinical Commissioning Group, NHS England or a local authority) identifies a local **need** for a service, sets out the **requirements** for that service, **procures** such a service,

Box 5F.3 Principles for commissioning identified by the Department of Health

Commissioning principles	Public health tool	See section
Population needs	Health needs assessment	1C.2
Local service gaps	Healthcare evaluation	1C.10
Equity	Health equity audit and equality impact assessment	1C.17
Evidence-based	Literature review and critical appraisal	6A.2
Partnerships	Change management analysis	5C.2
Value for money	Economic evaluation	4D.8

Source: Specialised Services Commissioning Transition Team, Securing equity and excellence in commissioning specialised services, 2012, Accessed online July 20, 2014 at http://www.commissioningboard.nhs.uk/files/2012/11/op-model.pdf.

and **monitors** its delivery. Commissioning is used because when it works well it

- Identifies local healthcare **needs**
- Exposes any **deficiencies** in the current provision
- Determines the level of **investment** required to address any unmet needs
- Favours healthcare services that are **cost-efficient**
- Ensures that unambiguous **agreements** are made between purchasers and providers
- Guides **workforce development**

Principles for commissioning

ENG The DH identifies six principles that should guide commissioners, each of which is associated with one or more tools from the public health armamentarium (see Box 5F.3).

5D covers the different commissioning arrangements in place internationally and in each of the nations in the United Kingdom.

Specialised commissioning

Random fluctuations in healthcare activity present a relatively larger risk to small commissioners than they do to large commissioners. This phenomenon is known as **volatility**. For example, in a GP practice list, a single patient with haemophilia requiring surgery might consume as many healthcare resources in a year as all other patients on the list combined. In order to cope with this volatility in overspending or underspending from one year to the next, commissioners can create a **risk pool**. This is a form of insurance for

Box 5F.4 Rationale for specialised commissioning

Interested party	Benefit of risk pooling and specialised commissioning
Patients	Improving access to rare services
Healthcare planners	Restricting the number of specialist centres so as to maintain high levels of expertise
Commissioners	Smoothing out risk volatility
Providers	Cash flow to support rare and expensive treatments
Specialists	Focus point for discussion about service development

commissioners in which overspending commissioners may access additional resources, subject to explicit criteria.

ENG In England, specialised commissioning is the responsibility of NHS England. The Advisory Group for National Specialised Services makes recommendations about the risk-sharing arrangements for rare or expensive conditions. This arrangement offers potential benefits to each of the groups listed in Box 5F.4.

5F.3 Methods for audit of healthcare spending

The purpose of financial audit is to provide an independent and objective opinion on the performance of organisation with regard to

- Financial control
- Risk management
- Governance

Internal audit

In order to maintain credibility, auditors must strive for integrity, objectivity, and confidentiality. A healthcare organisation may be audited by

- In-house audit teams
- In-house audit team with support from external contractors
- External 'whole-internal-audit' service

External audit

UK The National Audit Office (NAO) is an independent body that reports directly to parliament. One of its roles is to assess the efficiency and effectiveness with which public sector bodies use their resources. The NAO audits

- The DH resource account
- Accounts of DH arms length bodies
- Summarised accounts of NHS trusts
- Consolidated accounts of FTs [90]

Fraud detection

Fraud detection is, in general, a line-management issue rather than a direct responsibility of auditors. In England, the NHS Counter Fraud Service is charged with tackling all fraud and corruption in the NHS.

References

1. Belbin, R.M. (1996) *Team Roles at Work*. London, UK: Butterworth-Heinemann.
2. Belbin, M. (n.d) Belbin team roles. Belbin®. Accessed online March 23, 2014 at http://www.belbin.com/rte.asp?id=8.
3. Tuckman, B.W. (1965) Developmental sequence in small groups. *Psychol Bull* 63, 384–399.
4. The Happy Manager. Teamwork theory: Tuckman's stages of group development. Accessed online July 20, 2014 at http://www.the-happy-manager.com/articles/teamwork-theory/.
5. Handy, C.B. (1985) *Understanding Organizations* (Penguin Business) (3rd edn.). London: Penguin.
6. Pilowski, I. and Spence, N.D. (1977) Ethnicity and illness behaviour. *Psychol Med* 7, 447–452.
7. Janis, J.L. (1982). *Groupthink* (2nd edn.). Houghton Mifflin.
8. Amabile, T.M. (1998) How to kill creativity. *Harv Bus Rev* 76, 76–87.
9. Rogers, E. (1995) *Diffusion of Innovation* (4th edn.). New York: Free Press.
10. Dearing, J.W. (2009) Applying diffusion of innovation theory to intervention development. *Res Soc Work Pract* 19(5), 503–518.
11. Department of Health and the Rt Hon Earl Howe (2013) Increasing research and innovation in health and social care. Accessed online July 20, 2014 at www.gov.uk.
12. Humphries, D. and Hean, S. (2004) Educating the future workforce: Building the evidence about interprofessional learning. *J Health Serv Res Policy* 9, 24–27.

13. Department of Health (2000) *The NHS Plan: A Plan for Investment, a Plan for Reform*. London, UK: The Stationery Office. Available online at www.dh.gov.uk.
14. Department of Health (2002) *Getting Ahead of the Curve: A Strategy for Combating Infectious Diseases (including Other Aspects of Health Protection)*. London, UK: Department of Health. Available online at www.dh.gov.uk.
15. Covey, S.R. (1989) *The Seven Habits of Highly Effective People*. London, UK: Simon & Schuster.
16. Jessop, E. (2013) Effective meetings. In: Guest, C., Ricciardi, W., Kawachi, I., and Lang, I. Eds. *Oxford Handbook of Public Health Practice* (3rd edn.). Oxford: Oxford University Press, pp. 448–453.
17. Iles, V. (2005) *Really Managing Health Care*. Oxford, UK: Oxford University Press.
18. Stevenson, H. (undated) Leadership and Change: Some Writings of John Kotter. Accessed online March 23, 2014 at http://www.clevelandconsultinggroup.com/articles/leadership-and-change-writings-of-john-kotter.php.
19. Drucker, P. (1950) *The New Society: The Anatomy of Industrial Order*. New York: Harper.
20. Monroe (1935). Motivated sequence. Referenced in: Anon. 17.3 Organizing persuasive speeches. [Online]. Available at http://2012books.lardbucket.org/books/public-speaking-practice-and-ethics/s20-03-organizingpersuasive-speeches.html.
21. Fisher, R.U. and Ury, W.W. (1981). *Getting to Yes: Negotiating Agreement without Giving In*. Boston: Houghton Mifflin.
22. Forsyth, D.R. (2009) *Group Dynamics*, 5th edn. Pacific Grove, CA: Brooks/Cole.
23. Chapman, S. (2004) Advocacy for public health: A primer. *J Epidemiol Community Health* 58, 361–365.
24. Weber, M. (1958) *The Three Types of Legitimate Rule* (translation). Quoted in: *Tripartite classification of authority*. Wikipedia website at en.wikipedia.org/wiki/Tripartite_classification_of_authority. Berkeley, CA: University of California.
25. Binney, G. and Williams, C. (1995) *Leaning into the Future: Changing the Way People Change Organizations*. London, UK: Nicholas Brealey Publishing Ltd.
26. Stevenson, H. (n.d.) *Leadership and Change: Some Writings of John Kotter*. Accessed online March 23, 2014 at http://www.clevelandconsultinggroup.com/articles/leadershipand-change-writings-of-john-kotter.php.
27. Checkland (1980). *Systems Thinking, Systems Practice*. New York: Wiley.
28. Cancer services: Case for change. March 2010. http://www.londonhp.nhs.uk/wp-content/uploads/2011/03/Cancer-case-for-change.pdf; http://www.londoncancer.org/.
29. Iles, V. Briefing paper one: Systems thinking. Accessed online May 7, 2014 at http://www.reallylearning.com/Free_Resources/Systems_Thinking/systems_thinking.html.
30. The management centre (undated). Management thought leadership. Accessed online July 20, 2014 at http://www.managementcentre.co.uk/management-consultancy/thought-leadership.
31. Mind Tools. (2014) *The McKinsey 7S Framework: Ensuring That All Parts of Your Organization Work in Harmony*. Accessed online May 7, 2014 at http://www.mindtools.com/pages/article/newSTR_91.htm.
32. Handy (1976) Understanding organizations, London, Penguin. Summarised in: OpenLearn. (2014) Management: Perspective and practice, Section 3.5.2. Handy's four types of organisational cultures. Open University. Accessed online March 23, 2014 at: http://www.open.edu/openlearn/money-management/management/leadership-and-management/management-perspective-and-practice/content-section-5.5.2.
33. Barringer, B.R. and Harrison, J.S. (2000) Walking a tightrope: Creating value through interorganizational relationships. *J Manag* 26, 367–403.
34. Rosen, R. and Ham, C. (2008) *Integrated Care: Lessons from Evidence and Experience*. London, UK: Nuffield Trust.
35. Dunbar, R.I.M. (1992) Neocortex size as a constraint on group size in primates. *J Hum Evol* 22, 469–493.
36. Anon (2009) Primates on facebook. The economist. Accessed online July 20, 2014 at http://www.economist.com/node/13176775.
37. Mullins, L.J. (2005) The nature of leadership. In: Mullins, L.J. (ed.) *Management and Organisational Behaviour* (7th edn.). Harlow, UK: Financial Times/Prentice Hall.
38. Boaden, R., Harvey, G., Moxham, C., and Proudlove, N. (2008) *Quality Improvement: Theory and Practice*. Coventry, UK: NHS Institute for Innovation and Improvement. Accessed online March 23, 2014 at http://www.lj.se/info_files/infosida32905/quality_improvement_nhs.pdf.
39. Deming (1986). Summarised in: Boaden, R., Harvey, G., Moxham C., and Proudlove, N. (2008). Quality

Improvement:Theory and Practice. NHS Institute for Innovation and Improvement. [Online]. Available at http://www.lj.se/info_files/infosida32905/quality_improvement_nhs.pdf [Accessed: 23 March 2014].

40. Anon (undated) Quality and service improvement tools: Performance management. NHS Institute for Innovation and Improvement website, now NHS Improving Quality. Accessed online July 29, 2014 at http://www.institute.nhs.uk/quality_and_service_improvement_tools/quality_and_service_improvement_tools/performance_management.html.
41. Schonn (1998) Improvement: Theory and practice. http://www.lj.se/info_files/infosida32905/quality_improvement_nhs.pdf.
42. Goodwin, E. (2006) *Healthcare Management*. Maidenhead, UK: Open University Press. Chapter 11, p. 183.
43. Brownson, R.C., Seiler, R., and Eyler, A.A. (2010) Measuring the impact of public health policy. *Prevent Chron Dis* 7(4), A77. Accessed January 13, 2013 at http://www.cdc.gov/pcd/issues/2010/jul/09_0249.htm.
44. European Commission (undated) Health strategy: Policy. Accessed online July 20, 2014 at http://ec.europa.eu/health/strategy/policy/index_en.htm.
45. HM Government, Modernising government, The Stationery Office, March 1999.
46. Gilson, L. et al. (2012) Using stakeholder analysis to support moves towards universal coverage: Lessons from the SHIELD project. *Health Policy Plan* 27, i64–i76. doi:10.1093/heapol/czs007.
47. Glasgow, R.E., Vogt, T.M., and Bowls, S.M. (1999) Evaluating the public health impact of health promotion interventions: The RE-AIM framework. *Am J Public Health* 89(9), 1322–1327.
48. Kono, T. (1984) *Strategy and Structure of Japanese Enterprises*. London, UK: Macmillan.
49. Zahra, S.A. (1991) Predictors and financial outcomes of corporate entrepreneurship: An exploratory study. *J Bus Venturing* 6, 259–285.
50. Walt, G., Shiffman, J., Schneider, H., Murray, S.F., Brugha, R., and Gilson, L. (2008) "Doing" health policy analysis: Methodological and conceptual reflections and challenges. *Health Policy Plan* 23, 308–317.
51. Lasswell (1956). Summarised in: Walt, G. et al. (2008) "Doing" health policy analysis: Methodological and conceptual reflections and challenges. *Health Policy Plan* 23, 308–317.
52. Walt and Gilson (1994). Summarised in: Walt, G. et al. (2008) "Doing" health policy analysis: Methodological and conceptual reflections and challenges. *Health Policy Plan* 23, 308–317.
53. Kingdon (1984). Summarised in: Walt, G. et al. (2008) "Doing" health policy analysis: Methodological and conceptual reflections and challenges. *Health Policy Plan* 23, 308–317.
54. Baumgartner and Jones (1993). Summarised in: Walt, G. et al. (2008) "Doing" health policy analysis: Methodological and conceptual reflections and challenges. *Health Policy Plan* 23, 308–317.
55. Sabatier (1999). Summarised in: Walt, G. et al. (2008) "Doing" health policy analysis: Methodological and conceptual reflections and challenges. *Health Policy Plan* 23, 308–317.
56. Walt's (1994). Summarised in: Walt, G. et al. (2008) "Doing" health policy analysis: Methodological and conceptual reflections and challenges. *Health Policy Plan* 23, 308–317.
57. Osman, F.A. (2002) Public policy making: Theories and their implications in developing countries.
58. Fair society healthy lives. *The Marmot Review*, February 2010. http://www.instituteofhealthequity.org/projects/fair-society-healthy-lives-the-marmot-review.
59. Department of Health (undated) Modernisation of health and care. Accessed online July 20, 2014 at http://healthandcare.dh.gov.uk/guide-system.
60. Green, A. (2007) *An Introduction to Health Planning for Developing Health Systems*. Oxford, UK: Oxford University Press, 2007.
61. Welsh Assembly Government (2009) Explanatory Memorandum to the Local Health Boards (Establishment and Dissolution) (Wales) Order 2009. Accessed online July 20, 2014 at http://www.assemblywales.org/sub-ld7452-em-e.pdf.
62. National Services Division, National Services Scotland (2012) Available at http://www.nsd.scot.nhs.uk/index.html.
63. Davies, P. (2007) *The NHS in the UK 2007/08: A Pocket Guide*. The NHS Confederation: London, UK.
64. Delamothe, T. (2008) Founding principles. *BMJ* 336, 1216.
65. NI Direct Government Services (2014) Prescription charges. Accessed online July 20, 2014 at http://www.nidirect.gov.uk/prescription-charges.
66. Gilson, L. and Raphaely, N. (2008) *Health Policy Plan* 23(5), 361–368. doi:10.1093/heapol/czn021.
67. Klein, R. (2006) *The New Politics of the NHS: From Creation to Reinvention*. Oxford, UK: Radcliffe Publishing Ltd.

68. The NHS Confederation (2007) *The NHS in the UK 2007/08: A Pocket Guide*. London, UK.
69. NICE (2012) How NICE clinical guidelines are developed: An overview for stakeholders, the public and the NHS (5th edn.). Accessed online July 20, 2014 at http://publications.nice.org.uk/how-nice-clinical-guidelines-are-developed-an-overview-for-stakeholders-the-publicand-the-nhs-pmg6f/nice-clinical-guidelines.
70. Holder, R. and Thorlby, R. (2013) The new NHS in England: Structure and accountabilities. The Nuffield Trust. Accessed online July 20, 2014 at http://www.nuffieldtrust.org.uk/talks/slideshows/newstructure-nhs-england.
71. NHS Choices (2013) Get involved in the NHS. Accessed online July 20, 2014 at http://www.nhs.uk/NHSEngland/thenhs/about/Pages/getinvolved.aspx.
72. Donaldson, L.J. (2001) Professional accountability in a changing world. *Postgrad Med J* 77, 65–67.
73. National Clinical Assessment Service website. Accessed online July 20, 2014 at http://www.ncas.nhs.uk/about-ncas/.
74. Department of Health (2012). News story: Chief Medical Officer revalidated as doctor. Accessed online July 20, 2014 at http://www.dh.gov.uk/health/2012/12/chief-medical-officer-revalidated-as-doctor/.
75. General Medical Council revalidation website. Accessed online July 20, 2014 at http://www.gmc-uk.org/doctors/revalidation.asp.
76. Faculty of Public Health revalidation pages. Accessed online July 20, 2014 at http://www.fph.org.uk/revalidation.
77. Levinson, D.R. (November 2010) Adverse events in hospitals: National incidence among medicare beneficiaries. Washington, DC: US Department of Health and Human Services. Available at http://oig.hhs.gov/oei/reports/oei-06-09-00090.pdf.
78. http://www.midstaffsinquiry.com/index.html.
79. NHS Litigation Authority (March 2012) Solicitors' risk management reports on claims: Analysis and annual review 2010/11. http://www.nhsla.com/Pages/Home.aspx.
80. Blunt, I. and Bardsley, M. (2012) Use of patient-level costing to increase efficiency in NHS trusts. The Nuffield Trust. Accessed online July 20, 2014 at http://www.nuffieldtrust.org.uk/sites/files/nuffield/120920_use_of_patient-level_costing_full_report.pdf.
81. Monitor (2012) Costing patient care: Monitor's approach to costing and cost collection for price setting. http://www.monitor-nhsft.gov.uk/sites/default/files/Costing%20Patient%20Care%20201112%20%20FINAL_0.pdf.
82. Yorkshire and Humber Health Intelligence. PCT CCG Spend and Outcome Factsheets and Tool (SPOT). Public Health England. Accessed online July 20, 2014 at http://www.yhpho.org.uk/spot.
83. http://www.monitor-nhsft.gov.uk/sites/default/files/publications/Introduction_to_SLR_screenview.pdf.
84. HFMA (professional body for healthcare finance professionals) website. Accessed online July 20, 2014 at www.hfma.org.uk.
85. Brambleby, P., Jackson, A., and Stewart, I. Using programme budgeting and marginal analysis to deliver quality, innovation productivity and prevention. Report. Accessed online July 20, 2014 at http://www.rightcare.nhs.uk/downloads/third_annual_pop_review.pdf.
86. Brambleby, P. and Fordham, R.J. (2003) What is PBMA? Evidence-based-medicine. http://www.medicine.ox.ac.uk/bandolier/painres/download/whatis/pbma.pdf.
87. Charlesworth, A., Davies, A., and Dixon, J. (2012) Reforming payment for health care in Europe to achieve better value. Nuffield Trust, London, UK, pp. 9, 15. Accessed online March 23, 2014 at http://www.nuffieldtrust.org.uk/sites/files/nuffield/publication/120823_reforming-payment-for-health-care-ineuropev2.pdf.
88. http://www.institute.nhs.uk/world_class_commissioning/pct_portal/cquin.html.
89. Specialised Services Commissioning Transition Team (2012) Securing equity and excellence in commissioning specialised services. Accessed online July 20, 2014 at http://www.commissioningboard.nhs.uk/files/2012/11/op-model.pdf.
90. The National Audit Office website. Health and social care section. Accessed online July 20, 2014 at http://www.nao.org.uk/sector/health_and_social_care.aspx.
91. Department of Health (October 2012) Choice and competition—The Health and Social Care Act 2012. Factsheet. http://www.dh.gov.uk/health/files/2012/06/C4.-Fact sheet-Choice-andcompetition-270412.pdf.
92. NAO/Department of Health (2011) The procurement of consumables by NHS acute and foundation trusts. Report by the Comptroller and Auditor General. http://www.nao.org.uk/publications/1011/nhs_procurement.aspx.

Section 6

SKILLS TESTED IN THE PART A MFPH EXAMINATION

Sections 1 to 5 of this book have covered the knowledge basis of public health. However, public health specialists also require a broad range of skills in order to function effectively. These skills encompass research (design and interpretation of studies), the manipulation of information (data processing, presentation, and interpretation), and communication.

Skills cannot be learned through reading but instead require application and practice. However, we hope that the tips, formulae, and principles presented in Section 6 will help trainees as they develop these abilities.

6A

Research Design and Critical Appraisal

The ability to design and appraise research is a fundamental public health skill. In offering advice about study design, there is a **balance** to be struck between meeting a **scientific ideal** and the **pragmatics** of conducting the study. Your effectiveness will depend on being able to sell the benefits of a good study method coupled with the **diplomacy** of being able to recognise what is achievable given the realities of running a health service.

The steps involved in conducting a research study begin with an initial idea, followed by the development of a research question and hypothesis, through to the design and conduct of the study. Some of the early priorities will be to consider which individuals to include in the **research team** based on their skills and personality types, as well as the **ethical dimensions** and how the research will be **funded**.

6A.1 Skills in the design of research studies

Key steps in the design of a research study are listed in Table 6A.1.

When designing a study, it is imperative to consider the target audience for the results:

- To whom will the results be addressed?
- How do you intend to communicate with each audience?
- How much will communications cost?
- What do you expect to be the results of your communications?

Table 6A.1 Designing research studies

Stage of the design process	Details	
State the aim of study	Estimating **parameters** of risk. Determining whether there is an **association** between an exposure and an outcome. **Evaluating** an intervention, such as new treatment.	
Hypothesis	An assumption to be tested by conducting the study.	
Choose an appropriate study design	*'How common is this?'*	Prevalence studies such as **surveys**, **ecological** or **descriptive studies**.
	'What caused this?' (particularly for rare disease)	Case–control studies.
	'What effect does this have?' (How does the level of the risk factor affect the outcome?)	Cohort studies.
	'What happens if …?' (test the hypothesis by applying the intervention and observing the outcome)	Interventional/experimental studies, such as an RCT.
	'What or why?' (To explore phenomena, perceptions, and subjective experiences)	Qualitative studies.
Planning	Consider what **resources** are available. Ensure that the study is **ethical**.	
Choose study populations, sampling strategies, and allocation methods	Use **comparison** groups as controls (see Section 1A.7). **Sampling** methods (see Section 1A.25). **Allocation** (see Section 1A.26).	
Measures to reduce errors (see Sections 1A.9, 1D)	**Chance** (sample size, power). **Bias** (randomisation, blindness, standardisation, etc.). **Confounding** (restriction, matching, stratification). *Qualitative studies:* **credibility, plausibility, reflexivity** (rigorous methods, triangulation, researchers' perspective).	
Exposure measurement in the context of observational research	Attention to aspects of **data collection** and processing (including coding, data entry, cleaning, quality control).	

6A.2 Critical appraisal

Ability to critically evaluate papers, including the validity of the use of statistical techniques and the inferences drawn from them.

Critical appraisal is the **systematic process** of assessing and interpreting evidence. It involves judging a paper or study with regard to three factors:

1. **Validity** (Could the findings be explained by chance, bias, or confounding?)
2. **Results** (Are the statistical methods sound?)
3. **Relevance** (Are the findings useful to your organisation?)

A guiding principle when conducting a critical appraisal is that *'just because a study has been published, does not necessarily make it true'*. It is crucial to balance your appraisals: they must be neither overly deferential to the study authors nor too harshly critical.

Critical appraisal frameworks

Frameworks are useful when critically appraising research papers to ensure that all relevant aspects of a study are evaluated.

Here, we describe a generic framework for evaluating any form of study, followed by specialist frameworks for evaluating interventional and observational studies, systematic reviews and meta-analyses, economic evaluations, and qualitative studies.

Generic framework

While different features need to be appraised depending on the type of study design, there are some aspects that are common to all studies (Table 6A.2).

Table 6A.2 Summary of critical appraisal frameworks

Stage	Aspects to appraise	Mnemonic
Start	Summary Aim Population/setting	'Start Appraising Papers'
Middle *(this section depends on the study design)*	**Intervention/observational studies** 1. Methods (internal validity) 2. Result	'Most Research'
	Systematic reviews 1. Study identification/selection 2. Study descriptions 3. Analysis 4. Result	'Select Systematically And Review'
	Economic evaluations 1. Alternatives 2. Design 3. Costs and consequences 4. Effectiveness established 5. Analysis and results	'Appropriately Designed Cost Effectiveness Analyses'
	Qualitative studies 1. Theoretical perspective 2. Data collection 3. Findings	'Translate Deeper Findings'
End	External validity Discussion Relevance	'End Discussing Relevance'

Interventional and observational studies (Table 6A.3)

Table 6A.3 Critical appraisal framework for interventional and observational studies
('SAP MR EDR')

Stage	Aspects to appraise
Start	**Summary** • Type of study and subject • Journal, date • Authors, conflict of interest, funding • Ethics
	Aim • Clearly focused question • Important and relevant • What the study adds to the current literature
	Population/setting • Including exclusion criteria

Middle	**Methods** (internal validity)
	• Design
	  • Appropriateness
	• Sample
	  • Size
	  • Allocation/recruitment
	  • Loss to follow-up
	• Intervention/exposure
	  • Clear, validity, reliability
	• Outcome
	  • Clear, validity, reliability
	• Analysis
	  • Appropriate statistics, intention to treat, adjustments, etc.

	Result
	• Chance
	  • *p*-values, confidence intervals, type 1 error (number of tests), type 2 error (power)
	• Bias
	  • Selection/measurement
	• Confounding
	  • Check baseline characteristics, adjustments, randomisation
	• Truth

Table 6A.3 (*Continued*) Critical appraisal framework for interventional and observational studies **('SAP MR EDR')**

Stage	Aspects to appraise
End	**External validity** (generalisability) • Based on population/setting, internal validity
	Discussion • Discussion of limitations • Conclusions justified?

	Relevance
	• Applicability
	  • To my population/policy/public health (PH) practice
	• Reproducibility
	  • Costs/staff/resources/sustainability

Systematic reviews/meta-analyses (Table 6A.4)

Table 6A.4 Critical appraisal framework for systematic reviews/meta-analyses **('SAP SSAR EDR')**

Stage	Aspects to appraise
Start	**Summary** • Type of study and subject • Journal, date • Authors, conflict of interest, funding • Ethics
	Aim • Clearly focused question • Important and relevant • Exposure/intervention and outcome clearly described
	Population/setting • Including exclusion criteria

Middle	**Study identification/selection**
	• Process clearly described
	  • Permits repeat review
	• Identify all relevant studies
	  • Multiple bibliographical databases, reference list, personal contact with experts, unpublished, non-English

(*continued*)

Table 6A.4 (*Continued*) Critical appraisal framework for systematic reviews/meta-analyses **('SAP SSAR EDR')**

Stage	Aspects to appraise

	• Eligibility criteria
	  • Clearly defined a priori, participants, interventions/exposures, outcome
	• Quality assessed
	  • Clear/appropriate criteria, >1 assessor (inter-rater reliability)

	Study descriptions
	• Description of studies
	  • Have the studies been well described (e.g. in a table), anything missing?
	• Quality of studies
	  • Comment on the quality of the studies included

	Analysis
	• Heterogeneity
	  • Were the studies similar? If not, were reasons for variations explored to test for statistical heterogeneity?
	• Measure of effect
	  • What does it mean, appropriate? Check correct? Crude/adjusted
	• Results combined
	  • Reasonable to do so? (Yes if results were similar; no if heterogeneous) How? (weighting, etc.)
	• Publication bias
	  • Assessed? (e.g. funnel plot)

End	**External validity** (generalisability) • Based on population/setting, internal validity
	Discussion • Discussion of limitations • Conclusions justified?

	Relevance
	• Applicability
	  • To my population/policy/PH practice
	• Reproducibility
	  • Costs/staff/resources/sustainability

Critical appraisal of economic evaluation (Tables 6A.5 and 6A.6)

Table 6A.5 Critical appraisal framework for economic evaluations (**'SAP ADCEA EDR'**)

Stage	Aspects to appraise
Start	**Summary** • Type of study and subject • Journal, date • Authors, conflicts of interest, funding • Ethics
	Aim • Clearly focused question • Important and relevant • Was it designed for a specific decision, who by?
	Population/setting Including exclusion criteria

Middle	**Alternatives**
	• Comprehensively described
	    • Who did what to whom, where, and how often?
	• Appropriate comparator(s)
	    • Normally should include current practice

	Design
	• Type of economic evaluation
	    • CUA, CEA, CBA, etc.
	• Type of analysis
	    • Based on an RCT or simulation model

	Costs and consequences
	• Perspective
	    • All relevant perspectives (e.g. societal, healthcare, patient) and all relevant costs/consequences included
	• Time horizon
	    • Should be long enough to capture all major costs/consequences
	• Measured accurately
	• Valued credibly
	    • Non-monetary/monetary valuation (e.g. how were QALYs calculated)
	• Discounting

(continued)

Table 6A.5 (*Continued*) Critical appraisal framework for economic evaluations **('SAP ADCEA EDR')**

Stage	Aspects to appraise
	Effectiveness established • Validity of effectiveness data

	Analysis and results
	• Incremental
	  • Should show incremental costs and benefits of one over the other
	• Sensitivity analysis
	  • Are conclusions robust to uncertainty in parameter/model

End	**External validity** (i.e. generalisability) • Based on population/setting, internal validity
	Discussion • Discussion of limitations • Conclusions justified?

	Relevance
	• Applicability
	  • To my population/policy/PH practice
	• Reproducibility
	  • Costs/staff/resources/sustainability

Table 6A.6 Critical appraisal framework for qualitative studies **('SAP TDF EDR')**

Stage	Aspects to appraise
Start	**Summary** • Type of study and subject • Journal, date • Authors, conflict of interest, funding • Ethics

	Aim
	• Important research question
	  • Pragmatically and theoretically useful, advances knowledge
	• Appropriate for qualitative study
	  • That is exploratory/open questions

	Population/setting • Researchers' relationship to population/setting also given

Table 6A.6 (*Continued*) Critical appraisal framework for qualitative studies **('SAP TDF EDR')**

Stage	Aspects to appraise
Middle	**Theoretical perspective of the researcher** • For example, positivist, realist, interpretivist

	Data collection and analysis
	• Data collection approach
	  • Suited to the study population and the research question
	• Appropriate sampling strategy
	  • Clearly described
	• Data collection method
	  • Focus groups, interviews, observation, etc.; who collected the data?
	• Data collection tools
	  • Described or included
	• Analytical approach stated
	  • Thematic, grounded theory, framework, etc.
	• Transparent analytical process
	  • All steps and coding frameworks described

	Findings
	• Original data given
	  • For example anonymised quotes
	• Clear and concisely described
	  • Structured in themes, data clearly labelled and support the themes
	• Credible
	  • Approaches to verification given (e.g. triangulation, peer review, debriefing); contradictory data discussed; researchers' role(s) considered

End	**External validity** (generalisability) • Setting and context • Relevance of the study population/setting to generating wider knowledge, theory

	Discussion
	• Reflexivity discussed
	  • Researcher's preconceptions, subjectivity
	• Conclusions justified?
	  • Data provided that support the researchers' themes?

	Relevance • Applicability • To my population/policy/public health practice

Sources: Adapted from Cohen, D. and Crabtree, B., *Ann. Fam. Med.*, 6(4), 331; CASP, 10 questions to help you make sense of qualitative research, http://www.casp-uk.net/wp-content/uploads/2011/11/CASP_Qualitative_Appraisal_Checklist_14oct10.pdf, 2010; Tong, A. et al., *Int. J. Qual. Health Care*, 19(6), 349, doi: 10.1093/intqhc/mzm042, http://intqhc.oxfordjournals.org/content/19/6/349.long

Critical appraisal of statistical techniques

You may not be familiar with the exact statistical analysis used in the paper that you are appraising. However, this need not be intimidating: simply interpret the statistical test in terms of its *p*-value and the confidence interval.

Other issues to address when critically appraising statistical techniques include the following:

- Do the figures in the **tables add up**?
- Was a **power** calculation used?
- Were **multiple comparisons** made without using the Bonferroni correction or similar?
- Were confidence intervals given?
- Was a ***p*-value** quoted for null results?
- Was the **absolute risk reduction** quoted (not simply the relative risk reduction)?
- Can you suggest an **alternative statistical test** that might have been used?

6A.3 Drawing conclusions from research

Ability to draw appropriate conclusions from quantitative and qualitative research.

In the context of the MFPH Part A examination, ask yourself: Why was this research paper included in today's examination? Are there any traps? Are there any conclusions or inferences that should *not* be drawn? Are there any biases or fundamental flaws? Think of all the possible explanations other than the orthodox.

Conclusions drawn from research should clearly state whether the findings support or refute the hypothesis posed. The public health relevance of the findings can then be described by considering whether they

- Justify or prove the **effectiveness** of a programme
- Serve to refine an **existing theory**
- Can be used to develop a **new theory**

The *BMJ* (bmj.bmjjournals.com/advice/sections.html) recommends that conclusions should be structured as follows:

- Statement of **principal findings**
- **Strengths** and **weaknesses** of the study
- Strengths and weaknesses in **relation to other studies**, discussing important differences in results
- **Meaning** of the study: possible explanations and implications for clinicians and policymakers
- **Unanswered questions** and **future research**

6B

Drawing Conclusions from Data

6B.1 Drawing conclusions from data

Ability to sort and manipulate data and to draw appropriate conclusions from quantitative and qualitative data.

A fundamental skill for all public health specialists is the ability to handle data and to draw appropriate conclusions. Sometimes, public health specialists may need to present data that they themselves have collected and analysed. At other times, it requires a critical review of the conclusions and data presented by others.

Summary statistics and graphical techniques can be used to highlight trends and to make comparisons within quantitative data. For example, frequencies may be illustrated using a bar chart or a pie chart (for categorical data) or using a histogram (for continuous data).

Transforming raw data into meaningful information

See also Sections 1B.9 and 1B.10.

Well-presented tables, figures, and graphs enable the reader to identify patterns and to draw contrasts in the data that would otherwise not be immediately apparent.

Tables

When displaying data in tables, aim to follow the following rules:

- Sort in a **meaningful order** (e.g. largest to smallest rather than random or alphabetical order).
- **Label** the table correctly: rows and columns (with units), together with the title for the table itself.
- Two **significant figures** or **decimal places** generally provide sufficient information for the reader.
- **Rates** are often more useful than numbers for comparing data (but the denominators must be comparable).

Graphs

When generating graphs, follow the principles of clarity, simplicity, and transparency (see Box 6B.1).

Which graph to use?

See also Section 1B.8.

Table 6B.1 provides guidance as to the choice of graph for different circumstances.

Common pitfalls in graphical display

There are several ways in which a poor graphical display can cloud or distort the message that it intended to convey. These shortcomings include the following:

- *'Chart junk'* (i.e. unnecessary graphics or text on charts)
- Overuse of 3D or complex graphical designs that obfuscate the main message and may bias the presentation (e.g. items at the back of a 3D chart appear smaller than those at the front)
- Incorrect or insufficient labelling
- Scaling problems
    - Too small to see trends
    - No zero
    - Distorted scales (see the 'gee-whiz' graph in Figure 6B.1)

Box 6B.1 Principles for choosing an appropriate graph

Principle	Details
Clarity	Label the graph (title, axes, units) completely but succinctly. Use scales appropriately: fill as much of the graph's space with data. Maintain convention by starting the axes of the graph from zero. Ensure that the colour or pattern of lines or bars clearly differentiates each category.
Simplicity	Consider Edward Tufte's **ink-to-data** ratio by using the least ornate format of data to convey the message (i.e. choose a table rather than a bar chart, a bar chart rather than a pie chart, etc.). Use few gridlines. Use 3D designs only where a 2D design would be inappropriate. Be selective with content: only include relevant data.
Transparency	Provide a source and date for the data wherever possible. If the data have been transformed (e.g. divided into categories or calculated as percentages), then provide the raw data as well.

- Spurious comparisons (e.g. unequal denominators; numbers provided rather than rates)
- Too many data points
- Too few data points

Example 1: The effects of scaling on data presentation ('gee-whiz' graphs)

Depending on how the data in Figure 6B.1 are presented, the effectiveness of the New Year diet plan can appear to be very different.

Example 2: Choosing appropriate graphical design formats

See Table 6B.2.

Drawing conclusions from data displays

See also Appendix A.

When presented with data, it is tempting to focus immediately on the detail. However, it is generally better to describe observations in a logical order, such as the following:

- What **type** of display (chart/plot) is it?
- What **information** is it attempting to show? (title, x and y axes, and scale)
- What **shapes** do you observe? (e.g. bell?, skewed?, linear increase?, sharp increase or spike?, J and S shapes?)
- What **similarities and differences** do you notice?
    - Range of data—highest/lowest
    - Trends
- How do you **interpret** what you see? Are there alternative explanations?
- What **caveats** would you note?
    - Quality of the presentation (simplicity, clarity, transparency)
    - Quality of data handling, manipulation
    - Comprehensiveness of the data (other information that you would need to strengthen your interpretation).

See Box 6B.2.

Data analysis packages

For both quantitative and qualitative data, statistical packages are widely used to accelerate the process of data manipulation and display (see Table 6B.3). However, the effectiveness of such software still relies on a fundamental understanding of what the data mean.

Table 6B.1 Summary of display graphs

	Type of display	Strengths	Weaknesses
Any data	Table	Displays details of the data that would be lost in charts or text	Difficult to visualise relationships and trends
Categorical data	Pie chart	Displays proportions Easily understood, popular in lay materials (e.g. newspapers)	Sometimes difficult to gauge the size of pie slices by eye Difficult to compare proportions across two pie charts
	Bar graph 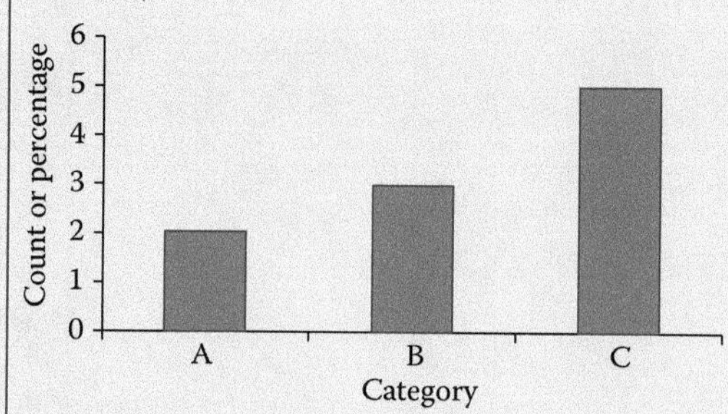	Summarises large amounts of data in a visual form Trends and relationships easy to visualise Relatively simple; so, accessible to a range of audiences	Scaling effects (i.e. when one variable is much greater than others, this reduces the scale of the graph and therefore makes it difficult to visualise small changes in other variables)
Univariate numerical data	Box and whisker 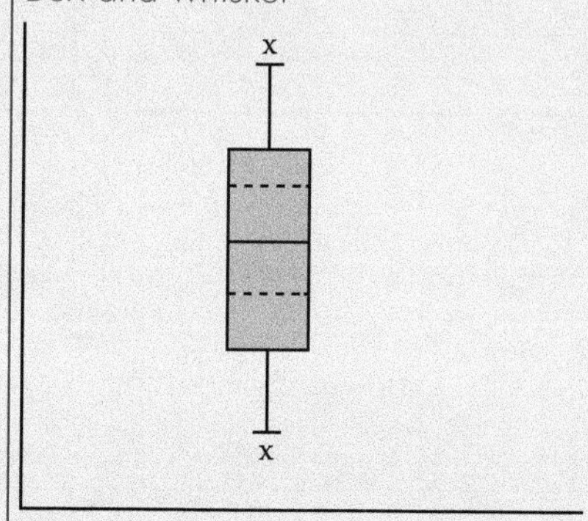	Median and range of data points easily identifiable Useful for comparing two or more sets of data	Relatively complex; not readily accessible to a wide range of readers Exact values are not retained
	Histogram 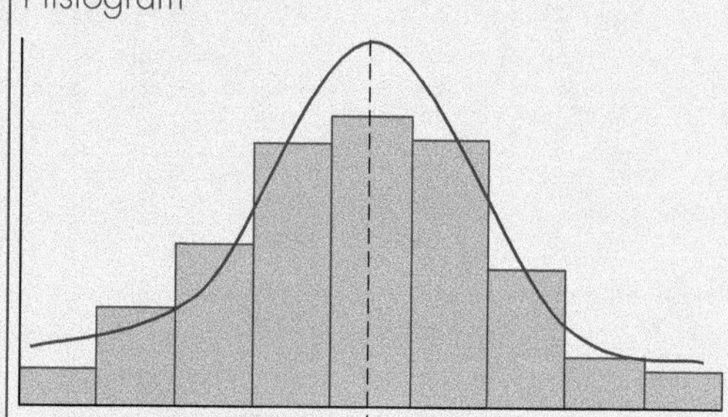	Illustrates the shape of the frequency distribution (e.g. symmetrical or skewed)	Does not display exact numbers, only category bands

(continued)

Table 6B.1 (*Continued*) Summary of display graphs

	Type of display	Strengths	Weaknesses
Bivariate numerical data	Line graph 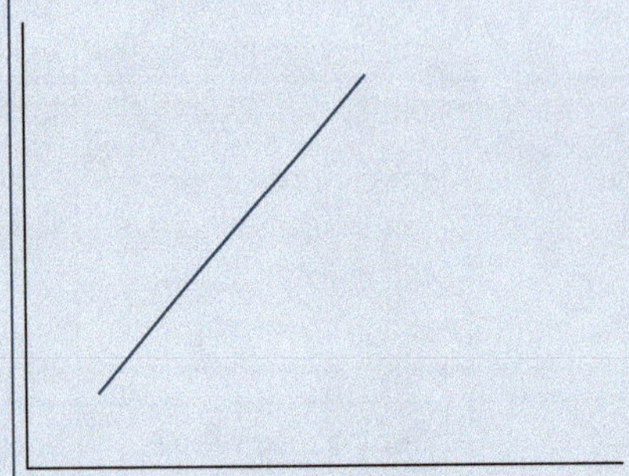	Clearly displays the relationships between a dependent variable and an independent variable Displays trends (e.g. changes over time)	Temptation to extrapolate beyond data points Difficult to distinguish between lines (particularly if printed on black and white or poorly photocopied) Scaling effects can bias the results (e.g. on a 0–100 scale, a change of two points looks small, whereas on a scale of 30–40, a change of two points looks large)
	Scatterplot 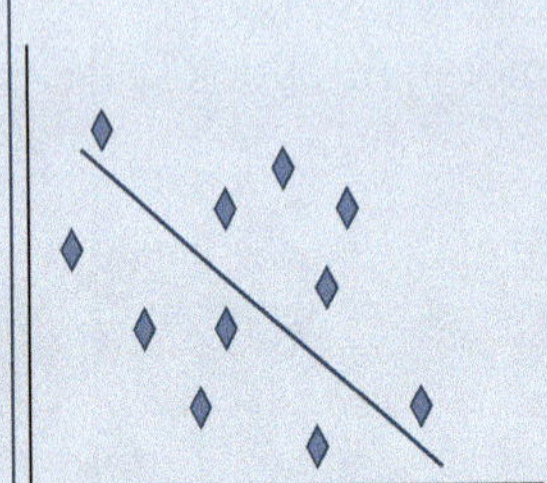	Shows minimum, maximum, and outliers Illustrates the relationships between variables	Hard to visualise results, trends, and relationships for large datasets

Table 6B.1 (*Continued*) Summary of display graphs

	Type of display	Strengths	Weaknesses
Other	Flowchart 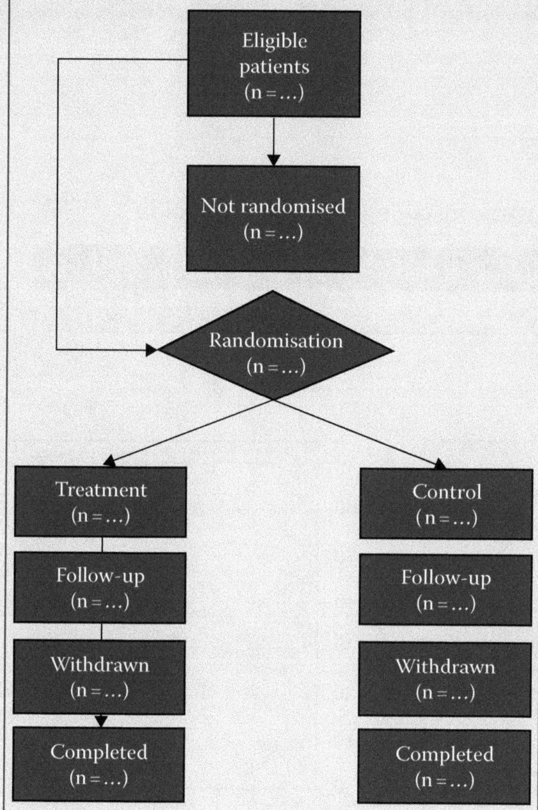	Illustrates a series of steps in a procedure, decision, or other stepwise process Essential in RCTs to show the proportion of original units of analysis retained by the end of the study	Potential to oversimplify processes or procedures
	Maps Qualitative: mind maps/organisational maps Coded mapping (e.g. MapInfo)	Shows relationships between areas Allows rates to be compared between and among regions and countries	Potential to distort (e.g. large rural areas with small populations appear bigger on a map than small urban areas with a high population density)

Individual's weight by week following new year diet plan

	1 Jan	8 Jan	15 Jan	22 Jan	29 Jan
Weight (kg)	73	72.5	72	70	69.5

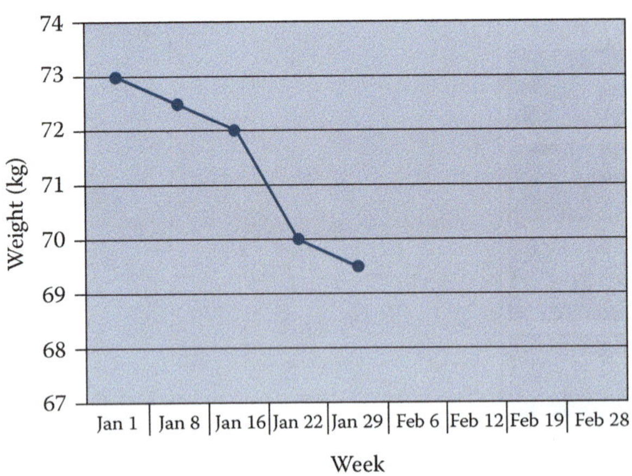

'Gee-Whiz'-amplified change
Most of the y-axis scale is missing (67–74 kg)
2 months shown: x-axis compressed, relative to vertical

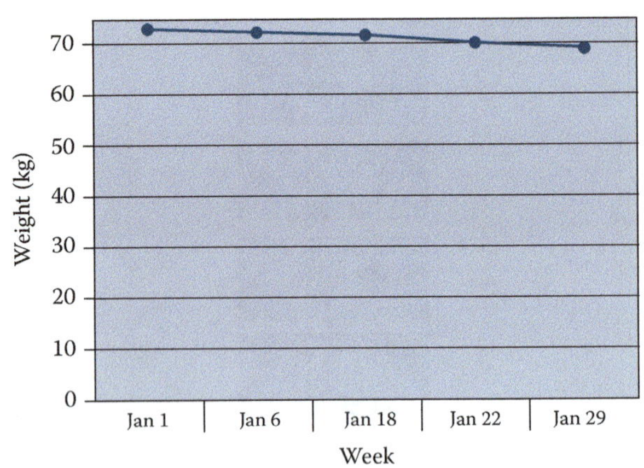

Normal scaling—reduced change
All of the scale is shown (y-axis 0–75 kg)
x-axis only 1 month

Figure 6B.1 Illustration of how the Gee-Whiz graph amplifies change.

Table 6B.2 Choosing a graphical design format

Choosing the right methods for displaying data

Area	Ethnicity (%) White	South Asian	African/Caribbean
A	81	6.1	3.2
B	63	21	6.0
C	42	45	11

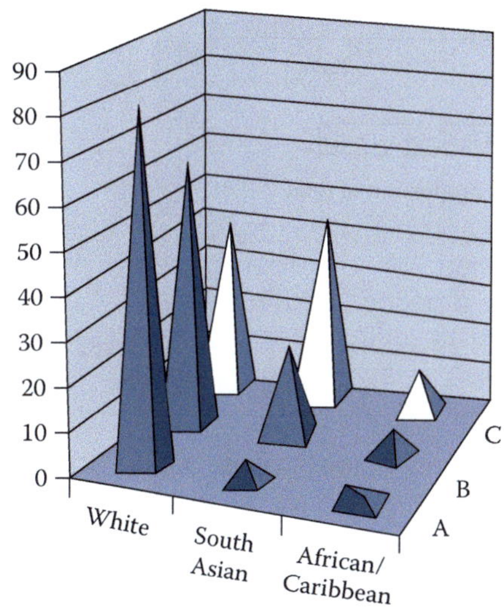

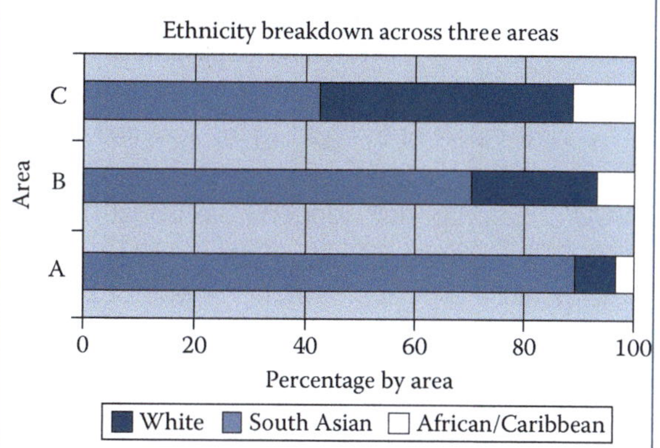

	Weaknesses	Strengths
Design	3D, complex design Takes up more space, confuses message	2D, simple design Enables easy comparison of relative population constituents
Labelling	No title No label or units on *y*-axis, obtrusive labelling of *x*-axis	Title describing what the graph shows Axes labelled with units Legend at the bottom of graph, taking up least room possible
Scaling	Size disparity between categories: difficult to see relative differences in each ethnic category, cannot read off the values	Scale appropriate for category sizes—enables comparison between three areas

Box 6B.2 Example: Interpreting a line graph

GP registered patients (15–75 years) with a recorded BMI of 30 or over

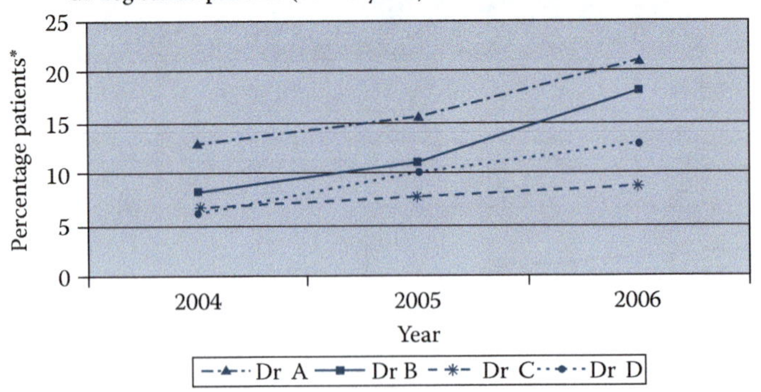

*Registered patients with recorded BMI 30+ as a proportion of total GP registered population.

This is a line graph, showing the proportion of patients registered with four different general practices with a recorded BMI of over 30 kg/m^2 (clinically obese) in a 3-year period (2004–2006).

In all practices, the proportion of patients considered clinically obese rose between 2004 and 2006. In 2004, the proportion ranged from about 6% in Dr D's practice to 14% in Dr A's practice. In 2006, the proportion ranged from just under 9% in Dr C's practice to 21% in Dr A's practice.

The increase was approximately linear for Dr C's practice, with an increase of roughly 1% for each year. The increase was steeper in Dr D's practice in 2004–2005 than in 2005–2006. In contrast, the increase for Dr A's and Dr B's practices was greater in 2005–2006 than in 2004–2005.

The graph indicates the following features:

- There appears to be a clear trend of growing obesity prevalence in all four practices.
- The proportion of obese patients varies by practice and this variation has increased since 2004, possibly indicating increasing health inequalities within the area.

However, the data should be interpreted with caution because of the following:

- The graph only indicates the proportion of patients registered with the GP with a recorded BMI of 30 kg/m^2 and above; therefore, it may simply be showing that the recording of BMI has increased. It would have been more useful to use a different denominator for the percentage calculations (e.g. people with a BMI 30 kg/m^2 as a percentage of all patients registered with the practice where BMI was recorded).
- The data have been divided into just two categories: a BMI of 30 kg/m^2 and above and a BMI below 30 kg/m^2. It would be helpful to have information on the raw values to find the range and the dispersal of BMI by practice over time.
- Only three years' worth of data are presented here; data from previous years would be helpful to forecast with greater confidence how the prevalence of obesity might change over time.

Table 6B.3 Statistical packages for different types of data

Type of data	Statistical packages
Qualitative	Packages such as ***NUD*IST, MaxQDA,*** and ***NVivo*** allow textual data to be searched and sorted. Segments of interest can be noted and marked with codes. The packages allow analyses to be performed on these codes, which can then be saved, exported, or subjected to further analysis.
Quantitative	Most data require processing prior to analysis. Data columns (i.e. variables) need to be checked for accuracy and may need to be re-arranged, re-coded, or re-ordered. Some tables may need to be combined with others, especially if the data are drawn from a relational database. Programs such as ***Microsoft Access***™ can do much of this analysis, although programming skill is required. A most versatile program, in terms of ease of use and the fact that it is to be found on most computers, is ***Microsoft Excel***™. This software is very useful for re-shaping and re-presenting data. Its graphs and tables are easy to produce, which is a particularly useful for novice users. In epidemiology, ***EpiInfo***™ can create questionnaires, store the data collected, then manipulate, analyse, and display the results. In general public health, the following statistical packages are often used: **SAS**™, **SPSS**™, and **STATA**™. The relative merits of these packages depend on the type of data, the analysis that needs to be performed, and the user's technical abilities and preferences.
Geographical	GISs such as ***MapInfo***™ offer a range of ways to manipulate and display information with a geographical component.

6C

Written Presentation Skills

6C.1 Written presentation skills

The ability to communicate clearly and effectively is a vital public health skill. Whether or not you communicate well can make the difference between your efforts leading to significant changes or gathering dust on a shelf. Always make sure that you have thought about each of the following three principles before committing pen to paper: **preparation**, **organisation,** and **customisation**.

Preparation

Before you start writing, consider the issues listed in Box 6C.1.

Organisation

Box 6C.2 sets out a number of ways to organise your writing.

Customisation

Make sure that your document addresses the purpose for which you were asked to write it. This process may involve rechecking with the person, team, or organisation that commissioned you to write it. Ensure that the **language** you use is appropriate for your audience. Aim for your writing to display the characteristics listed in Box 6C.3.

Conclusions

You should always **check** and then **summarise** what you have written by

- Referring back to the original instructions periodically: does what you have written meet the **original brief?**
- Although the executive summary will normally be at the start of your document, **write the summary last,** after reviewing what you have written. This delay should help ensure that the summary closely reflects the rest of the document.
- **Read what you have written**. Ideally, it is useful to leave written work a few days before checking and submitting it.
- Assuming you have written electronically, **use a spelling and grammar checker**. This tool is not a substitute for reading the document yourself, but it will pick up many errors and may suggest simpler sentence structures.
- Remove any embedded comments and tracked changes before submitting a document electronically.

Note: In an examination, it is questionable whether an extensive summary should be included because conclusions do not contain any new material and therefore may not attract new marks. Likewise, it is debatable whether or not to spend time checking what you have written.

Box 6C.1 Preparing for writing

Principle	Description
Brief	Why are you writing? What are your constraints (e.g. time, word count)?
Audience	Who is your intended audience? Different types of language, structures, and content will be appropriate for different audiences. Think about your audience in terms of their: • Familiarity with the subject matter • Education/understanding • Culture • Point of view

Note: In the MFPH Part A examination, candidates are tested on their written presentation skills. It is tempting in the examination setting to skimp on the amount of time you spend preparing the structure and presentation of your answers; however, to do so is a false economy.

Box 6C.2 Organising your writing

Method	Description
Structure	Use a **clear structure** for your written presentations (in the rest of this chapter some standard formats and structures for particular audiences and purposes are given).
Signposts	Add **signposting** paragraphs or sentences that explain to the reader how you have organised the text.
Subheadings	Use **subheadings** to help your reader navigate through your writing and to help you keep to the topic at hand.
Lists	Use **lists** and **bullets** interspersed throughout your prose.

Note: In an examination, it is absolutely vital to sketch out the structure of your answer before you start writing.

Box 6C.3 Writing for publication

Characteristic	Description
Clarity and **simplicity**	Use the simplest language appropriate for your audience: choose short words rather than long ones, keep sentences concise, prefer the active voice to the passive, aim to include 'flesh and blood' in every sentence (i.e. a person or character), begin each sentence with concepts that were introduced in the previous sentence, and place newer, more complex concepts to the end of each sentence.
Precision and **brevity**	Sometimes, technical language and abbreviations may be appropriate, but these should be defined at the first usage. Only use jargon if it provides a more precise way of expressing yourself in fewer words, and you anticipate that your audience will understand.
Neutral and **respectful language**	Avoid using words or phrases that could be construed as pejorative or insulting by some members of your audience. Common pitfalls include the term 'innocent victims' (implying that there are some guilty ones), defining groups by disease or characteristics (e.g. schizophrenics, diabetics, or insomniacs, as opposed to people with schizophrenia, diabetes, or sleeping problems), and sexist terms (e.g. workmen).

Note: In an examination, ensure that your writing addresses the question asked. Under pressure, it can be tempting to summarise all that you know about a subject or to adhere to a framework that you are comfortable with, whether it fits the question or not.

6C.2 Preparation of papers for publication

Before writing a paper, start the process by agreeing the main message (ideally in one sentence) and the order of the paper's authors. This clarity should help prevent conflicts later on in the process about the direction of the paper and any authorship disputes.

A paper should be structured along the lines shown in Box 6C.4.

The structure of a research paper is sometimes likened to the shape of a martini glass in cross section. The start of the introduction is analogous to the broad rim of the martini glass: it considers global issues. Over the course of the introduction, the focus becomes increasingly narrow. The methods section and the results section are represented by the narrow stem of the martini glass. Finally, the discussion is represented by the base of the glass, which begins with a narrow consideration of the additional contribution of the paper to the scientific paper and then broadens slightly (although not as broad as the rim of the glass) to consider potential implications for policymakers, clinical practice, and future research.

Submission process

Choose the journal carefully, ensuring

- Relevance to the subject
- Potential audience
- Impact factor

Box 6C.4 Structure for a typical journal article

Title

Keyword list

Used by the indexing and abstracting services (e.g. MeSH terms).

Abstract

(*Most journals specify a length, typically not exceeding 250 words*)

Principal objectives and scope of the investigation.

Summarise the results.

Principal conclusions.

Introduction

Context, background, literature review.

Why was there a need to conduct the study? Introduce pertinent literature.

Methods

Major study design elements:

- Sample
- Measurements
- Statistical models and testing

Include details of ethics approval.

Results

Combine the use of text, tables, and figures to condense data and highlight trends. Refer to the publisher's guidelines for preparing tables and figures.

Discussion (see also Section 6A.3)

Generalisations that can be drawn.

How the findings compare with the findings of others and with any expectations based on previous work.

Any theoretical or practical implications of your work.

Consider the limitations of work.

References

Check the publication's style.

The reference list should contain all references cited in the text; likewise, every reference list should appear in the text.

Use the reference format required by the publication (include with each reference details of the author(s), year of publication, title of article, name of journal or book, place of publication of books, volume, and page numbers).

Be consistent in the use of journal abbreviations.

Box 6C.4 (*Continued*) Structure for a typical journal article

Authorship

Order: Modern journals have strict rules regarding authorship and contributorship.

Acknowledgements

Grant-awarding body
Clerical support, etc.
Conflicts of interest

Most journals will have their own requirements on what they will accept for submission. When dealing with reviews

- Remain respectful of the editor and reviewers at all times.
- Organise the final version of the paper carefully before submission.
- Incorporate any helpful comments and resubmit, giving a point-by-point response to how you addressed all the reviewers' comments (including those comments you did not address).

If you are resubmitting an article to a different journal because of a rejection, then the article should be thoroughly redrafted and reformatted for the new journal. Goulding [4] summarises the main points to consider for different types of scientific publication.

6C.3 Presenting to different audiences

Preparation of material for different audiences, including expert and non-expert audiences; the media and information handling; and use of the media in advising the public about health services, disease prevention, and health promotion.

Slide presentations

PowerPoint™ is currently the most common way of delivering a professional presentation. For a presentation to be effective, it is important that the slides are produced in a format that is appropriate to the audience.

Producing effective slides

- Minimise the content per slide: 3–5 bullets, 5–6 words long (or use a simple graph, figure or picture)
- Ensure that the presentation is readable:
  - Font: size 20+; sans serif; high contrast with the background
  - Template consistent on all slides
  - Inconspicuous background colour and design
- Use slide animation sparingly, if at all

Preparation

Practice the presentation (e.g. audio or video recording).

Time its length.

Arrive early on the day and check that your presentation runs on the projector and computer or bring your own equipment.

Presentation

Talk to the audience not to the screen.

Use the slides as prompts: do not simply read off the screen or read from a script or presenter's notes.

Use a loud, low-pitched, slow voice (aim to speak at half the pace you would normally speak).

Combine with other formats (e.g. interact with the audience; include video; provide handouts).

Disseminating information

Press releases

General principles for press releases are described in Table 6C.1.

The format and content of a press release will vary to some extent depending on the issuing organisation and on the story itself. A standard layout is shown in Box 6C.5.

Interview briefings

Be clear about what **information** and what **impression** you want to leave with the audience. You should plan your own responses in advance and prepare for related issues—and topical matters—that may also be asked about. Always consider the **perspective** of the interviewer and that of the audience.

Organisations are likely to have their own format for briefings, but the following kinds of information will typically be generated in consultation with the **communications officer.**

Arrangements

- Interview for station/programme/presenter/newspaper
- Time
- Date
- Telephone/studio
- Live/pre-record

Key points

Identify **three** key points and ensure that they are

- In plain English and suitable for a general audience
- Short and memorable

Note that it is useful here to have *'bridging phrases'* handy. These acknowledge the question that was asked but also ensure that the key points are covered, for example, *'and this leads me on to…'* and *'…but the real issue is….'*

Background

- **Target audience** of radio station/newspaper, for example, ABC1 women, teenagers/young people, professional men.
- Agenda and **point of view** of the media (e.g. anti-/pro-public health issue?)
- Any other people due to be interviewed? Their viewpoint(s)?
- Topic(s) of the interview: some media will send through a list of questions/topics for the interview in advance if requested.

Submission

A submission from a civil servant to a minister should take the format shown in Box 6C.6.

Table 6C.1 Principles for press releases

Principles	Details
Information pyramid	Put the most important information at the beginning of the release, with less important material further down. (Imagine that the release could be 'cut' at any point from the bottom of the page upwards.)
Keep it short	Short **sentences** (~20 words). Short **paragraphs** (~2 or 3 sentences each). Short **release** (~2 pages in total, including notes to editors).
Active voice	Use the active, not the passive, voice (i.e. say *'Researchers found that …'* not *'It was found that …'*).
Non-technical language	Use lay terms wherever possible (e.g. use *'link'* not *'epidemiological association'*; use *'breathing'* not *'pulmonary'*).
Messages	Use the release to include **established public health messages** (e.g. effects of smoking).

Box 6C.5 Sample structure for a press release

Organisation

Date

Press release

Title, e.g. *New Research Links Smoking and Cot Death*

Embargoed until … hours, date (or for immediate release)

Subtitle (e.g. *'Reducing Parents' Smoking May Cut Baby Deaths'*)

Paragraph 1

Cover: **Who? What? Where? When?**

For example, *researchers (who) at X University (where) have linked cot deaths with smoking (what) in a paper published today* (when).

Paragraph 2

More details, answering '**how?**'

For example, *over 1000 families answered various questions about their lifestyle, health, and living conditions.*

Paragraph 3

More detail/**why?**

For example, *researchers believe the effects of smoking could be… or it is too early to understand why smoking has these effects.*

Paragraph 4

Quote from someone in authority or connected with the study

For example, *X Director of Public Health, Jane Smith, said, 'This could help reduce cot death …'*; or Professor John Smith, who led the study, said, 'This tells us something new about cot death'.

-ENDS-

Notes to editors:

- Contact details for more information.
- Background information: e.g. x babies die from cot death every year in the United Kingdom; smoking is the biggest preventable cause of death.

Social media

Sharing news as tweets, and information as blogs, is now a mainstream part of how public health professionals should disseminate information. These digital media require different communication styles from reports and press releases. For both tweets and blogs, it is important to

- Distinguish personal from professional social media activities (e.g. consider using a different account for professional and personal communications)
- Be mindful of information governance and corporate reputation in governing what information can be shared

Box 6C.6 Example structure for submission from civil servant to minister

To: [Minister]

From: [Author]
[Job title]
Clearance: [Senior official]
Date: February 15, 2013
Copy: [other officials]

Title

Issue

Recommendations

Background

Briefing

Costs

Annex A

Annex B, etc.

- Ensure your organisation has sufficient resources to commit to blogging or tweeting regularly and frequently and to respond to comments
- Have a second pair of eyes to read your output before you publish it

Tweets

Twitter is a microblogging service where users send and read text-based messages of up to 140 characters. Tweets are, by default, publicly available; however, it is possible to restrict access. Subscribers can opt to 'follow' individuals or organisations to receive tweets from them in their 'timeline'. Features of tweets include the following:

- Hashtags: Words or phrases prefixed with a '#' sign are used to index posts by topic.
- The '@' sign followed by a username is used for mentioning or replying to other users (if the @ sign appears at the start of a tweet, then only followers who also follow the person being referred to will see the tweet in their timeline; however, the tweet is still public and will appear in searches).
- RT: Indicates that the message has been reposted from another Twitter user (a retweet); MT indicates that the message has been modified (a modified tweet).

An LSE report [5] identified three styles of tweets: substantive, conversational, and middle ground. Table 6C.2 lists the pros and cons of each style.

Blogs

A blog is an online journal where readers can add their own comments. Blogs enable writers to express a more informal and personal perspective on an issue than is normally shared in a report. In their blog guidance, the DH Digital Team [6] identified the characteristics of effective blogs (see Table 6C.3).

Clark [7] describes a useful structure for writing a blog, based on the four P's of **promise**, **picture**, **proof,** and **push** (see Table 6C.4).

Table 6C.2 Three styles of tweets

Style	Features	Pros	Cons
Substantive	Tweets always in full sentences. Few abbreviations used, except shortened URLs. Must be independently understandable. Normally tweet is headline or 'taster' for a blog post, web article, or other piece of text. Solely professional or single topic. Team producing tweets often remains invisible.	Always make sense to all readers. Especially accessible when viewed in a combined stream of many tweets from different authors. Attracts followers with well-defined interests.	No conversational element, so can appear impersonal. Takes professional skill to write crisply and substantively.
Conversational	Tweets usually fragment from ongoing conversations with followers. Eclectic content, drawing on professional and personal life, commenting on current events, etc. Includes author photograph.	Conveys personality well. Attracts people who like this personality or culture (usually like-minded). Good at building 'community'.	Hard to follow and may not make sense to those not already involved in conversation in a Twitter feed. Eclectic contents make proportion of tweets not relevant to followers, leading some to unfollow over time.
Middle ground	Most tweets are substantive but some conversational. Goes beyond a 'corporate' focus without being too eclectic. Uses retweets to diversify/ enliven the tweet stream. Uses team photos and blog to identify team members.	Injects more personality or organisational culture into a professional approach. Most tweets are independently understandable.	Some conversational tweets will not make sense when read in combined tweet streams.

Table 6C.3 Characteristics of effective blogs

Characteristic	Description
Well signposted	Use self-describing titles and summaries.
Authentic	Always use your own words (even if based on a policy or briefing). Say things that only you could say.
Responsive	Moderate—and respond to—comments.
Targeted	Write about things that people are already talking about online.
Integrated	Connect your blog with other things you do (e.g. Twitter, guest articles elsewhere, interviews, speeches).

Table 6C.4 Structure for a blog (the four P's)

Element	Contents
Promise	Catch the reader's attention by explaining 'what is in it for them' (i.e. why they should spend the time reading to the end of your blog.
Picture	Paint a picture of the issue at hand using vibrant, descriptive language that is easy to digest. Use this section to hold the reader's emotional interest.
Proof	Provide facts and figures in this section to substantiate your claims (e.g. statistics, references, charts, third-party facts, testimonials).
Push	A call to action, which answers the original promise. For example, the action may be a change of behaviour or a change of opinion by the reader.

Correspondence

Letters

See Box 6C.7.

E-mails

E-mails combine the immediacy of face-to-face communication with the permanence of traditional written correspondence and the audience of broadcast media. When used well, e-mail can be invaluable. However, badly used e-mail is often ignored or may alienate the reader. The style and manner of e-mail correspondence (see Table 6C.5) can ensure that e-mails are effective and well received.

Style

Be **concise:** People receive hundreds or thousands of e-mails per month and can be impatient with unnecessarily long and uninterrupted text.

Be **sensitive**: The tone of communication implicitly conveyed through speech and even handwriting is lost in e-mails—it can be easy to offend through overly terse text or misplaced humor.

Retain the formality of traditional written correspondence when e-mailing people professionally:

Address people whose first name you have not been given as Ms, Mr, Dr, and Professor.

Follow rules of grammar, punctuation, and sentence structure.

Use conventional spellings, few abbreviations, no emoticons, or text language.

Suggested e-mail rules

The following rules should help you avoid some of the pitfalls of e-mail use:

- Consider helping your recipients by constraining yourself to two lines of text (the e-mail subject and the first line of the body of the e-mail), with the rest of the body of the e-mail serving as an appendix that the recipient may obtain additional details but only if interested.
- Avoid using the BCC field (except for mass e-mails; see the following).
- Avoid aggressive use of the CC field (i.e. avoid copying in a person's superior as a form of hostility).
- Reply within 24 hours wherever possible. **Never send an e-mail too hastily**.
- If responding to an offensive message, wait until you are calm enough to respond politely before sending a response or send a short message suggesting that you have a chat.
- Check the contents for errors.
- Observe good e-mail etiquette (see www.emailreplies.com).
- Never e-mail when intoxicated.
- Enable the 'undo send' function, if available (this function introduces a 10-s hold on all outgoing messages, during which the e-mail can be cancelled).

Box 6C.7 Sample structure for professional letters

Headed paper containing:
Organisation
Reply address

Date
Recipient address

Dear ...	***[title/name as they have written to you]***
Re:	**[subject of the letter]**
Paragraph 1	**Thank you for your letter of ....**
Paragraph 2	**Acknowledge concern/query ...**
	For example, 'I acknowledge that X is a particular issue ...'
Paragraph 3	**Background and evidence base for your point of view**
	For example, 'X services are provided currently ...'
Finish	**This is the current situation ...**
	We shall, of course, keep the situation under review.
Further contact	***Please contact me if I can be of further help.***

Yours sincerely*
Name, qualifications
Position

**Use 'Yours faithfully' for letters addressed to Dear Madam or Dear Sir.*

Table 6C.5 Rules for e-mail

Use always	Use sparingly
E-mail signature: Set as a template including the following: Disclaimer and confidentiality message (viruses, if received in error) Your full name and position Organisation name, telephone number, and postal address	**Attachments**: At best, unnecessary attachments are just ignored; at worst they could alienate recipients by clogging e-mail boxes or transmitting viruses.
Subject header: This can determine whether your e-mail is even opened. Good subject headers are concise but indicate what the message will contain. Ideally they should also give some insight into what the recipient needs to do.	**Urgent priority** (marks e-mails as '!'): The recipient is unlikely to respond any quicker to these e-mails if there is no obvious reason for its use.
BCC for mass mailings: Ensure that recipients do not need to scroll down a list of names before the message (write your own e-mail address in the To: field and all other names in the Bcc field).	**Reply to all**: Ensure that e-mails are sent only to those people who need to see them.
Spell checker	**Formatting and graphics**: Hypertext markup language (HTML) formats (e.g. font styles, bullets, tables) may not be retained when sent to different systems.

Strategy document

A standard framework for strategy documents is as follows:

Current position (identify issues)—**Where are we now?**
Future priorities and objectives (including targets, evidence base)—**Where do we want to be?**
Strategy (include time table, implementation)—**How are we going to get there?**
Monitoring and evaluation—How will we know we are there?

Consider using the '1,2,24 rule' (i.e. start with a one-page summary, followed a two-page executive summary, then a maximum of 24 pages for the body of the text, followed by appendices).

Report to management

General principles

Keep the report to around four sides of A4 maximum.
Why is this paper being written, and **why now**?
Main points only: You need to make it clear what exactly it is that you are asking the management to decide.
Intersperse text with **bullet points**.
Use **subheadings** to break up the text.

A standard layout is shown in Box 6C.8.

Box 6C.8 Sample structure for management report

Example: Standard report template
Report to: *Name of management board*
Report from: *Name, position, department*
Title: *Covering the main subject of the paper in non-technical language*
Date:
Purpose: *What the board should do: i.e. for information, for approval of recommendations, for discussion*
Executive summary (and recommendations if appropriate)
5–7 sentences summarising the report.
Enough information needs to be included for someone to read the executive summary only.
Background
Set out the context.
What is known from policy and/or research.
Issue under question.
Heading(s) specific to subject
Consider the audience:
Lay members (use non-medical language, outline relevant medical principles)
Responsibility of the board (e.g. if commissioning, consider cost and contracting issues)
Recommendations/options
Make clear:
Who is responsible for implementing what
Timescales involved
Resource implications of options

References

1. Cohen, D. and Crabtree, B. (2008) Evaluative criteria for qualitative research in health care: Controversies and recommendations. *Ann Fam Med* 6(4), 331–339.
2. CASP (2010) 10 questions to help you make sense of qualitative research. http://www.casp-uk.net/wp-content/uploads/2011/11/CASP_Qualitative_Appraisal_Checklist_14oct10.pdf.
3. Tong, A., Sainsbury, P., and Craig, J. (2007) Consolidated criteria for reporting qualitative research (coreq): A 32-item checklist for interviews and focus groups. *Int J Qual Health Care* 19(6), 349–357. doi: 10.1093/INTQHC/MZM042. http://intqhc.oxfordjournals.org/content/19/6/349.
4. Goulding, N. (2003) *How to Prepare and Write for a Scientific Journal*. www.wolfson.qmul.ac.uk/epm/students/ssm7/ssm7medauth.pdf.
5. Anon (2011) Academic tweeting: finding the appropriate tweeting style for your project. Accessed online July 20, 2014 at http://blogs.lse.ac.uk/impactofsocialsciences/2011/10/04/academic-tweeting-styles/.
6. Wood, S. (2013) Blogging guidance. Accessed online July 20, 2014 at http://digitalhealth.dh.gov.uk/blogging-guidance/.
7. Clark, B. (2008) The four "P" approach: A persuasive writing structure that works. Copy blogger. Accessed online July 20, 2014 at http://www.copyblogger.com/4ps/.

Appendix A

Revision Tips

The revision tips presented here are focused on the UK MFPH Part A examination, although the principles of examination technique will apply more broadly.

The UK MFPH Part A examination is notorious for its low pass rate: barely one candidate in four passes at some sittings. The elaborate marking algorithm penalises candidates who do not perform consistently well in all questions. Accordingly, we advise you to make sure that:

- Your knowledge of the syllabus is **broad** rather than deep
- You divide your time in the examination **proportionately** across the questions' sub-questions based on the marks that are available

Examination Structure

UK Passing the examination (known formally as the 'Part A Examination for Membership of the Faculty of Public Health of the Royal Colleges of Physicians of the United Kingdom') entitles you to apply for the following:

- Diplomate membership of the Faculty of Public Health (DFPH)
- Entry to the Part B examination (the Objective Structured Public Health Examination or 'OSPHE')—success in which leads to full MFPH

Although the Part A examination actually consists of four papers (one each morning and afternoon over two consecutive days), the Faculty's marking scheme refers simply to papers I and II, one for each day.

Day 1

Session	Paper	Duration	Description	Details	Marks	Timing
a.m.	**Paper Ia**	2½ h	Short answer questions (SAQs)	Research methods (epidemiology, statistics, qualitative research, health information sources), health promotion, and health protection	60	6 questions in 150 min = 25 min per question
p.m.	**Paper Ib**	1½ h	SAQs	Medical sociology, social policy, health economics, and organisational management of healthcare	40	4 questions in 90 min = 22½ min per question

Day 2

Session	Paper	Duration	Description	Details	Marks	Timing
a.m.	**Paper IIa**	2½ h	Critical appraisal and discussion	Candidates are provided with a journal paper to read (usually from the *BMJ*). Questions include composing a structured abstract of the paper, critically appraising the paper and then addressing more general questions on the topic.	50	50 marks in 150 min = allow approximately 1 hour to read and digest the paper, then roughly 20 min per 10 marks
p.m.	**Paper IIb**	1½ h	Data interpretation	Candidates are provided with evidence in the form of raw data, tables of data, maps, or graphs. Questions involve interpretation of these data. Answers (which may include statistical manipulation) may be numerical, graphical, multiple choice, or short answer (short paragraphs or sentences).	50	5 questions (50 marks) in 90 min = 18 min per question

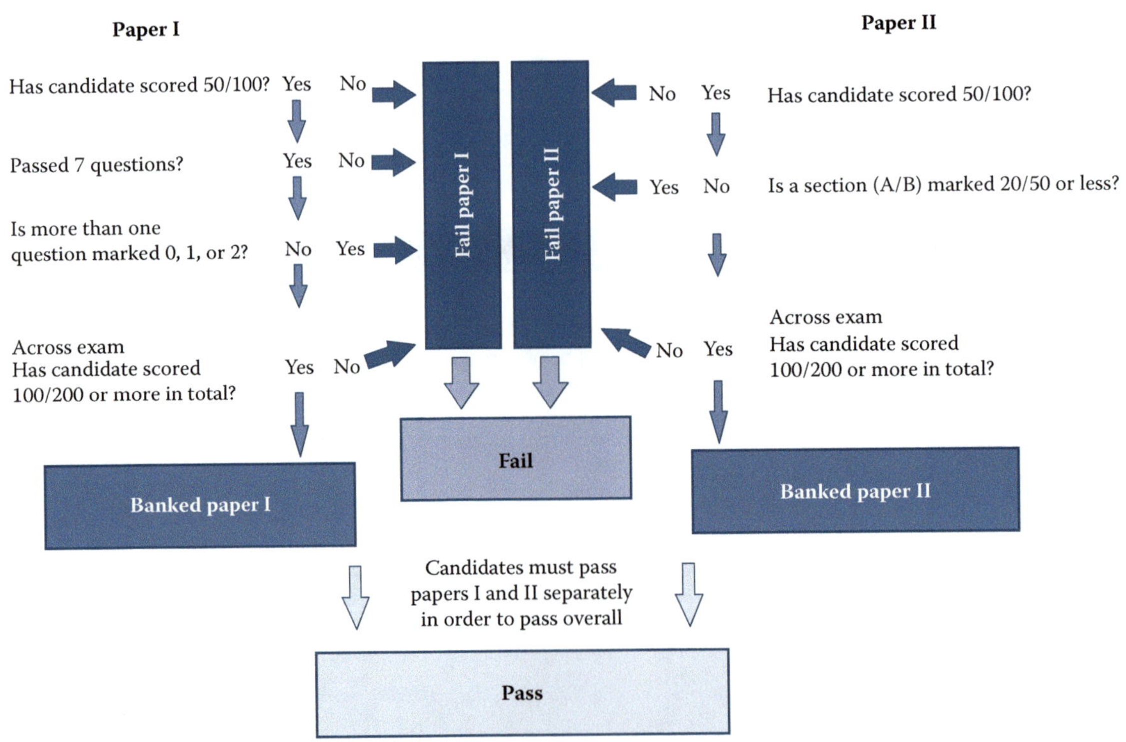

Figure A.1 MFPH Part A pass/fail algorithm. (Reproduced from www.fph.org.uk/uploads/marking%20algorithm%20new.ppt.)

Each of the two papers carries 100 marks, so that the examination is marked out of 200 in total. There is a complex marking algorithm containing several hurdles (see Figure A.1). A candidate who stumbles on any of these hurdles will fail the examination.

In order to pass the examination, a candidate must pass both paper I and paper II. However, if a candidate passes only one of the papers but also obtains an overall score of at least 100/200, then that paper can be **banked**. Once a paper has been banked, a candidate needs only to attempt the remaining paper when resitting the examination on a subsequent occasion.

In practice, the intricacies of the pass/fail algorithm are irrelevant, and the bottom line is that you must avoid doing badly in any question.

Revision

Clearly, the amount of time you will need for revision will depend on your prior knowledge and experience and on your personal revision style. That said, most successful candidates seem to devote at least 4–6 months to revision for this examination. A good way to gauge how much work you will need to do is to familiarise yourself with the syllabus and with one of the past papers and examiners' comments. However, we would advise you not to look at the most recent paper until a week before the exam, when you can use it as a mock examination to be sat under self-imposed examination conditions. Table A.1 presents a suggested revision schedule that worked for us and that you might want to use or adapt to your personal revision style.

Table A.1 Suggested revision schedule

Revision phase	Topic	Details
Initial	Syllabus Sample past paper	Read the **syllabus** and scan through the contents of this book. Read a sample **past paper** (not the most recent) and the associated examiners' **comments** to gauge the required standard.
Early	Epidemiology and statistics	Ensure that you are familiar with all of the epidemiological components of the syllabus. **Epidemiology** and **statistics** are the backbone of the MFPH Part A examination and are tested not only in the epidemiology questions in paper Ia but also throughout paper II. Study Section 1 of this book and read the recommended epidemiology text by Charles Hennekens (detailed in Table A.2).
Mid	Cover the whole syllabus	Study the rest of this book. Consult the further reading as recommended in Table A.2. Attend a critical appraisal workshop (such as those run by **CASP** UK (www.casp-uk.net), which is crucial for paper IIa).
	Past papers	Again, setting aside the most recent past paper, work your way through the previous five or six past papers as follows: For each question, write down the **introductory sentence** that you would use and the **essay structure** that you would employ. Compare what you have written with the examiners' key points and comments.

(continued)

Table A.1 (*Continued*) Suggested revision schedule

Revision phase	Topic	Details
		Note that recent past paper IIb questions are no longer available on the Faculty of Public health website, so this paper is harder to prepare for. There are a few specimen questions on the Faculty of Public Health website; however, these are best left until later on in your revision. In order to help prepare for this paper, some regions run mock exams using a bank of questions that they have collated. It may also be useful to practise some of the pre-2005 paper IIb questions: although the structure of this paper has changed, many of the skills remain the same.
Late	Context	You can add weight to your answers by including material and examples from the following sources: Selected editorials from the last few months' editions of the ***BMJ*** (see Dr Edmund Jessop's weekly reading list [www.edmundjessop.org.uk]). Items from the **websites** of the following organisations: King's Fund (www.kingsfund.org.uk), Nuffield Trust (www.nuffieldtrust.org.uk), Food Standards Agency (www.food.gov.uk), Office for National Statistics (http://www.ons.gov.uk), National Institute for Health and Clinical Excellence (www.nice.org.uk), Care Quality Commission (www.cqc.org.uk), Health Protection Agency (www.hpa.org.uk), Department of Health (www.dh.gov.uk), and the World Health Organization (www.who.int).
Week before	Mock paper	One week before the exam, you should attempt the most recent past paper in 'real time' (i.e. at the same time as you will be sitting the examination next week) and under full **exam conditions**. Write your answers longhand and use only the materials that will be available to you in the examination itself (http://www.fph.org.uk/part_a_on_the_day). For this mock examination, use the few specimen paper IIb questions that are provided on the Faculty of Public Health website [2]
	Finalise	Consolidate and review your revision notes.
	Short-term memory	Memorise the following: Question timings/marks-per-minute rates for each paper Statistical formulae (see Appendix B) Key definitions (infant mortality, etc.)

We know from personal experience that this book contains more than enough information to pass the MFPH Part A. The following books were useful for us for addressing uncertainties (Table A.2).

Table A.2 Further reading

Subject area	Further reading
Epidemiology	Hennekens C, Buring J (1987) *Epidemiology in Medicine*. Philadelphia, PA: Lippincott Williams & Wilkins
Statistics	Swinscow TDV, Campbell MJ (2002) *Statistics at Square One*. London, UK: BMJ Books Campbell MJ (2001) *Statistics at Square Two*. London, UK: BMJ Books Kirkwood BR, Sterne JAC (2003) *Essential Medical Statistics*. Blackwell Science
Health information	Health and Social Care Information Centre. Accessed online July 20, 2014 at http://www.hscic.gov.uk
Health promotion	Nutbeam D, Harris E (2004) *Theory in a Nutshell: A Guide to Health Promotion Theory*. Maidenhead: McGraw-Hill Education
Environmental public health	Chapter within Donaldson LJ, Scally G (2009) *Essential Public Health*, 3rd edn. Radcliffe Publishing
Communicable disease	Hawker J et al (2012) *Communicable Disease Handbook*, 3rd edn. Oxford, UK: Blackwell Science
Medical sociology	Scambler G (2008) *Sociology as Applied to Medicine*, 6th edn. Philadelphia, PA: WB Saunders
Qualitative research	Green J, Browne J (2005) *Principles of Social Research (Understanding Public Health)*. Milton Keynes: Open University Press
Health economics	Guiness L, Wiseman V (2011) *Introduction to Health Economics (Understanding Public Health)*. Milton Keynes: Open University Press Fox-Rushby J, Cairns J (2005) *Economic Evaluation (Understanding Public Health)*. Milton Keynes: Open University Press
Healthcare management	Iles V (2005) *Really Managing Health Care*. Oxford: Oxford University Press
Critical appraisal	Critical Appraisal Skills Programme http://www.casp-uk.net/ Greenhalgh T *How to Read a Paper* BMJ series (http://www.bmj.com/about-bmj/resources-readers/publications/how-read-paper)
Public health practice	Pencheon D et al. (2006) *Oxford Handbook of Public Health Practice*, 2nd edn. Oxford, UK: Oxford University Press
Writing skills	Williams JM, Colomb GG (2010). *Style: the Basics of Clarity and Grace*, 4th edn. New York: Longman

Examination Technique

Unfortunately, the examination rarely starts exactly at the published time: a delay of 5–10 min is usual. This delay can make the timing of questions rather tricky, so you will need to spend the first minute or two of the exam calculating the exact times at which you should start each question. Write down these times alongside each question on the question paper so that you keep on track. Note that the short answer questions (SAQs) are of different durations in paper Ia (25 min each) and paper Ib (22½ min each).

You need to remain acutely aware of the time throughout the examination. During the MFPH Part A examination, we suggest you regard your watch as the equivalent of the rearview mirror in a driving test: force yourself to keep looking at it very frequently. This is the only way to ensure that you allow a proportionate amount of time to each question and sub-question.

Paper I

As the questions in all parts of paper I are compulsory, and marked by separate examiners, there is little to be gained from reading through the whole question booklet at the start. Instead, we would suggest treating each SAQ as a mini exam and then starting each new question afresh at the calculated time that you have written down.

Use the first 5 minutes of each SAQ for planning. We advise that you use this time to do the following:

- Read and reread the question, underlining the keywords
- Brainstorm the question (i.e. write down the key points that you think the examiners are expecting you to cover, together with any 'gems' that you can throw in from your own work experience or from your revision, particularly the contextual material that you may have read in the later stages of your revision)
- Choose and write down what structure you will use to answer the question (either one of the structures listed in Appendix B or a bespoke structure that you develop for that particular question)
- Read the question one more time to check that you have not missed anything
- Craft the first sentence of your answer very carefully: first impressions count
- There is generally no need for a conclusion.

Note that where a question asks you to answer in relation to a 'country of your choice', you are expected to state the name of that country explicitly at the beginning of your answer.

Paper IIa

In contrast to paper I, you should read through all of the questions as soon as you are allowed to turn over the paper. This is because the questions build on each other and therefore provide an indication of the examiners' line of thought.

We would advise you to set aside the first **hour** to read and digest the study that you are being required to appraise. We suggest that you follow Dr Edmund Jessop's advice (see www.edmundjessop.org.uk/partI_main.doc) of reading the following parts of the paper first:

- Title
- Last paragraph of the introduction
- First paragraph of the discussion
- Last paragraph of the discussion

These four sections will provide you with the gist of the paper, and you should try to make sure that this overview is completely clear in your mind before you read any further.

You can then use one of the frameworks described in Chapter 6A to structure your critical appraisal.

Paper IIb

There tends to be a significant time pressure for this paper, so ensure you spend only 18 min per question. You should ensure that you have memorised the statistical techniques outlined in Appendix B and that you have a systematic approach to describing data (see Chapter 6B). Medically qualified candidates will be familiar with the standard way to report a chest radiograph, namely:

- Type of image
- Name and date of birth of the patient
- Date of examination
- Striking features
- Systematic approach to bones, soft tissues, zones of the lungs, etc.

For example, the report may read, 'This is a postero-anterior chest radiograph of Mr David Jones (DOB 24/7/46) taken on 14 June 2006. The most striking abnormality is a left-sided pneumothorax. The bones appear normal....'

You should adopt a similar methodical approach to describing whatever data source you are asked to describe in paper IIb—paying particular attention to any axes, units, or denominators shown.

Technique for Short-Answer Questions

For each SAQ, you must convince the examiners that you understand:

- What exactly the question is asking
- Why this question is being asked today (i.e. why it is important to contemporary public health)
- How to set about tackling the question in a logical fashion

We would encourage you to approach each SAQ by covering these three points. Always begin with a carefully constructed sentence that teases out the issues in the question and explains why they are important to the world of public health today. Next, set out the structure that you are going to adopt to answer the question (i.e. the answer framework).

You should then proceed to answer the question, writing out and underlining the individual headings contained in your box as you go along.

Aim for a clear writing style that follows the advice of the *Economist's Style Guide*, by

- Using short, snappy sentences
- Avoiding trite turns of phrase
- Steering clear of unnecessary jargon

The examiners encourage you to employ the *rationed use of bullet points, tables, and diagrams* to illustrate your answers. You should aim to include relevant examples and to name any eponymous theories or structures that you use.

Example (January 2006, Paper Ia, Question 1): Describe how you would undertake a formal survey to determine the prevalence of angina in a local area of a developed country (population 100,000), e.g. the United Kingdom

Angina is important in public health because

- *It is an indicator of unmet need in relation to the treatment of ischaemic heart disease (currently the commonest cause of death in developed countries).*
- *In most cases, it is treatable either medically or through revascularisation (surgically or percutaneously).*
- *Differences in its prevalence can be used to compare inequalities in access to healthcare within and across populations.*

1. *Definitions (setting, angina, formal survey)*
2. *Steps: for undertaking a formal survey*
   Obtaining a sampling frame
   Obtaining a sample
   Assessing the presence of angina
   Calculating the prevalence
3. *Strengths and weaknesses of method chosen*

Definitions

I shall conduct this survey in the relatively deprived inner-London borough of Tower Hamlets, United Kingdom. Although there are many types of angina (e.g. Ludwig's angina, Prinzmetal's angina), for the purpose of this study, angina will be defined as stable angina of cardiac origin, specifically ...

References

1. www.fph.org.uk/uploads/marking%20algorithm%20new.ppt.
2. Anon (undated). Part A marking algorithm powerpoint slide. Faculty of Public Health. Accessed online July 20, 2014 at http://www.fph.org.uk/part_a_results_and_feedback.

Appendix B

Core Statistical Techniques

This appendix lists the statistical techniques that candidates should remember and be able to perform in the UK MFPH Part A examination.

Screening

In order to make calculations relating to screening, data should first be placed in a 2 × 2 table with the results of the screening test in the rows and the true disease status (or gold standard) in the columns.

		Truth (Gold Standard) +	Truth (Gold Standard) −		
Test result	+	*a*	*b*	*a* + *b*	→ PPV
	−	*c*	*d*	*c* + *d*	→ NPV
		a + *c*	*b* + *d*		
		↓	↓		
		Sensitivity	Specificity		

Sensitivity

Ability of a test to detect all those people with the disease in the screened population (i.e. probability of testing positive if diseased):

$$\text{Sensitivity} = \frac{a}{a+c}$$

Specificity

Ability of a test to identify correctly all those free of the disease in the screened population (i.e. probability of testing negative if normal):

$$\text{Specificity} = \frac{d}{b+d}$$

Positive predictive value (PPV)

Proportion of people testing positive who truly have the disease:

$$\text{PPV} = \frac{a}{a+b}$$

Negative predictive value (NPV)

Proportion of those testing negative who are truly disease-free:

$$\text{NPV} = \frac{d}{c+d}$$

Numbers Needed to Treat

NNT is the number of patients that needs to be treated for one person to benefit (i.e. the lower the better) NNT is used in intervention studies:

$$\text{NNT} = \frac{1}{\text{Absolute risk reduction}}$$

Note: The absolute risk reduction is the same as excess risk (i.e. the risk difference):

$$\begin{aligned}&\text{Absolute risk reduction}\\&\quad = \text{Risk of disease in treatment group}\\&\qquad - \text{Risk of disease in controls}\end{aligned}$$

If the treatment or exposure is harmful (e.g. if you are looking at side effects as the outcome), then calculate the NNH instead.

Relative Risk

The most commonly used measures of relative risk in epidemiology are the **risk ratio**, **rate ratio**, and **odds ratio**. Other relative risks include the **standardised mortality ratio** (see Chapter 1A.5) and the **hazard ratio** (see Chapter 1B.18).

Risk ratio

$$\text{Risk ratio} = \frac{\text{Risk of disease in exposed}}{\text{Risk of disease in unexposed}}$$

Rate ratio

$$\text{Rate ratio} = \frac{\text{Incidence rate in exposed}}{\text{Incidence rate in unexposed}}$$

Odds ratio

In order to calculate odds ratios, the results of the study are normally presented in a 2 × 2 table, for example,

	Case	Control	
Exposed	*a*	*b*	*a* + *b*
Unexposed	*c*	*d*	*c* + *d*
	a + *c*	*b* + *d*	*a* + *b* + *c* + *d*

The odds of a disease is the number of cases in a group divided by the number of non-cases in a group:

$$\text{Odds} = \frac{\text{No. of cases}}{\text{No. of non-cases}}$$

So, in the previously presented 2 × 2 table, the odds of disease in the exposed is *a*/*b*.

The odds ratio can be calculated based on the odds of the disease (in any study design) or based on the odds of exposure (in case–control study):

$$\text{OR} = \frac{\text{Odds of disease in exposed}}{\text{Odds of disease in unexposed}}$$

$$= \frac{\text{Odds of exposure in cases}}{\text{Odds of exposure in controls}}$$

So, in the previously presented 2 × 2 table,

$$\text{OR} = \frac{a/b}{c/d} = \frac{a/c}{b/d}$$

In a case–control study, we cannot directly calculate the incidence (risk or rate) because the subjects were selected on the basis of their disease status, not on the basis of their exposure. We can, however, calculate the odds of exposure and thus the odds ratio.

If a case–control study is appropriately designed and the disease is rare, then the odds ratio provides an estimate of the risk ratio or the rate ratio.

Note: The odds ratio is calculated differently for paired data (see section on McNemar's test).

Attributable Fraction

Attributable risk (risk difference)

This is the risk of disease in the exposed group that can be considered attributable to the exposure, after taking account of the risk of the disease that would have occurred anyway:

$$\text{AR} = R_e - R_0$$

where

R_e is the risk in the exposed group
R_0 is the risk in the unexposed group

Attributable fraction (aetiological fraction/attributable risk %)

Proportion of disease among the exposed that is attributable to the exposure:

$$\mathrm{AF} = \frac{\mathrm{AR}}{R_e} = \frac{R_e - R_0}{R_e}$$

Population attributable risk

This is the excess risk of disease in the total study population that is attributable to the exposure:

$$\mathrm{PAR} = R_t - R_0$$

where
R_t is the risk in the whole population
R_0 is the risk in the unexposed group

Population attributable fraction (population attributable risk %)

This is the proportion of disease in the study population that is attributable to the exposure (and could potentially be eliminated if the exposure were eliminated):

$$\mathrm{PAF} = \frac{\mathrm{PAR}}{R_t} = \frac{R_t - R_0}{R_t}$$

Note: Risks or rates can be used for all of these measures.

Note: All of these attributable measures assume that the association is causal.

Standard Error and Confidence Intervals

Variance

Variance of a sample: $s^2 = \dfrac{\sum (x-\bar{x})^2}{(n-1)}$

Note: Variance is in units².

Standard deviation

Standard deviation of a sample: $s = \sqrt{\dfrac{\sum (x-\bar{x})^2}{(n-1)}}$

Note: Standard deviation takes the same units as x.

Standard error

Standard error measures how precisely a population measure (e.g. mean/proportion/rate) is estimated by a sample measure (i.e. the amount of variability in the sample measure).

The method of calculating the standard error depends on the type of outcome:

Standard error of a sample mean (normal distribution)

For a single mean

$$\mathrm{se} \approx \frac{s}{\sqrt{n}} \approx \sqrt{\frac{s^2}{n}}$$

(*As we rarely know the population standard deviation, the sample standard deviation 's'* is used instead)

For the difference between two means

For a large sample,

$$\mathrm{se} \approx \sqrt{\frac{s_1^2}{n_1} + \frac{s_0^2}{n_0}}$$

For a small sample (e.g. <60),

$$\mathrm{se} \approx s_p \sqrt{\frac{1}{n_1} + \frac{1}{n_0}}$$

where $s_p = \sqrt{\dfrac{(n_1-1)s_1^2 + (n_0-1)s_0^2}{(n_1+n_0-1)}}$

(for paired data, calculate difference between each pair and then treat as a single sample or single mean)

Standard error of a sample proportion (risk) (binomial distribution but approximated by the normal distribution)

For a single proportion p

$$se \approx \sqrt{\frac{p(1-p)}{n}}$$

(*As we rarely know the population risk, the sample proportion 'p'* is used instead)

For the difference between two proportions

$$se \approx \sqrt{\frac{p_1(1-p_1)}{n_1} + \frac{p_0(1-p_0)}{n_0}}$$

Standard error of a count (Poisson distribution)

$$SE \approx \sqrt{\mu}$$

where μ is the mean count [number of occurrences].

Confidence intervals

General formula for a 95% confidence interval (CI):

$$95\% \text{ CI} = \text{Estimate} \pm 1.96 \text{ SE}$$

(whether the estimate is a mean, difference between means, regression coefficient …)

If we had a small sample for a mean/difference in means, we would use the t distribution instead of the normal distribution and use the t value for a 5% two-tailed test (instead of 1.96); however, the distribution tables are not currently provided in the Part A MFPH examination.

Interpretation of 95% CI

Example: 95% CI (3, 7)

There is a 95% chance that the true estimate (e.g. mean) in the population lies somewhere between 3 and 7. Alternatively, we can say that there is only a 1-in-20 chance that the true estimate in the population lies outside the interval between 3 and 7.

X^2 Test for a 2x2 Table

Used when there is a binary exposure and a binary outcome. (**Note:** χ^2 is also used for categorical variables.)

Steps involved are as follows:

1. Arrange the data you are provided with in a 2 × 2 contingency table—this gives the 'observed' values, O:

	Outcome Yes	Outcome No	
Exposed (/intervention)	a	b	$a + b = v$
Unexposed (/control)	c	d	$c + d = w$
	$a + c = x$	$b + d = y$	$a + b + c + d = z$

2. Create a second 2 × 2 table, this time with the values you would expect if the null hypothesis were true, by keeping the row and column totals the same (i.e. the same proportions of each outcome in the exposed and unexposed group):

	Outcome Yes	Outcome No	
Exposed	$\frac{x}{z} \times v$	$\frac{y}{z} \times v$	v
Unexposed	$\frac{x}{z} \times w$	$\frac{y}{z} \times w$	w
	x	y	z

3. Calculate the χ^2 statistic using the observed values, O, for each cell in step 1 and the expected values, E, for each cell in step 2:

$$\chi^2 = \sum \frac{(O-E)^2}{E}, \quad (\text{d.f.} = 1)$$

(degrees of freedom, d.f. = $(r - 1) \times (c - 1)$; so for a 2 × 2 table, d.f. = $(2 - 1) \times (2 - 1) = 1$)

4. Calculate the corresponding p-value. In the Part A MFPH examination, candidates are not provided with distribution tables so remember the following:

χ^2 of $1.96^2 = 3.84$ corresponds to $p = 0.05$

Therefore, $\chi^2 > 3.84$ corresponds to $p < 0.05$ (i.e. 'statistically significant at the 5% level').

McNemar's X^2 Test

McNemar's test is used with paired binary data (e.g. an individually matched case–control study or repeat measures of the same variable in each participant).

In such cases, you must *avoid* presenting the data as you would in an unmatched study (e.g. unmatched case–control study):

	Case	Control	
Exposed	a	b	a + b
Unexposed	c	d	c + d
	a + c	b + d	a + b + c + d

Instead, present the data in *pairs* with the cases in the rows and controls in the columns:

		Controls		
		Exposed	Unexposed	
Cases	Exposed	q	r	q + r
	Unexposed	s	t	s + t
		q + s	r + t	q + r + s + t

q = Both exposed
r = Case exposed Control unexposed
s = Case unexposed control exposed
t = Both unexposed

so each cell represents a set of matched pairs rather than individuals). Note that the total $(q + r + s + t)$ should be half the sample size.

The data of interest are the discordant pairs (i.e. r and s). These pairs are used to calculate the odds ratio:

$$\text{OR} = \frac{r}{s}$$

And the p-value using McNemar's test

$$\text{McNemar's } \chi^2 = \frac{(r-s)^2}{r+s}, \quad (\text{d.f.} = 1)$$

As with χ^2, McNemar's $\chi^2 > 3.84$ corresponds to $p < 0.05$ (i.e. 'statistically significant at the 5% level').

See example in 1B.14.

Standardisation

Direct standardisation

Study rates are applied to standard population:

1. Identify a standard population (e.g. one of the populations being compared, their average or total, or an outside standard population).
2. Apply the age-specific rates in the study (or other variable-specific rates) to the weighting of the standard population (i.e. age-specific rate times size of standard population in that age band).
3. Sum the values to give the expected deaths in the standard population.
4. Divide by the total standard population to give the 'age-standardised rate' (i.e. a weighted average).

Indirect standardisation

Standard rates are applied to study population (e.g. when the study population does not have age-specific rates):

1. Identify a standard population with stratum-specific death rates (e.g. age-specific death rates). The standard population may be one of the populations being compared, their average or total, or an outside standard population.
2. Apply these standard death rates to the study population to obtain the expected number of deaths for each stratum.
3. Add up the expected stratum-specific deaths to give the total number of expected deaths.
4. Calculate the SMR based on the actual (observed) total number of deaths in the study population and the expected number of deaths (calculated in step 3):

$$\text{SMR} = \frac{\text{Observed deaths}}{\text{Expected deaths}} \times 100\%$$

CI for standardisation (estimated)

For standardised mortality rates or ratios (or indeed any other binary events), the numerator is a count. For direct standardisation, the count is the expected deaths in the standard population (calculated in step 3 previously), and for indirect standardisation, it is the observed deaths. The CIs of the count can be calculated based on the Poisson distribution, for which the standard error is $\sqrt{\text{count}}$. The upper and lower CIs of the count can then be converted back into rates or ratios. Accordingly, the calculation involves the following two steps:

1. Calculate the 95% CI for the count:

$$95\% \text{ CI} = \text{Count} \pm (1.96\sqrt{\text{count}})$$

2. Then convert these into upper and lower CIs for the
   a. Standardised rate (direct) by dividing by the total standard population
   b. SMR (indirect) by dividing by the expected number of deaths

Note: While more accurate methods exist, these are more complicated. The previously mentioned approach provides a good estimation and is a commonly used method that can be applied quickly in the Part A examination.

Weighted Averages

A weighted average is an average in which each quantity is assigned a weight. These weightings determine the relative importance of each quantity on the average. The importance of a quantity may be represented by the size of a group (e.g. size of an age band in direct standardisation, sample size of a study in meta-analysis) or by another factor such as the variance (which also takes into account the size of a sample).

The weighted average is then calculated as follows:

$$\text{Weighted average}, e = \frac{\sum (w_i \times e_i)}{\sum w_i}$$

where

e is an estimate (e.g. a mean or an OR)

e_i is the value of the estimate for each study (or stratum) i

w_i is the weighting for each study (or stratum)

As mentioned, there are several potential ways of weighting a study or a group, including the following:

1. Weight of a study (w_i) is simply the study (or stratum) size (e.g. size of an age band in direct standardisation).
2. A common method of weighting used in meta-analysis is the inverse variance method.
   Weight of a study (w_i) is the inverse of the variance of the measure of effect of that study:

   $$w_i = \frac{1}{s_i^2}$$

   where s_i^2 is the variance of the measure of effect for study i.
3. Mantel–Haenszel weights are sometimes used in meta-analysis or when adjusting for confounding using the Mantel–Haenszel method for controlling for confounding.

Appendix C

Answer Frameworks

A recurrent gripe in the examiners' comments is that candidates tend to lack structure to their answers. To avoid this issue, candidates must ensure that without exception, every word that they write in the examination fits into some form of explicit structure.

Candidates can structure their answers either by using one of the frameworks in the following discussion or by using a custom-made framework developed by the candidate for a particular question during the examination. Either way, the candidate should make it explicit to the examiners what framework is being used (e.g. by drawing a box at the start of each answer and writing the framework for that answer inside the box). The contents of the box should be repeated as headings within the answer, and these headings should be underlined.

Paper I Frameworks

We begin by presenting a number of generic frameworks, followed by frameworks that candidates may use for more specialist questions relating to needs assessment, healthcare evaluation, health impact assessment, the epidemiology of a particular disease, environmental health, health protection, health promotion, and health information, policy, and management.

Generic frameworks

The three structures detailed in Tables C.1 to C.3 can be used either as the **stand-alone framework** for an entire question (especially if none of the more specific frameworks fits) or alternatively as the **subheadings** within another framework.

Table C.1 Generic framework 1: How would you implement...

'**DTOSC**'	
Define/describe	*Key points in question.*
Team	*Who will be involved?*
Operational aspects	*Practicalities (set up meeting; who would you contact; what you would do in real life), staff, equipment, finance, timing.*
Strategic aspects	*Management, governance, guidelines, targets, policies, etc.*
Communication	

Table C.2 Generic framework 2: Write short notes on...

'**DAP ADE**'	
1. Describe/define	
2. Application/uses	
3. PH importance	H^4AE, any topical issues (see Generic framework 3)
4. Advantages	
5. Disadvantages	
6. Example/current issues	

Table C.3 Generic framework 3: Roles of public health

'H⁴AE'
1. **H**ealth improvement
2. **H**ealth protection
3. **H**ealth services
4. **H**ealth intelligence
5. **A**cademic
6. **E**quity/inequalities

Needs assessment (Tables C.4 to C.6)

Table C.4 Framework for health needs assessment

'PPRE'	
1. Profiling (situation analysis) • Health problem identification • Size/distribution/determinants • Current services	Approaches (epidemiological/comparative)
2. Prioritising (interventions options appraisal) • Stakeholders' views • EEE_AAA (Maxwell) • Resource implications	
3. Recommendations/implementation plan	Roles, resources, timescales, barriers, strategy
4. Evaluation (of health gains)	*Process/outcome indicators*

Table C.5 Needs for a population group/health effects of a risk factor

'PP SS'	
Physical health • Prevention • Lifestyle • Primary care • Specialist	For example, immunisations, screening For example, smoking, drugs, sex
Psychological	
Social	*Employment, education, housing*
Special groups	*Pregnancy/children/infants*

Table C.6 Needs for a disease

Epidemiological	Definition Numbers Current setup Alternative setups
Comparative	Other places Gold standard
Corporate	Central government Health authority

Healthcare evaluation (Tables C.7 and C.8)

The names of Maxwell or Donabedian should be quoted if their frameworks are used.

Donabedian	
Structure	Staff numbers Staff qualifications Bed capacity
Process	Admissions Procedures
Outcomes	Survival Quality of life

The Maxwell 6	
'A^{3}E^3'	
A	Access Acceptability Appropriateness
E	Equity Efficiency/economy Effectiveness

Table C.7 Steps of evaluation

'PD³RA'	
1. Purpose	Formative/process/outcome
2. Dimensions	*Maxwell (EEEAAA)*
3. Data	Measures to use for dimension, sources, quantitative/qualitative
4. Design/methods	Study design, confounding
5. Reporting	
6. Action	

Table C.8 Performance monitoring (ongoing evaluation)

'HAD EPO'	
Health improvement	*PH indices (mortality/morbidity)*
Access (equity)	*Wait times, geographic equity*
Delivery (appropriate/effective care)	↑*Effective interventions,* ↓*ineffective, EBM*
Efficiency	*For example, cost per case*
Patient experience	*Surveys, complaints, etc.*
Outcomes of healthcare	*Audit, readmissions, mortality, QoL, safety, etc.*
Assess all of these in terms of average levels and inequalities.	

Health impact assessment (Table C.9)

Table C.9 Health impact assessment framework

'SSAREM'	
1. Screening (is HIA necessary?)	Wider determinants, lifestyles, health/social services
2. Scoping	Detail needed, who to involve
3. Appraisal	Positive/negative; burden, inequalities; evidence, risk assessment
4. Recommendations/reporting	Maximise positive and mitigate negative impacts, alternatives
5. Engaging decision-makers	
6. Monitoring/evaluation	Effect on decision, impact on population health

Epidemiology of specific diseases (Table C.10)

Table C.10 Epidemiology of non-communicable diseases

Classified **I**n **T**ime, **P**lace, **P**erson, **C**heck	
1. **C**linical features	
2. **I**mportance	Incidence/severity/cost/screening/other PH importance
3. **T**ime	Secular trend—last 50 years, more recent
4. **P**lace	Within the United Kingdom, the United Kingdom versus Europe, famous places
5. **P**erson ('ASS EOLF'): (1) Age (2) Sex (3) SES (4) Ethnicity (5) Occupation (6) Lifestyle (7) Familial/genetic	
6. **C**auses/risk factors	Any risk factors not already mentioned

Environmental health (Tables C.11 and C.12)

Table C.11 Factors affecting health + where to take action

WHO 'DPSEEA' framework	
Driving force	*For example, population growth*
Pressure	*For example, traffic*
State	*For example, PM10 emissions*
Exposure	*For example, inhalation of PM10*
Effect (health outcome)	*For example, mortality*
Actions (at all levels)	

Table C.12 Risk management

Risk assessment ('HDE')	
Hazard identification	
Dose-response assessment	*Based on research*
Exposure assessment	*Field measurements of level of exposure*
Risk management ('ECCM')	
Evaluation (of risk)	*Compared with standards/guidelines*
Communication (of risk)	*So neither frightened nor apathetic*
Control/prevention	*(Including legislation—licences, taxes, etc.)*
• Source	For example, substitution, engineering controls, regulation
• Path	For example, exhaust ventilation, acoustic treatment of walls
• Person	For example, PPE, education/training of workers
• Secondary prevention	
Monitoring (of risk)	*Surveillance, detection systems, reporting*

Health protection (Tables C.13 to C.16)

Table C.13 '**CCDCs D**o **H**elp **T**o **C**ontrol **C**holera'

Confirm outbreak exists	*Information collection, comparison with expected*
Confirm diagnosis	*Specimens*
Case **D**efinition	*Time/place/person/symptoms; possible/probable/confirmed*
Count cases	
Describe data	*Time(epidemic curve)/place/person*
Generate **H**ypothesis	*Pathogen, source, transmission*
Test hypothesis	*Cohort/case-control/?microbiology*
Control/prevention measures	*Throughout*
Communication/report	*Healthcare professionals, local authority, WHO, European Centre for Disease Prevention and Control, the press and the public*

Table C.14 Epidemiology and control of an infection

'**ACE D**octors **R**eact **T**o **S**almonella **C**onfidently'	
Agent	
Clinical features	
Epidemiology (time/place/person) • Time • Place • Person ('**ASS EOLF**') (1) Age (2) Sex (3) SES (4) Ethnicity (5) Occupation (6) Lifestyle (7) Familial/genetic	Seasonal and secular time trends Within the United Kingdom, the United Kingdom versus Europe, famous places
Diagnosis (laboratory test)	
Reservoir	
Transmission	
Surveillance	Laboratory reports, notifications, vaccine coverage
Control ('PGS CCS')	

Table C.15 Control of infection

'**PGS CCS**'
Prevention • **G**eneral • **S**pecific
Case
Contacts
Source

Table C.16 Emergency planning

'**APP DRR**'	
Assess risks	
Prevention	*Source/path/person, legislation, regulations, education and awareness.*
Preparedness	*Information (sites, chemical information, health sector capacity), response plan, training.*
Detection + alert	*Detection systems, surveillance, alert channels.*
Response	*Terminate release/prevent spread/limit exposure, PH response, communication.*
Recovery	*Victim support, risk assessment, investigate cause, prevent recurrence.*

Health promotion (Tables C.17 to C.21)

Table C.17 Developing Health Promotion Programme

'**AS ROME**'
Assess need (and determinants)
Stakeholder analysis/engagement
Resources
Objectives/aims (and targets)
Methods (evidence for effective interventions)
Evaluation

Table C.18 Determinants of health

Dahlgren and Whitehead health policy rainbow
'**SLSLS**'
5. **S**ocioeconomic/cultural/environmental conditions
4. **L**iving + working conditions (education, work, housing, water/sanitation, food, healthcare)
3. **S**ocial + community influences
2. **L**ifestyle factors
1. **S**ex, age, constitutional factors

Table C.19 Health field concept (LALONDE)

1. Genetic predisposition
2. Individual behavioural and lifestyle factors
3. Health services
4. Environmental circumstances

Table C.20 Methods of health promotion/PH interventions

'LESS'	
Legislative • Fiscal (tax/subsidies) • Bans • Regulation	
Empowering (information) • Education • Media • Social marketing	
Socio-environmental • Community development • Facilities • Transport/urban planning, etc.	 For example, sports facilities, workplace initiatives For example, prioritising pedestrians/cyclists
Specific interventions • Behavioural (individual/group) • Medical • Helplines	 For example, *CBT, motivational interviewing* For example, NRT, vaccination, needle exchange, screening

Table C.21 Dahlgren and Whitehead framework for action

1. Strengthening individuals	*Empowering, recognising barriers*
2. Strengthening communities	Community development and regeneration
3. Improving access to services	*Inverse care law, food desserts*
4. Encouraging macroeconomic + social change	↓ *Income inequalities*

Health information (Tables C.22 and C.23)

Table C.22 Routine health information sources

'**D**ata **M**anagement **M**akes **R**outine **N**umbers **P**erfect'
1. **D**emographic/social (including births, ethnicity)
2. **M**ortality
3. **M**orbidity • Hospital • Primary care (including prescribing) • Disease specific (registries, notifiable infections, vaccine coverage, screening rates, etc.) • Others: surveys
4. **R**isk factors (health status) • Surveys • Synthetic estimates from surveys • GP data (CPRD, QOF) • Smoking cessation clinic
5. **N**on-health service • Council (crime, education, employment, environment, housing, benefit, transport, social care) • Police, fire service • Food supply data
6. **P**rivate sector (e.g. Experian [supermarkets, etc.])

Table C.23 Uses of data

'BCHR'	
Burden	Incidence/prevalence of a disease or risk factor Mortality Disease severity Health need
Comparisons	Time trends Benchmarking against other areas Comparisons within population subgroups (including inequalities) Identifying unwarranted variation
Health services	Assessing current provision Planning Commissioning Service improvement
Research and evaluation	Service evaluation Research Clinical audit Performance management

Policy (Table C.24)

Table C.24 Policy formation/implementation

'A PIE'	
1. **A**genda setting	Problem/pressure for change →broad goals
2. **P**olicy formulation (alternative proposals) • Review evidence + consult experts • HIA on each option • Barriers • Stakeholder consultation	*Incremental > major changes* To local implementation
3. **I**mplementation • Interpretation • Organisation • Application	Top-down/bottom-up/principal–agent theory Translation of policy into admin directives Routine administering of service
4. **E**valuation	+ revised agenda setting

Organisations and management (Tables C.25 to C.31)

Table C.25 Describing an organisation—Mckinsey's 7S

Shared values	*Guiding concepts/goals (policy/vision)*
Strategy	*Long-term plan to achieve vision*
Structure	*For example, functional, divisional, matrix*
Staff	*How many + type (e.g. doctors, nurses)*
Skills	*Of staff*
Systems	*Procedures—monthly/annual planning cycle, etc.*
Style(culture)	*Handy: power, task, role, person*

Table C.26 Stakeholder analysis

'**I AM**'	
Identification	*Internal/external stakeholders*
Assessment	*Influence (power) versus interest*
Manage + monitor	*Depending on influence/interest*

Table C.27 Functions of management (Fayol)

'**POC³**'	
Plan	
Organise	
Command	
Coordinate	
Control	*As in receive feedback and make adjustments*

Table C.28 Change management

1. Current situation	McKinsey's 7S + DEPESTELI, stakeholder analysis
2. Need for change	*SWOT, vision*
3. Drivers + resistors	Lewin force-field analysis
4. Communicate vision	Promote the change; leadership
5. Implement	Diffusion model (early adopters), staff (Maslow's hierarchy of needs)
6. Monitor + evaluate	*Effects of the change*

Table C.29 ADKAR change management model

Awareness (of need for change)	*For example, results of SWOT, focus groups, newsletters*
Desire (to support/participate in change)	*For example, sell benefits, listen/respond to concerns*
Knowledge (of how to change)	*For example, info, training programmes*
Ability (to implement the change)	*For example, support, feedback, be a role model*
Reinforcement (to sustain the change)	*For example, communication, feedback, incentives*

Table C.30 Strategy development (4-step model)

1. **Where are we now?**—situation analysis • HNA • Benchmarking • McKinsey's 7S, DEPESTELI, SWOT, stakeholder analysis
2. **Where do we want to get to?**—future direction/target • Vision, aims, objectives (SMART)
3. **How are we going to get there?**—options appraisal/implementation • Consider results of HNA + other evaluations (e.g. econ eval) • Route map • Force field, other change management steps
4. **How will we know when we have got there?**—monitoring + evaluation • Including key performance indicators

Table C.31 Commissioning/prioritising

'**PPPE**'	
1. **Profiling** (situation analysis) • HNA • Current services	
2. **Prioritising** (interventions, options appraisal) • Stakeholders' views • EEE_AAA (Maxwell) • Resource implications	*For example, PBMA*
3. **Procuring services**	
4. **Evaluation** (of health gains)	

Paper II Frameworks

Frameworks for answering Paper II questions relate to epidemiology, critical appraisal, and communication skills.

Epidemiology (Table C.32)

Table C.32 Reasons for an association

1. Chance
2. Bias
3. Confounding
4. Underlying trend
5. Reverse causation
6. Causal association

Critical appraisal

See Chapter 6A.2 for critical appraisal frameworks for different study designs.

Communication skills (Tables C.33 and C.34)

Abstract (taken from *BMJ*)
Objective
Design
Setting
Participants
Intervention
Outcome measures
Results
Conclusions

Table C.33 Report/briefing paper

'**A P**lanned **B**riefing **S**aves **L**ooking **C**rummy'	
1. **A**ppropriate language	
2. **P**urpose	
3. **B**ackground/introduction • Importance of issue • Scientific—what is already known Policy: any government policies/NICE guidelines, etc.	
4. **S**ummary of study (brief, not redoing critical appraisal) • Key findings • Key strengths/weaknesses • Generalisability • What it adds	
5. **L**ocal implementation • Likely views of HCPs, public/pts, ethical issues • Requirements for staff, equipment, buildings • Cost and cost-effectiveness	Pragmatic (not unrealistic), pilot
6. **C**onclusions and recommendations	

Table C.34 Letter

'**AT SOLO**'	
1. **A**ppropriate language	
2. **T**hank for interest and acknowledge local situation/concern	
3. **S**ummary of findings (brief, not redoing critical appraisal) • Key points • Key limitations • Practical issues reimplementation	
4. **O**ther interventions/other factors to consider	
5. **L**ocal application of findings/implementation	*Pragmatic (not unrealistic), pilot*
6. **O**ffer further discussion	

Appendix D

Last-Minute Revision

In the examination, you will need to quote certain standard criteria, classic studies, and key names in order to demonstrate your knowledge of the speciality of public health. We suggest that you use the following lists as a starting point for creating your own lists, which you then memorise prior to the examination.

Top Fives

Epidemiology

	Concept	More information in chapter
John Snow [1]	Epidemiological method: cholera and Broad Street pump	5D
Richard Doll and Austin Bradford Hill [2]	Doctors' cohort: smoking causes lung cancer	2B
Archie Cochrane [3]	Evidence-based medicine	1A
David Barker [4]	Risk of coronary heart disease in adults is linked to in utero development	2A
Geoffrey Rose [5]	Population-based prevention and the prevention paradox	2H

UK public health policy UK

	Concept	More information in chapter
Chadwick [6]	Sanitation and health	5D
Tudor Hart [7]	Inverse care law	1C
Black et al. [8]	Health inequalities are growing in the United Kingdom and are linked to social class	2I
Acheson [9]	Reducing health inequalities under the new labour government	2I
Wanless [10]	Economic case for investing in public health	2I

Health promotion: Frameworks

	Concept	More information in chapter
Tannahill [11]	Health promotion = overlapping spheres of protection, prevention, and education	2H
Lalonde [12]	Health field concept	2H
Dahlgren and Whitehead [13]	Policy rainbow	2H
Evans and Stoddart [14]	Health field model	2H
Diderichsen and Hallqvist [15]	Social determinants	2H

Health promotion: Models

	Concept	More information in chapter
Hochbaum [16]	Health belief model	2H
Bandura [17]	Social learning	2H
Prochaska and DiClemente [18]	Stages of change	2H
Beattie [19]	Dimensions of health promotion: authoritative—negotiated; individual—collective	2H
Ewles and Simnet [20]	Health field concept	2H

Sociology

	Concept	More information in chapter
Talcott Parsons [21]	The sick role	4A
Edwin Lemert [22]	Primary and secondary deviance	4A
Erving Goffman [23]	Stigma; institutionalisation	4A
Ivan Illich [24]	Iatrogenesis	4A
Emile Durkheim [25]	Social integration and suicide	2B
John Rawls [26]	Social justice	4C

Management

	Concept	More information in chapter
Donabedian [27]	Health service quality: structure–process–outcome	1C
Maxwell [28]	Health service quality: access, equity, efficiency, effectiveness, economy, appropriateness, acceptability	1C
Belbin [29]	Team roles	5A
Maslow [30]	Hierarchy of needs	5A, 5B
Handy [31]	Organisational types	5A

Key Studies

Study design examples

Study design	Example	Participants	Major finding(s)	More information
RCT	**Women's health initiative** (2003)	64,500 women over 15 years	Contrary to observational study evidence, HRT does *not* protect against CHD	Wassertheil-Smoller S et al. (2003). *JAMA* 289:2673–2684
Cohort	**Whitehall** (1967 onwards)	Whitehall I: 18,000 male civil servants Whitehall II: 10,000 male and female civil servants	Risk of death from CHD linked to social status/ employment grade	www.ucl.ac.uk/ whitehallII
Case–control	**UK Childhood Cancer Study** (1999)	*Cases*: records of 30,000 children with cancer *Controls*: children matched for age, sex, area of birth	Proximity to powerlines at birth linked to childhood leukaemia	Draper G et al. (2005) *BMJ* 330:1290
Cross-sectional	**Health Survey for England** (annual)	6000 adults + 3000 children (in 2004—random selection and boosted sample in high-minority ethnic group areas)	Prevalence of risk factors and health behaviours, e.g. fruit and vegetable consumption	www.ic.nhs.uk/ pubs/healthsurvey 2004ethnicfull/ hse2004vol1/file
Case reports	***Pneumocystis jiroveci* pneumonia (PCP) in Los Angeles** (1981)	Five homosexual men aged 29–36	Abnormal epidemiology of PCP, early sign of emergence of AIDS	www.cdc.gov/ MMWR/preview/ mmwrhtml/june_5. htm

Effects of diet on health

	Study design	Major finding(s)	More information
North Karelia (1972–1982)	Intervention (before/after): residents of North Karelia	Altering lifestyle (including saturated fat intake), reduced CHD mortality	Chapter 2E
Framingham (1948–)	Cohort: 5000 residents of Framingham, MA	Factors affecting risk of CHD include cholesterol	www.nhlbi.nih.gov/about/framingham/index.html
Seven Countries (1958–1970)	Ecological cohort: 11,000 men aged 40–59 in 7 countries in Europe and the United States	Link between unsaturated fat and lower risk of death from CHD	Chapter 2E
Intersalt (1988)	Cross-sectional: 10,000 men and women	Dietary salt levels linked to blood pressure	Chapter 2E
UK Women's Cohort (1993–)	Cohort: 35,000 women in the United Kingdom	Exploring links between diet and cancer	www.leeds.ac.uk/medicine/ceb/NutEp/ukwcs/publications.htm

Other Revision Lists

Screening: UK national screening committee summary UK

The **condition**	An **important health problem.** Epidemiology and natural history understood. Cost-effective primary prevention interventions implemented first.
The **test**	**Simple, safe, precise, and validated.** Distribution of test values in the target population should be known and a cut-off level defined and agreed. **Acceptable** to the population. Policy on diagnostics for individuals with a positive test and choices available. Criteria to select mutations to be covered by screening.
The **treatment**	**Effective treatment** exists for patients identified through early detection. Early treatment has better outcomes than late treatment. Agreed criteria for which individuals to be offered treatment and what should be offered. Providers prepared to manage patients before programme starts.
The **programme**	**Reduces mortality or morbidity.** Where screening aimed solely at providing "informed choice," test accurately measures risk and provides valuable information readily understood by the individual being screened. Complete programme clinically, socially, and ethically acceptable to health professionals and the public. **Benefit outweighs harm** (physical and psychological). Value for money. **Managing and monitoring** arrangements in place. Adequate resources available—staffing and facilities for testing, diagnosis, treatment, and programme management. Other options for managing the condition considered. Evidence-based **information for potential participants** explaining screening consequences. Anticipate public pressure for widening eligibility criteria. Decisions about screening parameters should be justifiable to the public.
More information	Chapter 2C www.nsc.nhs.uk/pdfs/criteria.pdf Wilson and Jungner [32]

Causation and association

Bradford Hill 'Viewpoints' for Studying Causation [33] (see Section 1A)

Strength	High relative risk or odds.
Consistency	Similar results from several studies in different populations.
Specificity	Single cause produces a single effect.
Temporality	Cause must precede effect.
Biological gradient	Dose–response curve.
Plausibility	Biologically acceptable or relevant reason for the cause to produce effect.
Coherence	Does not conflict with current knowledge.
Experimental	Introduction or removal of putative cause leads to change in effect.
Analogy	Consistent with previous experience in similar situations.

Choice of statistical tests

Figures D.1 to D.4 illustrate appropriate tests for particular types of outcome variables. Reproduced with permission from Kirkwood and Sterne [34].

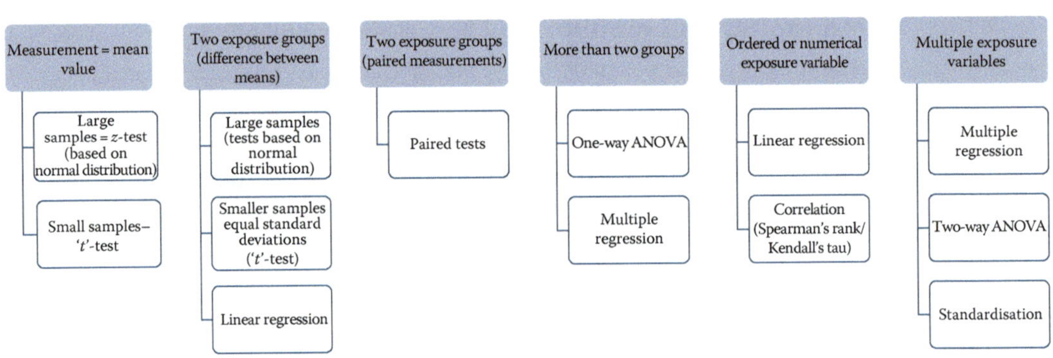

Figure D.1 Numerical outcome variable.

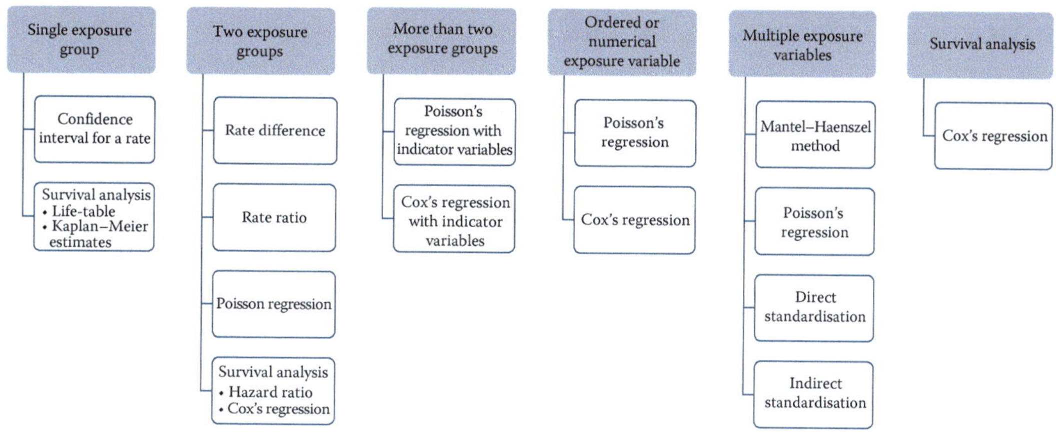

Figure D.2 Rates and survival times.

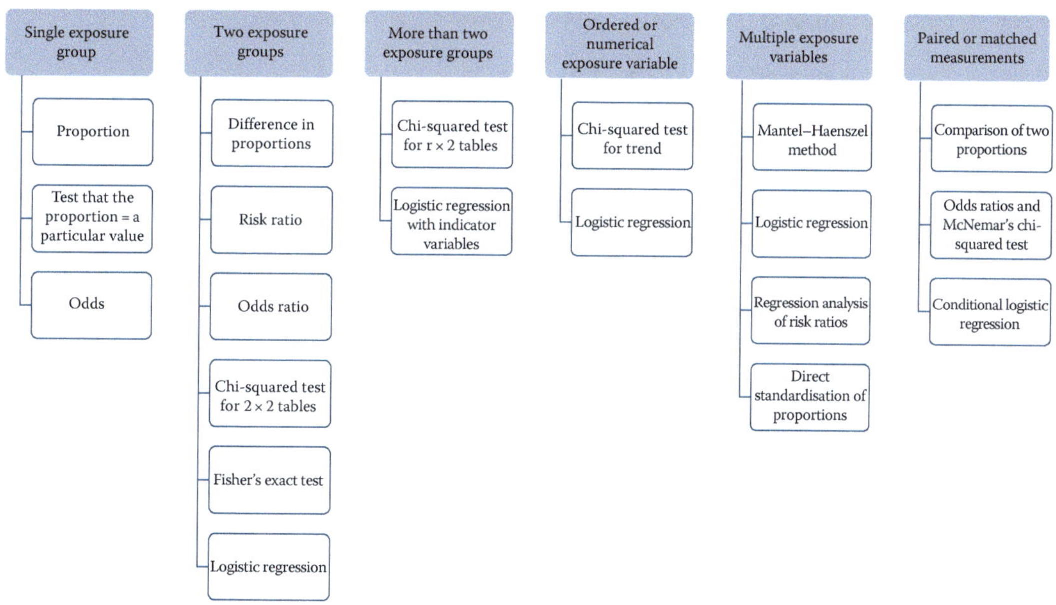

Figure D.3 Binary outcome variable.

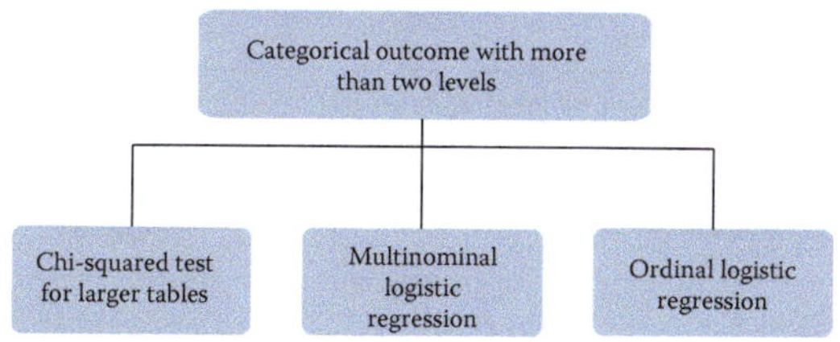

Figure D.4 Categorical outcome with more than two levels.

Mnemonics (Tables D.1 to D.8)

Table D.1 Epidemiology of noncommunicable diseases

'**C**lassified **I**n **T**ime, **P**lace, **P**erson, **C**heck'
1. **C**linical features
2. **I**mportance
3. **T**ime
4. **P**lace
5. **P**erson **C**auses/RF

Table D.2 'CDDCs DHTCC'

'**CCDC**s **D**o **H**elp **T**o **C**ontrol **C**holera'
Confirm outbreak exists
Confirm diagnosis
Case **D**efinition
Count cases
Describe data
Generate **H**ypothesis
Test hypothesis
Control/prevention measures
Communication/report

Table D.3 Epidemiology and control of an infection

ACE Doctors **R**eact **T**o **S**almonella **C**onfidently
Agent
Clinical features
Epidemiology (time/place/person)
Diagnosis (lab test)
Reservoir
Transmission
Surveillance
Control (PGS CCS)

Table D.4 Developing health promotion programme

'AS ROME'
Assess need (+ determinants)
Stakeholder analysis/engagement
Resources
Objectives/aims (+ targets)
Methods (evidence for effective interventions)
Evaluation

Table D.5 Routine health information sources

'**D**ata **M**anagement **M**akes **R**outine **N**umbers **P**erfect'
1. **D**emographic/social
2. **M**ortality
3. **M**orbidity
4. **R**isk factors (health status)
5. **N**on-health service
6. **P**rivate sector

Table D.6 Policy formation/implementation

'A PIE'
1. **A**genda setting
2. **P**olicy formulation (alternative proposals)
3. **I**mplementation
4. **E**valuation

Table D.7 Stakeholder analysis

'I AM'
Identification
Assessment
Manage + monitor

Table D.8 Belbin's team roles

'ICE FIRST'
Implementer/company worker
Coordinator/chair
Evaluator/monitor
Finisher/completer
Innovator/plant
Resource investigator
Shaper
Team worker

References

1. Snow, J. (1855) *On the Mode of Communication of Cholera*. London, U.K.: John Churchill, pp. 1–38. Available online at www.ph.ucla.edu/EPI/snow/snowbook.html.
2. Doll, R. and Hill, A.B. (1954) The mortality of doctors in relation to their smoking habits: A preliminary report. *BMJ* 228, 1451–1455.
3. Cochrane, A.L. (1972) *Effectiveness and Efficiency: Random Reflections on Health Services*. London, U.K.: Nuffield Provincial Hospitals Trust. Reprinted in 1999 for Nuffield Trust by the Royal Society of Medicine Press, London, U.K.
4. Barker, D. (2003) The midwife, the coincidence, and the hypothesis. *BMJ* 327, 1428–1430.
5. Rose, G. (1992) *The Strategy of Preventive Medicine*. Oxford, U.K.: Oxford University Press.
6. Chadwick, E. (1842) The sanitary conditions of the labouring population. Self published.
7. Hart, J.T. (1971) The inverse care law. *Lancet* 1, 405–412. Available online at www.sochealth.co.uk/history/inversecare.htm.
8. Black, D., Morris, J.N., Smith, C. et al. (1980) Inequalities in health: Report of a research working group (Black Report). London, U.K.: Department of Health and Social Security. Available online at www.sochealth.co.uk/history/black.htm.
9. Acheson, D. (1998) Independent inquiry into inequalities in health report. London, U.K.: TSO. Available online at www.archive.official-documents.co.uk/document/doh/ih/ih.htm.
10. Wanless, D. (2004) *Securing Good Health for the Whole Population*. London, U.K.: HMSO.
11. Tannahill, A. (1985) What is health promotion? *Health Educ J* 44, 167–168.
12. Lalonde, M. (1974) A new perspective on the health of Canadians: A working document. www.phac-aspc.gc.ca/ph-sp/phdd/pdf/perspective.pdf.
13. Dahlgren, G. and Whitehead, M. (1991) *Policies and Strategies to Promote Social Equity in Health*. Stockholm, Sweden: Institute for Futures Studies.
14. Evans, R. and Stoddart, G. (1990) Producing health, consuming resources. *Soc Sci Med* 31, 1347–1363.
15. Diderichsen, F. and Hallqvist, J. (1998) Social inequalities in health: some methodological considerations for the study of social position and social context. In: Arve-Parès, B. (ed.) *Inequality in Health—A Swedish Perspective*. Stockholm, Sweden: Swedish Council for Social Research, pp. 25–39.
16. Hochbaum, G.M. (1958) Public participation in medical screening programs: A socio-psychological study. PHS publication No. 572. Washington, DC: US Government Printing Office.
17. Bandura, A. (1977) *Social Learning Theory*. New York: General Learning Press.
18. Prochaska, J.O. and DiClemente, C.C. (1984) Self-change processes, self-efficacy and decisional balance across five stages of smoking cessation. In: *Advances in Cancer Control—1983*, Denver, CO. New York: Alan R. Liss, Inc.
19. Beattie, A. (1991) Knowledge and control in health promotion: A test case for social policy and social theory. In: Gabe, J., Calnan, M., and Bury, M. (eds.) *The Sociology of the Health Service*. London, U.K.: Routledge.

20. Ewles, L. and Simnet, I. (1995) *Promoting Health: A Practical Guide* (3rd rev. edn.). London, U.K.: Ballière Tindall.
21. Parsons, T. (1951) *The Social System*. New York: Free Press.
22. Lemert, E.M. (1967) *Human Deviance, Social Problems and Social Control*. London, U.K.: Prentice Hall.
23. Goffman, E. (1963) *Stigma: Notes on the Management of Spoiled Identity*. London, U.K.: Prentice-Hall.
24. Illich, I. (1975) *Medical Nemesis: The Expropriation of Health*. London, U.K.: Marian Boyars.
25. Durkheim, E. (1897) *Le Suicide*. Paris, France: Alcan.
26. Rawls, J. (1971) *A Theory of Justice*. Cambridge, U.K.: Harvard University Press.
27. Donabedian, A. (1966) Evaluating the quality of medical care. *Milbank Mem Fund Q* 44, 166–206.
28. Maxwell, R.J. (1984) Quality assessment in health. *BMJ* 288, 1470–1472.
29. Belbin, R.M. (1996) *Team Roles at Work*. London, U.K.: Butterworth-Heinemann.
30. Maslow, A.H. (1943) A theory of human motivation. *Psychol Rev* 50, 370–396.
31. Handy, C.B. (1987) *Understanding Organizations* (Penguin Business) (3rd edn.). London, U.K.: Penguin.
32. Wilson, J.M. and Jungner, G. (1968) *Principles and Practice of Screening for Diseases*. Geneva, Switzerland: WHO.
33. Hill, A.B. (1965) The environment and disease: Association or causation? *Proc Roy Soc Med* 58, 295–300.
34. Kirkwood, B. and Sterne, J. (2003) *Essential Medical Statistics* (2nd edn.). Oxford, U.K.: Blackwell Science.

Index